THIRD 3 EDITION

Case Studies in

CRITICAL
CARE
NURSING

A GUIDE FOR APPLICATION AND REVIEW

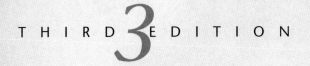

THIRD **3** EDITION

Case Studies in

CRITICAL CARE NURSING

A GUIDE FOR APPLICATION AND REVIEW

SHEILA DRAKE MELANDER, RN, DSN, ACNP-C, FCCM
Professor of Nursing
University of Tennessee Memphis
Memphis, Tennessee
Cardiovascular Acute Care Nurse Practitioner
Owensboro, Kentucky

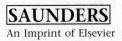
SAUNDERS
An Imprint of Elsevier

SAUNDERS
An Imprint of Elsevier

The Curtis Center
Independence Square West
Philadelphia, Pennsylvania 19106

NOTICE

Pharmacology is an ever-changing field. Standard safety precautions must be followed, but as new research and clinical experience broaden our knowledge, changes in treatment and drug therapy may become necessary or appropriate. Readers are advised to check the most current product information provided by the manufacturer of each drug to be administered to verify the recommended dose, the method and duration of administration, and contraindications. It is the responsibility of the licensed prescriber, relying on experience and knowledge of the patient, to determine dosages and the best treatment for each individual patient. Neither the publisher nor the author assumes any liability for any injury and/or damage to persons or property arising from this publication.

Previous edition copyrighted 2001.

International Standard Book Number 0-7216-0344-0

Executive Publisher: Barbara Nelson Cullen
Developmental Editor: Julie Vitale
Publishing Services Manager: Catherine Jackson
Project Manager: Anne Gassett Konopka
Designer: Amy Buxton

Printed in China

Last digit is the print number: 9 8 7 6 5 4 3 2 1

Cinda Alexander, MSN, CCRN, CNRN, CNOR, CRNFA
Tri-State Neurological
Evansville, Indiana
Subarachnoid Hemorrhage with Aneurysm; Head Trauma and Subdural Hematoma; Epidural Hematoma

Sharon West Angle, RN, BSN, MSN
Director, Shore Memorial School of Practical Nursing, Corporate Director of Compliance and Quality
Shore Health Services, Inc.
Nassawadox, Virginia
Acute Respiratory Distress Syndrome

Connie Cooper, RN, BSN, MSN
Assistant Professor
DePaul University
Nursing Department
Chicago, Illinois
Acquired Immunodeficiency Syndrome

Phyllis Ann Egbert, MSN, RN, ACNP-C, CNN
Clinical Instructor/Lecturer
Vanderbilt University
School of Nursing

Research Coordinator/Nurse Practitioner
Vanderbilt University Medical Center
Nashville, Tennessee
Chronic Renal Failure and Renal Transplantation

Linda K. Evinger, RN, MSN, C-OGNP
Instructor
School of Nursing and Health Professions
University of Southern Indiana
Evansville, Indiana
Esophageal Varices; Drug Overdose

Judith A. Halstead, RN, MSN, DNS
Professor of Nursing and Director of Undergraduate Nursing Program
School of Nursing and Health Professions
University of Southern Indiana
Evansville, Indiana
Pulmonary Contusion

Roberta E. Hoebeke, RN, PhD, FNP, APRN, BC
Assistant Professor of Graduate Nursing
University of Southern Indiana
School of Nursing and Health Professions
Evansville, Indiana

Family Nurse Practitioner
Tulip Tree Family Health Center
Fort Branch, Indiana
Cardiogenic Shock and Anterior Wall Myocardial Infarction

W. Gale Hoehn, RN, MSN
Instructor
University of Southern Indiana
School of Nursing and Health Professions
Evansville, Indiana
End of Life Issues

Joan E. King, RN, PhD, ACNP, ANP
Program Director for the Acute Care Nurse Practitioner Program
Associate Professor of Nursing
Vanderbilt University School of Nursing

Acute Care Nurse Practitioner
Vanderbilt Preanesthesia Evaluation Center
Nashville, Tennessee
Heart Failure; Abdominal Aortic Aneurysm; Blunt Abdominal Trauma

Judi Kuric, PhD, MSN, RN, APRN, BC, CRRN-A, CNRN
Assistant Professor
University of Southern Indiana
School of Nursing and Health Professions
Acute Care Nurse Practitioner
HealthSouth Tri-State Rehabilitation Hospital
Evansville, Indiana
Gastrointestinal Tract Bleeding

Alice Lowe, RN, BSN
Deaconess Hospital
Evansville, Indiana
*Percutaneous Transluminal Coronary Angioplasty and Thrombolytic Therapy in
   Myocardial Infarction*

Sheila Drake Melander, RN, DSN, ACNP-C, FCCM
Full Professor of Nursing
University of Tennessee Memphis
Memphis, Tennessee

Cardiovascular Acute Care Nurse Practitioner
Owensboro, Kentucky
Percutaneous Transluminal Coronary Angioplasty and Thrombolytic Therapy in Myocardial Infarction; Non–Q-Wave Myocardial Infarction; Pulmonary Contusion; Chronic Obstructive Pulmonary Disease with Pneumonia; Acute Respiratory Distress Syndrome; Acute Renal Failure

Amy Reese Ramirez, RN, BSN, MSW, MSN, FNP-C
Family Nurse Practitioner
St. Mary's Hospital
Deaconess Hospital
Evansville, Indiana
Non–Q-Wave Myocardial Infarction; Acute Renal Failure

Katherine B. Riedford, RN, BSN, MSN, DNS
Instructor of Psychiatric/Mental Health Nursing
University of Southern Indiana
Evansville, Indiana
Drug Overdose

M. Lynn Rodgers, RNC, MSN, CCRN, CNRN, ACNP-BC
Acute Care Nurse Practitioner
Deaconess Hospital
Evansville, Indiana
Coronary Artery Bypass Graft; Carotid Endarterectomy; Peritonitis; Sepsis/Septic Shock

Lynn Smith Schnautz, RN, MSN, CCRN, CCNS
Clinical Nurse Specialist
Deaconess Hospital
Evansville, Indiana
Cardiac Trauma and Cardiac Tamponade; Disseminated Intravascular Coagulation

Mary Jane Swartz, RN, MSN, APRN, BC
Professor Associate of Science in Nursing
Ivy Tech State College
Evansville, Indiana
Hypertensive Crisis/Emergency

Colleen R. Walsh, RN, MSN, ONC, CS, ACNP-C
Faculty, Graduate Nursing
School of Nursing and Health Professions
University of Southern Indiana
Evansville, Indiana
Adrenal Crisis; Syndrome of Inappropriate Secretion of Antidiuretic Hormone;
Diabetic Ketoacidosis; Multiple Organ Dysfunction Syndrome

Mary Ann Wehmer, RN, MSN, CNOR
Nursing Instructor
School of Nursing and Health Professions
University of Southern Indiana
Evansville, Indiana
Pulmonary Embolism

Ann H. White, RN, PhD, MBA, CNA
Associate Professor of Nursing
University of Southern Indiana
Evansville, Indiana
Acute Pancreatitis; Burns

Jennifer Basler, RN, MSN, CCRN
Clinical Nurse Specialist for Cardiovascular Services
Appleton Medical Center
Appleton, Wisconsin

Barbara Chamberlain, MSN, RN, CNS, CCRN
College of Nursing and Health Professions
Drexel University
Philadelphia, Pennsylvania

Louise M. Diehl-Oplinger, RN, MSN, CCRN, APRN, BC, CLNC
Staff Development Instructor
Warren Hospital
Phillipsburg, New Jersey

Kristine M. L'Ecuyer, RN, BSN, MSN, CCNS
Director of Continuing Nursing Education
School of Nursing
Saint Louis University
St. Louis, Missouri

Cecilia J. Maier, MS, RN, CCRN
Assistant Professor
Mount Carmel College of Nursing
Columbus, Ohio

Erika M. Schwelnus, RN, MSN, APN, CNP
Rush Presbyterian-St. Luke's Medical Center
College of Nursing
Rush University
Chicago, Illinois

Leslie Rachell Toney, RN, BSN
PN Instructor
Wes Watkins Technology Center
Wetumka, Oklahoma

Tamara M. Ware, RN, MSN, BC, OCN
Shepherd College
Shepherdstown, West Virginia

ACKNOWLEDGMENTS

I'd like to take this opportunity to thank specific people in my life who have supported me throughout the publishing process of this text. I'd like to begin by thanking the talented contributors of the case studies. Without each contributor, whose expertise is clearly reflected through each of their case studies, this project would not have been possible.

I would also like to thank the three most important people in my life: my husband Chuck, and my two children, Ryan and Matthew. I want to take this moment to tell you how much I appreciate your continuous patience, love, and support. God truly blessed me when he brought my husband and my children into my life.

Sheila Drake Melander

Knowledge is of the past, wisdom is of the future.
Vernon Cooper

It has been said that knowledge is knowing facts, but wisdom is knowing what to do with facts. We are often very good at knowing facts. Much of our testing and evaluation focuses on knowing facts. Measurement of the ST segment and the action and indications of amiodarone are important facts to know in caring for critically ill patients. However, so much of what it is that nursing does goes beyond facts and acquiring knowledge. What we do and how we react in nursing is determined not only by what we know but also by what we bring to the situation. We use our cognitive and affective skills to focus on a problem and thereby increase the probability of a positive outcome. In other words we use critical thinking.

This case study book offers the reader the opportunity to gain wisdom, to know what to do with facts, and reach a level beyond knowledge. The case studies allow the reader to do more than problem solve, they also develop critical thinking, a vital skill for nurses today and in the future. Critical thinking can identify ways to not only solve but also prevent problems. It helps the learners maximize their potential and efficiency in order to make an optimal contribution to their patients and their profession.

How better to develop the necessary skill of critical thinking than to provide an active, experiential learning through case studies? The cases presented are actual practice-based scenarios. They allow the reader to analyze reality-based data about a patient situation and then challenge the reader with questions about the nursing care for that patient. Answers for the scenario-based questions are provided for comparison but also to challenge the reader to explore options, analyze controversies, and consider going beyond the initial response, providing a link to other learning resources.

These case studies can be useful in the classroom for nursing students but they also challenge experienced nurses to expand their knowledge by exploring facts, considering possibilities, examining explanations, and relying on reason. For example, a preceptor could use the cases to assist with orientation of the novice critical care nurse, using the book to develop goal-directed purposeful and reasoned thinking processes. This critical thinking can then be applied to the clinical situations that are seen every day.

The world around us is changing in quantum leaps. Nursing needs highly developed critical thinking skills that will help us adapt to new situations, make competent decisions, and foster lifelong learning. This text is a tool to help us obtain those skills so needed in acquiring wisdom in nursing for now and for the future.

Mary G. McKinley, RN, MSN, CCRN
Past President, AACN
Critical Connections
Maxwell Centre
Wheeling, West Virginia

Case Studies in Critical Care Nursing was compiled with the intent of capturing actual patient data from various critical care settings. The data were then placed into scenarios that recaptured patient events as they actually occurred. Patient scenarios were sought that represented common diagnoses seen in six body systems—respiratory, cardiovascular, renal, neurologic, gastrointestinal, and endocrine—and in multisystems. The 33 chapters include five new case studies that we hope will add to the students' body of knowledge. The cases are grouped according to body systems for quick reference. Each case was compiled with one goal in mind: to create a tool for use with critical care students that provides a true perspective of patient needs in the critical care setting. Students can study actual patient situations and apply critical thinking skills in discussions of current treatment modalities, effectiveness of treatments and medications prescribed, alternative care options, the necessity for diagnostic tests ordered, and the impact of hemodynamic values on patient care and the "real-life" necessity for hemodynamic monitoring.

The case study application text represents a different approach to education of critical care nurses. In each scenario, students follow the patient from entrance into the health care setting through his or her discharge from the acute care setting. Students are challenged to use critical thinking skills to accurately answer the case study questions that accompany each case and provide solutions to the patient's problem. Students can then study answers to those same questions written by the author of the chapter. Students should then be well versed in current diagnostic procedures, laboratory data requirements, pharmacologic needs, and treatment modalities for that particular disease entity.

This text is appropriate for the baccalaureate or graduate student and for use in the hospital setting in critical care training. It may also serve as a review tool for nurses preparing for the CCRN® examination. The answers to the case study questions provide a detailed account of each disease studied. Educators can choose the questions appropriate for the student's level or can adapt their expectations of the depth of the student's answers.

Health care needs are quickly changing, and we must prepare nurses to change and adapt with the health care system. Students who are challenged to think critically while still in the classroom setting can translate those skills into the clinical care setting to better meet the changing needs of the critically ill patient. It is hoped that this text will increase students' knowledge of the needs of the critically ill patient and enhance education in the clinical setting.

Sheila Drake Melander

CONTENTS

CARDIOVASCULAR ALTERATIONS

1

Percutaneous Transluminal Coronary Angioplasty and Thrombolytic Therapy in Myocardial Infarction

Alice Lowe, RN, BSN
Sheila Drake Melander, RN, DSN, ACNP-C, FCCM

CASE PRESENTATION

Mr. Johnson, a 54-year-old, began having chest pain 1 hour after supper, while he was at work. He described the pain as a "grabbing pressure" located midsternally. He rated the pain at "about 2" on a scale of 1 to 5. He stated that the pain radiated down his left arm and through to his back. He was transported to the emergency department (ED) by ambulance. On admission Mr. Johnson was pale and diaphoretic and complained of shortness of breath (SOB). He denied nausea or vomiting. In the ED, unstable angina was diagnosed and tests to rule out myocardial infarction (MI) were initiated. He had experienced chest pain for 1 hour upon arrival in the ED at 8:13 PM.

The patient reports no previous episodes of chest pain or pressure. He has smoked two packs of cigarettes daily for 25 years. His mother died of Alzheimer's disease, and his father died of cancer. He has no family history of heart disease.

On initial examination the patient did not exhibit jugular venous distention, the carotid arteries were 2+/4 without bruits, and the point of maximum impulse was located at the fifth intercostal space, midclavicular line. Normal S_1 and S_2 sounds were auscultated with an S_3 present. No S_4 sound or murmurs were heard. There were vesicular lung sounds with scattered wheezes, but no crackles were heard. No edema was present, and bowel sounds were normal.

Diagnostic data at admission were as follows:

BP	140/90 mm Hg	**Sao$_2$** 95% with oxygen 4 L/min	
HR	92 bpm and regular	per nasal cannula	
Respirations	32 breaths/min	**Height** 173 cm	
Temperature	36.9° C (98.5° F)	**Weight** 104 kg	

The 12-lead electrocardiogram (ECG) findings at 8:15 PM were as follows:

- Normal sinus rhythm (NSR) with frequent premature ventricular contractions (PVCs) and three- to four-beat runs of ventricular tachycardia (VT)
- ST-segment elevation in leads I, aV$_L$, and V$_2$ through V$_6$ (3 to 4 mm)

- ST-segment depression in leads III and aV$_F$
- Q waves in V$_2$ through V$_4$

The chest x-ray film revealed slight cardiomegaly with mild congestive heart failure (CHF).

The echocardiogram findings were as follows:

- Trileaflet aortic valve with normal openings
- Normal mitral configuration with normal opening of mitral valve diastole and normal coaptation in systole
- Normal right atrium and right ventricle
- Thin layer pericardial effusion (mostly posterior)
- Left ventricular ejection fraction 25% to 30%
- Mild mitral valve regurgitation

Cardiac enzyme measurements were as follows at admission and on day 1:

	Admission 2013	Admission 2400	Day 1 0400
CK (U/L)	254	7357	5638
CK-MB (%)	10	>300	>300
Troponin I (ng/ml)	3.5	>50	>50

In the ED, Mr. Johnson's chest pain was unrelieved after three sublingual nitroglycerin (NTG) tablets. Morphine sulfate 5 mg intravenous push (IVP) was administered, resulting in a small decrease in pain.

After evaluation of the initial laboratory results, presenting symptoms, and the ECG, the diagnosis was an extensive anterolateral MI. Mr. Johnson was assessed for contraindications to thrombolytic therapy. The patient was considered a candidate for thrombolytic therapy, and administration of tissue plasminogen activator (tPA) was started immediately. An NTG drip (50 mg/250 ml in 5% dextrose in water [D5W]) was started at 20 µg/min (6 ml/hr). A heparin bolus of 8000 U was given, and a drip was begun at 10 ml/hr (1000 U/hr). Metoprolol titrate (Lopressor) 5 mg IVP was given every 5 minutes three times (total 15 mg) and an enteric-coated aspirin was administered. After the NTG and heparin drips were started, the patient's pain was relieved. He was then transferred to the coronary intensive care unit (CICU).

In the CICU Mr. Johnson's chest pain returned. He rated it as 4 on a scale of 1 to 5. His blood pressure was 96/60 mm Hg, and he began having ST-segment elevations in the anterior leads along with six- to eight-beat runs of VT. Three sublingual NTG tablets were given, followed by 4 mg of morphine intravenously, but the pain did not decrease. Mr. Johnson was sent to the catheterization laboratory for emergency angiography and possible angioplasty.

The angiogram showed 90% blockage of the left anterior descending (LAD) artery. An emergency rescue angioplasty (percutaneous transluminal coronary angioplasty [PTCA]) was performed, but the artery continued to reocclude, so a coronary stent was inserted. While the PTCA was performed, 23,000 U of heparin and 500,000 U of urokinase were given as an intracoronary injection. Mr. Johnson became hypotensive, tachycardic, pale, cool, and diaphoretic. His arterial blood oxygen saturation (SaO$_2$) dropped to 86%, and he was placed on a mechanical ventilator with a 100% non-rebreather mask. He continued having runs of VT; therefore a 100-mg bolus of lidocaine was given and a lidocaine drip (2 g/500 ml of D5W) was started at 2 mg/min. A dopamine (Intropin) infusion was started at 2 µg/kg/min and was gradually increased to 4 µg/kg/min. A dobutamine (Dobutrex) drip was started at 5 µg/kg/min. An abciximab (ReoPro) bolus of 0.25 mg/kg was administered followed by an infusion at 21 ml/hr (which will continue for 12 hours). A pulmonary artery (Swan-Ganz) catheter was placed to monitor for CHF and cardiogenic shock. An intraaortic balloon pump (IABP) was inserted in the right groin to stabilize Mr. Johnson's blood pressure (BP), decrease the workload of the heart, and improve cardiac output. Upon return to the CICU, Mr. Johnson was free of pain.

His vital signs and hemodynamic readings were as follows:

BP	133/59 mm Hg	**RAP**	10 mm Hg
HR	90 bpm	**PAS**	42 mm Hg
Sao$_2$	99% with 100% non-rebreather mask	**PAD**	22 mm Hg
ECG	NSR with occasional PVCs	**MAP**	31 mm Hg
		PAWP	22 mm Hg

Findings from an ECG on the day of admission post-PTCA (11 PM) were as follows:

- NSR, T wave inverted in aV$_R$
- ST segment elevated in leads I, aV$_L$, and V$_2$ through V$_6$ (1 to 2 mm)

Findings from an ECG on postadmission day 1 (6:50 AM) were as follows:

- NSR, ST segment almost baseline
- Q waves in V$_2$ through V$_6$
- Inverted T waves, leads V$_2$ through V$_6$
- aV$_R$ T waves now upright

Mr. Johnson's lidocaine drip was discontinued the next day. The heparin drip was discontinued and the arterial line, IABP, and pulmonary artery catheter were removed on day 2. He was started on enoxaparin (Lovenox) 100 mg subcutaneously twice a day. On day 3 his dopamine, dobutamine, and NTG drip were tapered and discontinued. He was released to the cardiac progressive step-down unit on day 4. On day 6 he was released to home. He was instructed in outpatient cardiac rehabilitation, smoking cessation, and a prudent heart diet. He was sent home with prescriptions for diltiazem (Cardizem) 30 mg three times daily, captopril (Capoten) 6.25 mg three times daily, ticlopidine (Ticlid) 250 mg twice daily, metoprolol (Lopressor) 25 mg twice daily, and NTG tablets as needed. Mr. Johnson was also instructed to take an aspirin every day.

PERCUTANEOUS TRANSLUMINAL CORONARY ANGIOPLASTY AND THROMBOLYTIC THERAPY IN MYOCARDIAL INFARCTION

QUESTIONS

1. Describe angina pectoris and discuss the difference between chronic stable angina, unstable angina, and Prinzmetal's angina.

2. Define CAD and discuss associated risk factors.

3. Describe an acute myocardial infarction (AMI) and its effects on the heart and lifestyle.

4. List the symptoms of an AMI.

5. What is the significance of the following heart sounds: S_3, S_4, and a murmur?

6. What do crackles auscultated during lung sound assessment signify?

7. Discuss the use of cardiac enzymes and their normal values. What laboratory values would be indicative of an AMI for Mr. Johnson?

8. What is the significance of Mr. Johnson's ST-segment changes?

9. Why was an echocardiogram done?

10. What are the desired pharmacologic effects of NTG?

11. Why was Mr. Johnson given an aspirin in the ED? Explain the use of abciximab (ReoPro), ticlopidine (Ticlid), and aspirin therapy for Mr. Johnson.

12. Discuss the pharmacologic actions of heparin and enoxaparin (Lovenox) and the indications for use with a patient with an AMI.

13. Discuss the pharmacologic effects of morphine.

14. Describe what a β-blocker is and the rationale for Mr. Johnson receiving this medication.

15. Why was Mr. Johnson given lidocaine?

16. tPA is a thrombolytic agent. Discuss the effects of a thrombolytic agent and why it was used for Mr. Johnson initially rather than angioplasty.

17. What are the contraindications for tPA?

18. What is a PTCA?

19. What made Mr. Johnson a candidate for PTCA? What are the potential complications for a patient undergoing PTCA?

20. What is a stent and why was it used on Mr. Johnson?

21. What do the readings from the pulmonary artery catheter tell the nurse about Mr. Johnson?

22. What is cardiogenic shock? What symptoms did Mr. Johnson exhibit?

23. What are the therapeutic effects of dopamine (Intropin) at low, moderate, and high dosages?

24. What are the therapeutic effects of dobutamine (Dobutrex)?

25. What advantage does an IABP offer Mr. Johnson?

26. What significance does the IABP have in relation to the tPA and urokinase given previously?

27. Mr. Johnson was sent home with a prescription for diltiazem (Cardizem). Why would a patient with heart disease be given a calcium channel blocker?

28. Why was Mr. Johnson sent home with a prescription for captopril (Capoten)?

PERCUTANEOUS TRANSLUMINAL CORONARY ANGIOPLASTY AND THROMBOLYTIC THERAPY IN MYOCARDIAL INFARCTION

QUESTIONS AND ANSWERS

1. Describe angina pectoris and discuss the difference between chronic stable angina, unstable angina, and Prinzmetal's angina.

Angina pectoris (chest pain) is a symptom of myocardial ischemia resulting from an imbalance in the oxygen demand and the oxygen supply. "Angina is usually manifested when the coronary artery occlusion is equal to or greater than 75% of the lumen" (Becker, 1999, p. 204). Patients with angina describe a sensation of pressure, heaviness, burning, gas, or squeezing in the chest area. The pain can radiate to the neck, jaw, shoulders, arms, or hands (Urden et al, 2002).

Etiologic Factors for Angina Pectoris

Atherosclerotic heart disease, hypertension, aortic valve disease, anemia, arrhythmia, thyrotoxicosis, shock, CHF, and coronary artery spasm are the etiologic factors associated with angina pectoris.

Chronic Stable Angina

Chronic stable angina is a stable pattern of chest pain with the same frequency, severity, duration, and precipitating factors (exercise or exertion) that have not changed in the past 2 months (Alexander et al, 1998; Becker, 1999).

Unstable Angina

Unstable angina is (1) new-onset chest pain in patients who have never had anginal symptoms or (2) pain that is suddenly different (more intense, more frequent, brought on by less effort, or different in character) in patients who have had stable angina. The pain may be steady or it may be intermittent. It lasts longer than 15 minutes and is not relieved by NTG or rest. Unstable angina is a medical emergency. About 1 of 10 people with it develop AMI. This pain usually signifies that the patient has some CAD, and it should be evaluated. Chest pain that is not relieved with rest and NTG in 15 minutes should be evaluated in the ED (Alexander et al, 1998; Goldman & Bennett, 2000).

Prinzmetal's (Variant) Angina

The angina occurs without an increase in effort or stress and without warning. The pain occurs about the same time every day, commonly at bedtime or upon awakening. The pain is believed to be caused by vasospasm of the coronary artery. With Prinzmetal's angina, the ECG will show ST-segment elevations with pain and disappear when the pain is gone (Becker, 1999; Goldman & Bennett, 2000).

2. Define CAD and discuss associated risk factors.

CAD (coronary artery disease) is subintimal deposition of atheromas in the large and medium-sized arteries serving the heart. Atherosclerosis is the name for plaque buildup (cholesterol, calcium, and other minerals) in the coronary arteries. Once the artery's lumen is reduced to less than 50%, it is considered significant CAD. When the blood flow is severely reduced by atherosclerosis, a clot can form as blood trickles through the narrowed vessel, causing a sudden, complete stoppage of blood flow (Alexander et al, 1998; Becker, 1999; Goldman & Bennett, 2000).

The following are unmodifiable risk factors for CAD:

1. *Heredity:* CAD tends to run in families. Some families have narrow coronary arteries; others have tendencies toward hyperlipidemia, hypertension, or other risk factors.

2. *Age:* CAD is more prevalent in older age groups. The incidence of AMI increases with age.
3. *Sex:* Men have a higher incidence of CAD earlier in life, but after women go through menopause (and lose the protective benefits of estrogen), the risks for CAD are about the same.
4. *Race:* White men die more often from CAD than do nonwhite men, and white women die slightly less often from CAD than do nonwhite women (Becker, 1999; Goldman & Bennett, 2000; Urden et al, 2002).
5. *Socioeconomic status:* A new report identifies low socioeconomic status as an unmodifiable risk factor. A number of mechanisms may explain this. First, risk factors for atherosclerosis, such as smoking, hypertension, obesity, and sedentary lifestyle, are higher in people with low socioeconomic status. Second, some of these risk factors, as well as psychosocial responses to stressors, may increase exposure to CAD triggers in these groups. Finally, these groups have less access to care (Alexander et al, 1998, p. 1186).

Modifiable risk factors for CAD are as follows:

1. *Hypertension:* Systolic BP more than 160 mm Hg or diastolic greater than 95 mm Hg increases the risk of CAD two to three times.
2. *Diabetes mellitus:* Diabetic patients have a two times higher incidence of CAD than those without diabetes.
3. *Cigarette smoking:* "Smoking increases heart rate and causes vasoconstriction, thereby impairing oxygen transport by the blood and increasing myocardial oxygen demand. Smoking also facilitates atherosclerosis by making the endothelium more porous" (Becker, 1999, p. 203). Smokers have a two to six times higher risk of death from CAD than nonsmokers.
4. *Hyperlipidemia:* Hyperlipidemia is the leading risk factor responsible for atherosclerosis. Serum levels of cholesterol less than 200 mg/dl are associated with minimal risk of CAD. High levels of triglycerides (>160 mg/dl) and low-density lipoproteins (>160 mg/dl) as well as low levels of high-density lipoproteins (<35 mg/dl) contribute to CAD.

The following factors contribute to CAD:

1. *Obesity:* Morbid obesity has been shown to be positively associated with an increased risk of CAD. In addition, it also contributes to the development of hypertension and diabetes.
2. *Sedentary lifestyle:* A positive correlation exists between a sedentary lifestyle and CAD (Alexander et al, 1998; Lessig & Lessig, 1998; Goldman & Bennett, 2000).

3. Describe an acute myocardial infarction (AMI) and its effects on the heart and lifestyle.

An MI occurs when there is a blockage of the coronary artery that causes necrosis of the cells of an area of the heart muscle as a result of oxygen deprivation. In most patients it is the result of severe atherosclerotic narrowing of one or more of the coronary arteries. Rarely, an MI can occur in the absence of coronary artery narrowing if there is a marked disparity between myocardial oxygen supply and demand. Cocaine abuse has been implicated as a possible cause of such a disparity (Becker, 1999). Infarctions are usually the result of an obstruction, the etiology of which can be caused by thrombosis, plaque rupture, dissection, or myocardial vasospasm. During an AMI the diminished blood flow to the heart can force the myocardium to shift from aerobic to anaerobic metabolism. This results in less efficient energy production, lactic acid buildup, intracellular hypokalemia, intracellular acidosis, intracellular hypernatremia, and interference with the release of calcium from the sarcoplasmic reticulum (Goldman & Bennett, 2000).

The patient who has suffered an AMI may have an area of the heart that no longer functions or functions in a diminished capacity. The effects on the patient vary with the extent of the heart muscle affected. A severe MI can decrease the ejection fraction (amount of blood pumped from the heart with each beat) to 15% to 20% (normal, 60% to 70%), an amount that could cause disability. Patients with severely limited left ventricular (LV) function suffer from SOB and weakness with even small activities of daily living.

4. List the symptoms of an AMI.

The symptoms vary with each patient. Patients may describe the symptoms as simply "indigestion" or a burning sensation that radiates from the midchest to the jaw. The hallmark symptom of an AMI is chest pain. The pain is typically in the middle of the chest behind the sternum, and does not improve with NTG or rest. It usually lasts longer than 15 minutes. Other symptoms include an uncomfortable pressure, crushing, heaviness, squeezing, fullness, tightness, aching, constriction, or an oppressive feeling. The pain may radiate to the jaw, to the shoulders, through to the back, or down the arms or hands (Goldman & Bennett, 2000; Urden et al, 2002).

5. What is the significance of the following heart sounds: S₃, S₄, and a murmur?

The third heart sound, S_3, may indicate heart failure. It is an early diagnostic sound. The sound is generated from vibrations produced during rapid filling of the ventricles in patients with ventricular dysfunction and overfilled ventricles (as in CHF). It can also be a normal variant in individuals up to 30 years of age. It is a lower-frequency pitch that often can be detected best with the patient in the left lateral decubitus position and in conditions in which the venous return is increased. It is best heard at the apex with the bell of the stethoscope.

The fourth heart sound, S_4, is a low-pitched presystolic sound. It is secondary to a forceful atrial contraction into a ventricle that has decreased compliance. Chronic ischemia, ventricular hypertrophy, cardiomyopathy, and idiopathic hypertrophic subaortic stenosis are some of the conditions in which an S_4 may be heard. It can be heard best at the apex in the left lateral decubitus position with the bell.

A murmur is a turbulence in the blood flow; it can be caused by a ruptured papillary muscle, valvular disease, or mitral and aortic insufficiency. Assessment should always include auscultation of heart sounds of the patient with an MI. A patient without a murmur on admission who develops one may have ruptured the papillary muscle (Goldman & Bennett, 2000).

6. What do crackles auscultated during lung sound assessment signify?

Crackles signify that the heart is not handling the workload efficiently. It suggests LV failure or decreased LV compliance. "If the blood does not leave the left ventricle, the fluid will back up into the lungs and cause congestive heart failure. This can be exhibited by shortness of breath, dyspnea, or crackles on auscultation of the lung fields. If this condition is allowed to persist, then the patient may develop a productive cough of frothy, pink sputum resulting from pulmonary edema" (Becker, 1999).

7. Discuss the use of cardiac enzymes and their normal values. What laboratory values would be indicative of an AMI for Mr. Johnson?

Creatine Kinase (CK) (50 to 180 U/L)

CK is an indicator of damage to the heart. It is released when a muscle is damaged. CK is an enzyme found in the heart, skeletal muscle, and brain. It consists of three isoenzymes: mm, found in the skeletal muscles; MB, found in the cardiac muscles; and BB, found in the brain tissues. Damage to any of these tissues causes the release of CK into the serum. The isoenzymes are then used to further differentiate the damaged tissue.

CK-MB (<5%)

After injury CK and its MB isoenzymes are released into the blood at a predictable rate. Within 4 to 8 hours, serum levels rise above normal limits, indicating tissue destruction. A peak of 5 to 15 times the baseline is reached within 12 to 24 hours; the level returns to normal within 2 to 3 days (Becker, 1999; Goldman & Bennett, 2000). Because of the exclusivity of the MB isoenzymes present in the cardiac muscle, serum MB elevations greater than 3% are definitive in the diagnosis of MI. After cardiac surgery, MB elevations greater than 7% indicate MI.

Troponin (<0.3 ng/ml)

Troponin, a protein that helps regulate heart muscle contraction, can be isolated in the serum and is a sensitive indicator of MI. The troponin protein actually consists of three separate proteins: troponin I, T, and C, each with a different function. "Cardiac troponins T and I are not found in significant levels in the blood of healthy adults, so the presence of those troponins in the serum is an indication of the death of myocardial tissue" (Murphy & Berding, 1999). After MI, troponin T rises in the serum and correlates with the amount of tissue damaged. Troponin T is measurable in the serum within 3 to 5 hours of symptom onset, peaks at about 72 hours, and remains detectable in the blood for up to 14 days. The presence in the blood for up to 2 weeks provides a diagnostic advantage to patients who have delayed seeking treatment for their symptoms (Murphy & Berding, 1999). Cardiac troponin I levels begin to increase 3 hours after myocardial ischemia occurs, peak at 14 to 18 hours, and remain elevated for 7 to 10 days (Antman et al, 1996; Murphy & Berding, 1999). A cardiac troponin I level of at least 0.4 ng/ml when a patient with unstable angina is first evaluated predicts an increased risk of short-term mortality, probably because it permits the diagnosis of non–Q-wave MI that one might have overlooked by sampling only for CK-MB. With progressively higher levels of cardiac troponin I, the risk of mortality increases, presumably because the amount of myocardial necrosis increases. Measuring cardiac troponin I is therefore useful in evaluating patients with unstable angina (Antman et al, 1996; Goldman & Bennett, 2000; Urden et al, 2002).

Myoglobin (<120 µg/ml)

Myoglobin is a heme protein that is found in all striated muscle fibers, which account for about 2% of both skeletal and cardiac tissue mass. The small molecular weight of myoglobin allows it to be released rapidly from muscle tissue when the tissue is damaged. This release of myoglobin is particularly important when one is trying to determine whether cardiac muscle has been damaged. Because myoglobin escapes rapidly from damaged myocardial cells, it can be detected as soon as 2 hours after an AMI, with peak serum levels occurring in 3 to 15 hours (Murphy & Berding, 1999; Goldman & Bennett, 2000).

Mr. Johnson had an initial CK value of 254 U/L, CK-MB of 10%, and troponin I of 3.5 ng/ml. All of these are suggestive of AMI.

8. **What is the significance of Mr. Johnson's ST-segment changes?**

The ST segment represents the resting phase between ventricular depolarization and repolarization. Thus it is normally neutral or isoelectric, that is, near baseline on the ECG. ST-segment shifts (elevations or depressions) associated with myocardial cell injury may be the result of an inability of the affected cells to maintain their normal intracellular polarity during the resting phase.

The T wave represents repolarization of the myocardium and is normally positive (upward deflection) in all of the 12 leads except V_1 and sometimes III and V_2. T-wave inversions may reflect ischemia or it may reflect an MI. T-wave inversion associated with AMI may persist for several days and is associated with ischemia.

Pathologic Q waves are greater than 0.04 second deep and usually greater than 0.03 second wide. Q waves normally occur in leads III and aV_F and are likely to disappear with deep inspiration or position change (Goldman & Bennett, 2000; Urden et al, 2002).

An AMI evolves in three stages:

1. *Ischemia:* Ischemia results from a temporary interruption of the myocardial blood supply. It is the least acute stage of tissue hypoxia and is often reversible with little or no permanent

cell death if prompt intervention increases blood supply to the myocardium or reduces oxygen demand. Its characteristic ECG change is T-wave inversion, a result of altered tissue repolarization.

2. *Injury:* Injury to myocardial cells results from a prolonged interruption of blood flow. Its characteristic ECG change is ST-segment elevation.

3. *Necrosis:* Infarction results from an absence of blood flow to myocardial tissue, leading to necrosis. The ECG shows pathologic Q waves, reflecting abnormal depolarization in damaged tissue or absent depolarization of scar tissue (Goldman & Bennett, 2000).

Inferior MI (Leads II, II, and aVF)

The right coronary artery supplies the inferior myocardium and lower third of the interventricular septum. Infarction of these surfaces is best reflected in the inferior leads. Because the infarcted tissue on the inferior surface no longer depolarizes, opposing forces become dominant, and current traveling away from the positive pole is visible as a new Q wave.

Anterior MI (Leads V_1 through V_6)

The LAD supplies the anterior ventricular myocardium and upper two thirds of the septum. Infarction in this area is best seen in leads V_1 through V_6. The result is smaller or absent R waves. Loss of R waves in V_2 through V_4 indicates necrosis of the anteroseptal surface; loss of R waves in V_2 through V_6 indicates extensive anterior or anterolateral infarction.

Lateral MI (Leads I, aV_L, V_5, and V_6)

The circumflex artery and the diagonal branches of the LAD supply the lateral myocardium. Infarction in this area is best seen in leads I, aV_L, and V_5 and V_6.

Posterior MI (Leads V_1 and V_2)

The mid- and posterior-marginal branches of the circumflex artery supply the posterior wall of the heart. The process of infarction here can sometimes be seen in leads V_1 and V_2 as ST-segment depression, reversal of the T-wave polarity, or initial R-wave upswing that is wider than normal.

On Mr. Johnson's ECG, the elevations in leads I, aV_L, and V_1 through V_6 signify that anterolateral injury is present. The Q waves in leads V_1 through V_4 could be from a previous MI or could represent some necrosis in the anterior portion of the myocardium. The ST-segment depression in leads III and aV_F signifies reciprocal changes of the damage in the anterior leads (Bucher & Melander, 1999; Goldman & Bennett, 2000; Urden et al, 2002).

9. **Why was an echocardiogram done?**

Echocardiograms use ultrasound waves to obtain and display images of cardiac structures. This test is performed to rule out aortic valvular disease, idiopathic hypertrophic subaortic stenosis, or other structural malformations. It can also help determine the extent to which LV wall motion has been affected and to estimate ejection fraction (Becker, 1999; Goldman & Bennett, 2000).

10. **What are the desired pharmacologic effects of NTG?**

Nitrates decrease the myocardial oxygen demand in patients with fixed obstructive CAD and coronary vasospasm. NTG is a vasodilator that increases venous capacitance. It relaxes vascular smooth muscle, thereby reducing blood pressure by generalized vasodilation. Both of these actions lower peripheral resistance against which the heart must pump, decreasing preload. Decreases in preload lead to an increase in cardiac output. Nitrates also decrease systemic arterial pressure and afterload, which may result in hypotension. The combined effects reduce the preload on the heart and help relieve chest pain (Lessig & Lessig, 1998; Green, 2003).

11. Why was Mr. Johnson given an aspirin in the ED? Explain the use of abciximab (ReoPro), ticlopidine (Ticlid), and aspirin therapy for Mr. Johnson.

Antiplatelet therapy, specifically aspirin, is now standard therapy for unstable angina and treatment after an MI. The American Heart Association (1999) recommends the use of aspirin in patients who have experienced an MI, unstable angina, ischemic stroke, or transient ischemic attacks. The primary mechanism accounting for the benefit is believed to be related to irreversible inhibition of the cyclooxygenase pathway in platelets, blocking formation of thromboxane A_2 and thromboxane A_2-induced platelet aggregation. This inhibition is complete with small doses of aspirin. It is strongly recommended that all patients with AMI receive nonenteric-coated aspirin, 160 to 325 mg, to chew and swallow as soon as possible after the clinical impression of evolving AMI is formed, and whether or not thrombolytic therapy is to be given. The dose should be repeated daily by mouth indefinitely (Cairns et al, 1998; Green, 2003). The adverse effects of aspirin are related to bleeding, particularly gastrointestinal.

Ticlopidine (Ticlid) is given in 250-mg doses twice a day. It is also an antiplatelet agent, but unlike aspirin, it does not block cyclooxygenase but interferes with the platelet activation mechanism mediated by adenosine diphosphate (ADP) and with transformation of the fibrinogen receptor glycoprotein IIb/IIIa into its high-affinity state. It can be associated with diarrhea, rash, reversible neutropenia, thrombocytopenia, and liver function abnormalities. It takes approximately 2 weeks of treatment before the full benefit of ticlopidine is achieved (Alexander et al, 1998; Cairns et al, 1998; Green, 2003).

Abciximab (ReoPro) is a platelet glycoprotein IIb/IIIa receptor inhibitor with proven efficacy in the management of ischemic coronary syndromes (Casserly et al, 1998). Abciximab is started during the PTCA and is most often used as adjunctive therapy to intracoronary stent implantation (Hasdai et al, 1998). It is administered as an intravenous bolus of 0.25 mg/kg followed by an infusion at a rate of 10 µg/min for 12 hours. This regimen results in greater than 80% receptor occupancy and inhibition of platelet aggregation induced by ADP. The drug can be found on platelets as long as 15 days after its discontinuation (Cairns et al, 1998; Green, 2003).

Eptifibatide (Integrilin) is another antiplatelet agent. It works by preventing the binding of fibrinogen, von Willebrand factor, and other adhesive ligands to glycoproteins IIb/IIa. The recommended regimen consists of a bolus ranging from 90 to 250 µg/kg followed by an infusion at rates of 0.5 to 3 µg/kg/min. It is recommended for use in patients with acute coronary syndrome, including patients who are to be managed medically and those undergoing PTCA. It has been shown to decrease the rate of a combined endpoint of death, new MI, or need for urgent intervention (Key Pharmaceuticals, 1998; Green, 2003).

There is a striking reduction in adverse outcomes in patients treated with inhibitors of the platelet glycoprotein IIb/IIIa receptor as an adjunct to angioplasty and combined with thrombolytic therapy (GUSTO IIb, 1997).

There are also recommendations for patients undergoing balloon angioplasty or atherectomy alone who cannot tolerate aspirin to be treated with clopidogrel 300 mg oral loading dose, followed by a daily dose of 75 mg prior to the procedure. This has as well been postintervention if a stent has been placed with great success to prevent restenosis.

12. Discuss the pharmacologic actions of heparin and enoxaparin (Lovenox) and the indications for use with a patient with an AMI.

During an AMI there is a hypercoagulability that leads to blood cells "sticking together." This can increase the closure of arteries and lead to a more severe MI. The anticoagulant effects of heparin and enoxaparin (Lovenox) keep the blood thinner and prevent clotting. This can help the blood travel arteries that are very narrow with atherosclerosis.

Heparin is an anticoagulant. It inhibits activated factors IS, S, SI, and XII, which are involved in the conversion of prothrombin to thrombin, thereby reducing clot formation. At low dosages it prevents the conversion of prothrombin to thrombin. At higher dosages, it neutralizes thrombin, preventing the conversion of fibrinogen to fibrin and thus

If the volume ejected decreases, the heart rate will increase as a compensatory mechanism to maintain the same cardiac output. If the heart rate is unable to maintain the same level of cardiac output, blood pressure will drop" (Becker, 1999). The determinants of cardiac output are preload, afterload, contractility, and heart rate. Therapy can be implemented to affect each of the determinants of cardiac output to achieve optimum heart function.

Preload

Preload is defined as the volume of pressure generated at end-diastole. LV preload is recorded as the pulmonary artery wedge pressure (PAWP). A normal PAWP is between 6 and 12 mm Hg. The PAWP can be used to monitor the relative extent of pulmonary congestion. A PAWP of 18 to 20 mm Hg is considered moderate congestion, and a PAWP of greater than 30 mm Hg is acute pulmonary edema. Right ventricular preload is recorded as the central venous pressure or the right atrial pressure; normal is 2 to 7 mm Hg.

Afterload

Afterload is defined as the impedance to the ejection of blood from the ventricle. It is the resistance that the ventricle must overcome to eject blood in a forward direction. The two determinants of afterload are (1) the volume and mass of blood ejected from the ventricle and (2) the compliance and total cross section of the vascular space into which the blood is ejected.

Right ventricle afterload is recorded as peripheral vascular resistance (PVR). The normal PVR is 150 to 250 dynes/sec/cm^{-5}. LV afterload is systemic vascular resistance, the normal of which is 800 to 1500 dynes/sec/cm^{-5}.

Medications that decrease the systemic vascular resistance (SVR) include nitroprusside, hydralazine, and captopril. Dobutamine may also be used to decrease the SVR by increasing the cardiac output. Medications that increase the SVR include dopamine, epinephrine, norepinephrine, and phenylephrine (Lessig & Lessig, 1998).

Ranges of normal values for hemodynamic parameters are as follows:

RAP	1-7 mm Hg	**PAWP**	6-12 mm Hg
RVP		**MAP**	70-105 mm Hg
Systolic	15-25 mm Hg	**SVR**	800-1500 dynes/sec/cm^{-5}
Diastolic	0-8 mm Hg	**PVR**	150-250 dynes/sec/cm^{-5}
PAP		**CO**	4-8 L/min
Systolic	15-25 mm Hg	**CI**	2.5-4.5 L/min/m^2
Diastolic	8-15 mm Hg	**SV**	60-130 ml/beat

22. What is cardiogenic shock? What symptoms did Mr. Johnson exhibit?

Cardiogenic shock is when the body's needs for oxygen are not met for a prolonged period. The body begins to compensate for the decreased oxygen supply by increasing the heart rate, stroke volume, and contractility. However, as the condition continues, these compensatory measures result in cardiac decompensation. The patient begins to show signs of shock: low blood pressure, increased or decreased heart rate, and decreased oxygen saturation. Auscultation of rales signifies that the patient is developing CHF or pulmonary edema. The patient may have a decreased level of consciousness, diaphoresis, nausea, and vomiting. This condition is critical and must be addressed immediately.

Mr. Johnson had an S$_3$ with wheezes on auscultation and his chest radiograph showed some CHF before angioplasty. After PTCA, his pulmonary artery systolic pressure was 42 mm Hg, his pulmonary artery diastolic pressure was 22 mm Hg, and his PAWP was 22 mm Hg. His SaO$_2$ dropped to 86%, requiring mechanical ventilation with a 100% nonrebreather mask. All of these represent moderate congestion of the lungs. He became hypotensive, tachycardic, pale, cool, and diaphoretic. These are typical signs of cardiogenic shock. After the PTCA, an IABP was placed to help decrease the workload of the heart and ease the cardiogenic shock. Therapy with dobutamine (Dobutrex) was started to increase his blood pressure and cardiac output.

23. What are the therapeutic effects of dopamine (Intropin) at low, moderate, and high dosages?

Dopamine has α- and β-adrenergic effects as well as dopaminergic effects. At low dosages of 1 to 2 µg/kg/min, it increases renal and mesenteric blood flow. At moderate dosages of 2 to 10 µg/kg/min, its positive inotropic effects increase cardiac output, blood pressure, and cerebral blood flow. At dosages greater than 10 µg/kg/min, dopamine exhibits pure α stimulation, causing peripheral vasoconstriction (with increased SVR and afterload) and loss of renal and mesenteric dilation. Dopamine is indicated to treat hypotension in shock states not caused by hypovolemia (LeFever-Key & Hayes, 1997; Lessig & Lessig, 1998).

24. What are the therapeutic effects of dobutamine (Dobutrex)?

Dobutamine (Dobutrex) stimulates β-receptors in the heart. It is a direct-acting positive inotropic agent. It increases stroke volume and cardiac output by increasing contractility and decreasing SVR (Lessig & Lessig, 1998; Green, 2003).

Cardiogenic shock can be the result of a "stunned myocardium," a situation in which the heart does not work very well because the muscle is still in a state of shock from the decreased blood supply during the MI. Dobutamine can increase the cardiac output and stroke volume by increasing the heart's contractility, thereby decreasing the workload of the heart.

25. What advantage does an IABP offer Mr. Johnson?

The purpose of the IABP is to decrease myocardial oxygen demand by decreasing myocardial workload, to increase coronary perfusion, and to decrease afterload. An IABP can prevent cardiogenic shock, limit infarct size, and limit myocardial ischemia (Lessig & Lessig, 1998). For Mr. Johnson, the IABP was used because of cardiogenic shock after an AMI and refractory chest pain after administration of tPA.

To place an IABP, a balloon catheter is inserted via the femoral artery into the descending thoracic aorta. The inflation and deflation of the balloon are synchronized with the patient's ECG. The balloon is inflated during diastole, which augments diastolic pressure and increases coronary blood flow and myocardial oxygen supply. The result is improved myocardial contractility. The balloon is deflated just before systole, creating a vacuum effect. This helps the ventricle empty its contents more fully, reducing the LV end-diastolic pressure. In addition, deflation in systole reduces the afterload for the left ventricle, decreasing its myocardial oxygen requirements (Lessig & Lessig, 1998; Goldman & Bennett, 2000).

26. What significance does the IABP have in relation to the tPA and urokinase given previously?

Potential complications associated with the use of an IABP are (1) ischemia of the limb distal to the insertion site, (2) dissection of the aorta, (3) thrombocytopenia, (4) septicemia, and (5) infection at the insertion site (Lessig & Lessig, 1998; Goldman & Bennett, 2000). A common complication of IABP therapy is bleeding of the insertion site. The patient usually receives heparin (except after coronary artery bypass graft surgery) during the course of treatment with IABP, and this potentiates the bleeding.

Mr. Johnson, who has received tPA and urokinase, has an extremely high risk of bleeding at the insertion site of the IABP. The insertion site, pulses in the left radial artery, peripheral pulses, urine output, and level of consciousness need to be checked every 15 minutes for the first 2 hours, then every 30 minutes for 2 hours, and then at least hourly.

27. Mr. Johnson was sent home with a prescription for diltiazem (Cardizem). Why would a patient with heart disease be given a calcium channel blocker?

Calcium channel blockers decrease the entry of calcium into smooth muscle and dilate coronary arteries and peripheral arterioles. Vasodilation of the coronary arteries provides an increase in coronary blood flow and oxygen supply. Arteriolar vasodilation in peripheral circulation produces a reduction in afterload and reduces myocardial oxygen demand. This decreases systemic blood pressure, total peripheral resistance, and afterload of the heart. Platelet aggregation may be inhibited and bleeding prolonged (Alexander et al, 1998; Green, 2003). Examples of calcium channel blockers include diltiazem (Cardizem), nifedipine (Procardia), and verapamil (Calan).

28. Why was Mr. Johnson sent home with a prescription for captopril (Capoten)?

Captopril (Capoten) is an angiotensin-converting enzyme (ACE) inhibitor. ACE inhibitors block the conversion of angiotensin I to angiotensin II. Angiotensin II is a potent vasoconstrictor. The goal is to decrease the patient's blood pressure and afterload without causing an increase in heart rate or a change in cardiac output. Studies have shown that patients who exhibit LV dysfunction have improved mortality and morbidity rates from major cardiovascular events when these drugs are used (Becker, 1999; Goldman & Bennett, 2000; Green, 2003). ACE inhibitors are continued for 4 to 6 weeks after MI.

PERCUTANEOUS TRANSLUMINAL CORONARY ANGIOPLASTY AND THROMBOLYTIC THERAPY IN MYOCARDIAL INFARCTION

References

Alexander, R. W., et al. (1998). *Hurst's the heart* (9th ed.). St Louis: McGraw-Hill Health Professions Division.

American Heart Association. (1999). *Your heart* [WWW document]. http://www.americanheart.org/catalog/Heart catpage16.html.

Antman, E. M., et al. (1996). Cardiac-specific troponin I levels to predict the risk of mortality in patients with acute coronary syndromes. *The New England Journal of Medicine, 335,* 1342-1349.

Aversano, T. (1998, September). Primary angioplasty in the treatment of acute myocardial infarction. In R. D. Bahr (Chair), *The strategy of chest pain units (in emergency departments) in the war against heart attacks: Proceedings of the First Maryland Chest Pain Center Research Conference,* Dearborn, MI [WWW document]. www.aspen.newc.com/chestpain/clinicalinformation/maryland/aversano.html.

Becker, D. (1999). Coronary artery disease. In L. Bucher & S. Melander (Eds.), *Critical care nursing* (pp. 201-225). Philadelphia: W. B. Saunders.

Braunwald, E., Zipes, D., & Libby, P. (Eds.). (2001). *Heart disease: A textbook of cardiovascular medicine* (6th ed., Vols. 1 and 2). Philadelphia: W. B. Saunders.

Bucher, L. & Melander, S. (Eds.). (1999). *Critical care nursing.* Philadelphia: W. B. Saunders.

Cairns, J. A., et al. (1998). Antithrombic agents in coronary artery disease. *Chest, 114* (Suppl. 5), 611-628.

Casserly, I. P., et al. (1998). Usefulness of abciximab for treatment of early coronary artery stent thrombosis. *American Journal of Cardiology, 82,* 981-984.

Erbel, R., et al. (1998). Coronary-artery stenting compared with balloon angioplasty for restenosis after initial balloon angioplasty. *The New England Journal of Medicine, 339,* 1672-1678.

Global Use of Strategies to Open Occluded Coronary Arteries in Acute Coronary Syndromes (GUSTO IIb). (1997). A clinical trial comparing primary coronary angioplasty with tissue plasminogen activator for acute myocardial infarction. *The New England Journal of Medicine, 336,* 1621-1627.

Goldman, L. & Bennett, J. (2000). *Cecil textbook of medicine* (21st ed.). Philadelphia: W. B. Saunders.

Green, S. (2003). *Tarascon's pocket pharmacopoeia.* New York: Tarascon Publishing.

Gulanick, M., Bliley, A., Perino, B., & Keough, V. (1998). Recovery patterns and lifestyle changes after coronary angioplasty: The patient's perspective. *Heart & Lung, 27,* 253-262.

Gurfinkel, E., Fareed, J., Antman, E., Cohen, M., & Mautner, B. (1998). Rationale for the management of coronary syndromes with low-molecular-weight heparins. *American Journal of Cardiology, 82,* 151-181.

Hasdai, D., et al. (1998). Abciximab administration and outcome after intracoronary stent implantation. *American Journal of Cardiology, 82,* 705-709.

Holmes, D. R., Jr. (1999, January). Coronary stenting: A revolution in cardiology. *Cardiology Today,* www.todayin-cardiology.com/199901/editorial.ASP.

Holubkov, R., et al. (2002). Angina 1 year after percutaneous coronary intervention: A report from NHLBI registry. *American Heart Journal, 144*(5), 826-833.

Key Pharmaceuticals, Inc. (1998). Product information: Integrilin. Kenilworth, NJ.

Lessig, M. L. & Lessig, P. M. (1998). The cardiovascular system. In J. G. Alspach (Ed.), *American Association of Critical-Care Nurses: Core curriculum for critical care nursing* (5th ed.). Philadelphia: W. B. Saunders.

Lundergan, C., Reiner, J., & Ross, A. (2002). How long is too long? Association of time delay to successful reperfusion and ventricular function outcome in acute MI: The case for thrombolytic therapy before planned angioplasty for acute myocardial infarction. *American Heart Journal, 144* (3), 456-462.

Murphy, M. J. & Berding, C. B. (1999). Use of measurements of myoglobin and cardiac troponins in the diagnosis of acute myocardial infarction. *Critical Care Nurse, 19*(1), 58-66.

Popma, J., et al. (2001). Antithrombotic therapy in patients undergoing percutaneous coronary intervention. *Chest 119* (1 Suppl.), 321-336.

Shavelle, D., Parsons, L., Sada, M., French, W., & Every, N. (1999). Is there a benefit to early angiography in patients with ST-segment depression myocardial infarction? An observational study. *American Heart Journal, 143*(3), 488-496.

Tcheng, J. E. (1996). Glycoprotein IIb/IIIa receptor inhibitors: Putting the EPIC, IMPACT II, RESTORE, and EPILOG trials into perspective. *American Journal of Cardiology, 78,* 35-40.

Topol, E. J. (1998). Coronary-artery stents—gauging, gorging, and gouging. *The New England Journal of Medicine, 339,* 1702-1703.

Urden, L. D., Stacy, K. M., & Lough, M. E. (Eds.). (2002). *Thelan's critical care nursing: Diagnosis and management* (4th ed.). St. Louis: Mosby.

Zidar, J. P. (1998). Low-molecular-weight heparins in coronary stenting (the ENTICES trial). *American Journal of Cardiology, 82*(Suppl. 5B), 29-32.

2

Coronary Artery Bypass Graft

M. Lynn Rodgers, RNC, MSN, CCRN, CNRN, ACNP-BC

CASE PRESENTATION

Mr. Cates, a 57-year-old moderately obese man, had a 3-month history of progressive typical anginal chest pain. He reported that the symptoms first occurred with heavy exertion and involved what he described as a "heaviness" in his chest. The symptoms were promptly relieved with rest. Over the past weeks he had been experiencing increasingly frequent episodes of chest pain accompanied by diaphoresis. The episodes had become more prolonged, and he had experienced one episode of pain occurring at rest after a heavy meal. Mr. Cates was moderately obese and had a 20-year history of hypertension, which was being treated with an ACE inhibitor. A 12-lead electrocardiogram (ECG) showed atrial fibrillation with rapid ventricular response, another long-term problem for which he took amiodarone and warfarin (Coumadin). Other risk factors in Cates's history include hypercholesterolemia (350 mg/dl) that decreased to 190 mg/dl with dietary modifications and treatment with atorvastatin (Lipitor). Mr. Cates also took aspirin, 325 mg, every day. He also had a 30-year, two-packs-a-day smoking history, which continued up to the present. Mr. Cates previously had surgery for a bilateral inguinal hernia repair, cholecystectomy, and arthroscopic surgery on his left knee. He had rheumatic fever as a child. He also gave a history of problems with gastric reflux and was currently taking pantoprazole (Protonix).

Mr. Cates was evaluated by his family physician after a prolonged episode of chest pain. The results of an ECG were unremarkable; however, in view of the progression of his symptoms, he was referred to a cardiologist. Mr. Cates underwent an exercise stress treadmill examination with a Adenosine Myoview scan. The stress test was terminated after 3.2 minutes because he developed anterior chest pain and 2 to 2.5 mm ST-segment depression in ECG leads V_1 through V_4. Sublingual nitroglycerin times two was required to completely relieve his chest pain. The myoview scan revealed two areas of reversible defects in the anterior wall of the left ventricle. An echocardiogram was also performed that demonstrated severe mitral stenosis. The decision was made to proceed with cardiac catheterization to further delineate the extent of disease. Cardiac catheterization revealed the following:

- Severe triple-vessel coronary artery disease was found with significant left main stenosis of 70%.
- The left anterior descending coronary artery (LAD) had 99% obstruction.
- The right coronary artery (RCA) had 90% (dominant) obstruction.
- The first obtuse marginal ramus (OM1) had 80% obstruction.
- The aortic valve was normal without significant stenosis or regurgitation; however, the mitral valve showed moderate stenosis with vegetative debris.

- The left ventricular end-diastolic pressure (LVEDP) was 7 mm Hg before injection and 14 mm Hg after dye injection. The left ventricular ejection fraction was estimated to be within the normal range at 55%.
- Mild to moderate hypokinesia was seen in the anterior wall.
- The left internal mammary artery was found to be of good caliber and available for a conduit.

Because of the critical stenosis of the left main coronary artery, the presence of severe triple-vessel disease, and mitral valve stenosis, angioplasty was not an option. Urgent coronary artery revascularization was scheduled for the next morning, with bypass grafts proposed to the LAD coronary artery, diagonal artery, RCA, circumflex coronary artery, and OM1 as well as mitral valve replacement and possible Maze procedure. Immediately after the catheterization, Mr. Cates developed severe (rated as a 9 on a 1 to 10 pain scale) anterior chest pain with radiation to the left arm. He became diaphoretic, and his systolic blood pressure fell to 90 mm Hg. He was given intravenous (IV) nitroglycerin and an infusion of dobutamine (Dobutrex) at 3 µg/kg/min to stabilize his condition. Because of the left main artery stenosis, an intraaortic balloon pump (IABP) was inserted via the left femoral artery. Excellent augmentation was obtained with a 2:1 setting, and all pain was relieved. The next morning cardiac surgery was performed, using the left internal mammary artery to bypass the LAD, with separate saphenous vein grafts placed to the LAD, diagonal artery, OM1, and RCA. Atrial and ventricular pacing wires were placed. The IABP was left in place and was used before and after the bypass. The surgery was uneventful, and Mr. Cates was admitted to the open-heart recovery area 6 hours after initiation of anesthesia.

On admission to the open-heart recovery area, the following data were obtained from Mr. Cates:

BP	110/70 mm Hg (via arterial line)
HR	110 bpm (sinus tachycardia)
Respirations	10 breaths/min (ventilation with IMV 10)
Temperature	35.1° C (95.2° F)
PAP	25/8/18 mm Hg (systolic, diastolic, mean)
PCWP	7 mm Hg
Cardiac index	2.3 L/min/m^2 (cardiac output: 4.2 L/min)
SVR/SVRI	1500 dyne/sec/cm^{-5}/814 dyne/sec/cm^{-5}/m^2

A chest x-ray film confirmed correct placement of the pulmonary artery (Swan-Ganz) catheter, endotracheal tube, and nasogastric tube.

The following laboratory data were obtained:

Hgb	10.3 g/dl
Hct	31%
Glucose	220 mg/dl
K$^+$	3.2 mmol/L
Mg$^+$	1.5

The following ventilator settings were used:

IMV	10
V$_T$	750 ml
Fio$_2$	100%
PEEP	5 cm

Arterial blood gas measurements showed the following:

pH	7.30
Po$_2$	156 mm Hg
Pco$_2$	46 mm Hg

HCO₃⁻   16 mmol/L
Sao₂   96%

The following lines were placed:

- Right radial arterial line
- Swan-Ganz (pulmonary artery) catheter in the right subclavian vein
- Endotracheal tube (oral)
- Nasogastric tube via the left nares to low continuous suction
- Peripheral IV line via a #19 angiocatheter in the left forearm
- Chest tube in mediastinum, which drained 150 ml since placement
- Foley catheter
- IABP

Mr. Cates's urinary output values were as follows:

- Produced 300 ml of urine during bypass
- Produced 250 ml since termination of bypass

The following drugs were given via drip:

- Dobutamine (Dobutrex) 5 µg/min
- Nitroglycerin 15 µg/min

CORONARY ARTERY BYPASS GRAFT

QUESTIONS

1. Discuss the pathophysiology of coronary artery atherosclerosis. Include a discussion of risk factors associated with the development of this disease. How does Mr. Cates fit the profile of the "typical" patient who has coronary artery bypass graft (CABG) surgery?

2. Explain the purpose of nuclear scanning and include a discussion of Mr. Cates's findings and how these led to the decision to proceed with cardiac catheterization.

3. What are the indications for CABG surgery? What is the mortality rate for CABG surgery? Why was angioplasty not considered as an option for Mr. Cates?

4. Discuss the significance of left main coronary artery stenosis.

5. Mr. Cates requested that the surgeon perform the "new" minimally invasive surgery and drill holes in his heart. Discuss minimally invasive direct coronary artery bypass graft (MIDCABG) surgery and transmyocardial revascularization (TMR) and their applicability to Mr. Cates's case.

6. How does valve surgery differ from CABG?

7. What is the Maze procedure, why is it done, and what are the nursing implications of this procedure?

8. Describe the cardiopulmonary bypass (CPB) machine and discuss myocardial protection during surgery. What are the potential complications associated with the CPB machine?

9. Discuss the mode of action of the IABP and the reason for its use in this case.

10. What other mechanical assist devices are used for a failing heart after open heart surgery?

11. Compare and contrast the use of the internal mammary artery and saphenous vein as conduits in CABG surgery. What are the relative benefits and concerns associated with each? What other conduits can be used?

12. What can be done in the future should Mr. Cates begin to have symptoms of coronary occlusion again?

13. Explain the purpose of the Swan-Ganz catheter in Mr. Cates. What are the potential complications associated with its use?

14. Describe the rationale for using dobutamine (Dobutrex) and nitroglycerin (Tridil) in Mr. Cates. Discuss how each of these drugs affects volume, preload, contractility, and afterload.

15. What other vasoactive drugs are used in the postoperative open heart patient and why?

16. Analyze the hemodynamic findings as presented and discuss therapy adjustments that might be necessary.

17. Based on the arterial blood gas results, are the ventilator settings correct? If not, what alterations would you recommend and why? What complications might be expected as a consequence of Mr. Cates's history of smoking?

18. What is the expected postoperative chest tube drainage in a patient after CABG surgery? Discuss autotransfusion as it relates to patients undergoing CABG surgery.

19. List appropriate nursing diagnoses that might be used in planning care for the patient after CABG surgery.

20. What other complications of open heart surgery can develop, and what measures are used to avoid or treat them?

21. Discuss lifestyle modifications that might be necessary after CABG surgery. What is the importance of a cardiac rehabilitation program in the recovery of the patient?

CORONARY ARTERY BYPASS GRAFT

QUESTIONS AND ANSWERS

1. **Discuss the pathophysiology of coronary artery atherosclerosis. Include a discussion of risk factors associated with the development of this disease. How does Mr. Cates fit the profile of the "typical" patient who has coronary artery bypass graft (CABG) surgery?**

   Atherosclerosis produces a hardening of the arteries or thickening of the arterial walls. Atherosclerosis generally is characterized by lipid deposits that can progress to partial or total obstruction of the lumen wall. Coronary arteries are particularly susceptible to atherosclerosis, which is most commonly seen in patients with a history of smoking, sedentary lifestyle, and high-fat diets (Urden et al, 2002). The exact cause is still unknown. There are basically two theories with widespread acceptance: the response to injury theory and the thrombogenic theory. The atherosclerotic lesion or plaque consists of elevated areas of fatty streaks, which are muscle cells filled with lipids and secondary deposits of calcium salts and blood products. Lipid levels of total cholesterol >200 mg/dl, low-density lipoprotein (LDL) >130 mg/dl, high-density lipoprotein (HDL) <50 mg/dl, and triglyceride >150 mg/dl are associated with an increased risk for development of coronary artery disease (Bucher & Melander, 1999; Ferri, 2001; Barron, 2003).

   Risk factors can be divided into two categories: modifiable and nonmodifiable. Nonmodifiable risk factors are uncontrollable and include age older than 55 years, gender (men have a greater incidence than women until menopause), family history of coronary artery disease, and race (African-Americans have a higher incidence than Caucasians). Modifiable risk factors are controllable and include hypertension (blood pressure >140/90 mm Hg), smoking, hyperlipidemia (increased low-density lipoprotein levels), obesity, stress, diabetes, and sedentary lifestyle (Bucher & Melander, 1999; Barron, 2003; Massie & Amidon, 2003).

   Mr. Cates's history fits the profile of a patient who has CABG surgery. He is moderately obese and has a 20-year history of hypertension. He also has hypercholesterolemia with a laboratory value of 350 mg/dl, which he initially attempted to modify through his diet, but had to resort to atorvastatin (Lipitor). Atorvastatin is a lipid-reducing agent that works by inhibiting enzymes that form cholesterol (Massie & Amidon, 2003). Mr. Cates also has a 30-year, two-packs-a-day smoking history and a family history positive for coronary atherosclerosis.

2. **Explain the purpose of nuclear scanning and include a discussion of Mr. Cates's findings and how these led to the decision to proceed with cardiac catheterization.**

   Several radioactive isotopes can be used in conjunction with either an exercise stress treadmill ECG or bicycle ergometer to differentiate between ischemia and infarction. The nuclear material is injected prior to exercise, and resting pictures are completed. When it is injected during peak exercise, normal heart cells will have more blood flow and activity than abnormal ischemic heart cells. Repeat nuclear scanning after exercise will reveal cold spots of perfusion defects due to decreased or absent blood flow and increased oxygen demand. Wall motor defects and heart pump performance are evaluated before and after exercise. A fixed abnormal defect may occur, which can indicate prior myocardial infarction. The myoview scan in this situation demonstrated an abnormal nonreversible cold spot that was the same before and after exercise. If a patient has normal results from a myoview stress study, there may be no need for a cardiac catheterization (Urden et al, 2002). However, 50% stenosis can exist before a nuclear stress test is "positive." Some acute myocardial infarctions occur with demonstrated stenosis of less than 50% due to plaque rupture and clot development (Wackers et al, 2001.)

Mr. Cates's stress myoview scan was terminated after 3.2 minutes when he developed severe anterior chest pain. The scan revealed two areas of reversible defects in the anterior wall of the left ventricle. Because of the test results, it was necessary to proceed with the cardiac catheterization for further evaluation of cardiac disease.

3. **What are the indications for CABG surgery? What is the mortality rate for CABG surgery? Why was angioplasty not considered as an option for Mr. Cates?**

More than 300,000 people in the United States undergo CABG surgery every year (Chen-Scarabelli, 2002). The following are indicators for CABG surgery (Gillinov & Loop, 2002; Lytle, 2002).

- Chronic stable angina refractory to medical therapy
- Significant left main coronary occlusion (>50%)
- Triple-vessel coronary artery disease
- Two-vessel coronary artery disease with angina and ischemia and a proximal anterior descending lesion
- Left ventricular dysfunction or proximal LAD disease
- Unstable angina
- Left ventricular failure (congestive heart failure or cardiogenic shock)
- Critical triple-vessel disease after thrombolytic therapy
- Postinfarction angina with multivessel disease
- Acute left ventricular aneurysm in patients with nonmechanical cardiogenic shock, if the patient's condition is stabilized
- Mechanical defects such as ventricular septal defects, mitral regurgitation (intermittent and persistent), and cardiac rupture with tamponade

Mr. Cates's diagnosis was severe triple-vessel disease with significant left main stenosis, both of which indicate the need for CABG surgery and rule out the need for angioplasty.

4. **Discuss the significance of left main coronary artery stenosis.**

The left main coronary artery supplies the apex, part of the lateral wall, the anterior wall, and two thirds of the septum. Because of the amount of myocardium that depends on blood supply from the left main coronary artery, significant stenosis of this artery or the proximal LAD places the myocardium at increased risk for myocardial infarction. CABG surgery involving the left main stem coronary artery is associated with higher hospital mortality of 13.6 % as reported by one study (Flameng et al, 2003). However, prompt surgical intervention in patients with left main coronary artery disease has been effective in increasing their 3-year survival rates to 85% or 90% compared with medical treatment rates of 65% to 69% (Gillinov & Loop, 2002).

5. **Mr. Cates requested that the surgeon perform the "new" minimally invasive surgery and drill holes in his heart. Discuss minimally invasive direct coronary artery bypass graft (MIDCABG) surgery and transmyocardial revascularization (TMR) and their applicability to Mr. Cates's case.**

Beating-heart or off-pump CABG surgery was first performed in 1967. With the development of the CPB machine, this method was abandoned in the mid-1970s. MIDCABG has had a resurgence since the early 1990s, and currently 20% of all CABG surgeries are performed in this manner (Chen-Scarabelli, 2002; Cheng et al, 2002). The MIDCABG is a type of heart surgery used to bypass blockages in one or two coronary arteries without use of the CPB. The procedure is most often used when the LAD needs to be revascularized, but an obstruction in the right descending coronary artery may also be accessed with this type of surgery. Obstructions in coronary arteries on the inferior and posterior portions of the heart are not amenable to this type of surgery. As the heart continues to beat, the distal anastomosis site on the myocardium is held motionless using a coronary artery stabilizer device. The proximal anastomosis site on the aorta is completed by applying a C-shaped clamp on part of the aorta that isolates the graft site from blood flow. If the internal mammary artery (IMA) is used, it is dissected from the chest wall and transected distally, freeing the end for anastomosis to the LAD or RCA. The proximal end of the IMA is left attached to the subclavian artery. The three major complications of CABG are related to median sternotomy, use of the CPB machine, and manipulation of the aorta. Use of MIDCABG can avoid these complications, and patients have shorter lengths of stay in the hospital with fewer complications (Chen-Scarabelli, 2002). There is a quicker return to normal activities and less morbidity associated with the surgery. For Mr. Cates, a MIDCABG is not the appropriate operation because of the complexity of his disease, the need for multiple bypass grafts and mitral valve surgery, and possible Maze surgery.

TMR is a method of creating 20 to 40 channels through the myocardium with a laser. Three theories have been suggested to explain the apparent clinical benefits of this procedure. The first theory attributes this benefit to the creation of myocardial holes or channels to allow blood to flow into ischemic areas. However, closure of these channels occurs soon after they are made, making this theory less likely. The second theory suggests that the created channels disrupt nerve fibers of the heart. Such denervation prevents nerve conduction of the sensations accompanying myocardial ischemia, and the patient does not feel the angina. The final and most accepted rationale for the benefits of TMR is that the procedure stimulates neorevascularization or angiogenesis. The irritation and inflammation of the laser channels stimulate the heart to grow microvascular structures that perfuse myocardial cells (Lytle, 2002). TMR is most often performed during open heart surgery with CABG and/or valve replacement as the channels are made from the epicardial to endocardial layers. TMR often results in less angina and a better quality of life for its recipients. A method of TMR performed from endocardial to epicardial layers via the standard cardiac catheterization procedure has also been done with mixed results (Urden et al, 2002). Both methods have a higher incidence of bleeding and cardiac tamponade (Gillinov & Loop, 2002).

6. How does valve surgery differ from CABG?

The aortic and mitral valves (AV; MV) are most frequently replaced during open heart surgery (Urden et al, 2002). Tricuspid and pulmonic valves are much less likely to require surgery. The AV and MV can both be replaced by biological tissue or mechanical valves. Biological tissue valves are either homogeneous or heterogeneous. Homogeneous valves are those that have been procured from brain-dead human donors and specially prepared for use. Heterogeneous tissue valves are either fashioned from bovine pericardium or obtained from porcine valves. Mechanical valves are of various types and consist of mechanical tilting disks that simulate valve activity. All types of artificial valves require incision into the myocardium with painstaking deployment and suturing into place. Proper valve size and placement are crucial. The MV can also be treated with commissurotomy in cases of mitral stenosis or with valve repair and annuloplasty with mitral regurgitation. During commissurotomy, fused valve leaflets are incised and/or calcium deposits are debrided to allow more valve mobility. With valve repair the annulus is tightened usually using a synthetic ring, and the size of the mitral valve is reduced. This allows the valve leaflets to close more completely (Braunwald, 2001).

Care of the patient with valvular surgery is similar to that of CABG, but some differences do exist. Patients with valve surgery generally have more dysrhythmias, bleeding, and stunned myocardium postoperatively (Braunwald, 2001). Most have temporary pacing wires placed as incisions into the myocardium, which can lead to disruption or inflammation of the electrical conduction structures. Bleeding and its associated complications are more likely with valve surgery. More surfaces in the heart have been disrupted, allowing more sites for bleeding. Because valve surgery frequently is accompanied by CABG, bypass pump time is increased. The myocardium is more likely to have poor contractility and low cardiac output and index. Longer bypass pump times are closely associated with more complications. Surgical mortality and length of hospital stay are often increased. Mortality for valve procedures is 4% to 5%, whereas valve procedures plus CABG have mortality rates of 7.6% (Flameng et al, 2003). Length of stay after valve surgery is generally longer than with CABG surgery alone, ranging from 5 to 9 days. Patients receiving mechanical valves must take lifelong anticoagulation with warfarin (Coumadin) to reduce thromboembolism (Adams & Antman, 2001). However, these mechanical valves are more durable and last longer. Those with biological tissue valves usually require anticoagulation for only a few weeks or months postoperatively. Biological tissue valves are selected for those patients that are older, cannot take anticoagulation, or are noncompliant with drug therapy. Younger women who anticipate childbearing could also receive a tissue valve to avoid anticoagulation during pregnancy (Zevola et al, 2002).

Interestingly, CABG and mitral valve procedures have recently been completed using robotic-assisted surgery. The Food and Drug Administration (FDA) approved robotic surgical systems for valve procedures in 2000, and IMA harvesting in 2001. Advantages of robotic-assisted cardiac surgery include earlier ambulation, smaller incisions, decreased pain levels, and reduced length of stay. In addition, operating time and personnel fatigue are reduced. Development of further technologies in cardiothoracic surgery is expected (Nifong et al, 2003; Reger & Janhke, 2003).

7. What is the Maze procedure, why is it done, and what are the nursing implications of this procedure?

The Maze procedure is a method of surgical interruption of the conduction pathways in the atria to correct atrial fibrillation unresponsive to medications. Patients unable to tolerate long-term anticoagulation required for atrial fibrillation may also be candidates for the Maze procedure. The atrial appendages are small extensions in the atria that are often responsible for the propagation of atrial fibrillation. These structures are surgically removed, and small cuts are made in the remaining atrial tissue to a Maze configuration. Reentry pathways are disrupted, and the sinoauricular (SA) impulse is directed to the atrioventricular (AV) node through the "maze." This allows restoration of a normal sinus rhythm and synchrony of the atria and ventricles. Bleeding may be increased due to the incisions into the heart. Temporary pacing wires are inserted as this surgical technique may result in bradycardia or asystole. If sinus rhythm is not eventually restored within the first 3 months of this procedure, a permanent pacemaker will be required (Massie & Amidon, 2003.)

8. Describe the cardiopulmonary bypass (CPB) machine and discuss myocardial protection during surgery. What are the potential complications associated with the CPB machine?

The CPB machine protects the heart with hemodilution, hypothermia, and anticoagulation (Chen-Scarabelli, 2002). The CPB machine diverts the patient's blood from the heart and lungs from the arrested heart's right atrium to a membrane oxygenator. Once in the oxygenator, carbon dioxide is given off and oxygen is bound to hemoglobin through diffusion. After arterialized with oxygen, the blood is returned to the systemic circulation through the aorta. This diversion creates a bloodless, motionless area in which to operate. The patient is systemically given heparin before initiation of the bypass pump to prevent clotting within the bypass circuit (Urden et al, 2002).

Myocardium protection during bypass surgery has been a concern from inception of this surgery. Experience has shown that the key to myocardium preservation is continuous myocardial hypothermia, as this decreases the need for oxygen by as much as 50% (Chen-Scarabelli, 2002). Myocardial hypothermia can be instituted by (1) lowering blood temperature via the heat exchanger on the CPB machine, (2) applying sterile saline slush to the heart and operative field, and (3) injecting cold cardioplegic solution directly into the coronary vessels by antegrade infusion in the coronary arteries and retrograde infusion via the coronary venous sinus. Cardioplegic solution consists of high levels of potassium, sodium bicarbonate, and glucose to stop the heart suddenly, prevent cellular acidosis, and provide energy for the myocardium. Oxygenated blood is frequently mixed with the car-

Table 2-1	*Potential Complications of Cardiopulmonary Bypass*
Causes	**Effects**
Third space losses, postoperative diuresis, sudden vasodilation (drugs, rewarming)	Intravascular fluid deficit (hypotension)
Decreased plasma protein concentration, increased capillary permeability	Third space losses (weight gain, edema) and subsequent relative hypovolemia
Hypothermia, increased systemic vascular resistance, prolonged cardiopulmonary bypass pump time, preexisting heart disease, inadequate myocardial protection	Myocardial depression (decreased cardiac output)
Systemic heparinization, mechanical trauma to platelets, depressed release of clotting factors from liver as a result of hypothermia	Coagulopathy (bleeding)
Decreased surfactant production, pulmonary microemboli, interstitial fluid accumulation in the lungs	Pulmonary dysfunction (decreased lung mechanics and impaired gas exchange)
Red blood cell damage in pump circuit	Hemolysis (hemoglobinuria)
Decreased insulin release, stimulation of glycogenolysis	Hyperglycemia (rise in serum glucose)
Intracellular shifts during bypass, postoperative diuresis secondary to hemodilution	Hypokalemia and hypomagnesemia
Inadequate cerebral perfusion, microemboli to the brain	Neurologic dysfunction
Catecholamine release and systemic hypothermia causing vasoconstriction	Hypertension

Data from Urden, L. D., Stacy, K. M., & Lough, M. E. (Eds.). (2002). *Thelan's critical care nursing: Diagnosis and management* (4th ed.). St Louis: Mosby.

dioplegic solution to help prevent myocardial hypoxia (Flameng et al, 2003). After an initial dose for diastolic arrest, intermittent infusion of cardioplegic solution approximately every 20 to 30 minutes is necessary for the maintenance of myocardial hypothermia and cardioplegic arrest. Myocardial hypothermic temperatures should remain between 12° and 20° C below normal to provide adequate protection (Chen-Scarabelli, 2002). Urden and associates (2002) outline potential complications from the use of the cardiopulmonary bypass machine in Table 2-1.

9. **Discuss the mode of action of the IABP and the reason for its use in this case.**

The IABP is used to increase coronary artery perfusion and support failing coronary circulation (Lorenz & Coyte, 2002; Urden et al, 2002). Indications for use of the IABP are as follows:

1. Left ventricular failure after cardiac surgery
2. Unstable angina refractory to medications
3. Recurrent angina
4. Complications of acute myocardial infarction including:
   a. Cardiogenic shock
   b. Papillary muscle dysfunction
   c. Ventricular septal defect
   d. Refractory ventricular arrhythmias

The IABP inflates during diastole and deflates before systole. Balloon inflation is timed by using the dicrotic notch, which denotes the closure of the aortic valve. The inflation forces blood forward and backward simultaneously. This increases coronary artery perfusion and decreases left ventricular afterload, the systemic vascular resistance the left ventricle pumps against. The forward flow also increases perfusion to the organs and the periphery, whereas the backward flow forces an increased amount of blood into the coronary arteries. The sudden deflation reduces the pressure in the aorta and decreases afterload, which decreases the workload of the heart (Massie & Amidon, 2003). Contraindications for using the IABP are severe aortic valve disease, inability to tolerate anticoagulation required, and severe tachycardia. The IABP was used in Mr. Cates after the catheterization, when he developed severe chest pain and his systolic pressure dropped to 90 mm Hg. Because of Mr. Cates's extensive left main coronary artery stenosis, the IABP did assist in increasing coronary artery perfusion, decreasing his afterload, and lessening the workload of the heart. Once the IABP was in place, all pain was relieved.

Crucial nursing care when a patient has an IABP are (Urden et al, 2002):

- Assessing for IABP migration and aortic dissection by monitoring bilateral upper and lower extremity perfusion and renal function
- Observing for bleeding as heparin is used to decrease thrombus formation on the IABP
- Detecting and treating rhythm disturbances because heart rate variations can alter timing of inflation and deflation
- Repositioning the patient carefully to prevent skin disruption and pulmonary atelectasis
- Protecting IABP placement and preventing artery shear by logrolling the patient, avoiding leg flexion, and maintaining head of bed elevation less than 30 degrees
- Reviewing timing of inflation and deflation to optimize augmentation of systolic function
- Providing adequate pain relief, emotional support, and sleep with medications and/or other measures

10. What other mechanical assist devices are used for a failing heart after open heart surgery?

Some patients with severe ventricular function are unable to be weaned off the extracorporeal bypass machine at the end of surgery in spite of aggressive inotropic therapy. An external ventricular assist device (VAD) can be used to assist the heart until the ventricles recover (Urden et al, 2002). Outflow cannulas are placed in the left atrium or left ventricle for left ventricular support and/or the right atrium for right ventricular support. Inflow cannulas are placed into either the aorta or femoral artery for the left ventricular assist device (LVAD) and the pulmonary artery for the right ventricular assist device (RVAD). Inflow and outflow cannulas are then attached to an external drive console. Anticoagulation with heparin is required. Console flow rates can be adjusted to 1 to 6 L/min to ensure adequate cardiac output until the ventricle(s) recover. Bleeding, infection, and device failure are all worrisome complications when using VADs. The VAD is also used as a bridge to transplantation in those patients with irreversible ventricular failure (Stahl & Richards, 2003; Bond et al, 2003; Cianci et al, 2003).

11. Compare and contrast the use of the internal mammary artery and saphenous vein as conduits in CABG surgery. What are the relative benefits and concerns associated with each? What other conduits can be used?

The conduits, or vessels, most commonly used today are the saphenous vein (SV) and the internal mammary (or internal thoracic) artery (IMA). Both conduits have been used successfully in surgical revascularization individually and in combination when multiple graft sites are necessary. Advantages for use of the saphenous vein include technical ease, decreased harvest time, and flexibility of the vein. However, because the SV has luminal valves, the vessel must be "reversed" to allow blood to flow to the heart in an unobstructed manner. By directing arterial blood in the direction opposite to that of the in situ SV, the valvular cusps are rendered nonfunctional. The patency rate for saphenous vein grafts is not as good as the IMA, being 87% at 1 year, 70% at 5 years, 81% at 10 years, and falling to 50% at 15 or more years (Lytle, 2002).

The internal mammary artery is viewed as the graft of choice for bypass of the LAD. Use of both internal mammary arteries in younger patients enhances revascularization results and increases survival rates and graft longevity (Gillinov & Loop, 2002). As reported by Lytle (2002) the patency rate of the internal mammary artery is 98% at 1 year, 96% at 10 years, and greater than 90% for up to 20 years. The absence of valves minimizes luminal turbulence, which reduces the risk of occlusion by thrombosis. Angiography has validated the ability of the internal mammary artery to dilate in response to increased demand. In addition only a distal anastomosis site is required if the IMA is left attached to the subclavian artery. Limitations include increased time needed for harvesting of the graft. Harvesting the IMA also requires extensive dissection from the chest wall, thus postoperative bleeding and chest wall discomfort are increased. The internal mammary artery may not be suitable as a conduit because of small size (especially in women), inadequate flow, or damage incurred during harvesting. In patients who have undergone chest wall irradiation, its use may also be limited. The internal mammary artery may be used as a pedicle or as a free graft (Adams & Antman, 2001).

Alternative conduits have been used successfully in patients who have had previous CABG surgery or whose IMAs or SVs are not usable (Urden et al, 2002). The gastroepiploic artery (GEA) that extends along the greater curvature of the stomach, and the inferior epigastric artery (IEA) originating from the left iliac artery, may be used as a pedicle or free grafts (Gillinov & Loop, 2002). The GEA and IEA are difficult to harvest and cannot be used on some coronary arteries due to anatomic limitations. An abdominal incision is required, and patients may have gastrointestinal complications after surgery with potential for intraabdominal bleeding (Lytle, 2002). The most commonly used alternative conduit, however, is the radial artery. It is easily harvested as a free graft, but collateral flow from the ulnar artery to the hand is required. Vasospasm of the alternative arterial grafts is more likely, and nitroglycerin and calcium channel blockers are required in the early postoperative period (Massie & Amidon, 2003).

12. What can be done in the future should Mr. Cates begin to have symptoms of coronary occlusion again?

Isolated vein graft and fibrous or intimal lesions that occur within 3 years of CABG surgery may be treated with percutaneous transluminal coronary angioplasty and stents. Complication rates are often high, and poor late results may occur. The AWESOME Trial from 1995-2000 studied patients with at least one prior CABG procedure to compare long-term survival of intervention by redo CABG or percutaneous coronary intervention (PCI). This study did reveal that PCI was a viable option for those patients with prior CABG. Mortality rates were lower in the PCI group at 1, 6, 12, and 36 months. However, those treated by redo CABG had less unstable angina and less need for repeat revascularization (Morrison et al, 2002). PCI and medical management may be the only option in those patients who are unable to have redo CABG surgery. Diffuse severe coronary atherosclerosis is best treated by reoperation if conduits are available. Reoperation is technically more difficult to do because of adhesions and scarring from the original surgery. Incidence of postoperative complications is greater, especially bleeding, and mortality rates are higher with repeated surgery. The incidence of reoperation is 3% at 5 years, 10% at 10 years, and 30% at 15 years (Gillinov & Loop, 2002). Currently 2% to 6% of CABG surgery is redo procedures (Czerny et al, 2003).

13. Explain the purpose of the Swan-Ganz catheter in Mr. Cates. What are the potential complications associated with its use?

Postoperative hemodynamic monitoring is needed for patients after CABG surgery so that vascular tone (preload and afterload), myocardial contractility, cardiac output, and volume or fluid balance may be monitored at the bedside. This is accomplished through use of a Swan-Ganz catheter. Postoperatively, patients may exhibit a low cardiac output because of preexisting heart disease, low volume from hemorrhage or third spacing, or prolonged time on the cardiopulmonary bypass machine (Gillinov & Loop, 2002). In most patients reduced preload is the cause of the reduced cardiac output. Less coming into the ventricle results in less going out of the ventricle. In addition, high systemic vascular resistance or increased afterload from vasoconstriction can further decrease cardiac output. Through use of the Swan-Ganz catheter, parameters can be assessed, and early intervention can be pursued to correct any postoperative problems (Urden et al, 2002).

The balloon-tipped Swan-Ganz catheter allows for measurements in the right atrium and pulmonary artery and indirect measurements of left atrial and ventricular function. The right atrial pressure (RAP) or central venous pressure (CVP) is measured through use of the proximal port opening just before the right atrium in the superior vena cava. This measurement reflects venous return to the right side of the heart and right ventricular function through central venous return and right ventricular end-diastolic pressure (RVEDP). Normal values for CVP vary from person to person; therefore, it is important to monitor the CVP trend along with the clinical picture. In general, values of 2 to 8 cm H_2O are considered within normal limits. The Swan-Ganz catheter also measures pulmonary artery pressures (PAP) and pulmonary capillary wedge pressures (PCWP), which are measured through the distal port opening in the pulmonary artery. Pulmonary artery systolic pressure represents pressures that are generated by right ventricular systole. The pulmonary artery diastolic pressure reflects LVEDP and is used as a measure of diastolic filling and left ventricular function or preload. The PCWP is measured by gently inflating the balloon at the end of the catheter, allowing pressure to be generated back through the lung vessels from the left side of the heart. It reflects the left atrial pressures and is used in the assessment of LVEDP as well. Direct left atrial pressure (LAP) measurement can be achieved through percutaneous insertion of a catheter directly into the left atrium during cardiac surgery and brought out of the chest wall to be connected to pressure-monitoring devices. This provides a continuous display of left atrium pressures, which can be used instead of inflating the balloon on the Swan-Ganz catheter to obtain a PCWP. LAP is the most accurate measurement of left ventricular preload and in the normal heart is the same as the LVEDP. Increased LAP or PCWP may be caused by decreased contractility, tachyarrhythmias, fluid overload, or mitral or aortic valve stenosis or regurgitation. Decreased levels may be caused by hypovolemia and possibly postoperative hemorrhage (Urden et al, 2002; Massie & Amidon, 2003) (Table 2-2).

14. Describe the rationale for using dobutamine (Dobutrex) and nitroglycerin (Tridil) in Mr. Cates. Discuss how each of these drugs affect volume, preload, contractility, and afterload?

Dobutamine (Dobutrex) is a synthetic catecholamine with mostly a β_1 effect. Dobutamine is more effective than dopamine for increasing myocardial contractility. It increases stroke volume and cardiac output by increasing contractility; it also decreases systemic vascular resistance and reduces the PCWP. Dobutamine is very effective in the treatment of heart

Table 2-2 *Normal Hemodynamic Readings*				
CVP		3 cm H_2O		
LAP		2 mm Hg		
	RAP	RVP	PAP	PCWP
Systolic	20-30 mm Hg	20-30 mm Hg		
Diastolic	1-5 mm Hg	10-20 mm Hg		
Mean arterial Hg	2-6 mm Hg	2-6 mm Hg	10-15 mm Hg	4-12 mm

failure, especially for patients who are hypotensive and cannot tolerate vasodilator therapy. Dobutamine does not have the renal vasodilating effect of dopamine, except indirectly as an effect of increased cardiac output. At low dosages, dobutamine can decrease blood pressure, especially if the patient is volume depleted. High doses of dobutamine can increase heart rate, thereby increasing myocardial oxygen consumption and possibly ischemia. A major advantage of dobutamine is its effect of reducing the PCWP or left ventricular preload, which is especially important in patients after surgery. Many physicians combine this drug with dopamine to maximize the renal blood flow and reduce the PCWP. An arterial line should be used to assess blood pressure. Dobutamine should be infused via a volumetric infusion pump. The range of dosage is 2.5 to 20 µg/kg/min but is usually started at 2 to 5 µg/kg/min and titrated on the basis of hemodynamic parameters (Massie & Amidon, 2003)).

Nitroglycerin (Tridil) is a nitrate and a direct smooth muscle relaxant. This drug produces smooth muscle relaxation, which causes decreased systemic vascular resistance (SVR). Hypotension may occur as a result of peripheral vasodilation. Patients may complain of headaches from the cerebral vasodilation. This pooling of blood in the systemic circulation decreases venous return and decreases preload. It is indicated for left ventricular failure, hypertension, angina pectoris, and congestive heart failure; it is also indicated after cardiac surgery. Patients should have an arterial line so that continuous blood pressure readings may be obtained. Nitroglycerin should be infused via a volumetric infusion pump for accuracy and safety. Usually, the IV infusion is started at 5 µg/min and titrated to the lowest amount that produces the desired effect. Often the combination of nitroglycerin and dobutamine allows for decreased SVR and increased cardiac output, resulting in increased blood pressure. Milrinone lactate (Primacor) can also be used for both these effects but with less control of each effect individually. Starting dose for milrinone is 50 µg/kg/min initial bolus followed by 0.375 to 0.75 µg/kg/min. These drugs should not be stopped suddenly but instead be tapered by reducing the flow every 15 minutes. During the tapering process the patient should be constantly observed for return of ischemic symptoms or hypertension (Urden et al, 2002).

15. **What other vasoactive drugs are used in the postoperative open heart patient and why?**

Other drugs can be used to affect preload, afterload, and myocardial contractility. Nitroprusside (Nipride) is used to decrease postoperative hypertension and/or elevated SVR similar to the use of nitroglycerin. Extensive catecholamine release by the body in response to empty ventricles during extracorporeal bypass (ECB) and hypothermic vasoconstriction can greatly increase SVR. By decreasing afterload, the workload of the ventricles is decreased and cardiac output improves. Starting dosage for nitroprusside is 0.5 to 2 µg/kg/min. Phenylephrine (Neo-Synephrine), dopamine, epinephrine, and norepinephrine (Levophed) infusions may be used when the SVR is low and hypotension is present. Vasodilation during rewarming, increased capillary permeability from histamine release during ECB that allows third spacing of intravascular fluid, and hypovolemia from bleeding and/or excess diuresis can lead to this low SVR and hypotension. Phenylephrine causes vasocontriction without unwanted tachycardia. Epinephrine is used to increase contractility of the heart and SVR thus increasing blood pressure. It is a potent α- and β-sympathetic nervous system stimulator that produces increased heart rates and should be used cautiously. Doses at 0.5 µg/kg/min are started and titrated upward to as high as 4 µg/kg/min until desired results are achieved without unwanted side effects. Low-dose dopamine at ≤3 µg/kg/min is used to improve cardiac output, thus increasing renal and mesenteric perfusion. Doses at 2.5 to 8 µg/kg/min produce mostly β-effects and cause increased myocardial contractility and blood pressure. High-dose dopamine at doses greater than 8 µg/kg/min produces mostly α-effects and causes profound vasoconstriction. A drug used as a last resort when other vasoconstricting drugs fail is norepinephrine (Levophed), a powerful vasoconstrictor because it has pure α-properties. It does not increase coronary artery perfusion pressure and increases myocardial oxygen consumption. Dosing starts at 0.02 to 0.04 µg/kg/min. Caution should be used when using norepinephrine or high-dose dopamine because renal perfusion and function can be decreased to the point of oliguria or even anuria. Use of any vasoconstricting drugs should be done through a central line if possible because infiltration of these powerful drugs can cause tissue ischemia and damage.

16. **Analyze the hemodynamic findings as presented and discuss therapy adjustments that might be necessary.**

The hemodynamic parameters that would be of concern are an increased heart rate at 110 bpm, blood pressure of 110/70 mm Hg, PCWP of 7 mm Hg, cardiac index of 2.3 L/min/m^2 body surface area, systemic vascular resistance of 1500 dyne/sec/cm^{-5} with an SVRI of 814 dyne/sec/cm^{-5}/m^2, and temperature of 35.1° C (95.2° F). These data indicate that the patient is "dry" and cold. When the patient begins to warm up after surgery, the vasodilation coupled with volume depletion could possibly cause the patient to "bottom out" hemodynamically. Administration of plasma expanders such as albumin, an increase in the rate of IV fluids, and an increase in vasoconstriction drugs may be necessary (Urden et al, 2002).

17. **Based on the arterial blood gas results, are the ventilator settings correct? If not, what alterations would you recommend and why? What complications might be expected as a consequence of Mr. Cates's smoking history?**

Mr. Cates's pH is in respiratory and metabolic acidosis, not uncommon immediately after open heart surgery. His PCO_2 value is high, and his HCO_3^- is low. His tidal volume is too low for his weight. Tidal volume is usually calculated at 8 to 10 ml/kg (Urden et al, 2002). By increasing his tidal volume to 1000 ml, the PCO_2 level will decrease and respiratory acidosis will most likely be corrected. Metabolic acidosis is common after CABG due to release of lactic acid from reperfusing peripheral tissue. Often improving respiratory ventilation will improve metabolic acidosis, but sodium bicarbonate may be required. In addition, his PO_2 levels are high, and a decrease in FIO_2 is warranted as well. Incrementally increasing the positive end-expiratory pressure (PEEP) to 7.5 cm H_2O, and to 10 cm H_2O if needed, while monitoring the blood pressure, would improve Mr. Cates's ventilation and allow even lower levels of FIO_2. Arterial blood gas measurements should be obtained in 1 hour to evaluate the patient's response to these changes and again prior to extubation (Chesnutt & Prendergast, 2003). Mr. Cates's extensive history of smoking may increase the difficulty level of weaning him from the ventilator postoperatively. He could develop increased secretions, which could alter oxygen exchange. Close monitoring of Mr. Cates's arterial blood gas results, vital signs, and airway secretions is necessary. Most patients after open heart surgery are extubated in less than 6 hours depending upon intraoperative events such as CPB time, preoperative lung function, comorbidities, and postoperative complications (Walthall & Ray, 2002).

18. **What is the expected postoperative chest tube drainage in a patient after CABG surgery? Discuss autotransfusion as it relates to patients undergoing CABG surgery.**

Urden and colleagues (2002) state that more than 500 ml of chest tube drainage in 1 hour or 300 ml in 2 consecutive hours after open heart surgery would be an indication to reenter the chest to assess the situation. Normal chest tube drainage should be no more than 100 to 150 ml/hr. One of the dangers of increased bleeding is cardiac tamponade. Autotransfusion is a mechanism in which the patient's own blood can be collected, filtered, and reinfused to minimize complications from using donor blood. Heparin or regional anticoagulants such as citrate phosphate dextrose or acid phosphate dextrose may be added to the autotransfusion collection system. Potential complications are coagulation problems, air embolism, hemolysis, cardiac tamponade, and sepsis. When these systems are used as autotransfusion mechanisms, it is necessary to remove all air and add a filter that will remove all clots before the blood is returned to the patient.

19. List appropriate nursing diagnoses that might be used in planning care for the patient after CABG surgery.

Nursing diagnoses for the patient after CABG surgery include the following (Bucher & Melander, 1999; Doering et al, 2002; Urden et al, 2002):

- Decreased cardiac output
- Ineffective airway clearance
- Ineffective breathing pattern
- Impaired gas exchange
- Altered tissue perfusion
- Activity intolerance
- Self-care deficit
- Altered body temperature, hypothermia
- Acute pain
- Altered sensory-perceptual deficit
- Altered thought processes
- Anxiety
- Fear
- Powerlessness
- Self-concept disturbance
- High risk for sexual dysfunction
- Fluid volume deficit
- High risk for fluid volume overload
- High risk for infection
- Impaired swallowing
- Impaired tissue integrity
- Altered oral mucous membranes
- High risk for constipation

20. What other complications of open heart surgery can develop, and what measures are used to avoid or treat them?

Most complications of open heart surgery are related to median sternotomy, use of CPB, and manipulation of the aorta and include the following (Chen-Scarabelli, 2002; Lorenz & Coyte, 2002; Lytle, 2002; Redeker & Hedges, 2002; Walthall & Ray, 2002):

Arrhythmias—Ventricular, Atrial Fibrillation, and Heart Block
- Correct K^+ and Mg^+ to high normal levels.
- Consider β-blockers, amiodarone, calcium channel blockers.
- Utilize temporary epicardial pacing.

Bleeding
- Consider fresh-frozen plasma, fibrinogen, cryoprecipitate, packed red blood cells, platelets.
- Administer aprotinin, aminocaproic acid (Amicar), desmopressin, or protamine.
- Apply PEEP.
- Reexplore the chest.

Cardiac tamponade
- Maintain chest tube patency—milk tubes for clots.
- Monitor for elevating and equalizing CVP, pulmonary artery diastolic pressure (PADP), and PCWP.
- Monitor for decreasing CO, blood pressure, and urine output.
- Observe for jugular vein distention (JVD), pulsus paradoxus, electrical alternans, and muffled heart sounds.
- Evaluate for increasing bleeding or sudden cessation of chest tube drainage.

Hypothermia
- Apply body-warming air blankets (BAIR Hugger).
- Apply warm blankets.
- Maintain warm recovery room temperature.
- Increase temperature of inspired ventilator gases.

Pulmonary complications
- Reverse neuroblockade at end of surgery.
- Plan for early extubation as possible within 2 to 6 hours postoperatively.
- Administer short-acting agents and minimize narcotic and benzodiazepines during ventilator weaning.
- Provide adequate pain medication after extubation to facilitate use of incentive spirometer, coughing, and activity.
- Get patient up to chair and ambulate within 12 to 24 hours postoperatively.
- Maintain chest tube patency.

Cardiogenic shock/Acute myocardial infarction (AMI)/myocardial stunning
- Assess for increased SVR and decreased cardiac output/cardiac index (CO/CI).
- Monitor cardiac enzymes—immediate postoperative rise is normal but values decrease sooner than with AMI.
- Observe for ECG changes indicating ischemia or infarction.
- Administer vasoactive drugs as ordered and indicated.
- Prepare for cardiac catherization and/or return to surgery.

Infection
- Monitor temperature→101° F (38.3 °C) persistently is not desirable.
- Normalize glucose levels with sliding scale or continuous insulin infusion.
- Perform sterile wound care with minimal wound manipulation.
- Administer antibiotics as ordered usually until chest tubes are removed.
- Monitor white blood cell count—large elevations are not unusual immediately postoperatively but should begin to trend downward.
- Obtain blood, urine, and sputum samples for culture and sensitivity.

Neurological deficits/psychological distress
- Assess level of consciousness and motor activity upon awaking from anesthesia.
- Reorient patient frequently and liberalize visitation.
- Maximize sleeping patterns.
- Control environmental stimuli to decrease sensory overload.
- Use pain, sedation, and antidelirium drugs as necessary and ordered.
- Remove restraints as soon as possible.

Renal dysfunction
- Maintain cardiac output and index.
- Administer fluids and diuretics as indicated.
- Monitor BUN and creatinine levels.
- Avoid antiinflammatory agents if renal insufficiency or failure is present.
- Prepare for dialysis or continuous renal replacement therapy (CRRT) as required.

GI dysfunction
- Remove nasogastric tube after extubation.
- Start clear liquids and advance diet as tolerated.
- Increase activity.
- Administer medications as ordered to decrease gastric secretions and increase peristalsis.
- Administer antiemetics and stool softeners as ordered.

21. **Discuss lifestyle modifications that might be necessary after CABG surgery. What is the importance of a cardiac rehabilitation program in the recovery of the patient?**

Patients who have had CABG surgery must maintain the regimen of care prescribed by their health care providers after they leave the hospital. Nurses in the critical care unit begin instructing the patient, and this process continues in the step-down units until the patient is discharged. Compliance is stressed in the areas of diet, exercise, medications, stress reduction, control of hypertension, and smoking cessation. Risk modification and continued medical therapy are necessary after CABG surgery because atherosclerotic involvement of saphenous vein grafts is a long-term major complication. Lipid abnormalities must be treated through drug administration or diet to reduce the chance of reoperation for coronary artery disease (Urden et al, 2002).

Spouses or significant others should be included in all teaching sessions when possible. Patients and families should be linked to a support group, as possible. Cardiac rehabilitation must continue after discharge not only for physical rehabilitation but also to provide a support group to assist in the maintenance of new lifestyle modifications. Often rehabilitation facilities provide support groups for spouses of patients who had CABG surgery to emphasize food preparation (low-fat, low-cholesterol, low-sodium diets) or exercise. Spousal support groups can be effective in dealing with fears and concerns of the group members. Continuing cardiac rehabilitation after hospital discharge is the key to recovery after CABG surgery. Participation in an inexpensive rehabilitation program involving simple calisthenics and graduated walking has been shown to significantly increase employment rates after surgery and improve overall quality of life (Ross & Ostrow, 2001; Urden et al, 2002).

CORONARY ARTERY BYPASS GRAFT

References

Adams, D. H. & Antman, E. M. (2001). Medical management of the patient undergoing cardiac surgery. In E. Braunwald, D. P. Zipes, & P. Libby (Eds.), *Heart disease*, 6th ed. Philadelphia: W. B. Saunders.

Barron, R. B. (2003). In L. M. Tierney, S. T. McPhee, & M. A. Papadakis (Eds.), *2003 current medical diagnosis and treatment*. New York: Lange Medical Books/McGraw-Hill Co.

Bond, A. E., Nelson, K., Germany, C. L., & Smart, A. N. (2003). The left ventricular assist device. *American Journal of Nursing, 103*(1), 32-41.

Braunwald, E. (2001). Valvular heart disease. In E. Braunwald, D. P. Zipes, & P. Libby (Eds.), *Heart disease* (6th ed.). Philadelphia: W. B. Saunders.

Bucher, L. & Melander, S. (Eds.). (1999). *Critical care nursing*. Philadelphia: W. B. Saunders.

Chen-Scarabelli, C. (2002). Beating-heart coronary artery bypass graft surgery: Indications, advantages, and limitations. *Critical Care Nurse, 22*(5), 44-58.

Cheng, W., et al. (2002). Off-pump coronary surgery: Effect on early mortality and stroke. *The Journal of Thoracic and Cardiovascular Surgery, 124*(2), 313-319.

Chesnutt, M. S. & Prendergast, T. J. (2003). Lung. In L. M. Tierney, S. T. McPhee, & M. A. Papadakis (Eds.), *2003 current medical diagnosis and treatment*. New York: Lange Medical Books/McGraw-Hill Co.

Cianci, P., Lonergan-Thomas, H., Slaughter, M., & Silver, M. A. (2003). Current and potential applications of left ventricular assist device. *The Journal of Cardiovascular Nursing, 18*(1), 17-22.

Czerny, M., et al. (2003). Coronary reoperations: Recurrence of angina and clinical outcome with and without cardiopulmonary bypass. *Annals of Thoracic Surgery, 75,* 847-852.

Doering, L. V., McGuire, A. W., & Rourke, D. (2002). Recovering from cardiac surgery: What patients want you to know. *American Journal of Critical Care, 11*(4), 333-343.

Ferri, F. F. (2001). *Practical guide to the care of the medical patient*, St. Louis: Mosby.

Flameng, W. J., Herijgers, P., Dewilde, S., & Lasaffre, E. (2003). Continuous retrograde blood cardioplegia is associated with lower hospital mortality after heart valve surgery. *The Journal of Thoracic and Cardiovascular Surgery, 125*(1), 121-125.

Gillinov, A. M. & Loop F. D. (2002). Coronary artery bypass surgery. In E. J. Toprol (Ed.), *Textbook of cardiovascular medicine*. Philadelphia: Lippincott Williams & Wilkins.

Lorenz, B. T. & Coyte, K. M. (2002). Coronary artery bypass graft surgery without cardiopulmonary bypass: A review and nursing implications. *Critical Care Nurse, 22*(1), 51-60.

Lytle, B. W. (2002). Coronary bypass surgery. In V. F., Fuster, et al: *Hurst's the heart* (10th ed.). St Louis: McGraw-Hill Health Professional Division.

Massie, B. M. & Amidon, T. M. (2003). Heart. In L. M. Tierney, S. T McPhee, & M. A. Papadakis (Eds.), *2003 current medical diagnosis and treatment*. New York: Lange Medical Books/McGraw-Hill Co.

Morrison, D. A., et al. (2002). Percutaneous coronary intervention versus bypass surgery for patients with medically refractory myocardial ischemia. *Journal of the American College of Cardiology, 40*(11), 1951-1954.

Nifong, L.W., et al. (2003). Robotic mitral valve repair: Experience with the da Vinci system. *Annals of Thoracic Surgery, 75,* 438-443.

Redeker, N. S. & Hedges, C. (2002). Sleep during hospitalization and recovery after cardiac surgery. *The Journal of Cardiovascular Nursing, 17*(1), 56-68.

Reger, T. B. & Janhke, M. E. (2003). Robotic cardiac surgery. *AORN Journal, 77*(1), 182-186.

Ross, A. C. & Ostrow, L. (2001). Subjectively perceived quality of life after coronary artery bypass surgery. *American Journal of Critical Care, 10*(1), 11-16.

Stahl, M. A. & Richards, N. M. (2003). Ventricular assist devices: Developing and maintaining a training and competency program. *The Journal of Cardiovascular Nursing, 16*(3), 34-43.

Urden, L. D., Stacy, K. M., & Lough, M. E. (Eds.). (2002). *Thelan's critical care nursing: Diagnosis and management* (4th ed.). St. Louis: Mosby.

Wackers, F. J., Soufer, R., & Zaret, B. L. (2001). SPECT nuclear. In E. Braunwald, D. P. Zipes, & P. Libby (Eds.) *Heart disease* (6th ed.). Philadelphia: W. B. Saunders/Harcourt Health Sciences Co.

Walthall, H. & Ray, S. (2002). Do intraoperative variables have an effect on the timing of tracheal extubation after coronary artery bypass graft surgery? *Heart and Lung, 31*(6), 432-439.

Zevola, D. R., Roffa, M., & Brown, K. (2002). Using clinical pathways in patients undergoing cardiac valve surgery. *Critical Care Nurse, 22*(1), 31-50.

3

Cardiogenic Shock and Anterior Wall Myocardial Infarction

Roberta E. Hoebeke, RN, PhD, FNP, APRN, BC

Mrs. Settles, a 50-year-old woman, came to the emergency department at 6:30 AM with a 2-hour history of crushing substernal chest pain radiating to the jaw, back, and subxiphoid area. She was mildly diaphoretic and slightly short of breath, and she complained of nausea. Her lungs had bibasilar crackles on auscultation. Heart sounds revealed the presence of an S_3 heart sound without murmurs. The initial chest x-ray film showed no abnormalities. Her initial vital signs were as follows:

BP	156/98 mm Hg	**Respirations**	30 breaths/min
HR	124 bpm	**Temperature**	37° C (98.6° F)

Mrs. Settles had a history of stable angina for an undetermined period. However, she revealed that for the past 3 weeks, she had experienced substernal pain radiating to the back every hour. Chest pain was relieved with sublingual nitroglycerin (NTG). There was a family history of a brother dying from a myocardial infarction (MI) and a sister with a history of three MIs. Mrs. Settles had a 30-year history of cigarette smoking and continued to smoke one pack of cigarettes a day. She has been taking the following medications:

- Aspirin 81 mg po qd
- Propranolol hydrochloride (Inderal LA) 80 mg po qd
- Isosorbide mononitrate (Imdur SR) 30 mg po qd
- Lisinopril (Zestril) 10 mg po qd

Upon arrival at the emergency department, intravenous (IV) NTG 50 mg in 250 ml of dextrose 5% in water (D5W) was started and titrated to Mrs. Settles's pain level and blood pressure. Mrs. Settles was also given morphine sulfate 2 mg via slow IV push, and oxygen at 6 L through a nasal cannula was started. The initial 12-lead electrocardiogram (ECG) revealed early Q waves and massive ST-segment elevation in leads V_1 to V_4. Initial baseline laboratory data results were as follows:

WBCs	13.9 mm³	**Myoglobin**	120 ng/L
Glucose	117 mg/dl	**K⁺**	4 mmol/L
Hgb	14 g/dl	**Troponin T**	0.0 μg/L
BUN	6 mmol/L	**Cl⁻**	103 mmol/L

The editor would like to thank Debra L. Harom for her contribution to this chapter in the second edition of *Case Studies in Critical Care Nursing*.

Hct	41.8%	**CK-MB**	1.8%
Creatinine	0.9 mg/dl	**CO_2**	24 mmol/L
Na$^+$	141 mmol/L	**Troponin I**	0.0 μg/L

Mrs. Settles was assessed and confirmed to be a candidate for thrombolytic therapy. A tissue plasminogen activator (tPA) bolus and infusion were given, and a weight-based heparin drip of 25,000 U/250 ml of D5W was started at 1200 U/hr. She was then transferred to the cardiac intensive care unit (CICU) at 8:30 AM.

Once the tPA infusion was complete, Mrs. Settles experienced pain relief and occasional premature ventricular contractions (PVCs). An echocardiogram revealed dyskinesia with the entire septum, apex, and anterior wall. The ejection fraction (EF) was 20%.

At 12:30 PM (4 hours later), enzyme and arterial blood gas levels were determined:

Myoglobin	150 ng/L	**Pco_2**	52.1 mm Hg
pH	7.261	**Troponin I**	5.2 μg/L
CK-MB	36%	**HCO_3^-**	22.4 mmol/L

Mrs. Settles was then given 60% oxygen via face mask, and her vital signs were as follows:

BP	140/100 mm Hg
HR	130 bpm
Respirations	34 breaths/min

Day 1

The next morning Mrs. Settles continued to complain of shortness of breath and restlessness with level 2 chest pain. Rales were auscultated throughout all lung fields. A chest x-ray film revealed increasing congestive heart failure (CHF) with pulmonary edema. Vital signs were as follows:

BP	100/60 mm Hg	**Respirations**	36 breaths/min
HR	128 bpm	**Urine output**	20 ml/hr for past 2 hr

Mrs. Settles was given dopamine (Intropin) at 5 μg/kg/min and dobutamine (Dobutrex) at 5 μg/kg/min. She was also given 40 mg of furosemide (Lasix) intravenously. The NTG drip was continued at the same rate as that when she was admitted to the CICU. Morning enzyme levels were as follows:

Myoglobin	63 ng/L	**Troponin I**	5.0 μg/L
CK-MB	24%	**Troponin T**	0.2 μg/L

A morning 12-lead ECG revealed resolution of the ST-segment elevation but development of a new left bundle branch block (LBBB). Mrs. Settles was given another 40 mg of furosemide intravenously. The dopamine drip was continued with the order to titrate to maintain systolic blood pressure of 100 mm Hg, and the dobutamine drip was continued at 5 μg/kg/min. Because Mrs. Settles continued to complain of chest pain despite the NTG drip, placement of an intraaortic balloon pump catheter (IABP) and a pulmonary artery catheter was done in the catheterization laboratory.

After her return to the CICU, Mrs. Settles's vital signs and hemodynamic values were as follows:

BP	90/60 mm Hg	**CO**	2.5 L/min
PCWP	22 mm Hg	**Respirations**	30 breaths/min
SVR	1800 dynes/sec/cm^{-5}	**CI**	1.5 L/min/m^2
HR	130 bpm		

The IABP was timed at 1 to 1. Mrs. Settles continued to receive dopamine 6 μg/kg/min (to maintain blood pressure) and dobutamine 5 μg/kg/min. The NTG drip was decreased to 1 µg/kg/min to reduce afterload. The urine output had increased to 150 ml/hr, and the patient was breathing easier and was less restless and more alert.

Day 2

The morning of the second day of her hospital stay, Mrs. Settles's vital signs and hemodynamic values were as follows:

BP	100/60 mm Hg	CO	3 L/min
PCWP	18 mm Hg	Respirations	28 breaths/min
SVR	1420 dynes/sec/cm^{-5}	CI	2 L/min/m^2
HR	110 bpm		

Her cardiac enzyme levels continued to return to normal, and the transient LBBB was gone. Urine output was 100 ml/hr, and the drips remained unchanged.

Day 3

The morning of the third day, Mrs. Settles was free of pain and had unlabored respirations. Oxygen was decreased to 4 L/min through a nasal cannula. Vital signs and hemodynamic values were as follows:

BP	100/60 mm Hg	CO	4 L/min
PCWP	14 mm Hg	Respirations	24 breaths/min
SVR	1250 dynes/sec/cm^{-5}	CI	2.1 L/min/m^2
HR	110 bpm		

The IABP settings were reduced to 2 to 1. The dopamine drip was decreased to 3 µg/kg/min, the dobutamine drip was reduced to 2 µg/kg/min, and the NTG drip was discontinued.

Day 5

By the morning of the fifth day, the vasoactive drips and the IABP were discontinued. Hemodynamic values were within normal range for Mrs. Settles, and her vital signs were as follows:

BP	110/60 mm Hg
HR	83 bpm
Respirations	22 breaths/min

Mrs. Settles was scheduled for an afternoon cardiac catheterization for follow-up after thrombolysis and her brief episode of cardiogenic shock.

CARDIOGENIC SHOCK AND ANTERIOR WALL MYOCARDIAL INFARCTION

QUESTIONS

1. What is the clinical presentation of a patient having an acute myocardial infarction (AMI)? Identify Mrs. Settles's clinical presentation to the emergency department.

2. How is a diagnosis of AMI determined? Identify the results for Mrs. Settles that confirmed the diagnosis of AMI.

3. What are the treatment goals for a patient with an AMI?

4. Discuss the role of thrombolytic therapy in a patient with an AMI. Include indications and contraindications for use of thrombolytics.

5. Discuss the role of nitrates, β-blockers, and angiotensin-converting enzyme (ACE) inhibitors in the patient with an AMI.

6. What complications are commonly seen after an MI? What are the most common complications seen with an anterior wall MI?

7. What significant 12-lead ECG changes are sometimes seen following an anterior wall AMI? What 12-lead ECG changes occurred with Mrs. Settles?

8. Define cardiogenic shock and why it occurs after an anterior wall MI. What is the prognosis for the patient with cardiogenic shock?

9. What are the hemodynamic parameters seen in the patient with cardiogenic shock in comparison with normal hemodynamic parameters?

10. Discuss the goals of pharmacologic management in cardiogenic shock. Which medications were used for Mrs. Settles?

11. What types of mechanical support devices can be used for patients in cardiogenic shock and why? Which type was used for Mrs. Settles? Identify any specific nursing responsibilities for the device chosen for Mrs. Settles.

12. What are the nursing diagnoses for the patient in cardiogenic shock after an anterior AMI?

CARDIOGENIC SHOCK AND ANTERIOR WALL MYOCARDIAL INFARCTION

QUESTIONS AND ANSWERS

1. **What is the clinical presentation of a patient having an acute myocardial infarction (AMI)? Identify Mrs. Settles's clinical presentation to the emergency department.**

   The clinical presentation of patients experiencing an AMI is composed of a variety of physical findings that are influenced by the severity and location of the infarct. Chest pain is the most common physical finding of an acute coronary syndrome or AMI, and is classically described as crushing or squeezing. The pain is retrosternal, lasts for approximately 20 minutes or more, and often radiates to the left shoulder or intrascapular region, neck, jaw, teeth, and down the ulnar aspect of the left arm (Sobel, 2000). Uncommonly the pain may consist of a dull aching or burning sensation in the epigastrium, and thus may be confused with indigestion. Although chest pain may be considered the key presenting symptom of AMI, it is not always present. A large prospective observational study of 434,877 patients with confirmed MI revealed that 33% were clinically silent on presentation to the hospital (Canto et al, 2000). The silent MIs occurred more frequently in women, those patients who were older, and patients with diabetes mellitus. According to Bucher and Melander (1999) and Sobel (2000), patients experiencing an AMI generally appear pale, diaphoretic, restless, anxious, and have a sense of impending doom. ECG patterns of patients with AMI may reveal symptomatic or asymptomatic bradycardia, tachyarrhythmias, ventricular ectopy, and/or atrioventricular blocks. Blood pressure may be elevated early on due to arterial vasoconstriction, normotensive, or hypotensive as a result of left ventricular dysfunction. Other cardiovascular findings include additional heart sounds, consisting of S_3, S_4, new murmurs, and/or pericardial friction rubs; and signs of CHF, including shortness of breath, frothy sputum, jugular venous distention, peripheral edema, and auscultated crackles in lung fields. Urine output and peripheral pulses may be diminished as a result of decreased cardiac output (CO). Gastrointestinal symptoms may include nausea and vomiting, which are more common with female patients. Neurologic findings may include confusion, syncope, and stroke, particularly in patients 85 years and older.

   Mrs. Settles's Clinical Presentation

   Mrs. Settles's clinical presentation included a 2-hour history of substernal crushing chest pain that radiated to the jaw, back, and subxiphoid area. Mrs. Settles was also diaphoretic and short of breath and complained of nausea. Auscultation of her lungs revealed bibasilar crackles, and heart sounds revealed the presence of an S_3 gallop. Her blood pressure was elevated at 156/98 mm Hg, and she was tachycardic with a heart rate of 124 bpm.

2. **How is a diagnosis of AMI determined? Identify the results for Mrs. Settles that confirmed the diagnosis of AMI.**

   Criteria established nearly three decades ago by the World Health Organization (WHO) have been the foundation for diagnosis of AMI (Boersma et al, 2003). According to the WHO definition, two of the three following criteria must be met for a confirmed diagnosis of AMI:

   1. ST-segment changes or new, pathologic Q waves must be present on the patient's ECG.
   2. The patient must have a clinical presentation of acute, severe, prolonged chest pain characteristic of AMI.
   3. The patient must have abnormally elevated serum levels of cardiac enzymes such as creatine kinase myocardial band (CK-MB), an isoenzyme of CK.

   However, since September 2000 a new definition of AMI was proposed by the joint committee of the European Society of Cardiology and the American College of Cardiology

(ESC/ACC) that included the use of troponins to diagnose AMI (Meier et al, 2002). Using these new criteria, elevated enzyme levels of CK-MB or troponin I or T, with either chest pain symptoms or ECG changes confirms the diagnosis of AMI.

Because the first criterion for diagnosis of AMI listed by WHO encompasses significant ECG changes, initial and serial ECGs are critical for diagnosis of an AMI (Bucher & Melander, 1999). Serial ECGs are important to obtain because only about half of all patients with AMI will have diagnostic changes on their initial ECG (Nagle & Nee, 2002). Therefore normal results from an initial ECG alone do not rule out the possibility of cardiac dysfunction.

A baseline 12-lead ECG should be done as early as possible once chest pain develops and continuous ECG monitoring should be initiated to track changes in the evolution of the AMI. ECG changes associated with an AMI include patterns of ST-segment and T-wave abnormalities and the development of pathologic Q waves in the area of infarct. These changes can develop over minutes to hours following the onset of symptoms, and continuous monitoring will help detect ST-segment, QRS, and T-wave abnormalities, even if the patient is not having symptoms. With ST-segment elevation AMI, ST-segment elevation of 1 mm or more above baseline is noted in the leads that face toward the infarcted area, accompanied by tall positive T waves. In the leads facing away from the infarcted area, reciprocal ST-segment depression may be seen. During the evolution of the AMI over hours to days, Q waves and T-wave inversion may develop. Pathologic Q waves are ≥0.04 second in duration and constitute 25% of the height of the R wave. Some changes, such as initial ST-segment depression and T-wave inversion, can be difficult to differentiate from myocardial ischemia without AMI. Because other conditions may produce ECG changes that can simulate an AMI, ECG changes must be evaluated in the context of the entire clinical picture (Sobel, 2000; Nagle & Nee, 2002). The clinical presentation, as described in question 1, helps establish the diagnosis of AMI. Although chest pain characteristics vary from person to person, it is a significant finding in the process of diagnosing an AMI.

Various cardiac serologic markers can be additional resources for early evaluation and diagnosis of an AMI. CK-MB has been the standard enzyme for AMI diagnosis for several years. Although CK-MB is the dominant isoenzyme of creatine kinase in the heart and is highly specific for myocardial tissue, timing of peak levels and return to normal levels limit the window of opportunity for diagnostic use (Nagle & Nee, 2002). The identification of three new markers—myoglobin, troponin I, and troponin T—has provided more sensitive indicators for diagnosing an AMI (Murphy & Berding, 1999). In a systematic review of the literature, Panteghini (2002) found that the combination of a rapid rising marker, such as myoglobin, and a marker that rises more slowly but is more cardiac specific, such as the cardiac troponins, significantly improves the accuracy of diagnosis of AMI when compared with CK-MB alone. A comparison of the four markers is provided in Table 3-1 (Plaut, 1998). The CK-MB has been the gold standard for many years, but it is also found in skeletal muscle and can be elevated by muscle trauma or disease. Although CK-MB starts to rise within the first 3 hours of the onset of an AMI, myoglobin rises faster (30 minutes to 2 hours) and is

Table 3-1 *Acute Myocardial Infarction Serum Markers*			
Marker	**Time Appears**	**Peak Time**	**Return to Normal**
Myoglobin	0.5-2 hr	5-12 hr	18-30 hr
Troponin I	3-6 hr	14-20 hr	5-15 days
Troponin T	3-6 hr	10-24 hr	10-15 days
CK-MB	3-8 hr	9-30 hr	2-3 days

Modified from Plaut (1998).
CK-MB, Creatine kinase myocardial band.
Note: These values depend on both the analytical method and the cutoff used.

more sensitive for AMIs with very early onset of symptoms (Murphy & Berding, 1999; Nagle & Nee, 2002). The CK-MB peaks in about 24 hours (range from 9 to 30 hours) and returns to normal levels in 48 to 72 hours after elevation, whereas the cardiac troponins provide a longer diagnostic window by remaining sensitive for up to 15 days. For patients who seek help 48 hours after onset of symptoms, the CK-MB peak can be easily missed. The cardiac troponins would be better indicators of myocardial damage for those patients seen with chest pain for longer than 48 hours. However, CK-MB may be the best indicator for reinfarction that occurs between 48 hours and 7 days after initial chest pain because of its time window of normal and peak levels.

Although not part of the WHO diagnostic criteria, a color-flow Doppler transthoracic echocardiogram is often used to confirm the infarction. Echocardiograms enable a physician to determine the extent of the MI by evaluating myocardial wall motion and ventricular performance. The sensitivity and specificity of detecting abnormal wall motion consistent with AMI with this diagnostic imaging technique exceeds 90%, especially for patients who have not had a previous MI (Sobel, 2000).

Mrs. Settles's Diagnostic Results That Confirmed the AMI Diagnosis

Mrs. Settles's 12-lead ECG showed Q waves and ST-segment elevation in leads V_1 to V_4, indicating an anterior wall MI. The baseline laboratory results indicated only elevated myoglobin, with the other cardiac enzyme levels within the normal range. By the sixth hour, CK-MB, troponin I, and troponin T enzyme levels were elevated abnormally, indicative of extensive damage to the myocardium. The echocardiogram revealed a significantly reduced EF of 20% and dyskinesia affecting the entire septum, apex, and anterior wall.

3. What are the treatment goals for a patient with an AMI?

"Time is myocardium and time is outcomes" (Gibson, 2001): The time to treatment is critical to patient outcomes. The closer the treatment is to the onset of AMI symptoms, the more optimistic the outcomes. Treatment strategies, such as reducing the time to reperfusion of the myocardium with thrombolytics or primary percutaneous transluminal coronary angioplasty (PTCA), are focused on the goal of preserving the myocardium and reducing mortality and morbidity (Bucher & Melander, 1999; Gibson, 2001; Meils et al, 2002). The goals for a patient with AMI are to limit the size of the infarct, support the heart during shock, relieve pain, and manage arrhythmias. Other goals include providing education concerning the diagnosis and necessary lifestyle changes needed to prevent another infarct.

4. Discuss the role of thrombolytic therapy in a patient with an AMI. Include indications and contraindications for use of thrombolytics.

Uncontroversial evidence from clinical trials has demonstrated that thrombolytics are the most effective reperfusion treatment for ST-segment elevation AMI (Ribichini & Wijns, 2002). Most AMIs result from thrombotic occlusion of fissured, unstable coronary atheromatic plaque. In more than 90% of patients with Q-wave AMIs, occlusive thrombi can be seen angiographically (Sobel, 2000). Thrombolytic therapy and early reperfusion have become a standard of care for treatment of AMIs. Thrombolytic therapy has the advantage of being widely available to patients, and there is less time delay to initiate treatment compared with primary angioplasty (Ribichini & Wijns, 2002).

Thrombolytic therapy should be initiated within 6 hours of symptom onset for the greatest benefit. The earlier therapy is initiated, the lower the mortality. An additional selection criterion is ECG evidence of ST-segment elevation of 1 mm or more in two contiguous leads. Thrombolytics appear to be most effective in patients younger than 75 years who are experiencing their first anterior wall MI. Absolute contraindications include active hemorrhage (except menses), history of a hemorrhagic stroke, known intracranial neoplasm, and suspected aortic dissection (Green, 2003). Relative contraindications include severe uncontrolled hypertension, current use of anticoagulants, pregnancy or recent delivery, recent trauma or major surgery (2 to 4 weeks), active peptic ulcer, and prolonged cardiopulmonary resuscitation longer than 10 minutes (Bucher & Melander, 1999; Urden et al, 2002). Available data from clinical trials support the use of primary angioplasty instead of thrombolytic therapy for high-risk patients and those with hemodynamic impairment who are ineligible for thrombolytic therapy (Ribichini & Wijns, 2002).

Concurrent therapies recommended with thrombolytic therapy are oral aspirin 165 mg to 325 mg daily and intravenous weight-based heparin (Lessig & Lessig, 1998; Fiorini, 2001). The benefit of aspirin is a significant reduction in early mortality associated with AMI. The benefits of heparin are early coronary artery reperfusion and reduction of coronary artery reocclusion from clots.

Reperfusion Strategies Used for Mrs. Settles

Mrs. Settles received thrombolytic therapy in the form of tPA. She had experienced pain for approximately 2 hours and had ECG evidence of ST-segment elevation in leads V_1 to V_4. Mrs. Settles was only 50 years of age and had no absolute or relative contraindications to thrombolytic therapy. Therapy with IV heparin was started concurrently with the tPA. She did not have any side effects from the thrombolysis except for reperfusion arrhythmias, which are expected.

5. Discuss the role of nitrates, β-blockers, and angiotensin-converting (ACE) inhibitors in the patient with an AMI.

Nitrates play a major role in treating patients with AMI. Nitrates dilate the large coronary arteries, prevent vasospasm, and increase coronary collateral blood flow to the ischemic myocardium, thus they are effective in managing pain and ischemic symptoms (Killip, 2000). Bucher & Melander (1999) suggests that NTG may trigger antiplatelet effects, reduce infarct size, and improve ventricular remodeling. Sublingual NTG decreases left ventricular filling pressure without significantly lowering systemic vascular resistance (SVR). Intravenous NTG reduces both left ventricular filling pressure and SVR. The resulting venous dilation from intravenous NTG may cause severe hypotension (Green, 2003). The goal in administering intravenous NTG is to reduce blood pressure by 10 to 20 mm Hg, but not to less than 80 to 90 mm Hg systolic, otherwise this may compromise coronary artery perfusion and aggravate myocardial ischemia (Killip, 2000).

β-Adrenergic–blocking agents decrease heart rate and blood pressure and thereby reduce cardiac workload and myocardial oxygen consumption. β-Blocker therapy within 12 hours of onset of infarction has been confirmed to decrease infarct size, prevent extension of the infarct, and reduce mortality from AMI (Bucher & Melander, 1999). When β-blockers are started with thrombolytics, reinfarction rates and recurrent ischemia are reduced. Intravenous metoprolol (Lopressor) or atenolol (Tenormin) should be started within 2 hours of infarct presentation for optimal effectiveness. β-Blockers are contraindicated in patients with bradyarrhythmias, hypotension, moderate to severe CHF, and certain pulmonary disorders such as severe chronic obstructive pulmonary disease and asthma (Green, 2003). Randomized clinical trials have demonstrated that β-blockers not only reduce morbidity and mortality in the acute phase of AMI (Killip, 2000), but also that they should be continued indefinitely in patients who have recovered from AMI (Boersma et al, 2003).

In Q-wave AMI, as many as 40% of patients have subsequent ventricular wall thinning and ballooning of the infarcted segment, which leads to reduced ventricular function (Killip, 2000). Results from several clinical trials have shown that ACE inhibitors preserve ventricular function, decrease the development of congestive heart failure (CHF), and have a favorable effect on ventricular remodeling post AMI (Boersma et al, 2003). Initially it is recommended that patients be started on an ACE inhibitor orally within the first 24 hours after thrombolytic therapy has been completed if blood pressure is stable (Killip, 2000). Begin with low-dose therapy (one quarter to one half the usual starting dose) and gradually increase the dose over 2 to 4 days. If ventricular dysfunction is not evident after 6 weeks, ACE inhibitors may be discontinued. For long-term management, if there is evidence of reduced ventricular function, ACE inhibitors should be continued indefinitely to reduce mortality and reinfarction risk (Boersma et al, 2003).

Nitrate, β-Blocker, and ACE Inhibitor Use for Mrs. Settles

Mrs. Settles received IV NTG for control of chest pain before the initiation of thrombolytic therapy. She had been receiving propranolol 80 mg po daily at home before this admission and was not given further β-blockade because of her pulmonary status during cardiogenic shock. She was taking an ACE inhibitor upon admission, and this therapy was continued throughout her hospital course. Her physician will likely continue nitrate, β-blocker, and ACE inhibitor therapy, as well as aspirin, because these drugs have proven value for the long-term medical management of AMI patients.

6. What complications are commonly seen after an MI? What are the most common complications seen with an anterior wall MI?

Complications after an AMI include the following, in order of occurrence: arrhythmias, heart failure, infarct expansion, left ventricular mural thrombus, pericarditis, cardiogenic shock, left ventricular aneurysm, and other structural defects (Bucher & Melander, 1999; Urden et al, 2002).

Anterior wall infarction results from proximal left anterior descending (LAD) artery occlusion and may sometimes involve the left main coronary artery. The distribution of this area involves important cardiac electrical and mechanical pumping structures. As a result, specific complications of an anterior wall AMI include tachyarrhythmias (sinus tachycardia, atrial fibrillation, atrial flutter, paroxysmal supraventricular tachycardia, ventricular tachycardia, and ventricular fibrillation), left ventricular dysfunction/pump failure, CHF, ventricular aneurysm, and other structural defects (Bucher & Melander, 1999; Urden et al, 2002).

In a recent study researchers assessed whether nonfatal 24-hour complications in patients with AMI receiving thrombolytic therapy could be predicted by calculating the sum of ST-segment elevation and depression (ST-segment deviation score) (Schreiber et al, 2003). Each patient enrolled in the study had a confirmed anterior or inferior AMI and was receiving thrombolytic therapy. *Nonfatal 24-hour complications* were defined as acute CHF or severe rhythm disturbances within 24 hours after the start of thrombolysis. The results showed that those who developed evidence of 24-hour complications had an ST-segment deviation score that was significantly higher than in patients without complications. Further analysis revealed that the ST-segment deviation score was an independent predictor of early complications in patients with both anterior MI and inferior MI. The conclusions of the study revealed that the ST-segment deviation score (the sum of all significant ST-segment elevations and depression on the 12-lead ECG greater than 1 mm from baseline) was superior to using the sum of ST-segment elevations alone in predicting the probability of 24-hour complications in patients with AMI after thrombolysis. This study may have an important effect on the further treatment of patients with AMI receiving thrombolytic therapy.

Mechanical complications after AMI have been predicted reliably in a recent research study by using C-reactive protein (C-RP) levels and lymphocyte counts within the first 96 hours of AMI (Widmer et al, 2003). *Mechanical complications* were defined as ventricular septal defect, papillary muscle rupture, and left ventricular free wall rupture. The results showed that prior to the mechanical complication, peak C-RP levels were significantly higher and relative lymphocyte counts were significantly lower than in control patients even though their creatine kinase (CK) levels did not differ. This study may also have an important influence on assessment data the nurse will monitor to help predict mechanical complications after AMI.

Mrs. Settles's Complications

Mrs. Settles experienced several life-threatening complications after her anterior AMI. She developed heart failure, as was noted by her dyspnea, crackles in all lung fields, S_3 gallop, and chest x-ray film that depicted pulmonary edema. She developed cardiogenic shock and a new LBBB the first day after her anterior AMI.

7. What significant 12-lead ECG changes are sometimes seen following an anterior wall AMI? What 12-lead ECG changes occurred with Mrs. Settles?

Most anterior AMIs are related to an occlusion of the LAD coronary artery. The LAD supplies blood to a large area of the left ventricle and almost all of the bundle of His and bundle branches of the ventricular conduction system. One of the most common ECG complications following an anterior AMI is the development of an LBBB (Bucher & Melander, 1999). A patient with LBBB has an increased risk for death from left ventricular failure, ventricular tachycardia, or ventricular fibrillation. However, early recognition and treatment can reduce mortality. Use of prophylactic temporary transvenous pacing followed by thrombolysis is the guideline recommended by the ACC and the American Heart Association (AHA) for new LBBB after AMI.

Other arrhythmias commonly seen with an anterior wall MI include sinus tachycardia, PVCs, premature atrial contractions, atrial tachycardia, atrial flutter, and atrial fibrillation. Intraventricular conduction disturbances include right bundle branch block (RBBB) and LBBB, and Mobitz II block progressing to complete atrioventricular block often occurs (Bucher, 1999).

Mrs. Settles developed LBBB the morning after admission to the hospital. If she had presented to the emergency department already in LBBB with chest pain and other symptoms suggestive of AMI, this could have made detection of her infarction more difficult. Failure to diagnose AMI in a patient with LBBB soon enough leads to delays in administering life-saving thrombolytic treatment. In order to look for diagnostic dynamic changes in ST segments, a recent study proposes that serial ECGs are needed that are *comparable* in precordial lead placement (Madias, 2002). According to Madias (2002), "Observations in daily practice and previous work suggest that significant alterations in the amplitude of ST-segment deviations are witnessed when variation of the sites of precordial lead recordings, by even 1.0 cm, is implemented" (p. 299). This has implications for nursing care. In order to ensure *comparable* serial ECG recordings in a patient with LBBB, the nurse should mark on the patient's chest wall where the electrodes should be attached and instruct the ECG technician to record all subsequent tracings using those marks.

Mrs. Settles's 12-Lead ECG Changes

Mrs. Settles experienced several rhythm disturbances during thrombolysis, which were expected. However, she did develop a transient LBBB with cardiogenic shock on her first day after the anterior AMI. The LBBB resolved without intervention by the third day.

8. Define cardiogenic shock and why it occurs after an anterior wall MI. What is the prognosis for the patient with cardiogenic shock?

Cardiogenic shock is defined by Jones and Bucher (1999) as "low cardiac output and hypotension with clinical signs of inadequate blood flow to the tissues" (pp. 47-49). Clinically, cardiogenic shock has been defined as a systolic blood pressure of less than 90 mm Hg for more than 1 hour that is (1) not responsive to fluid administration alone; (2) secondary to cardiac dysfunction; or, (3) associated with signs of hypoperfusion or cardiac index less than 2.2 L/min/m^2 (other investigators use 1.8 L/min/m^2 or less) and pulmonary capillary wedge pressure (PCWP) greater than 18 mm Hg (Hasdai et al, 2000). Cardiogenic shock occurs when the heart cannot maintain enough CO to meet the body's demands. The most common cause is MI, but other cardiac disorders such as end-stage cardiomyopathy, valvular heart disease, cardiopulmonary bypass, and cardiac tamponade may be the precipitating events. Cardiogenic shock usually develops in most patients within 48 hours of AMI. Clinical manifestations of cardiogenic shock include cool and clammy skin, alterations in level of consciousness, decreased peripheral pulses, and a low urinary output (Holmes, 2000).

Cardiogenic shock often follows a massive anterior AMI because of the link to the destruction of 40% or more of the left ventricle (Holcomb, 2002). The pathophysiologic process involved in cardiogenic shock is a self-perpetuating vicious cycle. Loss of cardiac muscle leads to decreased pumping ability of the ventricles and reduced stroke volume that causes a decreased CO. The decreased CO perpetuates a decrease in blood pressure and coronary perfusion, which causes progressive myocardial ischemia and cellular dysfunction. The incidence of cardiogenic shock after an anterior MI is 6% to 20% with a mortality rate of 75% to 90% (Jones & Bucher, 1999; Holmes, 2000).

The prognosis of patients with an anterior wall MI is significantly worse than that of patients with an inferior wall MI (Jones & Bucher, 1999). Patients with an anterior wall MI usually have a blockage in the LAD that generally involves greater myocardial damage than those with inferior wall infarction. Because the left ventricle is involved, the likelihood of heart failure or cardiogenic shock is much greater with an anterior wall MI.

9. What are the hemodynamic parameters seen in the patient with cardiogenic shock in comparison with normal hemodynamic parameters?

Hemodynamic parameters are severely altered in the patient with cardiogenic shock. CO and cardiac index (CI) are dramatically lowered. Tachycardia occurs as the body attempts to compensate for the drop in systolic blood pressure. The pulmonary artery catheter readings show an increase in the central venous pressure, the PCWP, and SVR, reflecting an increase in preload and afterload (Jones & Bucher, 1999). Cardiogenic shock can result in an SVR of 1800 dynes/second/cm^{-5} or greater (Holcomb, 2002).

In the assessment of the severity of cardiogenic shock, the CI is an effective parameter to provide hemodynamic information. A CI of less than 1.8 L/min/m^2 is indicative of cardiogenic shock. Clinical manifestations of hypoperfusion (as listed in answer 8) are observed when the CI is between 1.8 and 2.2 L/min/m^2. The body attempts to compensate for these changes by way of the sympathetic nervous system's release of epinephrine and norepinephrine. However, the results only cause the heart rate to increase and cause further peripheral vasoconstriction. Thus the complex activated mechanisms of cardiogenic shock dominate and normalization of the hemodynamic parameters is nearly impossible (Jones & Bucher, 1999).

Mrs. Settles's Hemodynamic Parameters

It is important to note that Mrs. Settles did not have a pulmonary artery catheter (PAC) placed initially because of thrombolysis. However, when she continued to have chest pain, a PAC was placed while she was in the catheterization laboratory. Mrs. Settles showed hemodynamic changes consistent with cardiogenic shock. On day 1 she had tachycardia (HR 130 bpm) and hypotension (BP 90/60 mm Hg). She also had signs of hypoperfusion: her CI was 1.5 L/min/m^2, SVR was 1800 dynes/sec/cm^{-5}, and PCWP was elevated at 22 mm Hg.

10. Discuss the goals of pharmacologic management in cardiogenic shock. Which medications were used for Mrs. Settles?

The two main goals in treating cardiogenic shock are to decrease the preload and afterload and optimize myocardial contractility. This presents a challenge pharmacologically because what supports one may be detrimental to the other. The use of multiple intravenous medications and drips in varying doses may need to be tailored for each individual with cardiogenic shock. The three main categories of drugs used for cardiogenic shock are diuretics, positive inotropic agents, and vasoactive medications. Although these pharmacologic agents may not alter mortality rates in some patients with cardiogenic shock, they will assist in maintaining vital organ perfusion while other interventions are used in an attempt to salvage the myocardium (Holcomb, 2002).

Diuretics

Even when patients have hypotension, a diuretic may be needed for fluid removal from the intravascular spaces. In cardiogenic shock, patients will experience decreased renal perfusion. Loop diuretics are the agents of choice for fluid removal in patients with decreased renal function (Green, 2003). A loop diuretic, such as furosemide (Lasix), in small amounts may provide enough diuresis to allow myocardial fibers to stretch more efficiently (Jones & Bucher, 1999). The better the myocardial stretch, the better the CO and blood pressure. Even small improvements such as this can make a major difference in the progression and resolution of cardiogenic shock. Hemodynamic monitoring is helpful in determining whether left ventricular pressures are elevated. Diuretics are given to patients with elevated filling pressures (too much preload) to reduce preload (Holmes, 2000).

Inotropes

Inotropes (positive) are used to increase the contractility of the heart. These include dobutamine (Dobutrex), dopamine (Intropin), and inamrinone (Inocor) (name changed from "amrinone" to avoid medication errors) (Green, 2003). These drugs may aggravate arrhythmias and increase myocardial oxygen demand, but they are essential for stabilization of the patient in cardiogenic shock.

Dobutamine stimulates β-adrenergic receptors, which leads to an improved CI, improved oxygen delivery, and reduced pulmonary artery pressure (PAP), PCWP, SVR, and pulmonary vascular resistance (Jones & Bucher, 1999; Rudis & Dasta, 2002). Unless the patient is hypotensive, dobutamine is the inotrope preferred for use in cardiogenic shock to increase cardiac index. An additional advantage of dobutamine is augmentation of diastolic coronary blood flow and collateral flow to ischemic areas of the heart. Dobutamine has minimal effects on myocardial oxygen demand and produces a better balance between oxygen supply and demand than other inotropes (Rudis & Dasta, 2002). Conventional dosing of dobutamine from 2 to 20 μg/kg/min produces optimal increases in myocardial contractility with very little increase in heart rate. At higher dosages (>20 μg/kg/min) tachycardia may result.

Dopamine is the agent of choice if hypotension is present (Jones & Bucher, 1999; Rudis & Dasta, 2002). However, dopamine effects are dose dependent. At low dosages (1 to 2 μg/kg/min), renal and mesenteric perfusion is increased while heart rate and blood pressure remain unaffected. In midrange dosages (2 to 10 μg/kg/min), dopamine stimulates both $β_1$- and α-adrenergic receptors, which increases CO and improves myocardial contractility. Dopamine will also produce a mild increase in the SVR and preload in midrange doses. At a dosage range above 10 μg/kg/min, peripheral arterial and venous vasoconstriction occurs, causing a significant increase in afterload and preload. Dopamine is usually given when hemodynamically significant hypotension occurs in the absence of hypovolemia. A disadvantage of dopamine is that cardiac workload increases without significantly increasing coronary blood flow (Rudis & Dasta, 2002). Even a therapeutic or midrange dosage of dopamine can stimulate $β_1$-receptors and increase heart rate, consuming myocardial oxygen supply (Green, 2003). The preferred inotropic therapy is the combination of dopamine and dobutamine at moderate dosages.

Inamrinone is a third inotrope that improves CO and PAP with little increase in myocardial workload (Jones & Bucher, 1999; Johnson et al, 2002). However, inamrinone works differently. It is a phosphodiesterase inhibitor that increases myocardial contractility without involving the sympathetic nervous system. It must be noted that although inamrinone has been studied extensively in patients with congestive cardiomyopathy, its efficacy for ischemic heart problems such as cardiogenic shock has not been validated and should be used with caution (Johnson et al, 2002). The maintenance infusion dosing range for inamrinone is 5 to 10 μg/kg/min, and total daily dose should not exceed 10 mg/kg (Green, 2003).

Vasoactive Agents

Vasoactive drugs such as sodium nitroprusside (Nipride) and nitroglycerin (Tridil) are given to improve the pumping action of the heart by decreasing both preload and afterload (SVR) (Jones & Bucher, 1999). In small doses, vasoactive agents can assist the failing heart in cardiogenic shock by reducing the workload of the heart. Vasoactive agents are not generally used initially in cardiogenic shock because they can cause hypotension, but may be used later in combination with inotropic agents (Holmes, 2000). Sodium nitroprusside increases CI and decreases venous pressure similar to dobutamine and inamrinone, even though it has no direct inotropic activity. It is used in patients who have a significantly elevated SVR. Sodium nitroprusside should be initiated in low doses (0.1 to 0.25 µg/kg/min) and increased in small increments (0.1 to 0.2 µg/kg/min) every 5 to 10 minutes as needed (Johnson et al, 2002). Nursing measures when administering intravenous sodium nitroprusside include protecting the IV minibag from light, usually with aluminum foil (Green, 2003).

Although IV NTG is not as strong an arteriolar vasodilator as sodium nitroprusside, it dilates coronary arteries, reduces coronary artery vasospasms, and increases coronary collateral blood flow to ischemic myocardium (Johnson et al, 2002). When given in combination with dopamine or dobutamine, it increases CI and decreases pulmonary artery occlusion pressure (PAOP). Intravenous NTG should be initiated in low doses (0.1 µg/kg/min) and increased every 5 to 10 minutes as necessary. Maintenance doses are usually from 0.5 to 3.0 µg/kg/min (Johnson et al, 2002). The nurse administering IV NTG should be aware that NTG migrates into polyvinyl chloride (PVC) IV tubing and therefore use lower doses when administering with non-PVC tubing (Green, 2003).

Mrs. Settles's Medications While in Cardiogenic Shock

Mrs. Settles was given the diuretic furosemide intravenously to reduce preload and enhance myocardial stretch and CO. Mrs. Settles was given dopamine and dobutamine at midrange dosages during cardiogenic shock for inotropic purposes. Her NTG drip was reduced to 1 µg/kg/min for afterload purposes, once her chest pain was relieved by the insertion of the IABP. The vasoactive drips were withdrawn by day 3.

11. **What types of mechanical support devices can be used for patients in cardiogenic shock and why? Which type was used for Mrs. Settles? Identify any specific nursing responsibilities for the device chosen for Mrs. Settles.**

The patient in cardiogenic shock may require the use of IABP counterpulsation. The intraaortic balloon is inserted into the femoral artery percutaneously and placed within the descending aorta just distal to the subclavian artery. The purpose of the IABP is twofold: to improve perfusion to the coronary arteries and to allow the heart muscle to rest. First the balloon inflates during ventricular diastole, which results in increased coronary artery perfusion. Second, deflation of the balloon occurs during ventricular systole, which decreases afterload or the workload of the heart. The triggering event for cycling can be either the R wave of the ECG, the upstroke of the arterial pressure waveform, or a pacemaker spike (Urden et al, 2002). Jones and Bucher (1999) state that 75% of patients who receive IABP therapy demonstrate clinical improvements in their condition. Recent studies have shown that the survival rate of AMI cardiogenic shock patients who received thrombolytic therapy in a community hospital and were transferred to a tertiary care center was 93% for those treated with IABP versus 37% for those who were not (Hasdai et al, 2000; Janin et al, 2000).

IABP counterpulsation is indicated for patients who need immediate reduction in cardiac workload and/or immediate increase in coronary blood flow. Examples include left ventricular failure after cardiac surgery, unstable angina refractory to medications, recurrent angina after AMI, and complications of AMI (cardiogenic shock, refractory ventricular arrhythmias, papillary muscle rupture/dysfunction with mitral regurgitation, and ventricular septal defect) (Urden et al, 2002). The desired outcomes of IAPB counterpulsation include stabilized hemodynamics in patients with cardiogenic shock and alleviation of myocardial ischemia in AMI patients. Contraindications to IABP use include aortic valve insufficiency, aortic aneurysm, severe peripheral vascular disease, coagulopathies, and end-stage heart disease not awaiting transplant (Christenson et al, 1999; Urden et al, 2002). The potential complications of IAPB therapy include lower extremity ischemia due to occlusion of the femoral artery or thromboembolism, balloon perforation, dissection of the aorta, displacement of the balloon catheter, thrombocytopenia, septicemia, and infection at the insertion site (Lessig & Lessig, 1998; Urden et al, 2002).

Other mechanical support devices used include ventricular assist devices (VADs) and extracorporeal membrane oxygenation (ECMO). Types of VADs include centrifugal, pneumatic, pulsatile, and electrical pulsatile. VADs may be implanted for extended periods and are used as a bridge to cardiac transplantation (Urden et al, 2002). The mechanical support device, ECMO, is used in children but is poorly tolerated in adults over long periods (Fuhrman & Hernan, 2000). Major complications such as biventricular failure, bleeding, and infection occur with VADs and ECMO. However, these mechanical devices can be a successful means of supporting patients experiencing cardiac failure who would otherwise die (Jones & Bucher, 1999).

Mrs. Settles's Mechanical Support Devices

Mrs. Settles required placement of an IABP because of unrelieved chest pain and development of cardiogenic shock. She tolerated the balloon pump well, and her hemodynamic values improved to allow weaning by day 3.

Specific Nursing Responsibilities with an IABP

Lessig and Lessig (1998) and Urden and colleagues (2002) identify specific nursing responsibilities when caring for a patient with an IABP:

- Maintain appropriate timing of IABP inflation and deflation by monitoring heart rate, heart rhythm, and mean arterial pressure every 15 minutes. Irregular heart rhythms and tachyarrhythmias will decrease IABP effectiveness. Maintenance of mean arterial pressure at 90 mm Hg may be supported with inotropic agents as needed. Auscultate between the second and third intercostal spaces for placement.
- Assess pulses in both feet (dorsalis pedis and posterior tibial) with a Doppler every hour and mark the location heard. Note the presence, quality, and any change from baseline assessment. Note changes in color, sensation, and temperature of lower extremities.
- Monitor the IABP insertion site every hour, noting any oozing or increase in bleeding/ hematoma. If bleeding, press 1 inch above the site, not directly over the site. Monitor platelet counts for thrombocytopenia. Note changes indicative of abnormal coagulation such as petechiae and guaiac-positive stools.
- Assess the left radial pulse versus the right radial pulse every 2 hours to monitor for migration of the IABP catheter. If the left radial pulse is absent or decreased, the left subclavian artery may be occluded by the catheter.
- Daily and as-needed chest x-ray films are crucial to check placement of the IABP catheter. Take chest x-ray films with the patient flat.
- Measure urine output every hour to monitor for migration of the balloon to the renal arteries. If urinary output decreases to less than 30 ml/hr, the renal arteries may be occluded by the catheter.
- Secure and check all IABP connections from the site of insertion to the connection with the external machine every hour.
- The patient will require education regarding the importance of keeping the affected extremity straight and minimizing leg movement. This may also require a soft restraint on the extremity and maintenance of the head of the bed at 15 degrees or lower to avoid flexion of the hip. These precautionary measures can prevent inadvertent IABP catheter migration.
- To prevent complications of immobility, turn the patient from side to side every 2 hours by logrolling.

- Monitor for IABP malfunction via external machine alarms. Most IABP machines fill, time, and troubleshoot automatically. However, if the IABP catheter is placed on standby for longer than 5 minutes, it must be programmed or be manually inflated/deflated slightly to prevent thrombus formation and possible occurrence of emboli.
- Teach the patient to report any pain in the back, leg, and/or chest, which may indicate a thromboembolism.
- Assess for signs of infection at the site with dressing changes per hospital protocol and monitor lymphocyte counts for signs of systemic infection.
- Observe for signs of improved cardiac output: pink skin and warmth, improved capillary refill time, improved urinary output, and improved mental status (if patient is not sedated).

12. What are the nursing diagnoses for the patient in cardiogenic shock after an anterior AMI?

Nursing diagnoses for patients in cardiogenic shock after an anterior AMI include the following (Lessig & Lessig, 1998; Jones & Bucher, 1999; Urden et al, 2002):

- Decreased cardiac output related to alterations in contractility
- Decreased cardiac output related to alterations in heart rate
- Fluid volume excess
- Altered renal, cerebral, cardiopulmonary, and peripheral tissue perfusion
- Altered comfort: pain related to myocardial ischemia during AMI
- Impaired gas exchange
- Risk for infection
- Altered nutrition, less than body requirements
- Ineffective individual and family coping related to anxiety and fear of death and the critical care environment
- Disturbed body image related to functional dependence on life-support equipment

CARDIOGENIC SHOCK AND ANTERIOR WALL MYOCARDIAL INFARCTION

References

Boersma, E., et al. (2003). Acute myocardial infarction. *The Lancet, 361,* 847-858.

Bucher, L., & Melander, S. (1999). Acute myocardial infarction. In L. Bucher, & S. Melander (Eds.), *Critical care nursing* (pp. 227-257). Philadelphia: W. B. Saunders.

Canto, J. G., et al. (2000). Prevalence, clinical characteristics, and mortality among patients with myocardial infarction presenting without chest pain. *JAMA, 283*(24), 3223-3229.

Christenson, J. T., Simonet, F., Badel, P., & Schmuziger, M. (1999). Optimal timing of preoperative intraaortic balloon pump support in high-risk coronary patients. *The Annals of Thoracic Surgery, 68*(3), 934-939.

Fiorini, D. M. (2001). The use of low-molecular-weight heparin in acute coronary syndromes. In P. G. Morton, D. Obias-Manno, & S. Apple (Eds.), *AACN clinical issues: Advanced practice in acute and critical care,* Vol. 12, No. 1 (pp. 53-61). Philadelphia: Lippincott.

Fuhrman, B. P. & Hernan, L. J. (2000). Congestive heart failure in infants and children. In W. C. Shoemaker, S. M. Ayres, A. Grenvik, & P. R. Holbrook (Eds.), *Textbook of critical care* (21st ed., pp. 1046-1050). Philadelphia: W. B. Saunders.

Gibson, M. C. (2001). Time is myocardium and time is outcomes. *Circulation, 104,* 2632-2634.

Green, S. M. (Editor-in-chief). (2003). *Tarascon pocket pharmacopoeia 2003 deluxe edition.* Loma Linda, CA: Tarascon.

Hasdai, D., Topol, E. J., Califf, R. M., Berger, P. B., & Holmes Jr., D. R. (2000). Cardiogenic shock complicating acute coronary syndromes. *The Lancet, 356,* 749-756.

Holcomb, S. S. (2002). Helping your patient conquer cardiogenic shock. *Nursing 2002, 32*(9), 32cc1-32cc6.

Holmes, D. R. (2000). Cardiogenic shock. In L. Goldman & J.C. Bennett (Eds.), *Cecil textbook of medicine* (21st ed., pp. 502-507). Philadelphia: W. B. Saunders.

Janin, Y., Vetrovec, G., & Hess, M. L. (2000). Interventional therapies for cardiogenic shock. In W. C. Shoemaker, S. M. Ayres, A. Grenvik, & P. R. Holbrook (Eds.), *Textbook of critical care* (21st ed., pp. 1037-1046). Philadelphia: W. B. Saunders.

Johnson, J. A., Parker, R. B., & Patterson, J. H. (2002). Heart failure. In J. T. DiPiro, R. L. Talbert, G. C. Yee, G. R. Matzke, B. G. Wells, & L. M. Posey (Eds.), *Pharmacotherapy: A physiologic approach* (5th ed., pp. 185-218). New York: McGraw-Hill.

Jones, K., & Bucher, L. (1999). Shock. In L. Bucher, & S. Melander (Eds.), *Critical care nursing* (pp. 1010-1035). Philadelphia: W. B. Saunders.

Killip, T. (2000). Treatment of myocardial infarction. In W. C. Shoemaker, S. M. Ayres, A. Grenvik, & P. R. Holbrook (Eds.), *Textbook of critical care* (21st ed., pp. 1018-1029). Philadelphia: W. B. Saunders.

Lessig, M. L., & Lessig, P. (1998). The cardiovascular system. In J. Alspach (Ed.), *American Association of Critical-Care Nurses: Core curriculum for critical care nurses* (5th ed., pp. 137-337). Philadelphia: W. B. Saunders.

Madias, J. E. (2002). Serial ECG recordings via marked chest wall landmarks: An essential requirement for the diagnosis of myocardial infarction in the presence of left bundle branch block. *Journal of Electrocardiology, 35*(4), 299-302.

Meier, M. A., et al. (2002). The new definition of myocardial infarction. *Archives of Internal Medicine, 162,* 1585-1589.

Meils, C. M., Kaleta, K. A., & Mueller, C. L. (2002). Treatment of the patient with acute myocardial infarction: Reducing time delays. *Journal of Nursing Care Quality, 17*(1), 83-89.

Murphy, M., & Berding, C. (1999). Use of measurements of myoglobin and cardiac troponins in the diagnosis of acute myocardial infarction. *Critical Care Nurse, 19*(1), 58-65.

Nagle, B. & Nee, C. (2002). Recognizing and responding to acute myocardial infarction. *Nursing 2002, 32*(10), 50-54.

Panteghini, M. (2002). Acute coronary syndrome: Biochemical strategies in the troponin era. *Chest, 122,* 1428-1435.

Plaut, D. (1998). Serum markers of cardiac cell damage. *American Medical Technologists Events CE Supplement, 15,* 210-215.

Ribichini, F. & Wijns, W. (2002). Myocardial infarction: Reperfusion treatment. *Heart, 88,* 298-305.

Rudis, M. I., & Dasta, J. F. (2002). Vasopressors and inotropes in shock. In J. T. DiPiro, R. L. Talbert, G. C. Yee, G. R. Matzke, B. G. Wells, & L. M. Posey (Eds.), *Pharmacotherapy: A physiologic approach* (5th ed., pp. 435-451). New York: McGraw-Hill.

Schreiber, W., et al. (2003). Prediction of 24-h, nonfatal complications in patients with acute myocardial infarction receiving thrombolytic therapy by calculation of the S-T segment deviation score. *Canadian Journal of Cardiology, 19*(2), 151-157.

Sobel, B. E. (2000). Acute myocardial infarction. In L. Goldman & J. C. Bennett (Eds.), *Cecil textbook of medicine* (21st ed., pp. 304-320). Philadelphia: W. B. Saunders.

Urden, L. D., Stacy, K. M., & Lough, M. E. (2002). *Thelan's critical care nursing: Diagnosis and management* (4th ed., pp. 395-494). St. Louis: Mosby.

Widmer, A., et al. (2003). Mechanical complications after myocardial infarction reliably predicted using C-reactive protein levels and lymphocytopenia. *Cardiology, 99*(1), 25-31.

4

Non–Q-Wave Myocardial Infarction

Amy Reese Ramirez, RN, BSN, MSW, MSN, FNP-C
Sheila Drake Melander, RN, DSN, ACNP-C, FCCM

CASE PRESENTATION

Mrs. Howard is a 70-year-old, 87.8 kg (194 lb) African-American with a history of insulin-dependent diabetes mellitus, hypertension, atherosclerotic peripheral vascular disease, cancer of the breast and uterus, and congestive heart failure. Mrs. Howard was seen at an outlying hospital with a complaint of chest pain and shortness of breath. Further questioning revealed that she had been having more frequent episodes of chest pain for the past week accompanied by shortness of breath.

The initial orders were as follows:

- >2 L of oxygen through a nasal cannula
- Intravenous (IV) line of normal saline started at a keep-open rate
- Cardiac monitor, which showed a normal sinus rhythm without ectopy
- 12-lead electrocardiogram (ECG)
- Immediate measurement of cardiac enzymes; repeat every 6 hours for 24 hours

Her diagnostic data on admission were as follows:

BP	190/94 mm Hg
HR	106 bpm
Respirations	32 breaths/min
CI	2.2 l/min/m^2
Troponin I	1.5 mg/L
CK	216 U/L
CK-MB	5.6%
LDH	400 U/L
AST (SGOT)	25 U/L
Myoglobin	95 ng/L

The ECG revealed ST-segment elevation in leads V_2 and V_3.

Mrs. Howard was given one sublingual nitroglycerin (NTG) tablet, which resolved her pain. She was admitted to the coronary care unit with the order to "rule out myocardial infarction [MI]."

Her serial cardiac enzyme levels continued to rise; values from the third set of cardiac enzyme measurements were the following:

CK	350 U/L
CK-MB	5.8%
Troponin I	5.3 µg/L
Myoglobin	125 ng/L
LDH	680 U/L
AST (SGOT)	52 U/L
CI	1.8 L/min/m^2

Day 2

Mrs. Howard had recurrent pain that was not eased with three NTG tablets, diaphoresis, and profound shortness of breath requiring intubation. An ECG demonstrated no change from the previous tracings. Mrs. Howard was then taken to the cardiac catheterization laboratory. Cardiac catheterization revealed the following:

- Ejection fraction of 35%
- 90% obstruction of the left anterior descending coronary artery
- 90% to 95% obstruction of the circumflex artery
- 80% obstruction of the right coronary artery

An intraaortic balloon pump was placed for control of Mrs. Howard's refractory chest pain, and a dopamine infusion of 3 µg/kg/min was started. NTG at 1.5 µg/ml and heparin at 800 U/hr were continued. At this time Mrs. Howard was transferred to another facility with the diagnosis of non–Q-wave MI and three-vessel disease with the need for emergency bypass surgery. Mrs. Howard subsequently underwent bypass surgery on day 3 and has done very well since that time.

NON–Q-WAVE MYOCARDIAL INFARCTION

QUESTIONS

1. What are the differences between a non–Q-wave MI and a transmural MI?

2. What methods are used in the diagnosis of non–Q-wave MIs?

3. Describe the characteristics of patients with the diagnosis of non–Q-wave MI.

4. Which pharmacologic agents may be used in the treatment of a non–Q-wave MI?

5. What are the current recommendations for the use of percutaneous transluminal coronary angioplasty (PTCA) and coronary artery bypass graft (CABG) surgery in the patient with a non–Q-wave MI?

6. Discuss extension of a non–Q-wave MI, including the time frame of occurrence and possible outcomes.

7. What are some nursing concerns for the patient with a non–Q-wave MI?

8. What are some nursing actions required for patients taking β-blockers (metoprolol and atenolol)?

9. What are the nursing implications for patients receiving thrombolytic therapy?

10. Develop a list of appropriate nursing diagnoses for the care of the patient with a non–Q-wave MI.

NON–Q-WAVE MYOCARDIAL INFARCTION

QUESTIONS AND ANSWERS

1. What are the differences between a non–Q-wave MI and a transmural MI?

The terminology used to classify non–Q-wave and transmural MIs has been debated. Traditionally the classification of a Q-wave MI indicated the involvement of all three layers of the heart muscle; therefore, it was labeled a transmural or full-thickness MI. When no abnormal Q waves were present, the area of necrosis was thought to be confined to the subendocardium; therefore, this was termed a nontransmural or partial-thickness MI. Research has found that classifying MIs as transmural or nontransmural is imprecise and should not serve as the basis for designing therapy (Braunwald et al, 2002). Bucher and Melander (1999) state that pathologic Q waves can be found in nontransmural infarctions, and normal Q waves can be located in transmural infarctions. Based on this information, the terms *Q-wave MI* and *non–Q-wave* MI are the most appropriate.

About 75% of patients initially presenting with ST-segment elevation will develop Q waves in the leads overlying the infarct zone, leading to the term Q-wave MI (Braunwald et al, 2002). In about 25% of patients presenting with ST-segment elevation, no Q waves develop but other abnormalities of the QRS are seen, such as diminution in R-wave height and notching or splintering of the QRS complex (Braunwald et al, 2002). Compared with Q-wave infarctions, non–Q-wave MIs are generally associated with less obstructive thrombi (Braunwald et al, 2002).

2. What methods are used in the diagnosis of non–Q-wave MIs?

The spectrum of clinical conditions ranging from unstable angina to non–Q-wave MI to Q-wave MI is referred to as acute coronary syndromes (Antman & Fox, 2000). Diagnosis of non–Q-wave MI is generally based on a combination of the patient's history, ECG findings, and laboratory results. The majority of non–Q-wave MIs present without ST-segment elevation. Patients presenting without ST-segment elevation are initially diagnosed as suffering either from a non–ST-segment elevation MI (NSTEMI) or unstable angina. Unstable angina and non–Q-wave MI are often considered together because they are not easily distinguishable from one another at the time of patient presentation (Antman & Fox, 2000). The distinction between NSTEMI and unstable angina is based on whether cardiac markers indicative of necrosis are detected in the blood (Antman & Fox, 2000; Braunwald et al, 2001).

The three major enzymes released into the blood at abnormal levels are creatinine phosphokinase, lactate dehydrogenase (LDH), and troponin. In the past, an isoenzyme of creatinine kinase (CK-MB) levels and LDH levels were the main diagnostic markers for myocardial injury. An elevated CK-MB value provides a sensitivity of 70% at 6 to 9 hours and 97% at 9 to 12 hours, returning to baseline after 48 to 72 hours (Ferri, 2002). Currently, the Task Force on the Management of Acute Coronary Syndromes of the European Society of Cardiology (Bertrand et al, 2002) and Braunwald and associates (2002) report the use of troponin T or I as the preferred and more reliable markers of myocardial necrosis. Troponin T and I are exclusively expressed in myocytes, thereby making them specific for myocardial damage (Bertrand et al, 2002). Troponin T and I are released 4 to 8 hours after the onset of myocardial necrosis, peak at 24 to 48 hours and decrease after 10 days, making them useful markers of late MI (>24 hours old) (Ferri, 2003). Troponin measurements are now replacing LDH as a late MI indicator (Ferri, 2003). Despite troponins' accuracy in identifying myocardial necrosis, not all myocardial necrosis is secondary to atherosclerotic coronary artery disease. Therefore Braunwald and colleagues (2002) recommend cardiac troponins to be used in conjunction with appropriate clinical features and electrocardiographic changes in establishing an accurate diagnosis. Bertrand and coworkers (2002) recommend obtaining troponin T or I levels on admission, and, if normal, repeated in 6 to 12 hours. Further recommendations include CK-MB and/or myoglobin measurements in patients with recent (<6 hours) onset symptoms as an early marker of MI and in patients with recurrent ischemia after recent infarction (<2 weeks) to detect another infarction (Bertrand et al, 2002).

3. Describe the characteristics of patients with the diagnosis of non–Q-wave MI.

Patients with non–Q-wave MI present with similar symptoms as those seen with Q-wave MI, including nausea, vomiting, diaphoresis, shortness of breath, generalized anxiety, and syncopal events (Tamberella & Warner, 2000). According to Braunwald and colleagues (2002), categorization of patients into those with Q-wave and non–Q-wave infarction should only be used as a crude guide to the extent of ventricular damage. Prognostic considerations must take into account other important factors, such as whether the ECG abnormality is due to a first infarct versus subsequent infarct, the location and size of infarction, patient comorbidities and demographic factors such as patient age. On average, patients with nontransmural infarcts have a more severe stenosis in the infarct-related coronary artery than do patients suffering from transmural infarcts. This finding suggests that a more severe obstruction occurring before infarction protects against the development of transmural infarction, perhaps by fostering the development of collateral circulation (Braunwald et al, 2002).

4. Which pharmacologic agents may be used in the treatment of a non–Q-wave MI?

The classification of Q-wave or non–Q-wave infarction has less prognostic meaning and should guide therapy to a lesser degree than clinical markers of risk, such as heart failure, recurrent chest pain, late ventricular arrhythmias, and persistent ST-segment depression (Rakel & Bope, 2003). Therefore initial care of the patient with a non–Q-wave MI includes the same regimen of care as that for the patient with a Q-wave MI: oxygen, cardiac monitoring, cardiac enzyme monitoring, and arrhythmia management.

Antiplatelet and antithrombin therapies are cornerstones in the management of non–Q-wave MI. Aspirin and fractionated heparin (enoxaparin) should be administered on admission after a non–Q-wave MI to decrease further thrombus formation (Bertrand et al, 2002). According to Antman and Fox (2000), clopidogrel is recommended for aspirin-intolerant patients, and it may be considered as a substitute for aspirin in those patients unresponsive to aspirin. In the Efficacy and Safety of Subcutaneous Enoxaparin in Non–Q-Wave Coronary Events (ESSENCE) trial, enoxaparin therapy significantly reduced the rates of recurrent ischemic events and invasive diagnostic and therapeutic procedures in the short term with sustained benefit at 1 year in patients with non–Q-wave MIs (Glys & Gold, 2000; Goodman et al, 2000). However, aspirin and heparin block only one of the pathways involved in platelet activation, leaving other thrombotic pathways unchecked. The critical role of platelets in thrombus formation along with the role of the platelet glycoprotein (GP) IIb-IIIa as the final common pathway for platelet aggregation led to the development of the GPIIb-IIIa inhibitors, abciximab, tirofiban, and eptifibatide (Glys & Gold, 2000). Studies have found the use of GPIIb-IIIa inhibitors to significantly reduce incidences of death, MI or urgent revascularization when used in both surgical intervention and medical treatment of non–Q-wave MI (Glys & Gold, 2000).

Other common pharmacologic interventions include nitrates, β-blockers, angiotensin-converting enzyme (ACE) inhibitors, and statins. Sublingual nitrates are indicated for most patients with an acute coronary syndrome because of their ability to enhance coronary blood flow by coronary vasodilation and to decrease ventricular preload by increasing venous capacitance (Braunwald et al, 2002). Sublingual nitroglycerin is contraindicated for patients with inferior MI and suspected right ventricular infarction or marked hypotension (systolic pressure <90 mm Hg) (Braunwald et al, 2002).

β-Blockers, by decreasing myocardial oxygen consumption, have been found to decrease infarct size, decrease arrhythmic death, modestly decrease all-cause mortality, and act as antianginal agents (Rakel & Bope, 2003). β-Blockers should not be used in patients with significant pulmonary edema, hypotension, or bradyarrhythmias. Studies have also demonstrated a significant reduction in mortality rate with the use of ACE inhibitors (Rakel & Bope, 2003). The proposed mechanism of action is inhibition of postinfarct ventricular remodeling. ACE inhibitors reduce angiotensin II levels and may protect the vasculature as evidenced by the HOPE trial in which patients with angina, stroke, or peripheral vascular disease and no history of MI or congestive heart failure had a significant reduction in mortality and all clinical outcomes with ACE inhibitors (Rakel & Bope, 2003). Rakel and Bope (2003) suggest starting ACE inhibitor therapy during the hospitalization unless the patient is hypotensive or has renal failure.

Studies have not demonstrated a reduction in mortality or combined cardiovascular events with calcium channel blockers, supporting the use of β-blockers as first-line agents unless they are contraindicated (Littrell & Kern, 2002). Calcium channel blockers can be considered in patients with refractory angina or atrial fibrillation with rapid ventricular response that is difficult to control (Rakel & Bope, 2003). More recently, studies have demonstrated the benefit of statins in reducing the mortality rate of post-MI patients by 33% when started several months after the cardiac event. Present National Center for Environmental Control (NCEP) guidelines recommend statins for post-MI patients if the lactate dehydrogenase level is greater than 100 mg/dl (Rakel & Bope, 2003).

5. What are the current recommendations for the use of percutaneous transluminal coronary angioplasty (PTCA) and coronary artery bypass graft (CABG) surgery in the patient with a non–Q-wave MI?

The use of invasive therapy in the patient with a non–Q-wave MI remains controversial. Risk stratification is utilized to determine treatment strategy. High-risk patients are those with recurrent ischemia, elevated troponin levels, major arrhythmias, hemodynamic instability, and diabetes mellitus. Currently, coronary angiography is recommended for higher risk patients. Revascularization via PTCA or CABG is determined based on these angiographic findings. Low-risk patients are those without ST-segment depression or elevation, no recurrent chest pain and no elevation of biochemical markers. A stress test is recommended. Patients with significant ischemia during stress testing should be considered for coronary angiography and possible revascularization (Bertrand et al, 2002).

6. Discuss extension of a non–Q-wave MI, including the time frame of occurrence and possible outcomes.

Non–Q-wave MI is less extensive and has a lower in-hospital mortality rate than Q-wave infarction but involves a greater percentage of jeopardized myocardium, leading to a higher incidence of reinfarction and recurrent angina after hospital discharge (Tamberella & Warner, 2000; Sabatine et al, 2002). Based on the Thrombolysis in Myocardial Infarction (TIMI) IIB and the ESSENCE trials, one third of myocardial infarctions and one half of deaths that occur in the first 6 weeks took place after the patient was discharged. The TIMI risk score has been used as a simple bedside tool for predicting early death and cardiac ischemic events for patients of unstable angina and NSTEMI. Seven patient characteristics are identified as being independent risk factors for subsequent cardiac complications. These include age ≥65 years, ≥3 traditional coronary artery disease risk factors, prior documented coronary artery stenosis >50%, ST deviation of ≥0.05 mV, ≥2 anginal events within the past 24 hours, aspirin use in the past 7 days, and elevated serum cardiac markers (Sabatine et al, 2002).

7. What are some nursing concerns for the patient with a non–Q-wave MI?

Nursing concerns for the patient experiencing a non–Q-wave MI are as follows:

- Patients must continually be assessed for any signs of chest pain or chest tightness, which could signal reinfarction or the development of unstable angina.

- Cardiac enzyme levels must be monitored closely and changes reported to the physician immediately.
- All regimens of care such as thrombolytic therapy and antithrombolytic medications should be explained to the patient.
- Before the patient is discharged with any prescribed medications, all possible side effects should be explained thoroughly.
- Cardiac rehabilitation should begin while the patient is still in the cardiac intensive care unit and should continue after discharge by a multidisciplinary cardiac rehabilitation team (Bucher & Melander, 1999).

8. What are some nursing actions required for patients taking β-blockers (metoprolol and atenolol)?

Nursing actions required for patients receiving IV or oral β-blockers include the following:

- Administer the IV dose slowly.
- Monitor the patient for symptomatic bradycardia, hypotension, and signs and symptoms of congestive heart failure and heart block.
- Instruct the patient to slowly change from a sitting or lying position to a standing position to avoid orthostatic hypotension.
- Monitor the patient for possible interactive effects with other medications, such as an additive effect on blood pressure in patients receiving other hypotensive medications.
- Consider the need for a reduced dosage in elderly patients and in patients with hepatic or renal impairment.
- Avoid abrupt cessation of drug, which may precipitate chest pain, ventricular arrhythmias, or Acute Myocardial Infection (AMI) (Bucher & Melander, 1999).

9. What are the nursing implications for patients receiving thrombolytic therapy?

Nursing implications for patients receiving thrombolytic therapy include the following:

- Identify potential candidates for thrombolytic therapy.
- Prepare patient by starting intravenous lines and obtaining baseline lab values and vital signs.
- Monitor the patient for physical signs of bleeding, including ecchymosis and petechiae; bleeding gums; blood in stool, urine, emesis, nasogastric drainage, or sputum; bleeding from the IV site; decreased blood pressure and increased heart rate; and changes in mentation.
- Observe for signs of reperfusion, including resolution of chest pain, early peaking of CK-MB enzyme levels, reperfusion arrhythmias, and normalization of the ST segments.
- Minimize bleeding potential by limiting unnecessary handling of patient, avoiding unnecessary injections, providing additional pressure at venipuncture and arterial puncture sites to ensure hemostatis.
- Provide patient education including information on the actions of thrombolytic agents, with emphasis on measures to minimize bleeding and bruising information (Urden et al, 2002).

10. Develop a list of appropriate nursing diagnoses for the care of the patient with a non–Q-wave MI.

Nursing diagnoses for the patient with a non–Q-wave MI include the following:

- Acute pain related to transmission and perception of cutaneous, visceral, muscular, or ischemic impulses
- Ineffective cardiopulmonary tissue perfusion related to decreased myocardial oxygen supply and/or increased myocardial oxygen demand
- Activity intolerance related to cardiopulmonary dysfunction
- Powerlessness related to lack of control over current situation
- Anxiety related to threat to biologic, psychologic, and/or social integrity
- Deficient knowledge: discharge regimen related to lack of previous exposure to information (Urden et al, 2002)

NON–Q-WAVE MYOCARDIAL INFARCTION

References

Antman, E. M. & Fox, K. M. (2000). Guidelines for the diagnosis and management of unstable angina and non-Q wave myocardial infarction: Proposed revisions. *American Heart Journal, 3,* 461-475.

Bertrand, M. E., et al. (2002). Management of acute coronary syndromes in patients presenting without persistent ST segment elevation. *European Heart Journal, 23,* 1809-1840.

Braunwald, E., Zipes, D. P., & Libby, P. (Eds.). (2002). *Heart disease: A textbook of cardiovascular medicine* (6th ed.). Philadelphia: W. B. Saunders.

Bucher, L. & Melander, S. (Eds.). (1999). *Critical care nursing.* Philadelphia: W. B. Saunders.

Ferri, F. F. (Ed.). (2003). *Ferri's clinical advisor: Instant diagnosis and treatment* (5th ed.). St. Louis: Mosby–Year Book.

Glys, K. & Gold, M. (2000). Acute coronary syndromes: New developments in pharmacological treatment strategies. *Critical Care Nurse, 20*(Suppl), 3-16.

Goodman, S. G., et al. (2000). Randomized trial of low molecular weight heparin (enoxaparin) versus unfractionated heparin for unstable coronary artery disease: One-year results of the ESSENCE Study. Efficacy and Safety of Subcutaneous Enoxaparin in Non-Q Wave Coronary Events. *Journal of the American College of Cardiology, 36,* 693-698.

Littrell, K. A. & Kern, K. B. (2002). Acute ischemic syndromes: Adjunctive therapy. *Cardiology Clinics, 20,* 159-175.

Rakel, R. E. & Bope E. T. (Eds.). (2003). *Conn's current therapy* (55th ed.). Philadelphia: W. B. Saunders.

Sabatine, M. S., et al. (2002). Identification of patients at high risk for death and cardiac ischemic events after hospital discharge. *American Heart Journal, 143,* 966-970.

Tamberella, M. R. & Warner, J. G. (2000). Non-Q wave myocardial infarction: Assessment and management of a unique and diverse subset. *Postgraduate Medicine, 107*(2): 87-93.

Urden, L. D., Stacy, K. M., & Lough, M. E. (Eds.). (2002). *Thelan's critical care nursing: Diagnosis and management* (4th ed.). St. Louis: Mosby.

5

Heart Failure

Joan E. King, RN, PhD, ACNP, ANP

CASE PRESENTATION

Sam Dukes, age 70 years, was admitted to the hospital after visiting his primary physician with complaints of having experienced general malaise for 3 to 4 days, shortness of breath, and abdominal pain. Initial assessment revealed bibasilar crackles, an audible S_3, and tachycardia. Mr. Dukes also informed the nurse of occasional epigastric pain, which he attributed to his "ulcer acting up."

Mr. Dukes's history includes hypertension and coronary artery disease (past examinations indicated an 80% blockage of the left anterior descending coronary artery and 60% blockage of the right coronary artery). He also has a history of a peptic ulcer. Following are his diagnostic data on admission:

BP	150/72 mm Hg
HR	102-123 bpm and irregular
Respirations	24-32 breaths/min
Temperature	37.3° C (99.2° F) tympanic
Height	175 cm
Weight	79 kg*
Urine	yellow and cloudy
Na$^+$	135 mmol/L
K$^+$	4.2 mmol/L
Hgb	11.8 g/dl
Hct	36.2%
AST (SGOT)	134 U/L
Cl$^-$	102 mmol/L
BUN	17 mg/dl
Glucose	120 mg/dl
Creatinine	1.2 mg/dl
LDH	705 U/L
CK	587 U/L

A chest x-ray film showed mild heart failure (HF) superimposed on chronic obstructive pulmonary disease (COPD) and chronic pulmonary parenchymal changes.

An electrocardiogram (ECG) revealed atrial fibrillation with a ventricular response of 112, no Q waves or ST-segment or T-wave changes.

---

*Mr. Dukes stated that his weight had increased approximately 3 kg (6.6 lb) during the past 3 days.

Shortly after admission Mr. Dukes's skin became cool and clammy. Respirations were labored, and he complained of abdominal pain. Upon physical examination Mr. Dukes was found to be diaphoretic and gasping for air, with jugular venous distention and a positive hepatojugular reflux and diminished bowel sounds. Bilateral crackles were present with an expiratory wheeze. Audible crackles were also heard with respirations. Mr. Dukes was placed in a high Fowler's position, and oxygen therapy of 4 L/min was initiated. It was noted that urinary output had been less than 30 ml/hr since admission.

Within 30 minutes Mr. Dukes showed further decompensation as he developed pulmonary edema. He was immediately transferred to the cardiac care unit (CCU) for aggressive diuretic therapy. Creatinine kinase myocardial band (CK-MB), an isoenzyme of CK, was confirmed at this time to be 4%.

Routine CCU orders were initiated, and the plan of care was briefly explained to Mr. Dukes. His heart monitor showed atrial fibrillation with a rapid ventricular response of 130. Furosemide (Lasix) 100 mg intravenously (IV) and digoxin 0.5 mg IV were administered. A Swan-Ganz catheter was inserted to monitor his hemodynamic parameters. His overall condition continued to deteriorate, and dobutamine (Dobutrex) 1 g in 250 ml of normal saline solution at 5 µg/kg/min was begun. Additional diagnostic data include the following:

BP	190/100 mm Hg
HR	130 bpm
Respirations	42 breaths/min
PAP	50/22 mm Hg
PAOP (PCWP)	24 mm Hg
CO	4.64 L/min
CI	2.34 L/min/m^2
CVP	19 cm H_2O
SVR	1810 dynes/sec/cm^{-5}
HCO$_3^-$	24 mmol/L
pH	7.46
Paco$_2$	31 mm Hg
Pao$_2$	80 mm Hg
Sao$_2$	96% (with 4 L of oxygen by nasal cannula)

At this point, Mr. Dukes's dobutamine drip was increased to 10 µg/kg/min. Administration of nitroprusside (Nipride) was initiated and titrated at 0.3 µg/kg/min. A dopamine drip was ordered to be on standby. An additional 200 mg of furosemide was administered IV, and a significant improvement in urinary output was obtained.

Within a short time, Mr. Dukes said that he found it "easier to breathe." Hemodynamic and laboratory results were as follows:

BP	140/90 mm Hg
HR	109 bpm
Respirations	24 breaths/min
PAP	30/10 mm Hg
PAOP (PCWP)	12 mm Hg
CO	5.5 L/min
CI	2.8 L/min/m^2
CVP	8 cm H_2O
SVR	1340 dynes/sec/cm^{-5}
HCO$_3^-$	25 mmol/L
pH	7.43
Paco$_2$	36 mm Hg
Pao$_2$	89 mm Hg
Sao$_2$	98% (with 4 L of oxygen by nasal cannula)

Over the next 2 days, Mr. Dukes's dobutamine and nitroprusside drips were discontinued, and he was given furosemide 160 mg twice daily, captopril 25 mg every 6 hours, and digoxin 0.125 mg daily. The heart monitor showed normal sinus rhythm, and an echocardiogram indicated an ejection fraction (EF) of 30%. Once stabilized Mr. Dukes was started on a low dose of carvedilol. The patient was transferred to the medical-surgical floor, and discharge planning, including patient and family teaching, was begun. Mr. Dukes was discharged 2 days later and was scheduled to be followed in the cardiology clinic 1 week after discharge where his treatment regimen was reassessed, and his β-blocker was gradually increased.

HEART FAILURE

QUESTIONS

1. Discuss the pathophysiology of HF.

2. Discuss the various classifications of HF.

3. Discuss Mr. Dukes's signs and symptoms that were consistent with HF.

4. Describe Mr. Dukes's predisposing risk factors for HF.

5. List the nursing diagnoses appropriate for Mr. Dukes's care.

6. Briefly define the following terms: cardiac output (CO), cardiac index (CI), central venous pressure (CVP), preload, afterload, pulmonary artery pressure (PAP), and pulmonary artery occlusive pressure (PAOP).

7. Describe the benefits of using a pulmonary artery catheter during HF.

8. Briefly describe the pathophysiology of pulmonary edema.

9. List the pharmacologic agents used in Mr. Dukes's care and explain their importance to his treatment.

10. Discuss long-term management of a patient with HF.

11. Discuss new drug therapies for HF that are on the horizon.

HEAR FAILURE

QUESTIONS AND ANSWERS

1. Discuss the pathophysiology of HF.

HF is a clinical syndrome that is defined as the inability for the heart to pump enough blood to meet the body's demands. The amount of blood pumped per minute is the CO, which is also defined as the product of the stroke volume times the heart rate. There are numerous causes of HF, including myocardial infarction, ischemic heart disease, dysrhythmias, hypertension, cardiomyopathy, and valvular dysfunction. Regardless of the cause, when the CO drops, compensatory mechanisms are activated. Initially the sympathetic nervous system (SNS) is stimulated, and the heart rate increases as well as force of contraction. SNS stimulation also produces vasoconstriction and hence increases afterload or systemic vascular resistance (SVR). The body's goal in increasing the SVR, or afterload, is to increase venous return to the heart. By increasing the venous return, the body is attempting to increase the preload, or the volume of blood that is present in the left ventricle at the end of diastole. The preload is also called the left ventricular end-diastolic pressure. The Frank-Starling law states that up to a point, the greater the preload, the greater the CO. However, after a critical point, increasing the preload will cause a decline in the CO. Physiologically this is attributed to the myocardial fibers providing the best CO when they are maximally stretched, but overstretching the fibers reduces the force of contracting and subsequently reduces CO. These four compensatory mechanisms (increase in heart rate [HR], increase in force of contraction, increase in SVR, and increase in preload) are all initial attempts by the body to increase the CO. At first, these compensatory mechanisms are beneficial but at the expense of an increase in myocardial oxygen consumption.

In addition to SNS stimulation to increase CO, the kidneys play a vital role in both the compensatory process and the further development of HF. When the CO drops, renal perfusion decreases, activating the renin-angiotensin-aldosterone system (RAAS). The RAAS activates the release of angiotensin II and aldosterone. The increased secretion of aldosterone leads to sodium retention. As the serum sodium level increases, secretion of antidiuretic hormone (ADH) is also stimulated, thus causing the kidneys to reabsorb more water. This combination of increase in sodium and water retention leads to a further increase in preload. The RAAS also results in the formation of angiotensin II, a powerful vasoconstrictor that attempts to increase the venous return to increase the preload. Aldosterone, ADH, and angiotensin II all work to try to increase the preload with the hope that an increase in preload will increase the CO. However, as previously stated, according to the Frank-Starling law, increasing the preload beyond the optimal point actually reduces the CO. In addition, just as SNS stimulation increases the SVR and hence the afterload, angiotensin II also contributes to an increase in the afterload and an increase in the heart's workload.

In both acute and chronic HF, these compensatory mechanisms become counterproductive. Increasing the preload, HR, and SVR begins to increase the workload on the heart, increase myocardial oxygen consumption, and decrease the CO. Current research has led to a further understanding of the dynamics of HF. A newer definition of heart failure states that HF is a neurohormonal imbalance resulting in a decrease in cardiac output as well as an increase in the systemic vascular resistance, and an increase in sodium and fluid retention. This theory of HF is called the neurohormonal model. This model supports the concept that prolonged SNS stimulation and an increase in angiotensin II and aldosterone secretion, and endothelial dysfunction cause direct changes in the myocardial fibers and myocytes. This results in a phenomenon known as *remodeling*, which leads to a further decrease in cardiac function (Piano et al, 2000; Futterman & Lemberg, 2001; McMurray, 2002).

Table 5-1 *Signs and Symptoms of Left- and Right-Sided Heart Failure*

Left-Sided Heart Failure	Right-Sided Heart Failure
Capillary refill >3 sec	Hepatomegaly
Orthopnea	Splenomegaly
Dyspnea, dyspnea on exertion	Dependent pitting edema
Nocturnal dyspnea	Venous distention
Cough with frothy sputum (pulmonary edema)	Hepatojugular reflux >1 cm
Tachypnea	Oliguria
Diaphoresis	Arrhythmias
Basilar crackles, rhonchi	Elevated central venous, right atrial, and right ventricular pressure
Cyanosis	Narrowing pulse pressure
Hypoxia, respiratory acidosis	Kussmaul's sign
Elevated pulmonary artery pressures	Murmur of tricuspid insufficiency
Elevated pulmonary artery occlusive pressures	Audible S_3 and S_4 heart sounds
Audible S_3 and S_4 heart sounds	Fatigue, weakness
Nocturia	Abdominal pain
Mental confusion	Anorexia
Weight gain	Chest radiograph shows enlarged right atrium and right ventricle
Fatigue, weakness, lethargy	Ascites
Murmur of mitral insufficiency	Weight gain
Chest radiograph shows enlarged left ventricle, left atrium and the presence of pleural effusion	
Narrowing pulse pressure	
Pulsus alternans	

Although the increase in sodium and fluid retention, vasoconstriction, and SNS stimulation are all initially compensatory mechanisms, over time they become maladaptive. When either the right or left ventricle can no longer handle the preload it receives, fluid begins to back up. When the left ventricle fails as a pump, fluid is backed up into the pulmonary bed, producing signs and symptoms such as shortness of breath, dyspnea on exertion, orthopnea, and as in Mr. Dukes's case, pulmonary edema. When the right ventricle fails, fluid is backed up into the systemic circulation, producing signs and symptoms such as elevated CVP, elevated jugular venous distention, hepatomegaly, ascites, anorexia, and peripheral edema (Table 5-1). Other signs and symptoms of heart failure are an S_3 gallop, anasarca, dysrhythmias, and a displaced point of maximal impulse (PMI) (Futterman & Lemberg, 2001).

2. Discuss the various classifications of HF.

HF can be classified in a number of different ways. Often HF is defined as left ventricular failure (LVF), right ventricular failure (RVF), or a combined failure. As stated, when the left ventricle fails initially, there is both a decrease in CO and a backup of fluid in the pulmonary bed. Signs and symptoms of LVF are rales or crackles, shortness of breath, dyspnea on exertion, orthopnea, paroxysmal nocturnal dyspnea, and pulmonary edema. As in the case presentation, hemodynamic changes seen with LVF are reduced CO, elevated SVR, and elevated pulmonary artery occlusive pressure also called the pulmonary capillary wedge pressure.

When the right ventricle fails, the blood backs up into the systemic circulation, producing elevated jugular venous distention, elevated CVP, hepatomegaly, ascites, anorexia, and pedal edema. Often, and especially with chronic HF, the patient will have signs and symptoms of both right-sided and left-sided heart failure.

A more current classification of HF is systolic versus diastolic heart failure. *Systolic heart failure* refers to the heart's inability to contract effectively. It is usually defined as an EF less than 35% to 40% (Midfred-LaForest, 2000; American College of Cardiology/ American Heart Association [ACC/AHA], Task Force 2001; Stanley & Prasun, 2002). Common causes of systolic dysfunction are coronary artery disease, hypertension, and idiopathic dilated cardiomyopathy (ACC/AHA, 2001). Diastolic heart failure implies that the heart can contract effectively, but the ventricle has an increased resistance to filling during diastole secondary to concentric hypertrophy, thus reducing the stroke volume (Futterman & Lemberg, 2001). *Diastolic failure* is usually defined as an EF of greater than 40%. Diastolic heart failure may be caused by cardiomyopathy (hypertrophic or restrictive), hypertrophy of the ventricle caused by hypertension, constrictive pericarditis, or impaired ventricular relaxation (ACC/AHA, 2001) As with right- and left-sided heart failure, it is possible to have combined diastolic and systolic dysfunction. To distinguish between diastolic and systolic heart failure, the clinician should use an echocardiogram to document the EF (Midfred-LaForest, 2000).

Documentation of systolic versus diastolic dysfunction is important because of the treatment ramifications. The cornerstone of therapy for systolic dysfunction is the use of a diuretic plus an angiotensin-converting enzyme (ACE) inhibitor and β-blocker therapy (Beattie, 2000; ACC/AHA, 2001). If the patient remains symptomatic, digoxin is also part of the treatment plan for systolic dysfunction. In addition, findings from the Randomized Aldactone Survical Study (RALES) indicate that the addition of spironolactone, an aldosterone antagonist, lowers the mortality by inhibiting the release of aldosterone (Chavey et al, 2001). Whereas many studies have focused on systolic dysfunction, fewer studies have dealt with diastolic dysfunction. Hence specific guidelines for the management of diastolic dysfunction are lacking. According to the ACC/AHA guidelines (2001) the recommended strategy for managing diastolic dysfunction is to focus on controlling blood pressure and heart rate, and reducing fluid retention through the use of β-blockers, ACE inhibitors, angiotension-receptor blockers, or calcium antagonists in order to minimize symptoms (p. 2111).

Although the terms *systolic* and *diastolic dysfunction* focus on the pathophysiologic alteration that leads to heart failure, there are two other classification systems used when discussing heart failure. The first classification system is the New York Heart Association (NYHA) functional classification. This system categorizes patients into four classes based on their severity of symptoms. Class I are patients without physical limitations. Class II are patients who are comfortable at rest, but ordinary activities may produce fatigue, angina, dyspnea or palpitations. Class III includes patients who are comfortable at rest but have marked limitations in physical activity. These patients become symptomatic with less than normal activity. Class IV are patients who are symptomatic even at rest. Any form of physical exertion produces symptoms for Class IV patients (Urden et al, 2002).

Another classification system has emerged that is meant to complement the NYHA classification system. This newer system, created by the ACC/AHA, is designed to capture both the evolution and the progression of the disease (ACC/AHA, 2001). The ACC/AHA guidelines categorizes patients into four stages or groupings, but the first two groupings represent patients who are asymptomatic. Specifically patients who are in Stage A are individuals who are at high risk for developing HF, but who presently do not have any heart disease and are asymptomatic. Stage B are individuals who have heart disease but who are still asymptomatic. Stage C are individuals who have heart disease and either are currently symptomatic, or have had symptoms of heart failure. Stage C parallels Class I, II, and III in the NYHA framework. Stage D are individuals who are refractory to therapy. These individuals parallel Class IV in the NYHA framework (ACC/AHA, 2001; Caboral & Mitchell, 2003).

Mr. Dukes presented with symptoms of both left- and right-sided heart failure. He has systolic dysfunction with an EF of 30%. At the time of discharge Mr. Dukes would be classified as Class II, and his ACC/AHA stage would be Stage C.

3. Discuss Mr. Dukes's signs and symptoms that were consistent with HF.

On initial assessment, Mr. Dukes complained of fatigue and shortness of breath. Physical findings revealed bibasilar crackles, an audible S_3, and tachycardia. These signs and symptoms indicate left-sided heart failure. Mr. Dukes's fatigue is related to his decreased CO. As his CO decreased, his SNS was activated and he became tachycardic. His heart also was in atrial fibrillation with a rapid ventricular response, which may have been either the cause or the result of his HF (Shapiro & Brundage, 2000). An audible S_3 indicates impaired filling during diastole. Mr. Dukes's increase in weight and his reduced urinary output represent activation of the RAAS and the subsequent release of aldosterone and ADH. Mr. Dukes's abdominal pain and positive hepatojugular reflux result from his right-sided heart failure with an increase in hepatic engorgement. His hypoactive bowel sounds indicate decreased gastric motility.

As Mr. Dukes's condition worsened, he became diaphoretic as a result of reduced CO and an increase in SNS stimulation. Hemodynamic changes included elevated blood pressure caused by SNS stimulation and elevated pulmonary artery pressures and pulmonary artery occlusive pressure caused by a backup of fluid into the pulmonary bed. The backup of fluid into the pulmonary bed also contributed to his labored respirations, dyspnea, and adventitious breath sounds. According to Braunwald and Goldman (2003), the development of rales correlates to a pulmonary capillary pressure of about 25 mm Hg. Elevated jugular venous distention and the presence of a hepatojugular reflux indicated right-sided heart failure as well. In addition, Mr. Dukes's SVR was elevated as a result of SNS stimulation and release of angiotensin II, and his cardiac index was reduced because of the combined failure of both his right and left ventricles. Mr. Dukes's EF of 30% indicated that his failure was systolic in nature as the result of his ventricles failing to contract effectively.

4. Describe Mr. Dukes's predisposing risk factors for HF.

Braunwald and Goldman (2003) stated that 1% to 2% of the Western population and approximately 5 million people in the United States have HF (Futterman & Lemberg, 2001; Stanley & Prasun, 2002). Mr. Dukes's predisposing risk factors for developing HF include his history of hypertension and his coronary artery disease. The existence of hypertension, which increases the workload on the heart, and documented blockages in the left and right coronary arteries indicate a potential for myocardial dysfunction resulting from ischemia and possible infarction. Also as previously stated, Mr. Dukes's atrial fibrillation could have been the result of his HF or an initial cause of his HF. In either event, the presence of his atrial fibrillation with a rapid ventricular response contributed to the reduced CO secondary to a loss of atrial kick and a decreased diastolic filling time. Additional risk factors to assess for are hyperlipidemia and diabetes mellitus. Hyperlipidemia is significant because it leads to the development of plaques and coronary artery disease. Diabetes also contributes to the development of coronary artery disease, thus placing the patient at risk for the development of HF.

Other predisposing factors that Mr. Dukes should be assessed for are (1) possible noncompliance with his antihypertensive therapy, (2) the possibility for either hypothyroidism or hyperthyroidism, (3) sleep apnea, (4) chronic anemia, and (5) a possible history of heavy alcohol intake (Stanley & Prasun, 2002). According to Braunwald and Goldman (2003), an intake of two drinks per day may be sufficient to exacerbate an already dysfunctional heart and lead to the development of HF (p. 314).

5. List the nursing diagnoses appropriate for Mr. Dukes's care.

According to Kotecki (1999), the following are appropriate nursing diagnoses for the patient with congestive heart failure (CHF):

- Decreased cardiac output related to ventricular damage, ischemia, and restriction
- Impaired gas exchange related to increase in pulmonary interstitial fluid secondary to decreased cardiac output

- Altered tissue perfusion, myocardial related to imbalance between oxygen supply and demand
- Fluid and electrolyte imbalance related to decreased cardiac output and aldosterone and ADH secretion and medication regimen
- Ineffective breathing pattern related to imbalance between oxygen supply and demand
- Fatigue related to imbalance between oxygen supply and oxygen demand
- Anxiety related to uncertain outcome
- Knowledge deficit related to new diagnosis and new medication regimen
- Ineffective coping related to health care demands of a newly diagnosed chronic illness

6. Briefly define the following terms: cardiac output (CO), cardiac index (CI), central venous pressure (CVP), preload, afterload, pulmonary artery pressure (PAP), and pulmonary artery occlusive pressure (PAOP).

CO is the amount of blood ejected from the heart per minute. It is the product of the stroke volume times heart rate (SV × HR). The normal CO is 4 to 8 L/min (Morelli, 1999).

CI is the cardiac output divided by the body surface area. It takes into account the patient's size or body surface area, and hence provides a more realistic indicator of cardiac function. The normal cardiac index is 2.5 to 4 L/min (Morelli, 1999).

CVP is the pressure in the right atrium. It reflects the pressure in the right side of the heart; thus as the pressure in the right ventricle increases with right ventricular failure, the CVP will increase. The normal CVP is 2 to 8 mm Hg (Morelli, 1999).

Preload is the volume of blood in the ventricle at the end of diastole. It is also called the *left ventricular end-diastolic pressure*. Clinically the preload is measured as the PAOP or the pulmonary capillary wedge pressure.

Afterload is the amount of work or resistance the ventricles must overcome to eject a given stroke volume. It is also referred to as SVR. The formula to determine the SVR is [(MAP – CVP)/CO] × 80. The normal SVR is between 800 and 1200 dynes/sec/cm^{-5} (MAP is mean arterial pressure).

SV is the amount of blood ejected per beat. The formula for determining the stroke volume is CO/HR. The normal stroke volume is 60 to 80 ml/beat.

PAP is the systolic and diastolic pressure within the pulmonary bed, in addition to the mean pulmonary pressure. The normal values are as follows (Morelli, 1999):

- Systolic PAP: 15 to 30 mm Hg
- Diastolic PAP: 8 to 15 mm Hg
- Mean PAP: 10 to 20 mm Hg

PAOP is the pressure in the pulmonary artery upon inflation of the balloon tip in a pulmonary artery catheter. The pulmonary arterial occlusive pressure reflects the preload or the left ventricular end-diastolic pressure. It is also called the pulmonary capillary wedge pressure. The normal PAOP is 8 to 15 mm Hg (Morelli, 1999).

7. Describe the benefits of using a pulmonary artery catheter during HF.

As stated, when the left and right ventricles begin to fail, fluid backs up into the pulmonary and systemic beds, respectively. Although signs and symptoms of HF are important in determining a patient's status, they are often not accurate enough to help monitor the patient during critical phases of treatment. The pulmonary artery catheter can provide more accurate data to determine the CO and CI, the PAOP, the PAPs, and the CVP. As stated in question 1, according to the Frank-Starling law, the greater the preload, the greater the CO up to a point. By using the pulmonary artery catheter and measuring the CO/CI and the PAOP simultaneously, one can plot the cardiac function curve and determine the appropriate preload for the most optimal CO. This allows the clinician to titrate intravenous fluid administration, use of diuretics, use of ACE inhibitors, and vasopressor therapy to provide the most optimal CO for a given patient.

8. Briefly describe the pathophysiology of pulmonary edema.

As stated in question 1, when the left ventricle fails as a pump, fluid is backed up into the pulmonary vasculature. When the pressure in the pulmonary vasculature exceeds 25 mm Hg or colloidal osmotic pressure, fluid begins to leak from the capillary bed into the interstitial spaces. When the buildup of pressure within the pulmonary bed is gradual, the lymphatic system is able to sequester the fluid away from the pulmonary bed (Braunwald & Goldman, 2003). However, when the increase in pressure is more acute, the fluid begins to leak into the alveoli. Classic signs and symptoms of pulmonary edema are extreme shortness of breath and respiratory distress, crackles, and pink frothy sputum. These signs and symptoms develop as the fluid begins to fill the alveoli and inhibit gas exchange, making the patient hypoxic. Also as the fluid crosses into the alveoli, capillaries rupture, making the sputum pink tinged. When arterial blood gas levels are measured, the patient's arterial oxygen pressure (PaO_2) will be usually less than 60 mm Hg.

9. List the pharmacologic agents used in Mr. Dukes's care and explain their importance to his treatment.

The cornerstone of drug therapy for CHF is a diuretic plus an ACE inhibitor and a β-blocker with digoxin added for patients who remain symptomatic (ACC/AHA, 2001; Futterman & Lemberg, 2001; McMurray, 2002). In patients such as Mr. Dukes who have a rapid onset of HF and the development of pulmonary edema, vasopressors such as dobutamine and dopamine may be added in addition to nitroprusside. Other medications that may be added to the protocol include nitroglycerin and morphine sulfate. Once Mr. Dukes is stabilized a β-blocker will be added to his therapy. If necessary, in order to reduce the effects of aldosterone, spironolactone can also be prescribed.

Mr. Dukes's specific medication regimen including potential therapies include:

Captopril (Capoten)

Based on the Cooperative North Scandinavian Enalapril Survival Study (CONSENSUS) and Studies of Left Ventricular Dysfunction Prevention (SOLVD-T) trials, the ACE inhibitor captopril is recommended for the treatment of HF because it produces vasodilation and blocks the RAAS (McMurray, 2002; McMurray & Pfeffer, 2002). By blocking the RAAS and inhibiting angiotensin II, captopril promotes vasodilation. Also by blocking the RAAS, aldosterone and subsequently ADH are inhibited and less fluid is retained. As the result of these actions, captopril reduces the preload and left ventricular filling pressures and moderately increases the CO. Long-term studies have indicated that captopril lessens symptoms and improves exercise tolerance (McMurray, 2002). Caution should be used when captopril is started because it may cause significant hypotension. A starting dose for captopril is 6.25 mg bid, which can be increased to 25 to 100 mg tid (Massie & Amidon, 2001; Nohria et al, 2002). In addition, because of the potential effects that ACE inhibitors have on renal function, the creatinine and potassium levels must be monitored closely.

Carvedilol (Coreg)

Carvedilol is a nonselective β-blocker. Studies, including the U.S. Carvedilol Heart Failure Study Group and the Carvedilol Prospective Randomized Cumulative Survival Study (COPERNICUS trial) indicate that the use of a β-blocker improves left ventricular function, increases survival rates by inhibiting remodeling and the processes that result in remodeling, including tachycardia, and increases force of contraction (Pritchett & Redfield, 2002). Presently the research indicates that patients respond better on a nonselective blocker agent, such as carvedilol, which blocks α-receptors as well as $β_1$- and $β_2$-receptors (Futterman & Lemberg, 2001; McMurray, 2002; Pritchett & Redfield, 2002). Because β-blockers are negative inotropic, they need to be titrated slowly after the patient has been stabilized with a diuretic and an ACE inhibitor (Chavey et al, 2001). Clinical guidelines for initiating β-blocker therapy include a systolic blood pressure greater than 85 mm Hg, a heart rate greater than 60, and no signs of sick sinus syndrome or heart block (Pritchett & Redfield, 2002). A beginning dose for carvedilol is 3.5 mg po bid (Midfred-LaForest, 2000).

Digitalis (Digoxin)

Digitalis is a cardiac glycoside that works by inhibiting the sodium-potassium pump. As a result, increased intracellular sodium is exchanged for extracellular calcium. The higher levels of intracellular calcium assist in increasing the force of the heart's contraction. Digitalis also inhibits atrioventricular conduction and is often used to decrease ventricular response to atrial fibrillation. Digoxin may be administered either orally or IV, but as in Mr. Dukes's case, when a rapid effect is desired to control atrial fibrillation, IV administration is preferred. Intravenously, the onset of digoxin's effect is 15 to 30 minutes, with a peak effect in $1\frac{1}{2}$ to 3 hours. Studies indicate that even a low serum blood level is therapeutic for HF patients (Michael & Parnell, 1998; Midfred-LaForest, 2000), thus even every other day dosing of digoxin is suggested (Nohria et al, 2002). However, because HF patients are frequently on a loop diuretic, which can cause hypokalemia, it is important that digoxin toxicity be avoided. Digoxin may also be prescribed for patients who are not in atrial fibrillation but still have symptoms of heart failure even after diuretic and ACE inhibitory therapy has been initiate. According to Stanley and Prasun (2002), whereas the research on digoxin does not indicate it reduces mortality, the use of digoxin has been correlated with a reduced number of hospitalizations and an improved exercise tolerance and quality of life.

Dobutamine (Dobutrex)

Dobutamine is a sympathomimetic that stimulates both β- and α-adrenergic receptors. However, dobutamine is more specific to β_1-adrenergic receptors (myocardium) than to β_2-adrenergic receptors (peripheral vessels and bronchioles). Although β-blocker therapy is part of the treatment modality for HF, sympathomimetic agents, such as dobutamine, are used to treat patients who are hemodynamically unstable or in cardiogenic shock (LeJemtel et al, 2003). At a dose of 2.5 to 10 μg/kg/min, dobutamine increases contractility, stroke volume, and CO (Kotecki, 1999). At doses greater than 10 μg/kg/min, β_2-adrenergic receptors are stimulated but not to the degree that β_1-adrenergic receptors are stimulated. Hence during the acute phase of Mr. Dukes's HF, dobutamine was added to his regimen to improve contractility and decrease afterload by producing some vasodilation.

Dopamine (Intropin)

Although dopamine was not used in Mr. Dukes's case, it is important to discuss its use and dose-related effects. At a low dose of 0.5 to 2 μg/kg/min, this inotropic agent increases renal perfusion, which aids in fluid elimination and preload reduction. At a dose of 2 to 10 μg/kg/min, β-adrenergic receptors are stimulated, increasing contractility, stroke volume, and heart rate. Doses greater than 10 μg/kg/min produce α-adrenergic effects that result in vasoconstriction, which increases blood pressure. At high dosage levels, however, this vasoconstriction leads to decreased renal perfusion (Kotecki, 1999). If dopamine had been added to Mr. Dukes's regimen, it would have been started at a low dosage to improve renal perfusion and hence increase the glomerular filtration rate and reduce fluid retention. Dopamine can also be used at moderate dosages to improve the force of contraction but at the expense of an increase in myocardial oxygen consumption. Consequently dopamine is often not the drug of choice for improving the CO.

Milrinone (Incor)

Milrinone is a phosphodiesterase inhibitor that may be used during an acute exacerbation of HF. Milrinone decreases or inhibits the breakdown of cyclic AMP resulting in an increase in myocardial contractility, and arterial and venous dilation. Short-term improvement may be seen related to its tendency to increase heart rate and contractility and thus increase the cardiac output. However, because these two factors also increase remodeling, milrinone may prove detrimental in the long run (Futterman & Lemberg, 2001). In this case study milrinone was not used because Mr. Dukes responded to furosemide, captropril, and dobutamine.

Furosemide (Lasix)

As stated, one of the cardinal features of HF is retention of fluid. According to ACC/AHA guidelines (2001) diuretics should be used for patients who have evidence of fluid retention. The goal is to return the patient to a euvolemic state, and then diuretics should be continued to prevent further fluid retention. Furosemide is a loop diuretic that has a rapid onset and is effective even in patients with severe renal insufficiency (LeJemtel et al, 2003). The dose for furosemide can range from 20 to 320 mg/day in either single or divided doses. Because Mr. Dukes was developing pulmonary edema and had evidence of the potential for poor gastric absorption, furosemide was administered IV. Complications that a clinician should be monitoring for are (1) volume depletion, (2) hypotension, (3) prerenal azotemia, and (4) hypokalemia, especially if digoxin is part of the medication therapy.

Nitroprusside (Nipride)

Nitroprusside is a potent venous and arterial dilator that reduces both preload and afterload and subsequently improves the CO. Nitroprusside is usually used only in the management of patients with acute decompensating HF (Futterman & Lemberg, 2001). Because nitroprusside can produce profound hypotension, the dosage is usually titrated according to the patient's blood pressure, and it is often used in conjunction with dobutamine or dopamine to maintain vascular tone while improving the CO.

Nitroglycerin Ointment

Nitroglycerin is both a venous and arterial vasodilator, and consequently it decreases both preload and afterload. According the ACC/AHA guidelines (2001), nitrates should be used only in patients who can not be given an ACE inhibitor because of hypotension or renal insufficiency (p. 2108). The standard dose is 12.5 to 50 mg (1 to 4 inches) every 8 hours; however, to prevent the development of tolerance to nitrates, an 8- to 12-hour drug-free period should be used (Massie & Amidon, 2001). When nitroglycerin is started, the dosage may need to be adjusted if hypotension or nitroglycerin-induced headaches develop.

Spironolactone (Aldactone)

Spironolactone is a potassium-sparing diuretic that competes with the aldosterone receptors at the collecting ducts and inhibits sodium retention. Although aldosterone is also implicated in the remodeling of the myocardium, inhibition of aldosterone through the use of spironolactone provides another avenue to reduce the remodeling process. In the Randomized Aldactone Evaluation Study (RACES trial) the use of spironolactone was associated with a 36% reduction in hospitalization and a 27% reduction in mortality (Piano et al, 2000). Initial dose is 25 mg/day, which may be increased to 50 mg/day. It is important to monitor the patient for hyperkalemia once this therapy is started.

10. Discuss long-term management of a patient with HF.

Readmission rates to acute-care facilities of 25% to 47% have been reported (Dunbar et al, 1998). Although frequent readmissions and exacerbation of a patient's HF result from a number of variables, insufficient patient and family education, inadequate self-monitoring and management, and noncompliance with dietary restrictions, medication regimens, and exercise recommendations have been cited as strong contributing factors. This is frequently discussed as "failure begets failure," implying that failure on the part of the patient to comply with a medical regimen results in a progression of HF (Pritchett & Redfield, 2002). These factors emphasize the importance of patient and family teaching and counseling to help the patient maintain the highest level of wellness possible and avoid rehospitalization. Broad areas that need to be addressed include medications, diet, fluid restriction, activities of daily living, exercise, smoking cessation, self-monitoring, and when to call a health care provider for progression of symptoms. In each of these categories various teaching strategies, including verbal and written communication, tapes (audio and video), and websites (if appropriate), should be used. Because HF is a chronic illness, these areas of content should be covered not only before discharge but also at each follow-up visit. Follow-up visits provide an excellent opportunity to reinforce appropriate behaviors and clarify misconceptions (Urden et al, 2002).

Specifically, the standard care for a patient with HF includes moderate dietary sodium restriction and a graduated exercise program along with the medication regimen (ACC/AHA, 2001). Massie and Amidon (2001) recommend restriction of sodium to 2 g per day and a graduated exercise program to increase exercise capacity. As with any patient, it is important to obtain a complete history, including dietary habits, use of over-the-counter medications, and exercise habits. By obtaining an accurate baseline, the clinician can individualize the patient teaching to maximize compliance. When teaching patients about dietary restrictions, the clinician must explain what sodium is and how to calculate sodium intake. This includes teaching patients not only to read labels but also learn what types of foods to avoid, such as canned or processed foods. In patients with more advanced HF, fluid restriction may be added. When fluid restriction is instituted, the patient and family must learn how to determine an accurate intake. The patient and family should also be cautioned that ice must be calculated into the patient's daily intake record.

Thorough patient teaching about the medication regimen is also critical. Patients need to know not only what their medications are and when to take them but also the possible side effects. In Mr. Dukes's case, it is important that he and his family have a complete understanding of the purpose of his digoxin, how to take his pulse, and what signs and symptoms may indicate digoxin toxicity. Also, because Mr. Dukes's medication regimen includes an ACE inhibitor, furosemide, and digoxin, his potassium levels need to be monitored carefully. In addition, Mr. Dukes needs to understand the purpose of his potassium supplements. Given his drug therapy, it would be advisable to counsel Mr. Dukes not to use a potassium-based salt substitute. Once Mr. Dukes has been stabilized, carvedilol is to be added to his treatment. It is important to teach the patient that carvedilol will need to be titrated very slowly over the next couple of weeks, and it may be at least 3 months before the positive benefits of the β-blocker are apparent (Pritchett & Redfield, 2002).

Self-management strategies should be taught to each patient. This includes the ability to assess changes in shortness of breath or dyspnea, to recognize paroxysmal nocturnal dyspnea (PND), new onset of orthopnea, changes in weight, pedal edema, abdominal distention (ascites), blood pressure changes, nausea, and fatigue. For elderly patients family members may be encouraged to note changes in mental status as a possible sign of an exacerbation of HF. Specifically, for weight changes, patients need to be taught to weigh themselves every day, on the same scales and at approximately the same time to be able to evaluate their fluid status. Patients need to be taught that a 2.2 lb increase in weight represents retention of 1 L of fluid. If a patient experiences a 2 lb increase in weight or greater over 1 to 2 days, he or she should be taught how to adjust the medication regimen appropriately, as well as how to modify diet and fluid intake. If patients and their families have doubts or if self-regulation fails, they need to know when and how to contact their clinician or practitioner.

When a nurse or practitioner sees a patient in the clinic for follow-up, the same guidelines apply. The clinician needs to monitor vital signs, weight, breath sounds, capillary refill, jugular venous distention, hepatomegaly, ascites, 12-lead ECG changes, digoxin level, and electrolyte levels (including K^+, Na^+, and creatinine). A focused history needs to be obtained to assess compliance with diet, medications, and exercise and any problems the patient may have developed. By working closely with the patient and family, the hope is that patients can achieve and maintain their desired quality of life and avoid rehospitalization.

11. Discuss new drug therapies for HF that are on the horizon.

Although the cornerstone of pharmacologic intervention for systolic dysfunction is a diuretic plus an ACE inhibitor, digoxin, and the use of a β-blocker, a number of recent studies support other potential therapies. Based on the pathophysiology of HF, new treatments are being explored. Focusing on reducing the RAAS stimulation, investigators have studied the use of angiotensin II receptor blockers (ARBs). Research on ARBs has focused on losartan. Losartan is a peripheral vasodilator, and it reduces SVR. It also decreases aldosterone secretion and release of norepinephrine. It has been demonstrated that losartan can improve left ventricular function in certain subgroups of patients with HF (Coodley, 1999). However, research indicates that ARBs are no more effective than ACE inhibitors, and it is recommended that they be used only in individuals who cannot tolerate an ACE inhibitor (Chavey et al, 2001).

Another new therapy is the use of brain natriuretic peptide (BNP) both as a marker of heart failure and as a therapy. BNP is a peptide that is secreted by the ventricle in response to fluid overload. It is possible to measure BNP blood levels, and correlate elevated blood levels with acute exacerbations (Futterman & Lemberg, 2001). BNP is also available for IV administration and is marketed as nesiritide (Natrecor). Nesiritide is recombinant BNP made for *Escherichia coli*. It has proven to reduce preload and afterload, and increase cardiac output in individuals who are experiencing an acute exacerbation. When compared with nitroglycerin, nesiritide improved hemodynamics more quickly than nitroglycerin (Publication Committee for the VMAC Investigators, 2002). Nesiritide may be given as a bolus or an IV infusion with an infusion dosage of 0.01 to 0.03 µg/kg/min. It begins to reduce PAOP within 15 minutes of infusion, and 95% of its effectiveness is reached within 1 hour of administration (Abernethy, 2002).

In terms of diastolic dysfunction, research is ongoing in order to determine better therapeutic management of patients with this form of HF. Focusing on calcium channel blockers, in the Prospective Randomization Amlodipine Survival Evaluation study and the Vasodilator Heart Failure Trial III, amlodipine and felodipine, respectively, were shown to be effective when used in combination with an ACE inhibitor in a selected group of patients (Michael & Parnell, 1998; Coodley, 1999). However, it is important to note that calcium channel blockers have been shown to be detrimental for patients who have a systolic dysfunction.

HEART FAILURE

References

Abernethy, D. (2002). Nesiritide. *Mosby GenRx Drug Guide*. St. Louis, Mosby, Inc. www.merckmedicus.com.

American College of Cardiology/American Heart Association Task Force. (2001). Guidelines for the evaluation and management of heart failure. *Journal of the American College of Cardiology, 38*(7), 2102-2113.

Beattie, S. (2000). Heart failure with preserved LV function: Pathophysiology, clinical presentation, treatment, and nursing implications. *The Journal of Cardiovascular Nursing, 14*(4), 24-37.

Braunwald, E. & Goldman, L. (2003). *Primary cardiology* (2nd ed.). Philadelphia: W. B. Saunders.

Caboral, M. & Mitchell, J. (2003). New guidelines for heart failure focus on prevention. *The Nurse Practitioner, 28*(1), 13-16, 22-24.

Chavey, W., et al. (2001). Guidelines for the management of heart failure caused by systolic dysfunction: Part II. Treatment. *American Family Physician, 64*(6), 1045-1054.

Coodley, E. (1999). Newer drug therapy for congestive heart failure. *Archives of Internal Medicine, 159,* 1177-1183.

Dunbar, S. B., Jacobson, L. H., & Deaton, C. (1998). Heart failure: Strategies to enhance patient self-management. *AACN Clinical Issues, 9*(2), 244-256.

Futterman, L. & Lemberg, L. (2001). Heart failure: Update on treatment and prognosis. *American Journal of Critical Care, 10*(4), 285-293.

Kotecki, C. (1999). Heart failure. In L. Bucher & S. Melander (Eds.), *Critical care nursing*. Philadelphia: W. B. Saunders.

LeJemtel, T., Sonnenblick, E., & Frishman, W. (2003) Heart failure: Diagnosis and management of heart failure. In Fuster, V. and Alexander, R. *Hurst's the heart*. New York: McGraw-Hill.

Massie, B. & Amidon, T. (2001). Heart. In L. M. Tierney, S. J. McPhee, & M. A. Papadakis (Eds.), *Current medical diagnosis and treatment*. Stamford, CT: Appleton & Lange.

McMurray, J. (2002). Heart failure in 10 years time: Focus on pharmacological treatment. *Heart, 88,* ii40-ii46.

McMurray, J. & Pfeffer, M. (2002). New therapeutic options in congestive heart failure: Part I. *Circulation, 105*(17), 2099-2106.

Michael, K. A. & Parnell, K. J. (1998). Innovations in the pharmacological management of heart failure. *AACN Clinical Issues, 9*(2), 172-191.

Mildred-LaForest, S. (2000). Pharmacology department: Pharmacotherapy of systolic heart failure: A review of recent literature and practical application. *The Journal of Cardiovascular Nursing, 14*(4), 57-75.

Morelli, P. (1999). Cardiovascular anatomy and physiology in failure. In L. Bucher & S. Melander (Eds.), *Critical care nursing*. Philadelphia: W. B. Saunders.

Nohria, A., Lewis, E., & Stevenson, L. (2002). Medical management of advanced heart failure. *Journal of the American Medical Association, 287*(5), 628-639.

Piano, M., Kim, S., & Jarvis, C. (2000). Cellular events linked to cardiac remodeling in heart failure: Targets for pharmacologic interventions. *The Journal of Cardiovascular Nursing, 14*(4), 1-23.

Pritchett, A. & Redfield, M. (2002). Beta blockers: New standard therapy for heart failure. *Mayo Clinic Proceedings, 77,* 839-846.

Publication Committee for the VMAC Investigators. (2002). Intravenous nesiritide vs nitroglycerin for treatment of decompensated congestive heart failure. *Journal of the American Medical Association, 287,* 1531-1540.

Shapiro, S. & Brundage, B. (2000). Cardiac problems in critical care. In F. Bongard, & D. Sue (Eds.). *Current critical care and diagnosis and treatment*. Stamford, CT: Appleton & Lange.

Stanley, M. & Prasun, M. (2002). Heart failure in older adults: Keys to successful management. *AACN Clinical Issues, 13*(1), 94-102.

Urden, L. D., Stacy, K. M., & Lough, M. E. (Eds.). (2002). *Thelan's critical care nursing: Diagnosis and management* (4th ed.). St. Louis: Mosby.

Online Resources:

Congestive Heart Failure. www.americanheart.org.

Facts about Heart Failure. www.nhlbi.nih.gov/health/public/heart/other/hrtfail.htm.

Guidelines for management of patients with heart failure caused by left ventricular systolic dysfunction: Pharmacological approach: www.hfsa.org/html.

6

Carotid Endarterectomy

M. Lynn Rodgers, RNC, MSN, CCRN, CNRN, ACNP-BC

CASE PRESENTATION

Mrs. Lee, age 62, has a history of coronary artery disease (CAD) and had four-vessel coronary artery bypass graft (CABG) surgery 4 years ago. Two years before her cardiac surgery she had a silent inferior wall myocardial infarction (MI). This MI was discovered during a routine physical examination, which included an electrocardiogram (ECG) that indicated Q waves previously undetected in leads II, III, and aV_F. She did not remember having any unusual episodes of chest pain before the discovery of the MI, other than her usual "indigestion." She had been doing well since her CABG surgery, but during the past 6 months, Mrs. Lee has had at least three transient ischemic attacks (TIAs).

The first TIA involved numbness of her left arm and leg, dizziness, and a headache. The second TIA was identical. The third TIA did not include a headache, but she did again have numbness of her left arm and leg and dizziness. Each episode lasted approximately 15 minutes. After the first TIA, Dr. Allen found bilateral bruits over the carotid arteries and bright yellow plaques of cholesterol (Hollenhorst plaques) on retinal examination. After obtaining these findings, he ordered a Doppler ultrasound of the carotid arteries and a computed tomography (CT) scan of the head to assist in determining the cause of the TIAs. The results of the Doppler ultrasound and the CT scan indicated bilateral carotid artery stenosis that was more severe on the right side. After treatment options were discussed with Mrs. Lee, a conservative medical approach was implemented. Aspirin (Bayer) 325 mg/day was started. She was already on lipid-lowering and hypertensive drug therapy.

After the second TIA, Dr. Allen encouraged Mrs. Lee to consider surgery, but she declined. After the third TIA, Mrs. Lee agreed to have a cardiac catheterization and an arch angiography. The cardiac catheterization revealed minimal (25%) occlusion of the right coronary artery. The remaining coronary vessels were 10% occluded. The two-vessel arteriogram report revealed bilateral carotid disease with 95% stenosis of the right internal carotid artery and 80% occlusion of the left internal carotid artery.

Intensive Care Unit Admission

After undergoing a right carotid endarterectomy, Mrs. Lee was admitted directly to the intensive care unit at 11:45 AM. Her initial postoperative vital signs and assessment revealed the following:

Height	162.5 (5 ft 5 in)
Weight	63 kg (140 lb)
BP	124/78 mm Hg
HR	80 bpm

Respirations	24 breaths/min
Temperature	36.8° C (98.2° F) (oral)

A clean, dry dressing was present over the right carotid area with a Jackson-Pratt (JP) drain in place. Her right neck area was slightly swollen.

The physician's orders were as follows:

- Cardiac monitor
- Continuous pulse oximetry
- Arterial line (A-line) for direct blood pressure (BP) measurement
- Oxygen at 2 L/min by nasal cannula
- 5% dextrose in 25% normal saline solution with 20 mEq potassium chloride (KCl) at 75 ml/hr
- Nitroprusside (Nipride) to keep BP below 140 (currently 10 ml/hr [33 µg/min] mixed as nitroprusside 50 mg in 250 ml of 5% dextrose in water)
- Complete blood count, basic metabolic profile, ECG, and chest x-ray film in the morning
- Morphine sulfate 1 to 4 mg intravenously qh prn for pain
- Oxycodone (Percocet) 1 to 2 tablets po q3-4h prn for pain
- Resume home medications when patient is able to swallow well
- Prudent heart diet as tolerated
- Head of bed elevated 30 degrees
- Neurologic checks every 15 minutes for 2 hours, every hour for 4 hours, every 2 hours for 6 hours, and then every 4 hours

At noon, 15 minutes after the initial assessment, the following data were obtained:

BP	172/92 mm Hg (cuff); 180/98 mm Hg (arterial line)
HR	68 bpm
Respirations	26 breaths/min
Temperature	37.2° C (98.9° F) (oral)

Breath sounds were clear, with a pulse oximetry reading of 96%. The trachea was midline with airflow auscultated over it. The ECG monitor revealed normal sinus rhythm at 68 bpm. The patient was easily aroused and oriented to person, place, and time. Handgrips were strong bilaterally with equal strength. Plantar flexion and dorsiflexion were intact. Mrs. Lee's speech was clear. Pupils were equal, round, and reacted to light. Cranial nerves were intact. Facial expressions were symmetrical. Shoulder shrugs were strong bilaterally.

Other tests revealed the following:

Glucose	80 mg/dl
BUN	11 mg/dl
Creatinine	0.9 mg/dl
Na$^+$	139 mmol/L
K$^+$	3.9 mmol/L
Cl$^-$	106 mmol/L
Hgb	12.3 g/dl
Hct	39.3%

Nitroprusside was increased to 15 ml/hr (50 µg/min).

CAROTID ENDARTERECTOMY

QUESTIONS

1. What is carotid artery disease? Briefly describe the anatomy of the cerebral circulation.

2. What is a stroke, and what factors relating to carotid artery disease contribute to development of a stroke?

3. What are the warning signs and symptoms of cerebral ischemia?

4. What medical and surgical therapy is available for carotid artery stenosis?

5. When should surgical treatment be selected over medical therapy?

6. Describe the surgical procedure for a carotid endarterectomy (CEA).

7. What new nonsurgical procedure is being used for carotid artery stenosis?

8. What nursing management does the patient with carotid endarterectomy require immediately postoperatively?

9. What neurologic complications can occur after carotid endarterectomy that should be immediately reported to the surgeon?

10. Discuss the blood pressure and heart rate changes that may occur in the early postoperative period after carotid endarterectomy.

11. Four hours after surgery, the nurse notices a hematoma around Mrs. Lee's incision site. What causes a hematoma after carotid endarterectomy, and what is the danger posed by this finding? What other complications could develop?

12. After surgery Mrs. Lee made good progress, the JP drain was removed, and she was discharged home the day after surgery. Discharge medications include nifedipine (Procardia) 20 mg orally every 8 hours and clopidogrel (Plavix) 75 mg daily. Describe the pharmacodynamics and clinical effects of these drugs.

13. What instructions should be given to Mrs. Lee before her discharge?

CAROTID ENDARTERECTOMY

QUESTIONS AND ANSWERS

1. What is carotid artery disease? Briefly describe the anatomy of the cerebral circulation.

Carotid artery disease occurs when atherosclerotic processes develop in the internal and external carotid arteries. Routine history and physical examination can reveal findings that are suspicious for carotid disease. A detailed history of neurologic symptoms can provide clues for suspicion of carotid artery disease (Dirks & Lough, 2003). Upon physical examination, the health care practitioner auscultates the areas over the carotid arteries while the patient holds his or her breath. The presence of a bruit or "swish" may indicate turbulence or increased blood flow due to intraluminal disruption (Urden et al, 2002). Carotid bruits are graded on a 1 to 4 scale dependent upon the intensity of the sounds. The most common diagnostic study to evaluate the carotid arteries is the noninvasive carotid duplex ultrasonography (Strandness, 2002). This test assesses artery blood flow and velocity by picking up sound generated by blood moving through the underlying vessels (Ricci & Knight, 2000). Cerebral angiography is performed by injecting a contrast material into one or more arteries to obtain radiographic visualization of the targeted circulation (Ferri, 2001). It is required in 10% of cases due to usual carotid anatomy, calcium deposits altering carotid duplex results, and disease outside the carotid bulb (Strandness, 2002). Preprocedure care involves premedication and signing of an informed consent. Postprocedure care involves checking the site for bleeding or hematoma formation. A major complication of this procedure can be a stroke caused by accidental dislodging of an atherosclerotic plaque from the artery wall or a clot formed at the end of the catheter or needle. However, risk for stroke or death during cerebral angiography is 1%. The brain receives 85% of its blood supply from the anterior circulation (bilateral carotid arteries) and 15% of its posterior blood supply from the posterior circulation (bilateral vertebral arteries). The common carotid arteries bifurcate extracranially into external and internal branches, with the external carotid artery carrying blood to the face and scalp and the internal carotid artery sending blood to the cerebral hemispheres. The internal carotid artery has four major intracranial branches: anterior cerebral artery, middle cerebral artery, ophthalmic artery, and posterior communicating artery (Black et al., 2001).

2. What is a stroke and what factors relating to carotid artery disease contribute to development of a stroke?

A stroke or cerebral vascular accident results from death of brain cells due to decreased blood flow to the brain. More than 750,000 strokes occur each year, and almost one third of these strokes are caused by a thromboembolic event originating from plaque in the carotid arteries (Urden et al, 2002). A narrow opening in the carotid artery can attract debris that traps blood clots that easily travel to the brain and cause total cerebral vessel occlusion. The obstruction usually occurs at the bifurcation of the common carotid artery and typically is a result of atherosclerosis. When fatty deposits are coated by fibrous tissue, a plaque develops, leading to stenosis. As this plaque increases in size, cerebral blood flow decreases. When the intimal lining of the artery is no longer intact, the plaque may become ulcerated or rupture and expose a roughened area. This, in turn, attracts more debris and can eventually lead to embolization. Cerebral blood flow decreases as the vessel narrows and the atheroma releases microemboli that travel to small cerebral arteries (Strandness, 2002). Emboli of platelet origin can precipitate vasospasm due to release of vasoactive substances such as thromboxane A_2, which creates more vasoconstriction. This further compromise to cerebral tissue leads to cerebral ischemia and infarction (Moore et al, 2000; Urden et al,

2002). Other causative factors include atherosclerosis, emboli, fibromuscular dysplasia, aneurysms, trauma, Takayasu's arteritis, and spontaneous dissection (Ferri, 2001).

3. What are the warning signs and symptoms of cerebral ischemia?

Patients with atherosclerotic carotid artery disease may present with cerebral vascular accident (CVA), TIA, reversible ischemic neurologic deficit (RIND), or be asymptomatic. Signs and symptoms of CVA can include weakness or numbness of the face, arm, or leg; loss of vision or dimness, usually in one eye; difficulty speaking or understanding speech; severe headache; and dizziness, unsteadiness, or falls (Ferri, 2001). A higher risk of CVA or death occurs with bilateral carotid occlusion, stenosis of the intracranial section of the ipsilateral internal carotid artery, and stenosis of the ipsilateral external carotid artery. If CVA signs and symptoms last from a few minutes or less than 24 hours, it is called a TIA. By definition, neurologic examination must be normal or baseline within 24 hours. During a TIA the neurologic deficit lasts 10 to 20 minutes and consists of contralateral hemiparesis and/or hemiparesthesia, visual changes, receptive and/or expressive aphasia, vertigo, syncope, headaches, and ataxia (Urden et al, 2002). A classic symptom of carotid TIA is transient spells of ipsilateral monocular blurring or blindness called amaurosis fugax. Amaurosis fugax is commonly referred to as a retinal TIA. Permanent damage is rarely associated with a TIA. When the presentation is the same for each attack, the cause is usually in the extracranial circulation, as patients with cardiac emboli tend to have variable symptoms. A RIND is a minor stroke that lasts more than 24 hours but usually eventually resolves. TIAs may occur for as long as 2 to 6 years prior to cerebral infarction.

4. What medical and surgical therapy is available for carotid artery stenosis?

Medical management of carotid stenosis and stroke prevention is smoking cessation, cholesterol reduction through diet and/or drug therapy, management of high blood pressure, glucose control for diabetic patients, and antiplatelet or anticoagulation medications such as aspirin, warfarin (Coumadin), ticlopidine (Ticlid), or clopidogrel (Plavix) (Gorelick et al, 1999; Urden et al, 2002). Some evidence supports the use of statin lipid-lowering medications to not only reduce lipid levels but also protect the endothelium by increasing nitric oxide and decreasing inflammatory responses (Vaughan, 2003). Also it is important to control thromboembolic cardiovascular abnormalities such as atrial fibrillation or flutter, valvular disease, and clotting disorders. Patient with these disorders that experience a TIA or stroke should have a transesophageal echocardiogram (TEE) to evaluate presence of mural thrombosis or valvular vegetation in the heart (Urden et al, 2002). In high-risk patients with diminished life expectancy, medical management of asymptomatic high-grade carotid stenosis is an accepted option (Erzurum et al, 2002).

A carotid endarterectomy is the surgical removal of an atheroma (fatty plaque) at the carotid bifurcation in an attempt to prevent stroke (Ballotta et al, 1999; Moore et al, 2000). Carotid endarterectomy is the therapy of choice in symptomatic patients with high-grade internal carotid artery stenosis. The goal is removal of the atherosclerotic plaque formation in an effort to prevent stroke. Because of Mrs. Lee's high-grade stenosis and history of TIAs, the surgical procedure is indicated as the best option for preventing stroke or CVA (Messina & Tierney, 2003).

5. When should surgical treatment be selected over medical therapy?

The North American Symptomatic Carotid Endarterectomy Trial (NASCET) has demonstrated that patients with more than 70% occlusion of the internal carotid artery would have a less than 6% surgical risk. Carotid endarterectomy would offer a clear benefit to these patients. The American Heart Association (AHA) agrees and includes those who have had a mild stroke within the previous 6 months (Gorelick et al, 1999; Kappelle et al, 1999; Nemoto, 1999). Other sources recommend surgical intervention for those patients with carotid stenosis greater than 50% and symptomatic or with carotid stenosis greater than 60% but asymptomatic (Abu Rahma et al, 2002; Strandness, 2002). Asymptomatic patients with less than 60% stenosis are most often treated medically. According to Ferri (2001) and Messina and Tierney (2003), there is less than 3% risk for those asymptomatic, 5% for those with TIA, 7% for those with stroke, and 10% for those with recurring stenosis. The following five clinical characteristics significantly increase a patient's risk with carotid endarterectomy: (1) surgery for CVA or TIA versus ocular ischemia alone (amaurosis fugax or retinal artery occlusion), (2) female sex, (3) age older than 75 years, (4) systolic BP greater than 180 mm Hg, and (5) a history of peripheral vascular disease. In most cases diabetes mellitus, angina, recent MI, or current smoking are not associated with higher surgical risk (Messina & Tierney, 2003).

6. Describe the surgical procedure for a carotid endarterectomy (CEA).

Carotid endarterectomy is the second most common cardiovascular surgery after coronary artery bypass grafting. After making an incision along the anterior area of the sternocleidomastoid muscle, the surgeon clamps the carotid vessel and removes the atherosclerotic plaque. If part of the vessel is also removed, a vein graft, polyester Dacron patch, or bovine pericardium patch is used to repair or replace the carotid artery (Biasi et al, 2002). Temporarily diverting blood around the operative vessel via a shunt is sometimes used to avoid disruption of cerebral perfusion. Continuous electroencephalograph (EEG) monitoring, cerebral pulse oximetry, and transcranial Doppler are often used to monitor for cerebral hypoxia and ischemia. Bilateral carotid endarterectomy surgery is not done due to greater risk for cerebral ischemia and infarct (Moore et al, 2000). Mrs. Lee will return for surgery on her remaining carotid stenosis at a later date, dependent upon her tolerance and recovery from the initial surgery and further symptoms from her remaining stenosis.

7. What new nonsurgical procedure is being used for carotid artery stenosis?

Carotid angioplasty and stenting (CAS) is a method of opening a stenotic area in the carotid artery similar to that used during coronary artery angioplasty and stenting (Strandness, 2002). CAS is performed in an interventional radiology or vascular laboratory suite. After anticoagulation with heparin and sometimes abciximab (ReoPro), the physician inserts femoral artery and vein sheaths. Angiography of the aorta and carotid arteries is performed, and an appropriate balloon-tipped catheter is selected. Once the balloon is positioned over the carotid stenosis, it is inflated slowly for up to 3 minutes to dilate the vessel and compress the plaque. After the vessel is maximally dilated, the catheter is removed and a stent is deployed to trap plaque and maintain lumen patency. Complications that may occur are bradycardia or asystole due to carotid baroreceptor pressure, bleeding, neurologic deficits including stroke, and airway obliteration from neck swelling. These complications are comparable to those of carotid endarterectomy. One study indicates CEA is cost effective when compared with CAS, related to the high cost of stents and higher stroke rate after CAS (Kilaru et al, 2003). Another study indicates that stroke death rate after CAS was 3% with a restenosis rate in 28 months of 6%, figures comparable to CEA (Gable et al, 2003). CAS was not recommended in the past, but as newer techniques decrease emboli development and stent costs decrease, CAS may be an effective nonsurgical option of treating carotid stenosis. The National Institutes of Health are sponsoring the Carotid Revascularization Endarterectomy Versus Stent (CREST) trial to evaluate the role of carotid balloon angioplasty and stenting (Strandness, 2002).

8. What nursing management does the patient with carotid endarterectomy require immediately postoperatively?

Nursing care for the patient with CEA includes (Urden et al, 2002):

- Observation for respiratory difficulties
- Provision of oxygen and oral suction equipment
- Frequent vital signs and neurologic assessment

- Maintenance of cardiac and arterial monitoring
- Maintenance of straight head alignment with no neck flexion
- Elevation of the head of bed (HOB) to decrease swelling if vital signs are stable
- Cold application to the operative site
- Observation for bleeding and/or hematoma
- Management of pain
- Administration of antiplatelet therapy

9. What neurologic complications can occur after carotid endarterectomy that should be immediately reported to the surgeon?

Cerebral ischemia and/or infarct can lead to neurologic deficits after surgery (Laman et al, 2002). Injuries to cranial nerves can also occur from intraoperative trauma (e.g., inadvertent transection, retractor injuries) and edema resulting in nerve compression (Urden et al, 2002). Cranial nerve damage occurs in 16% of patients undergoing carotid endarterectomy, but usually resolve; however, 1% to 4% do not (Nemoto, 1999). The presence of neurologic deficits and cranial nerve dysfunction should be determined before the patient is given any ice chips, water, or food. Once the gag reflex has returned, the patient should be given liquids only initially and cautiously when awake. The following should be reported to the physician (Urden et al, 2002):

- Ipsilateral vascular-type headaches
- Decreased level of consciousness, disorientation, or inability to follow commands
- Unequal, dilated, or sluggish pupils
- Motor weakness or hemiplegia
- Visual disturbances
- Respiratory or breathing pattern changes
- Dysphasia, dysarthria
- Seizures
- Widening pulse pressure (late and ominous sign)
- Cranial nerve dysfunction
- XII, hypoglossal (located under the carotid artery): inability to position the tongue midline
- X, vagus (laryngeal branch): hoarseness, loss of cough mechanism
- VII, facial (marginal mandibular branch): drooping of the lip ipsilateral to the surgery site
- XI, spinal accessory: inability to shrug shoulders and raise arms

10. Discuss the blood pressure and heart rate changes that may occur in the early postoperative period after carotid endarterectomy.

Frequent changes in BP often occur during the immediate postoperative period of carotid endarterectomy. Baroreceptors located in the carotid sinus may be disturbed during the surgical procedure, resulting in hypertension or hypotension. Hypertension usually occurs during the early postoperative period and generally lasts an average of 5 to 6 hours after surgery (Moore et al, 2000). One danger of hypertension includes rupture or oozing at the carotid vessel suture lines. Sustained hypertension can also increase the patient's risk for intracerebral edema, hemorrhage, and stroke. Sodium nitroprusside and nitroglycerin are vasodilators commonly used to maintain a patient's BP within 20 mm Hg of the patient's preoperative baseline (Blohme et al, 1999; Nemoto, 1999). Patients with chronic hypertension may develop reflex hypotension and/or bradycardia. Aggressive treatment with vasopressors and fluids is required because hypotension decreases cerebral blood flow and perfusion and may result in altered mentation and neurologic deficits. Bradycardia occurs due to manipulation of the vagal receptors during surgery (Urden et al, 2002). Atropine may be required because its parasympatholytic properties can reverse symptomatic bradycardia and should be kept at the patient's bedside.

11. **Four hours after surgery, the nurse notices a hematoma around Mrs. Lee's incision site. What causes a hematoma after carotid endarterectomy and what is the danger posed by this finding? What other complications could develop?**

Development of a hematoma or swelling is a serious, potentially life-threatening complication. A hematoma in the neck area can contribute to airway occlusion, tracheal deviation, or rupture of the operative vessel. The patient should be monitored for neck edema, bright red drainage from the incision site, decreased hematocrit, and hypotension. Such findings should be reported to the surgeon. In some cases the patient may need additional surgery for reexploration and evacuation of the hematoma (Nemoto, 1999; Ouriel et al, 1999; Moore et al, 2000). Stroke caused by embolization, thrombosis, or hemorrhage can occur. Postoperative MI as well can be a major complication of carotid endarterectomy. Mrs. Lee is a potential candidate for an MI due to her history of preexisting cardiovascular disease. MI occurs infrequently but is the most common cause of death after carotid endarterectomy (0.8% to 3%); the risk of MI is increased to 13% in patients with a history of angina (Moore et al, 2000).

12. **After surgery Mrs. Lee made good progress, the JP drain was removed, and she was discharged home the day after surgery. Discharge medications include nifedipine (Procardia) 20 mg orally every 8 hours and clopidogrel (Plavix) 75 mg daily. Describe the pharmacodynamics and clinical effects of these drugs.**

Calcium channel blockers and antiplatelet therapy are important for Mrs. Lee. Calcium channel blockers such as nifedipine relax vascular smooth muscle, specifically arterioles and veins, without causing orthostatic hypotension. Peripheral vascular resistance is decreased as well. Calcium channel blockers also reduce cardiac contractility and cardiac output in a dose-dependent fashion. Some research has indicated that calcium channel blockers may interfere with the development of atheromatous lesions (Strandness, 2002). The most important adverse side effect is cardiac depression, including cardiac arrest, bradycardia, atrioventricular block, and congestive heart failure. Minor toxic effects caused by calcium channel blockers include flushing, edema, dizziness, nausea, and constipation. Mrs. Lee should be taught how to take her pulse before taking this drug and to report a pulse of less than 50 bpm to her physician. Clopidogrel blocks the binding of adenosine diphosphate to platelets, preventing arterial and venous thrombosis. It results in a significant reduction of death caused by stroke compared with aspirin. Indigestion, nausea, vomiting, rash, and diarrhea are the most common adverse reactions (Ferri, 2001). Many patients stop taking this drug due to the approximate $3 per daily dose cost. Mrs. Lee should be encouraged to continue this medication and seek prescription assistance if needed rather than discontinue clopidogrel. In addition, Mrs. Lee should be instructed to report any persistent medication side effects to her physician.

13. **What instructions should be given to Mrs. Lee before her discharge?**

Surgeons have different discharge instructions, but most include variations of the following instructions. The patient should avoid sharp movements of the neck, excessive sneezing, coughing, lifting, or constipation. Any straining that could disrupt the vessel suture lines must be avoided. Nothing should be placed on the site that might cause injury or damage, and the head should be supported at all times (Urden et al, 2002). Driving is often delayed until the patient is seen by the surgeon in 2 weeks. Return to employment is dependent upon the patient's type of work and postoperative progress and can be relatively soon. The patient should contact the physician or go to the emergency department for any sudden change in neurologic status, excessive bleeding or swelling at the surgical site, fever greater than 101° F (38.3°C) or difficulty breathing or swallowing. Dressings may be removed upon discharge; however, some physicians may require a dressing and antibiotic ointment for up to 3 days postoperatively. Bathing or showering is usually allowed as long as direct water flow to the incision is avoided, and the incision is dried carefully.

CAROTID ENDARTERECTOMY

References

Abu Rahma, A. F., Thiele, S. P., & Wulu, J. T. (2002). Prospective controlled study of the natural history of asymptomatic 60%-69% carotid stenosis according to ultrasonic plaque morphology. *Journal of Vascular Surgery, 36*(3), 437-441.

Ballotta, E., Da Giau, G., Saladini, M., & Abbruzzese, E. (1999). Carotid endarterectomy in symptomatic and asymptomatic patients aged 75 years or more: Perioperative mortality and stroke risk rates. *American Vascular Journal, 13*(2), 158-163.

Biasi, G. M., Sternjakob, S., Mingazzini, P. M., & Ferrari, S. A. (2002). Nine-year experience of bovine pericardium patch angioplasty during carotid endarterectomy. *Journal of Vascular Surgery, 36*(2), 271-277.

Black, J.M., Hawks, J.H., Keene, A.M. (2001). *Medical-Surgical Nursing* (6th ed.). Philadelphia: W.B. Saunders.

Blohme, L., Sandstrom, V., Hellstrom, G., Swedenborg, J., & Takolander, R. (1999). Complications in carotid endarterectomy are predicted by qualifying symptoms and preoperative CT findings. *European Journal of Vascular and Endovascular Surgery, 17*(3), 213-218.

Dirks, J. & Lough, M. E. (2003). Cardiovascular clinical assessment. In L. M. Tierney, S. J. McPhee, & M. A. Papadakis (Eds.), *2003 Current medical diagnosis and treatment* (41st ed.). New York: Lange Medical Books/McGraw-Hill.

Erzurum, V. A., Littooy, F. N., Steffen, G., Chmura, C., & Mansour, M. A. (2002). Outcome of nonoperative management of asymptomatic high-grade carotid stenosis. *Journal of Vascular Surgery, 35*(4), 663-667.

Ferri, F. F. (2001). *Practical guide to the care of the medical patient.* St Louis: Mosby Co.

Gable, D. R., et al. (2003). Intermediate follow-up of carotid artery stent placement. *The American Journal of Surgery, 185*(2003), 183-187.

Gorelick, P. B., et al. (1999). Prevention of a first stroke: A review of guidelines and multidisciplinary consensus statement from the National Stroke Association. *Journal of the American Medical Association, 281*(12), 1112-1118.

Kappelle, L. J., Eliasziw, M., Fox, A. J., Sharpe, B. L., & Barnett, H. J. (1999). Importance of intracranial atherosclerotic disease in patients with symptomatic stenosis of the internal carotid artery. The North American Symptomatic Carotid Endarterectomy Trial. *Stroke, 30*(2), 282-286.

Kilaru, S., et al. (2003). Is carotid angioplasty and stenting more cost effective than carotid endarterectomy? *Journal of Vascular Surgery, 37*(2), 331-339.

Laman, D. M., Wieneke, G. H., von Duijn, H., & von Huffelen, A. C. (2002). High embolic rate early after carotid endarterectomy is associated with early cerebrovascular complications, especially in women. *Journal of Vascular Surgery, 36*(2), 278-283.

Messina, L. M. & Tierney, L. M. (2003). Blood vessels and lymphatics. In L. M. Tierney, S. J. McPhee, & M. A. Papadakis (Eds.), *2003 Current medical diagnosis and treatment* (41st ed.). New York: Lange Medical Books/McGraw-Hill.

Moore, W. S., Quinones-Baldrich, W., & Krupski, W. C. (2000). Carotid endarterectomy. In R B. Rutherford (Ed.), *Vascular surgery* (5th ed.). Philadelphia: W. B. Saunders Harcourt.

Nemoto, E. M. (1999). No absolutes in neuromonitoring for carotid endarterectomy. *Stroke, 30* (4), 895-897.

Ouriel, K., Shortell, C. K., Illig, K. A., Greenberg, R. K., & Green, R. M. (1999). Intracerebral hemorrhage after carotid endarterectomy: Incidence, contribution to neurologic morbidity, and predictive factors. *Journal of Vascular Surgery, 29* (1), 82-89.

Ricci, M. A. & Knight, S. J. (2000). The role of noninvasive studies in the diagnosis and management of cerebrovascular disease. In R. B. Rutherford (Ed.), *Vascular surgery.* Philadelphia: W. B. Saunders Harcourt.

Strandness, D. E. (2002). Noninvasive assessment of vascular disease (5th ed.). In E. J.Topol (Ed.), *Textbook of cardiovascular medicine* (2nd ed.). Philadelphia: Lippincott Williams & Wilkins.

Urden L. D., Lough, M. E., & Stacy, K. M. (2002). *Thelan's critical care nursing: Diagnosis and management* (4th ed.). St. Louis: Mosby-Year Book.

Vaughan, C. J. (2003) Prevention of stroke and dementia with statins: Effects beyond lipid lowering. *American Journal of Cardiology, 91*(4A), 23B-29B.

7

Abdominal Aortic Aneurysm

Joan E. King, RN, PhD, ACNP, ANP

Mr. Allen is a 65-year-old white male who presents to the emergency department (ED) with a chief complaint of a 3-day history of severe low back pain and new onset of severe abdominal pain accompanied by nausea and vomiting. Mr. Allen denies any history of recent back trauma or injury or any previous history of back pain. He rates his pain as an 8 on a 10-point scale.

Past Medical History

Mr. Allen reports that he has had hypertension for the past 10 years, but recently stopped taking his medication (enalapril [Vasotec]) because he thought his blood pressure was under control. His family history includes coronary artery disease (CAD), hypertension, and diabetes. His father died of a ruptured abdominal aneurysm at age 70.

Physical examination reveals a moderately obese gentleman who is in acute distress. Vital signs are as follows:

HR	106 bpm
Respirations	20 breaths/min
BP	180/110 mm Hg
Sao$_2$	95%

Breath sounds are clear bilaterally; bowel sounds are hypoactive. A midline palpable mass is noted 3 cm below the xphoid process. Radial and brachial pulses are strong bilaterally, but femoral, posterior tibial, and dorsalis pedis pulses are faintly palpable bilaterally. Capillary refill in the upper extremities is brisk (less than 3 seconds), whereas capillary refill in the lower extremities is greater than 3 seconds. Cranial nerves I through XII are intact and patient remains awake, alert, and oriented times three.

Mr. Allen's 12-lead electrocardiogram (ECG) indicated left ventricular hypertrophy but no ST or T-wave changes in any leads. Cardiac enzymes were not elevated. Chest x-ray revealed no widened mediastinum and no evidence of cardiopulmonary disease. Mr. Allen was immediately taken for a computed tomography (CT) scan with contrast, which revealed a 6.5 cm infrarenal abdominal aortic aneurysm. He was subsequently taken to the operating room for endovascular management of his abdominal aortic aneurysm (AAA).

ABDOMINAL AORTIC ANEURYSM

QUESTIONS

1. Define an AAA and distinguish it from an aortic dissection.

2. Discuss the pathophysiology of an AAA.

3. Discuss the presenting signs and symptoms of an AAA.

4. Discuss the risk factors associated with an AAA.

5. What diagnostic tests are used to confirm the diagnosis of an AAA?

6. Discuss the medical and surgical management of a patient presenting with an AAA.

7. Discuss the postoperative management of a patient who has had an AAA repair.

8. List the nursing diagnoses appropriate for a patient diagnosed with an AAA.

ABDOMINAL AORTIC ANEURYSM

QUESTIONS AND ANSWERS

1. Define an AAA and distinguish it from an aortic dissection.

An AAA is a localized dilation of the aorta below the level of the diaphragm, which is 50% greater than the normal diameter (Anderson, 2001). An AAA can lead to organ ischemia secondary to altered blood flow, but more important it can become a dissecting aneurysm and lead to rupture of the aorta. Abdominal aortic aneurysms are the thirteenth leading cause of death in the United States and have an 80% mortality rate (Jones et al, 2000; Anderson, 2001).

Whereas an AAA is a dilation of the aorta and a weakening of the muscular structure of the aorta (specifically the media or middle layer of the aorta), an aortic dissection is the result of a tear in the intima layer of the aorta that allows blood to become sequestered between the media layer and adventitia layer of the aorta. This forms a false lumen or what is termed a false aneurysm (Nauer, 2000). The false aneurysm or lumen can then dissect either antegrade or retrograde, or both (Finkelmeier & Marolda, 2001). Although an aortic dissection may involve an aortic aneurysm, all aortic aneurysms are not dissecting.

Classification of aortic dissection and aortic aneurysms is different. Aortic aneurysms are classified as either ascending or descending aneurysms, with descending aneurysms being further subdivided into thoracic aneurysms or abdominal aneurysms. Thoracic aneurysms are above the level of the diaphragm, and abdominal aneurysms are below the level of the diaphragm. In addition to the location, aneurysms are categorized as either fusiform or saccular. Fusiform is a circumferential dilation, and saccular is a saclike or ballonlike aneurysm that involves only a portion of the aortic wall (Nauer, 2000).

There are two classification systems available to categorize aortic dissections. The first is the DeBakey system, which divides aortic dissections into type I, which is from the ascending aorta beyond the subclavian artery; type II, which is from the ascending aorta proximal to the subclavian artery; and type III, which involves the descending aorta distal to the subclavian artery. The second classification is the Stanford system, which describes aortic dissections as involving either the ascending aorta or beyond (type A), or just the descending aorta (type B) (Finkelmeier & Marolda, 2001).

In this case study Mr. Allen is presenting with an infrarenal AAA, implying that the aneurysm is distal to the renal artery but proximal to the aortic bifurcation. An infrarenal AAA is the most common type of AAA, representing 65% of the AAAs (Anderson, 2001). The CT scan, performed with contrast, did not reveal any false lumen or dissection. Hence an aortic dissection was ruled out.

2. Discuss the pathophysiology of an AAA.

Previously the development of aortic aneurysms was thought to be secondary to atherosclerosis, but current theories indicate that it is the loss of elastin and collagen that leads to development of aortic aneurysms (Anderson, 2001). Specifically the aorta is composed of three layers of tissue. The intima is the innermost layer, the media is the middle layer, and the adventitia is the outermost layer. It is degenerative changes in the structure of the media that lead to the development of an aneurysm. Normally the media is composed of muscle cells, elastin, and collagen. Elastin is responsible for allowing the aorta to stretch and respond to pressure changes, and collagen fibers limit the aorta's degree of distention. Over time, degenerative changes, possibly secondary to increased enzymatic activity, elastin, and collagen are lost. This leads to a thinning of the media layer of the aorta, and allows the aorta to dilate. It is also possible that inflammation plays a role in the development of an aneurysm (Anderson, 2001).

There is also a possible genetic link to the development of an AAA. The incidence of an AAA in the general population is 4% to 5% for individuals older than the age of 50. However, if a first-line relative has an AAA, there is a 15% to 33% incidence of other family members also having an AAA (Anderson, 2001).

Regardless of the cause, as the media layer of the aorta becomes thinner, it allows the aorta to dilate and lose its normal integrity. Over time, many aortic aneurysms will grow or expand. Hence it is important once an aneurysm is detected to monitor its progression. Traditionally aortic aneurysms less than 5 cm in diameter are treated medically, whereas aortic aneurysms greater than 5 cm or aneurysms that have grown are treated surgically. The rationale is based on the probability that the aneurysm may rupture. Data support the larger the aneurysm, the greater the probability it will rupture. According to Cronenwett and colleagues (2000) aneurysms 5 cm or less have a 0.5% to 5% chance of rupturing per year, whereas aneurysms between 5 and 6 cm have a 3% to 15% chance of rupturing per year, and aneurysms between 6 and 7 cm have a 10% to 20% chance of rupturing per year. Mr. Allen's AAA was 6.5 cm, indicating that surgical intervention is recommended in an effort to prevent rupture of the aneurysm and possible death.

3. Discuss the presenting signs and symptoms of an AAA.

The presenting signs and symptoms of an AAA are highly variable. Many times a patient is asymptomatic, and an aneurysm is noted serendipitously, when either an abdominal x-ray or CT scan was obtained for another reason. Asymptomatic aneurysms may also be detected on routine physical examinations when a pulsating abdominal mass is noted in the area of the aorta. However, some individuals may present as Mr. Allen did with a history of back pain or epigastric pain that may radiate to the back or flank. Diminished pulses may also be present secondary to altered blood flow or the presence of a thrombosis. If an aortoenteric fistula develops or the patient develops ischemia of the bowel, the patient may present with GI bleeding. Other signs and symptoms include groin pain secondary to ureteral obstruction, venous thrombosis secondary to venous compressions, and nausea and vomiting secondary to compression of the bowel (Anderson, 2001). Generally the signs and symptoms of an AAA represent encroachment of the aneurysm on adjacent structures and the development of ischemia secondary to either compression or altered blood flow.

Signs and symptoms of a ruptured AAA include the presence of a pulsatile abdominal mass, sudden onset of severe abdominal pain, and hypotension (Anderson, 2001). It is important to quickly identify patients with a ruptured AAA and transport them to definitive care, because a ruptured AAA has a 50% or higher mortality rate if surgical intervention is delayed (Anderson, 2001).

4. Discuss the risk factors associated with an AAA.

Although the presence of a pulsatile abdominal mass, sudden onset of abdominal pain, and hypotension may lead the practitioner to an expedient diagnosis of a ruptured AAA, not all aneurysms present with such clarity. Therefore it is important to consider associated risk factors that may heighten a clinician's awareness that abdominal pain or back pain may represent symptoms of an AAA. A key factor to consider is the history of hypertension and the presence of an elevated diastolic pressure. Applying Laplace's law, the degree of tension on the arterial wall will be in direct proportion to the radius of the artery and the pressure within the artery (Anderson, 2001). With elevated diastolic pressures, the pressure within the aorta increases, which in turn increases the tension within the aorta. This cannot only lead to enlargement of the aorta but also increase the risk of rupture.

Another variable to consider is individuals who present with signs and symptoms of abdominal pain or back pain and who have recently stopped their antihypertensive medications. Again apply Laplace's law: if a patient has stopped his or her medication, and blood pressure is no longer under control, then the weakened area within the aorta is under more tension, and the aneurysm is more likely to either expand or rupture.

A history of chronic obstructive pulmonary disease (COPD) is also considered a red flag. It is felt that the increase in enzymatic activity within the pulmonary bed secondary to COPD may also increase the enzymatic activity within the aorta and weaken the integrity of the aorta (Anderson, 2001).

Other variables to consider are the patient's gender and age. Men are more likely to develop an aneurysm; the incidence of an AAA begins around age 50 and increases until the age of 80 (Anderson, 2001). Other associated risk factors are CAD, hyperlipidemia, smoking, and a positive family history of AAA. Less common risk factors associated with an AAA are Marfan's syndrome, aortitis, and trauma (Urden et al, 2002).

Although Mr. Allen did not report a history of COPD, he did state he had a 10-year history of hypertension and that he had recently stopped his enalapril (Vasotec). Both of these factors place Mr. Allen at a higher than normal risk for an AAA. Also Mr. Allen's age, gender, and family history place him at risk for the development of an AAA.

5. What diagnostic tests are used to confirm the diagnosis of an AAA?

In the past the gold standard for confirming the presence of an AAA was an angiography. In many instances, patients with an AAA are too acutely ill and require definitive diagnostic tests that can be performed more quickly. Therefore angiography is now limited to patient situations in which other vascular abnormalities need to be documented, such as additional peripheral vascular disease or renal stenosis.

Two other diagnostic tests that overcome the time limitation of angiography are CT with contrast and ultrasonography (US). US has the advantage of being readily available in most emergency departments, and it can be done at the bedside. However it does not provide the same level of detail that a CT scan with contrast does. With a CT scan the aneurysm can be easily identified, and the presence of a false lumen or aortic dissection can be identified. In addition, other data can be obtained concerning the status of the iliac artery and the size of the aorta, which are important variables in determining the most advantageous approach or surgical intervention (Schouchoff, 2000).

6. Discuss the medical and surgical management of a patient presenting with an AAA.

As mentioned, an AAA can be managed conservatively through medical management or surgical intervention. The deciding factor is the size of the aneurysm or if the aneurysm has recently expanded. The cutoff factor is 5 cm. For aneurysms 5 cm or less, medical management is considered appropriate. Medical management for individuals in this category includes controlling their hypertension and management of hyperlipidemia and any other modifiable risk factors.

For aneurysms greater than 5 cm or aneurysms that appear to be increasing in size rapidly, surgical correction is recommended. Surgical correction can be either an open abdominal procedure or a minimally invasive approach, called endovascular grafting. Both approaches consist of using a prosthetic graft to reestablish the integrity of the aorta and circumvent or isolate the aneurysm from arterial blood flow (Maldonado, 1996; Jones et al, 2000). While the endovascular approach is less stressful on the patient, and has a reduced length of stay, not all patients are candidates for this approach. One important factor is the specific location of the aneurysm and the involvement of any other arterial structures. For example, involvement of the renal arteries precludes the use of an endovascular approach.

For an open surgical approach, a midline abdominal incision is made starting at the xyphoid process. While the graft is being inserted, the aorta is cross-clamped and is secured both proximally and distally to the aneurysm. The cross-clamping is then released, the aorta is wrapped about the graft, and the abdominal incision closed. Whereas the open surgical approach provides direct visibility, there are a number of potential problems that can develop. These include infection, emboli formation, ischemia secondary to cross-clamping the aorta, and hemodynamic changes secondary to cross-clamping. The open surgical approach places the patient at risk for infection, not only from having a large abdominal incision but also for the potential of nicking the bowel during surgery. Emboli may be dislodged during the procedure as the result of either debris or dislodgement of an atherosclerotic plaque. Cross-clamping the aorta poses two problems. First, during the cross-clamping procedure there are pressure changes. Specifically as the aorta is cross-clamped the systolic pressure may become elevated and increase the systemic vascular resistance or afterload. This in turn can increase the workload on the heart and lead to myocardial ischemia if the heart cannot adjust to the increase in workload. Conversely, with the releasing of the cross clamps, the patient may become hypotensive and organ ischemia may follow. Organ ischemia is also possible during the cross-clamping process itself, because perfusion distal to the cross-clamping is impaired. This implies that the kidneys, intestines, and lower extremities are at risk for becoming ischemic during the procedure. Once the cross clamps are released, perfusion is reestablished, but toxins, particularly oxygen radicals, are released into the systemic circulation and can depress myocardial function. This phenomenon is reperfusion injury.

Because of the magnitude of the surgical procedure, patients who have had an open surgical repair of an AAA will be admitted to the surgical intensive care unit for at least 24 hours. They usually are intubated upon arrival, have at least one central line and a possible pulmonary artery catheter, an arterial line, and a Foley catheter. Close monitoring of these patients includes assessing for not only the possibility of hemorrhage from the graft site or excessive bleeding from the incision, but also renal failure, respiratory failure, and the possibility of loss of pulses distal to the graft secondary to microemboli from dislodged plaque. They are also monitored closely for any neurologic changes and the possibility for infection.

An alternative approach to the open surgical technique is an endovascular approach. Endovascular placement of a graft is done by threading a catheter and guidewire from a small incision in the groin into the femoral artery up into the aorta through the use of fluoroscopy. Once the site is appropriately located, the graft is deployed. Small hooklike structures on both the proximal and distal ends of the graft secure the graft to healthy tissue. Three major advantages to this technique are (1) it is a minimally invasive technique and requires a shorter surgical time, and subsequently less anesthesia; (2) cross-clamping of the aorta is not performed, thus limiting the possibility of organ ischemia and reperfusion injury; and (3) because a large abdominal incision is avoided, the patient is less likely to develop pulmonary problems postoperatively and require less pain medication. However, although there is a reduced incidence of major organ damage from either cross-clamping the aorta or manipulation of major organs during the surgery itself, the endovascular approach has a higher probability for embolic events. Because guidewires and catheters are used during the procedure, there is a 6% to 16% incidence of emboli being dislodged during the procedure (Schouchoff, 2000).

Another major complication of endovascular repair of an AAA is the development of an "endoleak." An endoleak is a leak around the graft site that can lead to sequestering of blood between the graft and the vascular wall and progress into an aortic dissection and rupture, impairment of the graft, or the development of a thrombosis. Endoleaks are classified as either primary or secondary. Primary endoleaks can occur intraoperatively up to 30 days postoperatively. If an endoleak develops intraoperatively, it may necessitate the need for an open surgical procedure to be performed. However, many endoleaks seal spontaneously and require no further intervention (Jones et al, 2000). Endoleaks that develop after 30 days are considered secondary leaks. These endoleaks are monitored carefully by sequential CT scans in order to evaluate their progression (Schouchoff, 2000).

In terms of postoperative management for patients having had an endovascular repair, the same assessment parameters are monitored as in the case of the more traditional open surgical approach. Cardiovascular assessments are essential, focusing on perfusion of the myocardial major organs and peripheral vasculature. However, many patients who have endovascular procedures are discharged within 24 to 48 hours postoperatively, and they do not require a stay in the intensive care unit. Mr. Allen's AAA was amenable to an endovascular approach, and he was discharged 24 hours after his repair.

7. Discuss the postoperative management of a patient who has had an AAA repair.

For patients who undergo either an open procedure or an endovascular procedure, the postoperative goals are to (1) prevent hemorrhage, (2) maintain the patency of the graft, (3) promote adequate perfusion to all organs, (4) prevent infection of the graft, and (5) prevent any secondary complications such as pneumonia. Patients who have undergone an open abdominal approach will be in the intensive care unit at least 24 hours. During that time hemodynamic monitoring will include monitoring both the arterial line and the pulmonary artery catheter or central line for signs of hypotension and hypertension. Because many of these patients are hypertensive preoperatively, they frequently require nitroprusside postoperatively to keep their systolic blood pressure within normal limits. Elevation in blood pressure for these patients places them at risk for bleeding from the graft site and potential hemorrhage. Also hypertensive episodes increase the systemic vascular resistance, which increases the workload on the heart and places the patient at further risk of possible myocardial ischemia. Hypotension is equally problematic. Hypotension from overcorrection of an elevated systolic blood pressure, excessive bleeding, or reperfusion injury places the patient's major organs at risk for further ischemic insults including the possibility of developing multiple organ dysfunction syndrome (MODS). Hypotension can also lead to graft failure by promoting the development of a thrombosis. Graft patency needs to be addressed in terms of patient positioning. Acute flexion over the graft area should be avoided in order to prevent any reduction in blood flow.

In order to ensure adequate perfusion to all organs it is imperative that the nurse monitor not only the blood pressure, cardiac output, and either the central venous pressure (CVP) or pulmonary artery occlusive pressure, but also the presence of ectopy, any ST or T-wave changes or tachycardia, alteration in level of consciousness, the urinary output (with a goal of 30 cc or more per hour), the presence or absence of bowel sounds, the abdominal girth and any increase in distention, abdominal pain or gastrointestinal (GI) bleeding, the presence or absence of peripheral pulses, as well as the ankle-arm index. The ankle-arm index is determined by taking the dorsalis pedis systolic pressure and dividing it by the brachial systolic blood pressure. The subsequent ratio reflects the degree of perfusion within the lower extremities. For example if the dorsalis pedis systolic pressure is 90 mm Hg and the brachial systolic blood pressure is 100 mm Hg, then there is 90% blood flow in the lower extremities. Because the patient is at risk for ischemia from cross-clamping and the possibility of emboli from dislodged plaque, assessing for perfusion in the lower extremities is essential. Other signs and symptoms of an ischemic event are the five P's (Schouchoff, 2000): paresthesia, pallor, pain, paralysis, and pulselessness. Thus motor function, altered sensation in the extremities, capillary refill, color, and pain should be assessed.

The last goal, which is specific to repair an AAA, is prevention of infection. The graft, which may be either Dacron or polytetrafluoroethylene (PTFE), is a foreign body, and it is at risk for becoming infected. Postoperatively the patient will be on antibiotics, and strict aseptic technique should be used when assessing the wound or intravenous (IV) insertion sites. Both the presence of a fever and elevation of white blood cells (WBCs) should be monitored. Discharge teaching with the patient and family should include the need for prophylactic antibiotic coverage for invasive procedures such as cystoscopies, colonoscopies, or even routine dental care in order to prevent any form of bacteremia that may infect the graft.

For the patient who has had an endovascular repair of an AAA, the same goals apply, but the patient most likely will not have a pulmonary artery catheter postoperatively. Rather he or she will have an arterial line and a central line. Although cardiac output and pulmonary occlusive pressures cannot be directly obtained, the CVP can be measured, and the same in-depth assessment of cardiac, peripheral vascular, renal, and GI function is performed in order to assess for either ischemia or possible embolization. Neurologic assessment is also vital to assess for a potential cerebrovascular accident. Specific to the endovascular approach is assessment of the femoral insertion site for the development of a hematoma, and possible reduced blood flow distally.

Thus whereas an AAA is an important diagnosis that needs close monitoring and surgical correction if larger than 5 cm, new surgical techniques have made it possible to endovascularly insert a graft without subjecting the patient to a large abdominal wound. This implies that the patient will be at a reduced risk for problems such as wound dehiscence, ileus, atelectasis, and restrictive abdominal pain. It also implies that the patient may not need postoperative ventilatory support or complex hemodynamic monitoring. However, it is vital that the clinician closely monitor the cardiac and peripheral vascular systems, as well as the patient's respiratory status and neurologic and renal function in order to ensure maximum recovery and prevent potential complications including embolization.

8. List the nursing diagnoses appropriate for a patient diagnosed with an AAA.

Nursing diagnoses for patients diagnosed with an AAA are as follows:

- Decreased cardiac output related to alterations in preload
- Acute pain related to transmission and perception of cutaneous, visceral, muscular, or ischemic impulses
- Ineffective peripheral tissue perfusion related to decreased peripheral blood flow
- Ineffective cardiopulmonary tissue perfusion related to decreased myocardial oxygen supply and/or increased oxygen demand
- Risk for infection: invasive procedures
- Anxiety related to threat to biologic, psychologic, and/or social integrity
- Ineffective renal tissue perfusion related to decreased renal blood flow
- Activity intolerance related to cardiopulmonary dysfunction
- Deficient knowledge: discharge regimen related to lack of previous exposure to information (Urden et al, 2002)

ABDOMINAL AORTIC ANEURYSM

References

Anderson, L. (2001). Abdominal aortic aneurysm. *Journal of Cardiovascular Nursing, 15*(4), 1-14.

Cronenwett, J., Krupski, W., & Rutherford, R. (2000). Abdominal aortic and iliac aneurysms. In R. Rutherford (Ed), *Vascular surgery* (5th ed., pp. 1246-1280). Philadelphia: W. B. Saunders Co.

Finkelmeier, B. & Marolda, D. (2001). Aortic dissection. *Journal of Cardiovascular Nursing, 15*(4), 15-24.

Jones, M., Hoffman, L., & Makarown, M. (2000). Endovascular grafting of repair of abdominal aortic aneurysm. *Critical Care Nurse, 20*(4), 38-51.

Maldonado, K. (1996). Care of patients after aortic aneurysm repair. *Journal of Post Anesthesia Nursing, 11*(1), 29-41.

Nauer, K. (2000). Acute dissection of the aorta: A review for nurses. *Critical Care Nursing Quarterly, 23*(1), 20-27.

Schouchoff, B. (2000). Endovascular aortic aneurysm repair: An alternative approach. *Critical Care Nursing Quarterly, 23*(1), 35-41.

Urden, L. D., Stacy, K. M., & Lough, M. E. (Eds.). (2002). *Thelan's critical care nursing: Diagnosis and management* (4th ed.). St. Louis: Mosby.

8

Cardiac Trauma and Cardiac Tamponade

Lynn Smith Schnautz, RN, MSN, CCRN, CCNS

CASE PRESENTATION

Jennifer Gardner, a 16-year-old 54 kg (120 lb) white female, is brought to the emergency department by ambulance following a motor vehicle accident. Emergency workers found her strapped into the passenger seat. It took workers more than 45 minutes to extricate her from the vehicle.

She is awake, alert, and oriented to person, place, and time when admitted via spinal board with cervical collar intact, on 2 L/min nasal cannula, with 16-gauge intravenous (IV) lactated Ringer's at 100 cc/hr. She is complaining of midsternal chest pain nonradiating of 2 to 3 on a pain scale of 1 to 5. The only visible marking are ecchymosis and redness across chest from seatbelt.

History reveals a healthy teenager who plays high school soccer. Vital signs on admission are as noted:

BP	140/80 mm Hg
HR	110 bpm
Respirations	26 breaths/min
Temperature	98.6° F (37°C)
Sao$_2$	97%-98%

Routine lab values reveal normal hemoglobin and hematocrit. Chest x-ray (CXR) was completed and reveals nondisplaced rib fracture on the right side. Electrocardiogram (ECG) reveals sinus tachycardia with no other abnormalities. Computed tomography (CT) scan and C-spine are completed and rule out any neurologic involvement. Morphine 2 mg IV is given along with naproxen (Naprosyn) for complaints of chest pain. Cervical collar and spinal board are removed and patient is admitted for 24-hour observation. After the initial 24 hours, it was decided that the patient should be admitted to the intensive care unit (ICU) for further monitoring and evaluation.

Admission to ICU

The patient is awake, alert, and oriented. Pain level is now a 1 with vital signs as noted:

BP	110/70 mm Hg
HR	118 bpm
Respirations	20 breaths/min

| **Temperature** | 98.6° F |
| **Sao₂** | 97% |

When assessing heart sounds the nurse notes distant, muffled heart sounds with the PMI slightly shifted to the left. Serial lab values 4 hours post-ICU admission reveal hemoglobin 11 and hematocrit 33.

The nurse contacts the physician regarding physical findings and lab results. The physician orders stat CXR, which reveals enlarged heart shadow. A subsequent echocardiogram reveals cardiac tamponade. Emergency pericardiocentesis is performed in the patient's room. Ms. Gardner is taken for emergency chest exploration to repair a small right ventricular tear and remove rib fragments. She has an uneventful recovery and is discharged home on the eighth postoperative day.

CARDIAC TRAUMA AND CARDIAC TAMPONADE

QUESTIONS

1. Define blunt cardiac trauma (BCT). State the etiology and pathophysiology of BCT.

2. What clinical presentation will patients with BCT display?

3. Discuss appropriate nursing diagnoses for a patient with BCT.

4. Outline Ms. Gardner's collaborative plan of care related to a diagnosis of BCT.

5. What complications may develop from BCT?

6. Define penetrating cardiac trauma (PCT). State the etiology and pathophysiology of PCT.

7. What clinical presentation will patients with a diagnosis of PCT display?

8. Discuss appropriate nursing diagnoses for a patient with PCT.

9. Outline Ms. Gardner's collaborative plan of care related to a diagnosis of PCT.

10. What complications may develop from PCT?

11. Define cardiac tamponade. State the etiology and pathophysiology of cardiac tamponade.

12. What clinical presentation will the patient with a diagnosis of cardiac tamponade display?

13. Discuss appropriate nursing diagnoses for a patient with cardiac tamponade.

14. Outline Ms. Gardner's collaborative plan of care related to a diagnosis of cardiac tamponade.

15. How should the nurse prepare Ms. Gardner for pericardiocentesis?

16. What complications may occur during a pericardiocentesis?

CARDIAC TRAUMA AND CARDIAC TAMPONADE

QUESTIONS AND ANSWERS

1. Define blunt cardiac trauma (BCT). State the etiology and pathophysiology of BCT.

Definition

Blunt cardiac trauma/injury is defined as blunt trauma to the heart causing ecchymosis and petechiae to develop in the myocardium (Dennison, 2000; Braunwald et al, 2001).

Etiology

Blunt cardiac trauma may be caused by acceleration/deceleration injury sustained in a motor vehicle collision (i.e., sternum hitting the steering wheel or dashboard, or shoulder strap of seatbelt); auto accidents (i.e., motorcycle collision), auto-pedestrian collision; kicking of chest by large animal (i.e., horse, cow, human); assault with a blunt instrument; industrial crush injury; explosion; and/or vigorous cardiopulmonary resuscitation (CPR) (Grif Alspach, 1998; Dennison, 2000; Urden et al, 2002). In Ms. Gardner's case the BCT was caused by the seatbelt.

Pathophysiology

Blunt trauma causes bruising or bleeding into the myocardium. Red blood cells extravasate around the myocardial fibers. Subpericardial and subendocardial myocardial fibers become edematous and may fragment. The right ventricle is usually the site of injury because it is directly under the sternum. Decreased right ventricular (RV) contractility causes an increase in right ventricular end-diastolic volume and decrease in right ventricular ejection fraction. Decreased RV ejection fraction causes decreased preload to the left ventricle. The ventricles accommodate this increase in volume by enlarging or dilating. Dilation of RV shifts the interventricular septum to the left, which compromises the left ventricular compliance. There is an increase in pulmonary vascular resistance causing an increase in right ventricular afterload, which further decreases right ventricular ejection fraction. Damage to cardiac valves may occur due to left ventricular pressures being higher (Dennison, 2000).

2. What clinical presentation will patients with BCT display?

Clinical Presentation

The clinical presentation of BCT varies from an asymptomatic patient without external signs of trauma to one in severe cardiac distress. Patients typically complain of the following symptoms: precordial angina-like chest pain (frequently increases with inspiration, cough, and movement, unrelieved by nitroglycerin but responsive to oxygen, antiinflammatory agents, or narcotics), sternal tenderness, shortness of breath (SOB), palpitations, and/or abdominal pain. Objectively the patient may display tachycardia, clinical indications of right ventricular failure (i.e., jugular venous distention [JVD], peripheral edema, and hepatomegaly). Ecchymosis may be present on the anterior chest (Dennison, 2000; Urden et al, 2002). Ms. Gardner presented with chest pain rated at level 2 to 3 on the pain scale and tachycardia.

Diagnostic

Serum creatine kinase myocardial band (CK-MB) and cardiac troponin may be positive depending on the severity of the injury. Twelve-lead ECG with right ventricular leads may display ST-segment changes, T-wave inversion, Q waves if coronary artery has been lacerated or thromboses, and/or prolonged QT interval. Commonly identified dysrhythmias may include premature atrial contractions, atrial fibrillation, atrial flutter, premature ventricular contractions, ventricular tachycardia, ventricular fibrillation, atrioventricular (AV) blocks, and bundle branch blocks. Echocardiography reveals decreased regional wall motion, increased end-diastolic wall thickness, and decreased RV ejection fraction (Dennison, 2000; Braunwald et al., 2001). Ms. Gardner's 12-lead ECG revealed sinus tachycardia without ectopy.

3. **Discuss appropriate nursing diagnoses for a patient with BCT.**

A variety of nursing diagnoses may be utilized for the patient with a medical diagnosis of BCT. Several examples include the following:

- Decreased cardiac output related to heart failure
- Cardiac tamponade and/or hemorrhage
- Risk for altered peripheral tissue perfusion related to emboli
- Impaired gas exchange related to pulmonary edema
- Activity intolerance related to heart failure

Additional nursing diagnoses would be based on patient presentation (Dennison, 2000).

4. **Outline Ms. Gardner's collaborative plan of care related to a diagnosis of BCT.**

The first priority in Ms. Gardner's care is to decrease myocardial oxygen demands by providing bed rest, supplemental oxygen to maintain SaO$_2$ of 95%, and anxiolytics as ordered. Ms. Gardner's pain needs to be treated with the use of narcotics, antiinflammatory agents, relaxation techniques, and alternative therapies. Treat dysrhythmias and other complications as they develop (Grif Alspach, 1998; Dennison, 2000).

5. **What complications may develop from BCT?**

Complications that arise from the development of BCT are covered in Box 8-1.

6. **Define penetrating cardiac trauma (PCT). State the etiology and pathophysiology of PCT.**

Definition

Penetrating cardiac trauma is defined as the puncture of the heart with a sharp object or rib (Dennison, 2000). In Ms. Gardner's case, the cause of the PCT was from a fractured rib.

Etiology

PCT results from a variety of etiologies that may include some type of force-inflicted injury. These may include incidences of violence (i.e., knife wound, gunshot wound, ice pick), industrial accident (i.e., falling on object), motorcycle collision with impalement of an object, sports injury, and/or crush injury (Dennison, 2000).

Pathophysiology

In PCT the heart has been punctured (usually right ventricle) with a sharp object or rib usually causing a cardiac contusion and/or laceration. Blood leaks into the pericardial space or into the mediastinum causing cardiac tamponade or shock (Dennison, 2000).

7. **What clinical presentation will patients with a diagnosis of PCT display?**

Clinical Presentation

Patients with a diagnosis of PCT may or may not complain of chest pain depending on their level of consciousness and extent of damages. Objectively a visible wound and/or bleeding may be seen. Hypotension, hypoperfusion-tachycardia, narrowed pulse pressure, tachypnea, cool skin, oliguria, restlessness, confusion, cardiac tamponade, hemothorax, and pneumothorax may be seen as well with PCT (Ferrera et al, 2001). Hemodynamic parameters will include decreased right atrial pressure, pulmonary artery pressure, and pulmonary artery occlusive pressure if hemorrhage has occurred (Lewis, 1999; Dennison, 2000; Ross & DeJong, 1999). Ms. Gardner complained of chest pain, associated with tachycardia and narrowed pulse pressure upon admission to the emergency department.

Box 8-1   **BCT Complications**

Cardiovascular Injuries	Myocardial Concussion
Cardiogenic Shock	Myocardial contusion
	Cardiac rupture
	Air embolus
	Traumatic aortic injury
	Aortic fistula
	Great vessel injury
	Ventricular rupture
	Cardiac tamponade
	Coronary artery thrombosis
	Valve rupture
	Conduction defects
	Heart failure
	Ventricular aneurysm
Pulmonary Injuries	Tracheal tear
	Bronchial tear
	Pneumothorax
	Pneumomediastinum emphysema
	Subcutaneous emphysema
	Hemothorax
	Pulmonary contusion
	Acute respiratory distress syndrome
Chest Wall	Rib fractures
	Flail chest
	Sternal fractures
	Thoracic spine fractures
Diaphragmatic Gastrointestinal	Esophageal injuries

(Data from Ferrera, P. C., Colucciello, S. A., Marx, J. A., Verdile, V. P., & Gibbs, M. A. [Eds.] [2001]. *Trauma management: An emergency medicine approach.* St Louis: Mosby.)

Diagnostic

Hemoglobin and hematocrit will be decreased (Dennison, 2000; Braunwald et al., 2001). Ms. Gardner's hemoglobin and hematocrit were slightly decreased 4 hours postadmission to ICU.

8. **Discuss appropriate nursing diagnoses for a patient with PCT.**

Nursing diagnoses related to PCT may include the following:

- Decreased cardiac output related to heart failure
- Fluid volume deficit related to hemorrhage, hypovolemic shock
- Impaired gas exchange related to pulmonary edema
- Activity intolerance related to heart failure
- Pain, anxiety, and knowledge deficit
- Risk of infection related to foreign body, trauma, and/or surgery (Dennison, 2000)

9. **Outline Ms. Gardner's collaborative plan of care related to a diagnosis of PCT.**

Initial goals of therapy should be to manage cardiopulmonary arrest by utilizing BLS and ACLS guidelines according to the American Heart Association. Control hemorrhage by applying direct pressure to the site if the object has been removed and the wound is bleeding. ***DO NOT REMOVE*** an impaled object; stabilize with IV bags and dressings. Assist with insertion of a chest tube for hemo- or pneumothorax. Assist with pericardiocentesis for cardiac tamponade. Improve oxygen delivery by applying 2 to 6 L/min of O_2 via nasal cannula to maintain SaO_2 of 95%. The patient may require intubation and mechanical ventilation. Insert two large-bore IV catheters and infuse normal saline or lactated Ringer's by rapid infusion until blood is available (may utilize colloids such as albumin, hetastarch, or dextran). Type and cross-match for blood transfusion and administer blood products as ordered. Assist in the preparation of exploratory thoracotomy (Dennison, 2000).

10. **What complications may develop from PCT?**

    Complications that may develop from PCT include hemorrhagic shock, cardiac tamponade, hemothorax, embolism, pneumothorax, and death (Ferrera et al, 2001).

11. **Define cardiac tamponade. State the etiology and pathophysiology of cardiac tamponade.**

    Definition

    Cardiac tamponade is defined as the accumulation of blood, effusion fluid, and/or pus in the pericardial space that compromises cardiac filling and cardiac output as a result of pressure building in a confined space (Dennison, 2000).

    Etiology

    See Box 8-2, Etiology of Cardiac Tamponade.

    Pathophysiology

    Cardiac tamponade is defined as the accumulation of fluid or blood (as little as 100 ml or as much as 2 L) in the pericardial space. Intrapericardial pressure rises to atrial and ventricular diastolic pressure, resulting in a fall in transmural cardiac pressure, which leads to inability of the heart to fill and pump. End-diastolic volume decreases, which results in decreased contractility, stroke volume, cardiac output, and shock (Knoop & Willenberg, 1999; Tsang et al, 1999; Dennison, 2000).

12. **What clinical presentation will the patient with a diagnosis of cardiac tamponade display?**

    Clinical Presentation

    The patient experiencing cardiac tamponade will complain of precordial fullness or pain, dyspnea, and a feeling of impending doom. Cardiac monitoring will display tachycardia or pulseless electrical activity (PEA). The patient my display Beck's triad: hypotension, distended neck veins, and muffled heart sounds, which are the classic signs of tamponade. Hemodynamics will reveal an increased right atrial pressure, pulmonary artery diastolic pressure, pulmonary artery occlusive pressure (usually within 5 mm Hg of each other), and a decrease in cardiac output and cardiac index (Tsang et al, 1999; Dennison, 2000; Urden et al, 2002). Ms. Gardner complained of chest pain, and the monitor revealed tachycardia with narrowed pulse pressure and distant heart sounds.

    Diagnostic

    Chest x-ray will review a widened mediastinum. An ECG may reveal ventricular dysrythmias, bradycardia, pulseless electrical activity, and/or electrical alternans (large and small QRS). An echocardiogram will display free space between the pericardium and the myocardium (Dennison, 2000; Braunwald et al, 2001).

Box 8-2   **Etiology of Cardiac Tamponade**

Acute Cardiac Tamponade	Blunt or penetrating cardiac trauma Postmyocardial infarction Pericarditis in the anticoagulated patient Cardiac rupture Post-CPR Electrical cardioversion Rupture of great vessels

Chronic Cardiac Tamponade	Malignancy
	Radiation therapy
	Connective tissue disease
	  Rheumatoid arthritis
	  Lupus erythematosus
	  Scleroderma
	Metabolic diseases
	  Renal failure
	  Hepatic failure
	  Myxedema
	Infections
	  Viral
	  Bacterial
	  Fungal
	Drugs
	  procainamide (Pronestyl)
	  hydralazine (Apresoline)
	  minoxidil (Loniten)
	  methyldopa (Aldomet)

Postoperative/Procedure Cardiac Tamponade Occurs within 2 weeks postsurgery or immediately postprocedure	Mediastinal chest tube occlusion or after removal of chest tubes After removal of epicardial pacing wires Perforation of the myocardium by transvenous pacemaker wires Invasive catheters Intracardiac injection Cardiac needle biopsy

(Data from Dennison, R. D. [2000]. *Pass CCRN!* [2nd ed.]. St Louis: Mosby.)

13. Discuss appropriate nursing diagnoses for a patient with cardiac tamponade.

Nursing diagnoses may include:

- Decreased cardiac output related to decreased preload and contractility
- Fluid volume deficit related to hemorrhage
- Pain/anxiety related to health alteration (Dennison, 2000; Braunwald et al, 2001)

14. Outline Ms. Gardner's collaborative plan of care related to a diagnosis of cardiac tamponade.

The first priority is to maintain airway, ventilation, oxygenation, and perfusion. BLS and ACLS guidelines should be followed. The patient may require intubation and mechanical ventilation. Circulating blood volume should be replaced with normal saline 200 to 500 ml over 10 to 15 minutes. Albumin, dextran, and blood products may also be required. Inotropes may be prescribed (Dennison, 2000).

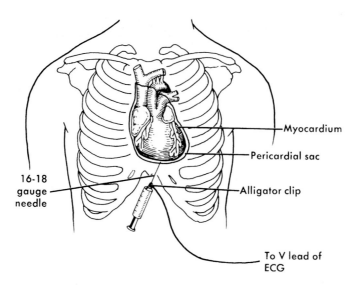

Figure **8-1.**   Pericardiocentesis. *(From Sheehy S. B. & Lenehan, G. P. [1999]. Manual of emergency care [5th ed.]. St Louis: Mosby.)*

15. How should the nurse prepare Ms. Gardner for pericardiocentesis?

Ms. Gardner should be placed in semi-Fowler's position and an ECG with limb leads should be applied. An ST-segment elevation will be seen when the needle attached to an alligator clamp touches the epicardium. Pain medication should be given prior to the pericardiocentesis procedure, and emergency equipment should be available. (See Figure 8-1.)

16. What complications may occur during a pericardiocentesis?

Ms. Gardner may experience laceration of the coronary artery or conduction system, myocardial puncture, pneumothorax, hemothorax, and dysrhythmias (Dennison, 2000).

CARDIAC TRAUMA AND CARDIAC TAMPONADE

References

Braunwald, E., Zipes, D. P., & Libby, P. (2001). *A textbook of cardiovascular medicine: HD.* (6th ed., vol. 2). New York: W. B. Saunders.

Dennison, R. D. (2000). *Pass CCRN!* (2nd ed.). St Louis: Mosby.

Ferrera, P. C., Colucciello, S. A., Marx, J. A., Verdile, V. P., & Gibbs, M. A. (Eds.). (2001). *Trauma management: An emergency medicine approach.* St Louis: Mosby.

Grif Alspach, J. (Ed.). (1998). *Core curriculum for critical care nursing.* Philadelphia: W. B. Saunders.

Knoop, T. & Willenberg, K. (1999). Cardiac tamponade. *Seminars in Oncology Nursing, 15*(3), 168-173.

Lewis, A. M. (1999, June). Cardiovascular emergency: Act quickly to help your patient through a crisis. *Nursing 99,* 49-51.

Ross, G. K. & DeJong, M. J. (1999, February). Pericardial tamponade: A young woman, kicked in the chest by her horse, exhibits signs of Beck's triad. *American Journal of Nursing, 99*(2), 35.

Tsang, T. S., Oh, J. K., & Seward, J. B. (1999, January). Diagnosis and management of cardiac tamponade in the era of echocardiography. *Clinical Cardiology, 22,* 446-452.

Urden, L. D., Stacy, K. M., & Lough, M. E. (Eds.). (2002). *Thelan's critical care nursing: Diagnosis and management* (4th ed.). St Louis: Mosby.

PULMONARY
ALTERATIONS

9

Pulmonary Embolism

Mary Ann Wehmer, RN, MSN, CNOR

CASE PRESENTATION

Lois Strange, a 62-year-old, was admitted to the hospital for an exploratory laparotomy for abdominal pain. The admission history and physical examination revealed a healthy white woman who smokes a pack of cigarettes a day. Mrs. Strange had no history of medical problems or abnormalities except for obesity and the absence from work with bed rest for the past week because of pain. She is married and has three children. She denied taking any medications except for hormone replacement therapy (HRT) and a multiple vitamin. Her preoperative diagnostic data were the following:

BP	160/84 mm Hg	RBCs	$5.0 \times 10^6/mm^3$
HR	77 bpm	WBCs	$5000/mm^3$
Respirations	16 breaths/min	Platelets	$148,000/mm^3$
Temperature	37.1° C (98.9° F)	PT	14 sec
Hgb	15 g/dl	PTT	40 sec
Hct	42%	Urine analysis	Normal

DAY OF SURGERY

Mrs. Strange's surgical procedure involved lysis of numerous adhesions and removal of the left ovary for an ovarian tumor. The tumor was sent for pathologic examination to rule out a malignancy. Results of the permanent pathologic report are pending. Mrs. Strange tolerated the general anesthesia and 2-hour surgical procedure without incident.

She was transferred to a medical-surgical floor from the postanesthesia care unit. Her vital signs remained stable. An intravenous (IV) infusion of 5% dextrose in 0.45% normal saline was infusing at 125 ml/hr, and she was to be given nothing by mouth (NPO). Her pain was managed with patient-controlled administration of morphine via a 2-mg bolus dose every 12 minutes for a maximum dose of 10 mg every hour. If postoperative nausea and vomiting occurred, she could receive ondansetron hydrochloride (Zofran) 4 mg IV every 3 to 4 hours.

Mrs. Strange was encouraged to try sitting in a chair the first postoperative day. While being assisted in a transfer from the side-of-the-bed sitting position to sitting in a chair at the bedside, Mrs. Strange experienced a lot of pain that resulted in nausea and vomiting. She was treated for the nausea and vomiting and returned to bed. Later that day she refused to get up because of her previous experience with pain and nausea.

Postoperative Day 2

Mrs. Strange's vital signs remained stable with the exception of the presence of a low-grade fever. Bowel sounds were hypoactive in all four quadrants, and because of nausea NPO status was continued, except for ice chips. Laboratory values remained normal with the exception of a slight decrease in the hemoglobin (12 g/dl) and increased at hematocrit (45%). Mrs. Strange continued to complain of incisional pain and nausea. She had experienced two episodes of vomiting. Mrs. Strange used her patient-controlled analgesia frequently and requested ondansetron for the nausea and vomiting. When encouraged to get out of bed, she responded, "I hurt too much and then throw up."

Postoperative Day 3

After the initial morning assessment, the registered nurse assisted Mrs. Strange to the bedside commode and then helped her return to bed. When the nurse checked on her later that morning, she found Mrs. Strange to be very restless and apprehensive. She was complaining of shortness of breath (SOB) and chest pain that worsened on inspiration. Upon assessment, her nurse found crackles in the left lower lobe, labored respirations, diaphoresis, and an erythematous, warm, and tender right calf with a dusky-colored lower leg and foot. Mrs. Strange's vital signs were the following:

BP	170/90 mm Hg	**Respirations**	36 breaths/min
HR	124 bpm	**Temperature**	37.8° C (100.1° F)

Mrs. Strange was placed in a semi-Fowler's position, and oxygen was started at 4 L/min through a nasal cannula. The physician was notified, and the stat orders of arterial blood gas (ABG) measurements, an electrocardiogram (ECG), ultrasound of the right leg, a chest x-ray film, and a Doppler study of the right leg were completed. Following are the results of these tests:

pH	7.52	**Chest x-ray Study**	Bibasilar
Paco$_2$	27 mm Hg	**ECG**	Sinus tachycardia
Pao$_2$	78 mm Hg	**Doppler Study**	Right DVT
Sao$_2$	95%		

A heparin bolus of 5000 U was administered, followed by a continuous infusion of 1400 U/hr. A ventilation-perfusion ($\dot{V}/\dot{Q}$) scan revealed perfusion defects of the left lower lobe with normal ventilation. A pulmonary embolism (PE) with deep vein thrombosis (DVT) in the right leg was suspected. Mrs. Strange was transferred to the intensive care unit and a pulmonary angiogram was performed that verified the diagnosis.

That evening Mrs. Strange's respiratory distress worsened, requiring intubation and mechanical ventilation. The following hemodynamic values were then obtained:

pH	7.58	**Sao$_2$**	80%
Paco$_2$	24 mm Hg	**PT**	17.1 sec
Pao$_2$	60 mm Hg	**PTT**	49.2 sec

PULMONARY EMBOLISM

QUESTIONS

1. Discuss the prevalence of venous thromboembolism (VTE) morbidity and mortality in the United States.

2. Discuss in detail venous thrombosis as the origin of PE.

3. Discuss other potential origins of PE.

4. Describe the risk factors and pathogenesis of PE with a DVT etiology.

5. Identify Mrs. Strange's risk factors.

6. What are clinical manifestations of DVT and PE?

7. Which manifestations did Mrs. Strange exhibit?

8. Describe the hemodynamic alterations that can occur as a result of PE.

9. What differential and diagnostic tests are available to determine the presence of a VTE event?

10. Which of Mrs. Strange's tests were positive for a VTE event?

11. Identify nursing diagnoses appropriate for management of Mrs. Strange's acute phase in the PE event.

12. Describe medical and nursing management for the prevention of a VTE event.

13. Describe nursing management during the acute phase of Mrs. Strange's PE event.

14. Describe nursing management after the acute phase of Mrs. Strange's PE event.

15. What guidelines are available for Mrs. Strange's anticoagulation therapy in the treatment of PE?

16. Compare the action and monitoring of low-dose unfractionated heparin (LDUH) and low-molecular-weight heparin (LMWH). Identify advantages of LMWH.

17. Identify new anticoagulants available in addition to LDUH and LMWH.

18. Explain the use of fibrinolytic therapy modalities in the management of PE.

19. Describe management of PE.

PULMONARY EMBOLISM

QUESTIONS AND ANSWERS

1. Discuss the prevalence of venous thromboembolism (VTE) morbidity and mortality in the United States.

Shorr (2002) identifies VTE as including PE and DVT. Feied (2003) identifies the U.S. PE clinically apparent morbidity to be estimated in excess of 780,000 cases annually and PE to rank as the third most common cause of mortality in hospitalized patients. Shorr (2002) states that PE is often not clinically apparent prior to death, but 30% of patients who develop PE will die as a result.

Feied (2003) notes that more than 600,000 DVT hospitalizations occurred in 2002 and many more occurred but were nonobstructing, caused no clinical manifestations, and thus were not diagnosed. The salient, nonspecific, and variant presentation clinical manifestation of VTE must be first and foremost in the clinical practitioner's mind to understand and provide newer options for prevention, diagnosis, and management. PE has consistently been found in 60% of hospital deaths. When prophylaxis was not used to prevent DVT in hospitalized patients, DVT incidence was 70% in postoperative fractured hip repair patients; 30% in intensive care patients; 20% in myocardial infarction, pulmonary, and cerebral vascular patients; and 15% in 1-week bed rest medical patients (Feied, 2003).

2. Discuss in detail venous thrombosis as the origin of PE.

One of the most common causes of PE is a dislodged DVT breaking free from the venous wall. The embolus travels through the right side of the heart into the main pulmonary artery and into the pulmonary circulation or until the clot blocks a segment of smaller diameter arteries. PE occurs in both lungs 65% of the time, in the right lung 25% of the time, and in the left lung 10% of the time (Rodgers, 1999). Chestnutt and Prendergast (2002) state that one half of asymptomatic PE patients are found to have a proximal DVT in the lower extremity 50% to 60% of the time. Lower extremity proximal deep veins are found in the popliteal and ileofemoral areas; lower leg distal deep veins are found in the calf. DVTs in the calf usually travel to the proximal veins before becoming emboli that travel into pulmonary circulation. A venous thrombus can occur from anywhere in the venous circulation. Many PEs occur in a salient manner or with variant clinical manifestations.

3. Discuss other potential origins of PE.

The etiology of a PE event is when anything flows from the larger venous lumen into a smaller pulmonary lumen, obstructing blood flow. Sources of PE include internal and external foreign bodies that are inadvertently introduced into the venous circulation.

Internal Sources of Foreign Bodies in the Venous Circulation

Fat emboli

Feied (2003) states that calf veins are the major source of fat emboli that occur with long bone and pelvic fractures, orthopedic and neurosurgery, and trauma. Pathophysiology occurs when the bone marrow releases fat globules that allow free fatty acid in venous circulation (Feied, 2002). Rodgers (1999) notes that clinical manifestations in other organs can occur before the emboli reach the pulmonary circulation; but bronchospasm and asthma-like symptoms are related to the vasoactive effects of the free fatty acid. Other manifestations include petechiae on the neck, anterior chest, axilla, and in the conjunctivae (Rodgers, 1999).

Right atrial or ventricular emboli

Sources of right atrial and ventricular emboli occur with flutter or fibrillation. Ineffective pumping action of the heart muscle leads to stasis of blood flow. When blood flow is stagnated, platelets contact the vessel wall lining and agglutinate to begin thrombus formation. With pressure or flow changes thrombi can travel down into pulmonary circulation.

Amniotic fluid emboli

Sources of amniotic fluid can occur with amniocentesis, abruptio placentae, active labor, or abortion when the amniotic fluid passes into the venous circulation. According to Lipchik and Presberg (2001), the pathophysiology of amniotic fluid in PE includes aminotic fluid or fetal particles circulating in the venous circulation that stimulate platelet aggregation, activate factor X, and/or another mechanism; or the aminotic fluid directly obstructs smaller pulmonary venous lumina. Clinical manifestations of PE from amniotic fluid may occur with a rapid onset of hyperemia, hypotension, and disseminated intravascular coagulopathy (DIC) (Lipchik & Presberg, 2001).

Tumor emboli

In 1865 Trousseau associated the development of VTE with the presence of an occult malignancy. Lipchik and Presberg (2001) state that when a healthy patient develops a DVT, look for a possible malignancy of the gastrointestinal tract, lung, breast, and renal and reproductive organs, or an occult malignancy. The pathophysiology of tumor emboli and PE is the increased production of thrombin effect by certain cancer cells (Lipchik & Presberg, 2001).

Thrombophlebitis

Feied (2003) predicts 10% of untreated hospitalized patients with superficial thrombophlebitis will develop PE with a 20% mortality complication rate. The pathogenesis of superficial thrombophlebitis occurs because the numerous inflamed perforating veins commune with the deep veins to transmit thrombi in the deep leg vein that travel to the pulmonary circulation (Feied, 2002).

Septic emboli

Sources of septic emboli occur most often with bacterial or viral infections. Examples include, but are not limited to, infected indwelling implants and catheters, obstetric/gynecologic surgeries, and acute infectious endocarditis. The pathophysiology of septic emboli and PE is that a clot of blood can become infected and break off to obstruct pulmonary circulation. Patients with PE from this origin are likely to have SOB, fever, hemoptysis, and a productive cough (Feied, 2002).

External Sources of Foreign Bodies in the Venous Circulation

Air emboli

Sources of air emboli can enter the venous circulation through central venous catheters, during neurosurgical head and neck procedures requiring a sitting position, vaginal insufflation, and pregnancy. The potential for air to enter the venous system exists when a venous tract is transected. In controlled situations such as cervical laminectomies and suboccipital craniotomies, an air-Doppler, arterial line, and central venous and/or pulmonary artery catheter is used for early detection of air entering the venous circulation. If an air embolus is suspected, attempts to prevent a PE from entering the pulmonary circulation include adding positive pressure ventilation, position change from sitting to left lateral position, and central line air emboli aspiration.

Catheter emboli

Sources of catheter emboli include both central venous and arterial catheters. The pathophysiology of the catheter as a foreign body PE includes secondary vascular wall injury. Mechanical and/or chemical trauma activates the coagulation cascade and the inflammatory process to set up for thrombi formation.

Other nonthrombotic emboli

Other sources of emboli entering the venous circulation may include any substances such as bile, vegetation growing on indwelling catheters, or stents; contaminated intravenous medications or irrigations; mercury; barium; and so on. The health care teams' vigilance to sterile technique is a priority in the technology of less invasive procedures in which tubes, drains, and irrigation are replacing the onetime open procedure closed by a primary incision to establish and protect the boundaries of membranes, tracts, and tissue.

4. Describe the risk factors and pathogenesis of PE with a DVT etiology.

Risk Factors and Pathogenesis

The Sixth American College of Chest Physicians Consensus Conference on Antithrombotic Therapy (ACCP) organized risk factors for DVTs and PE under one entity, venous thromboembolism (VTE) (Chesnutt & Prendergast, 2002). Risk factors may be reversible or nonreversible depending upon if they were inherited, acquired, or precipitated by a circumstance. VTE risk factors and pathogenesis was first explained by Virchow's 1856 theory consisting of three predisposing factors: venous stasis, vessel wall injury, and hypercoagulability.

Venous stasis

Venous stasis appears to be the most important factor of Virchow's triad that predisposes patients to PE (Urden et al, 2002). Decreased blood flow allows blood cells to contact the endothelial lining and collect clotting factors (Launius & Graham, 1998). Inherited, acquired, event-related conditions that disrupt venous blood return to the heart include immobility, dehydration, initial postoperative fluid shift, atrial fibrillation, decreased cardiac output, congestive heart failure, obesity, pregnancy, sickle cell disease, systemic lupus erythematosus, stroke, polycythemia, and sepsis. Rodgers states that immobilization of more than 7 days and obesity were identified as two of the top four risk factors for development of PE in hospitalized patients. PE occurs four times more often in the lower lobes of the lungs, where the blood flow is sluggish (Rodgers, 1999).

Vessel wall injury

When the venous intimal wall is injured, collagen is exposed to activate and aggregate platelets and factor III to form a fibrin plug or blood clot (Launius & Graham, 1998). Some causes of direct vessel injury include thrombus, surgical intervention, spontaneous rupture, bacterial or viral infections, hypoxia, and cholesterol plaque ulceration. DVT and postoperative status were identified as two of the top four risk factors for development of PE in hospitalized patients. Rodgers (1999) states that when phlebitis occurs with a DVT, an increased pooling of blood occurs at the inflamed site. Because the blood in deep veins is not rerouted, blood flow is further disrupted, which causes thrombi to attach to venous valves and increase the risk for VTE events. The frequency of PE that occurs with surgical procedures is identified as 40% with back and extremity procedures; 20% with head and neck procedures; 15.8% with abdominal procedures; and 9.4% with thoracic procedures (Rodgers, 1999).

Hypercoagulability

Hypercoagulability of blood or a low threshold for thrombus formation exists because of a release of cytokines that indirectly enhances thrombin's clotting activity (Rodgers, 1999). Patients with an inherited or acquired hypercoagulability condition usually have a secondary predisposition for hypercoagulability before a clinical significant thrombotic state develops (Launius & Graham, 1998). Sue and Vintch (2002) state that genetic conditions may include activated protein C resistance or factor V Leiden mutation, deficiency of antithrombin III, protein C, and protein S; fibrinolysis abnormalities; and prothrombin gene mutation (G20210A). Acquired conditions may include malignancy, estrogen use, pregnancy, polycythemia, lupus-associated anticoagulants, and DIC (Sue & Vintch, 2002).

According to Geerts and colleagues (2001), patients at risk for VTE events have multiple risk factors that are cumulative, which has a direct effect on VTE recurrence. Gallus and associates (2001) identified four risk categories for surgical patients according to the following data:

- Low-risk patient
  - Younger than 40 years, no additional risk factors, minor surgery
- Moderate-risk patient
  - Additional risk factors, minor surgery
  - 40 to 60 years, no additional risk factors, nonmajor surgery
  - Younger than 40 years of age, additional risk factors
- High-risk patient
  - Older than 60 years of age, nonmajor surgery
  - Additional risk factors, nonmajor surgery
  - Older than 40 years of age, major surgery
  - Additional risks, major surgery
- Highest-risk patient
  - Older than 40 years, major surgery, prior VTE, cancer, or molecular hypercoagulable state
  - Hip or knee arthroplasty
  - Hip fracture surgery
  - Major trauma
  - Spinal cord injury

5. Identify Mrs. Strange's risk factors.

Mrs. Strange's Risk Factors

- 62 years old
- Pack-a-day smoker
- Bed rest for 1 week preoperatively
- Obesity
- HRT
- High normal values preoperatively for blood pressure, hemoglobin (Hgb), hematocrit (Hct), red blood cells (RBCs), prothrombin time (PT), and activated partial thromboplastin time (apt)
- Pelvic surgical procedure lasting 2 hours
- Possible malignancy
- Postoperative pain and nausea/vomiting resulting in resistance to ambulate
- Slight decrease of Hct postoperatively to 45% related to postoperative dehydration (NPO status and vomiting)

6. What are clinical manifestations of DVT and PE?

When manifestations of DVT do occur, the most classic symptoms are asymmetry of the affected extremity with swelling, redness, and tenderness (Fedullo, 2000). Feied (2003) states that swelling, redness, and tenderness do not confirm or rule out the diagnosis of DVT and that the Homan's sign predictive reliance is not always accurate. Clinical manifestations of DVT occur only once obstruction of the vessel has occurred. Thrombi usually dislodge from the DVT 7 to 10 days after formation when the clot begins to dissolve.

When PE clinical manifestations are obvious, it is often after the patient makes a sudden movement with ambulation or has a vascular pressure change with straining, sneezing, or coughing (Rodgers, 1999). Clinical manifestations of PE vary greatly and are believed to be silent 50% of the time (Sue & Vintch, 2002). Hull, Pineo, & Raskob (2000) state that clinical signs and symptoms of PE such as dyspnea, pleuritic chest pain, hemoptysis, acute right-sided heart failure, and cardiovascular collapse can be difficult to distinguish from other respiratory and cardiovascular causes because the presentation is related to not only the size and number of emboli but also the patient's cardiopulmonary reserve. Fedullo (2000), states that the Pulmonary Embolism Prospective Investigation of Pulmonary Embolism Diagnosis (PIOPED) study identified findings of individual clinical manifestations differed from the clinical syndrome. In the individual signs and symptoms of patients with angiographically proven PE who had no preexisting pulmonary or heart disease, dyspnea was identified in 73% of patients, pleuritic chest pain that increased during inspiration was identified in 66% of patients, cough was identified in 33% of patients, lower extremity edema was identified in 28% of patients, and hemoptysis was identified in 13% of patients. The top clinical manifestations were hemoptysis, which occurred 65% of the time; isolated dyspnea, which occurred 22% of the time; and circulatory collapse, which occurred 8% of the time.

Rodgers (1999) notes that other clinical manifestations of PE may include the following:

- Wheezing related to bronchoconstriction
- Cyanosis and decreased breath sounds related to pleuritic chest pain and ventilation defects
- Hypotension related to ineffective sympathetic stimulation
- Accentuated pulmonic heart sounds and systolic murmurs related to ventricular compromise and increased pulmonary artery pressure
- Diaphoresis and tachycardia related to release of catecholamines
- Jugular venous distention and edema related to right-sided ventricular failure
- Phlebitis and fever related to inflammation

7. Which manifestations did Mrs. Strange exhibit?

Mrs. Strange's signs and symptoms were the following:

- Unexplained restlessness and apprehension after postoperative ambulation
- SOB and labored respirations
- Chest pain that worsened on inspiration
- Right calf pain with erythema, warmth, and tenderness and a dusky-colored leg and foot
- Crackles in the left lower lobe
- Diaphoresis

8. Describe the hemodynamic alterations that can occur as a result of PE.

Hemodynamic Alterations

PE can impair the ventilation and perfusion efforts of the pulmonary system by affecting the dead space, bronchi, and alveoli. Compensatory vascular shunting leads to pulmonary artery hypertension and right-sided ventricular failure. As the cardiac system is further compromised or the occlusion becomes massive, decreased cardiac output, right-sided ventricular failure, and pulmonary infarction can occur.

Increased Dead Space and $\dot{V}/\dot{Q}$ Mismatch

Feied (2003) states that alveolar-capillary gas exchange does not occur in alveoli distal to where the embolus lodges, and ventilatory efforts wasted on nonperfused alveoli is dead space.

Ventilation/perfusion ($\dot{V}/\dot{Q}$) mismatch occurs with the following:

- Diminished oxygen is available to local tissue (hypoxia).
- The blood being circulated to all body cells is low in oxygen (hypoxemia).
- Carbon dioxide cannot enter the affected alveoli (alveolar hypocarbia).
- The level of systemic carbon dioxide increases (hypercapnia).
- Varying degrees of hyperventilation increase the partial pressure of oxygen in arterial blood (PaO_2) but do not affect the alveolar-arterial (A-a) gradient elevation.

Bronchial Constriction

The bronchial constriction that occurs from alveolar hypocarbia causes ventilation to be shunted to perfused areas of the lung. Platelet aggregation at the site of the occlusion causes a release of thromboxane A_2 and serotonin that further constricts airways and the pulmonary artery (Rodgers, 1999).

Atelectasis

Atelectasis occurs after bronchoconstriction when the production of surfactant decreases proportionately with the length of time that alveoli are not perfused. Feied (2003) states that after a PE obstruction the alveolar surface, tension decreases within 2 to 3 hours, the production of surfactant is severely slowed within 12 to 15 hours, and surfactant production and alveolar type II cell nutrition are depleted, leading to atelectasis in 24 hours.

Pulmonary Arterial Hypertension

Urden and colleagues (2002) state that patients who have had a massive PE or obstruction of more than 50% of the pulmonary vascular bed are likely to demonstrate pulmonary hypertension. Pulmonary arterial hypertension is an ineffective but adaptive response of shunting blood from nonfunctional to functional alveoli. Hyperventilation occurs in an effort to perfuse and ventilate the lungs, which leads to increased pulmonary artery pressure and resistance (Urden et al, 2002).

Right-Sided Ventricular Failure

Lipchik and Presberg (2001) note that when pulmonary hypertension develops, the pulmonary artery diastolic-occlusive pressure gradient widens and right ventricle workload increases until right-sided ventricular failure occurs. A normal right ventricle compensates to systolic pressures of 65 mm Hg or a mean pulmonary artery pressure up to 40 mm Hg before right-sided ventricular failure results (Lipchik & Presberg, 2001).

The degree of systemic symptoms such as neck vein distention, peripheral edema, ascites, and hepatomegaly are directly related to the degree of right-sided heart failure. A decreased cardiac output leads to a decreased perfusion of the coronary arteries, brain, and kidneys (Rodgers, 1999). With decompensation of the right ventricle, a fixed-split P_2 heart sound may result from delayed closure of the pulmonic valve. A diastolic murmur from pulmonary insufficiency indicates further right-sided ventricular decompensation (Urden et al, 2002).

Feied (2003) states that chronic cor pulmonale can occur from a massive PE or from recurrent PE resulting in decreased elastic distention of vessels and thus impaired gas exchange in the pulmonary vascular system. Cardiac output demands increase related to the increase in the pulmonary artery pressure. The mortality rate from pulmonary hypertension is high and is usually fatal in several years (Feied, 2002).

Decreased Cardiac Output

Rodgers (1999) states that the right atrial pressure increases as blood backs up into the right atrium and the amount of blood entering the left ventricle decreases, resulting in decreased cardiac output. Two compensatory mechanisms responding to decreased cardiac output include an increased PaO_2 from increased ventilatory efforts and stimulation of the sympathetic nervous system, chemoreceptors, and baroreceptors. A normal pulmonary artery occlusive pressure in an acute PE event indicates normal left ventricular pressure (Rodgers, 1999).

Pulmonary Infarction

Pulmonary infarction (PI) occurs in 10% to 15% of PE events and usually is seen more often in patients with preexisting cardiopulmonary disease because of their extensive collateral circulation to the lungs. Hemoptysis may occur 24 to 48 hours after the PE event, which is not necessarily 24 hours from the clinical presentation of the PE. PI can cause changes in the pulmonary artery pressure and circulation that precipitate more PE events. Hemorrhage, effusion, fibrosis, and scarring result (Rodgers, 1999). Pulmonary resection may be required for large areas of necrosis or abscess.

9. What differential and diagnostic tests are available to determine the presence of a VTE event?

Swearingen and Keen (2001) state that baseline and differential diagnostic tests are conducted after assessment of the history and physical examination to determine etiology and distinguish VTE (DVT and PE) from other disease processes. Clinical manifestations of PE may appear similar to cardiovascular diseases (ischemic cardiac chest pain, pericarditis, or dissecting aortic aneurysm), pulmonary diseases (pneumonia, pleural effusion, or pleuritis), and gastrointestinal disorders (gastric or duodenal ulcer, gastritis, or esophageal rupture). Baseline and differential tests include the following:

- *Screening for thrombophilias.* According to Gossage (2003), if the patient is young and without risk factors, lab tests on the following should be assessed: protein C&S, antithrombin III, fibrinogen, factor V Leiden mutation, lupus anticoagulant, plasma homocysteine levels, anticardiolipin antibodies, and factors VIII and IX.
- *Lab tests.* Swearingen and Keen (2001) state that a lab workup should be performed before anticoagulant therapy is started. Lab workup should include baseline PT, International Normalized Ratio (INR), PTT, and platelet count. Feied (2003) states complete blood count (CBC), inflammation (WBCs and sedimentation rate), and hydration (Hgb and Hct) do not reflect changes specific or sensitive to PE.
- *Chest x-ray studies.* Feied (2003) notes that initial chest x-ray findings are not sensitive or specific for PE. Two findings that are associated with PE are (1) Westermark's sign, which is described as a sharp cutoff of collapsed veins distal to the embolism and a dilation of the pulmonary vessels proximal to the embolism; and (2) Hampton's hump, which is defined as a rounded or triangular infiltrate that lies adjacent to the diaphragm.
- *ECG.* Swearingen and Keen (2001) state that ECG changes are seen with pulmonary hypertension.
- *ABGs.* Ferri (2003) states that a decrease occurs in the PaO_2 and $PaCO_2$ and an elevated pH or respiratory alkalosis can be seen with PE.
- *A-a oxygen gradient.* According to Ferri (2003) the A-a oxygen gradient increases with the size of a PE. An increased A-a oxygen gradient does not confirm the diagnosis of PE, but an A-a oxygen gradient within normal limits does rule out a PE. The measure of oxygen gradient between the alveoli and arterial blood or A-a oxygen gradient is a more sensitive measure of the presence and extent of PE than the change of the PaO_2 (Ferri, 2003).
- Noninvasive imaging studies include ultrasound and Doppler studies to indicate blood flow by measuring sound waves reflected off RBCs and impedance plethysmography to measure electrical resistance changes as a blood pressure cuff deflates. I-fibrinogen leg scan tracks fibrinogen with a radioisotope once it has attached to a thrombus.
- A more sensitive, but invasive test for DVTs, is a venogram, which involves increased risks and adverse effects from the IV dye. Feied (2003) states color flow duplex ultrasound (US; B-mode ultrasound Doppler) is better than the venogram for femoral vein thrombus.
- *Pulmonary contrast venography.* Ferri (2003) states pulmonary angiography is the gold standard test for PE because it can detect small emboli, but it places the patient at risk for adverse reaction to the dye and is painful. The pulmonary vasculature is viewed under fluoroscopy after an iodine contrast medium has been injected via a peripheral catheter

threaded through the right side of the heart. Reliable signs of a PE include an abrupt termination of a pulmonary artery vessel or an intraluminal-filling defect.

- *Compression ultrasonography.* Ferri (2003) states the first choice of study for PE is the noninvasive compression ultrasonography, which has good sensitivity. This test is not recommended for visualizing proximal DVT and nonocclusive distal DVTs.
- *Transesophageal echocardiography (TEE).* Konstadt (1999) describes the use of TEE to differentiate an intraoperative PE from an acute cardiovascular collapse. A central PE that occurs in the main, right, or left pulmonary artery is associated with cardiovascular collapse and can be visualized with TEE.
- *Lung scintigraphy ($\dot{V}/\dot{Q}$ scan).* Swearingen and Keen (2001) states that pulmonary $\dot{V}/\dot{Q}$ scan is key to diagnosis of PE by detecting a mismatch between ventilation and perfusion. The $\dot{V}/\dot{Q}$ scan is performed (1) to differentiate PE from bronchogenic or lymphangitic carcinomas and congenital vascular abnormalities and (2) to determine the probability that a $\dot{V}/\dot{Q}$ mismatch exists. In the PIOPED study, lung scans were found to be sensitive and reliable in differentiating a normal $\dot{V}/\dot{Q}$ from a $\dot{V}/\dot{Q}$ mismatch. An even distribution of radiotracers for ventilation and perfusion throughout both lung fields without defects indicates normal perfusion and rules out PE. When ventilation tracers are normal in multiple segmental defects of abnormal perfusion, a $\dot{V}/\dot{Q}$ mismatch or a high probability for PE exists. An exception to the high reliability in the scan occurs in a patient who had a previous embolus with abnormal perfusion studies before scanning. When the scan does not fit into the high-probability or normal $\dot{V}/\dot{Q}$ groups, the scan is considered nondiagnostic and an investigation for a DVT should follow (Galvin & Choi, 1999).
- *D-dimer radioimmunoassay level.* Feied (2003) states D-dimer results from the breakdown from plasmin-mediated proteolysis of fibrin. An enzyme-linked immunosorbent assay (ELISA) is used to measure D-dimer levels. The D-dimer test is considered sensitive and specific for peripheral thrombi, but not so for PE. The D-dimer level may be used in combination with $\dot{V}/\dot{Q}$ scans (Langdale, 2002).
- *Fiberoptic and intravascular pulmonary ultrasound, digital subtraction angiography, and radiolabeled platelets*
- *Spiral CT and magnetic resonance imaging (MRI).* Langdale (2002) notes that CT imaging has a sensitivity of 94% and specificity of 96% for PE. Two disadvantages of the spiral CT scan are (1)it is not sensitive or specific for peripheral lesions, and (2)reliability of the test is radiologist experience-dependent. MRI angiography with gadolinium is sensitive and specific for both PE and peripheral lesions, but the MRI modality (pulse or angiography) is still under investigation and debated by radiologists (Langdale, 2002).

10. **Which of Mrs. Strange's tests were positive for a VTE event?**

Mrs. Strange's Positive Tests

Elevated vital signs were related to tissue hypoxia and compensatory efforts.

BP	170/90 mm Hg	**Respirations**	36 breaths/min
HR	124 bpm	**Temperature**	37.8° C (100.1° F)

Initial ABG measurements revealed respiratory alkalosis and the attempted response to blow off CO_2.

pH	7.52	**Pao$_2$**	78 mm Hg
Paco$_2$	27 mm Hg	**Sao$_2$**	95%

Later ABG measurements revealed alkalosis with a further drop in the Pao_2. The aPTT was within the therapeutic range for anticoagulation.

pH	7.58	**Sao$_2$**	80%
Paco$_2$	24 mm Hg	**PT**	17.1 sec
Pao$_2$	60 mm Hg	**aPTT**	49.2 sec

11. Identify nursing diagnoses appropriate for management of Mrs. Strange's acute phase in the PE event.

- Ineffective gas exchange
- Anxiety
- Ineffective breathing pattern
- Alteration in tissue perfusion
- Alteration in comfort: pain
- Risk for decreased cardiac output
- Risk for fluid volume excess
- Deficient knowledge

12. Describe medical and nursing management for the prevention of a VTE event.

Medical Management to Prevent VTE

The ASSP have made evidence-based recommendations for prophylactic treatment protocol because prevention has become the gold standard practice for high-risk patients of VTE (Geerts et al, 2001). Nutescu (2002) states that waiting to treat VTE has major ramifications in that the United States annual rates have been estimated at a VTE mortality rate of some 250,00 to 500,000 hospitalized patients and a long morbidity period for DVT patients with 20% to 30% emerging with a postthrombotic syndrome. Evaluation of risk factors is an important step in early diagnosis and treatment of VTE because more than 90% of patients have predisposing factors (Galvin & Choi, 1999). DVTs from the proximal leg veins and pelvis account for 90% of PEs (Brashers, 2002).

Knowledge of current guidelines for prophylaxis can be used for identifying at-risk patients. Guyatt and colleagues (2001) defined the grades of recommendations for antithrombotic agents for prophylactic treatment of VTE that were established at the Sixth American College of Chest Physicians Consensus Conference on Antithrombotic Therapy (ACCP). These grades were systematically rated according to the tradeoff between benefits versus risks and the methodologic strength of research supporting the recommendation guideline. A numerical value of 1 was given to a recommendation when the experts set the guideline for clinicians to offer as a treatment to the average patient. Grade 1 means that experts have strong confidence in the efficacy and benefits of the treatment outweighing the risk and costs. A Grade 2 recommendation was given if the tradeoff of benefit versus risk or cost was not as clear. Methodologic strength was graded on a scale of A, B, C+, or C based on the following criteria. Grade A recommendations were supported by randomized trials with consistent results. Grade B recommendations were founded on randomized trials with major methodologic weakness or inconsistent results. Grade C+ recommendations were based on generalizations from secure randomized trials or overwhelmingly compelling observational studies. Grade C was derived for other observations that may change when stronger evidence is available. (Guyatt et al, 2001).

Geerts and associates (2001) note the following recommendations for thromboprophylaxis in the following conditions.

General Medical Patients:

- Patients with risk factors for VTE: Grade 1A recommendation—LMWH or LDUH

General Surgical Patients:

- Low-risk patient: Grade 1C recommendation—early ambulation, no other prophylaxis
- Moderate-risk Patient: Grade 1A recommendation—LDUH, LMWH, intermittent pneumatic compression (IPC), graded compression elastic stockings (ES)
- High-risk patient: Grade 1A recommendation—LDUH or LMWH; Grade 2A recommendation—IPC or ES as alternative to pharmacologic prophylaxis in high risk for bleed patients

- Highest-risk patient: Grade 1C recommendation—LMWH or LDUH combined with IPC or ES; Grade 2C recommendation—postdischarge LMWH or perioperative warfarin (INR 2-3)

Gynecologic Surgical Patients:

- Brief surgeries for benign disease: Grade 1C recommendation—early ambulation, no other prophylaxis
- Major surgeries for benign disease: Grade 1A recommendation—LMWH or IPC started just prior to the procedure and continued several days postoperatively
- Major surgeries for malignancies: Grade 1A recommendation—routine prophylaxis with three daily doses of LDUH; Grade 1C recommendation—combination of LDUH plus IPC or ES or higher doses of LMWH

Urosurgery Patients:

- Transurethral or low-risk surgeries: Grade 2C recommendation—early ambulation, no other prophylaxis
- Major open surgeries: Grade 1B recommendation—routine prophylaxis LDUH, LMWH, ICP, or ES
- Highest-risk patients: Grade 1C recommendation—combination of LDUH or LMWH with ES and/or IPC

Orthopedic Surgery: (50%-60% of patients who have undergone total hip replacement [THR], total knee replacement [TKR], and hip fracture surgery without prophylactic thromboprophylaxis have a DVT detected by venography)

- Elective THR
  - Grade 1A recommendation—LMWH initiated 12 hours preoperatively or 12 to 24 hours postoperatively; warfarin initiated preoperatively or immediately postoperatively (INR 2-3).
  - Grade 1B recommendation—preoperative adjusted-dose heparin
  - ICP and ES used in combination with pharmacologic treatment provides supplemental protection
  - Extended prophylaxis—remains debatable: LMWH for up to 4 weeks postdischarge versus 9 to 14 days in hospital prophylaxis
  - Grade 2A recommendation—prophylaxis for at least 7 days and extended out-of-hospital LMWH prophylaxis for high-risk patients
- Elective TKR
  - Grade 1A recommendation—LMWH or adjusted-dose warfarin; Grade 1B recommendation—IPC as an alternative
- Hip Fracture
  - Grade 1B recommendation—LMWH or adjusted-dose warfarin; Grade 2B recommendation—LDUH as an alternative
- Arthroscopic Surgery
- No recommendations at this time; however, VTE has been demonstrated and anecdotally reported

Neurosurgery

- Intracranial surgery: Grade 1A recommendation—IPC with or without ES; Grade 1B recommendation—combined treatments of LMWH or LDUH prophylaxis with IPC or ES in high-risk patients may be more effective than either treatment used alone
- Acute spinal cord injury: Grade 1B recommendation—LMWH; Grade 2B recommendation—IPC and ES in combination with LMWH; Grade 1C recommendation—LMWH or warfarin in the rehabilitation phase

Trauma Victims

- Grade 1A recommendation—initiate LMWH in patients with identifiable risk factors as soon as safe and if no contraindications

- Grade 1C recommendation—if initiation of LMWH is delayed or contraindicated, consider IPC
- Grade 2C recommendation—consider inferior vena cava (IVC) filter placement with presence of DVT and contraindication of anticoagulation

Acute Myocardial Infarction

- Grade 1A recommendation—prophylactic or therapeutic subcutaneous LDUH or IV heparin
- Ischemic stroke (must exclude intracranial hemorrhage before starting pharmacologic thromboprophylaxis)
- Grade 1A recommendation—routine use of LDUH, LMWH, or danaparoid (a heparinoid) in patients with leg weakness

Nursing Management to Prevent VTE

DVT, postoperative status, immobilization more than 7 days, and obesity were identified as the top four risk factors for development of PE in hospitalized patients. Nursing management can affect the patient's immobility status related to illness, weakness, pain, and especially postoperative status.

While the patient is on bed rest:

- Change the patient's position every 2 hours while awake.
- Demonstrate and have patient return-demonstrate taking in a slow deep breath through the nose and holding for 5 seconds, then slowly exhaling through mouth to develop an effective pulmonary hygiene regimen.
- Facilitate moving the patient into a sitting position for 5 to 10 repetitions of pulmonary toileting every hour while awake to ventilate posterior bases of lungs.
- Provide an incentive spirometer if patient works better with biofeedback .
- Prepare patient for a cough at the end of the slow deep breaths by demonstrating and having the patient return-demonstrate splinting abdominal wound incisions with a folded blanket.
- Promote venous return from the lower extremities with proper placement and use of IPC and ES.
- Demonstrate and have patient return-demonstrate a pedaling motion with feet and circular ankle movement.
- Avoid placement of pillows under the legs or crossing of legs, which can impede blood flow in the lower extremities.
- Assess pain level on identified pain scale, provide analgesics with comfort measures, and evaluate effectiveness of pain management related to route of medication.
- Provide pharmacologic pain management.
- Follow up on pain coverage if current order is not adequate.
- Individualize nonpharmacologic pain management with measures such as a warm blanket, change of position, support with pillows, a kind word, soft hand, personal presence, music, quietness, light, low light, backrubs, healing touch, reiki, visualization, imagery, prayer, etc.
- Include the patient in the plan of care by explaining the physiologic and psychologic benefits of analgesia, rest, and healing.

To promote early ambulation and make early ambulation possible:

- Provide for a "win-win" situation by encouraging the use of analgesia before pain peaks and before initiating ambulation or increasing activities.
- Assist the patient in sitting up or sitting at bedside.
- Explain and talk through how the hospital bed can be adjusted to facilitate "getting out of bed."
- Supervise progression of activity to promote advancement.

Medical or Surgical Condition	Recommendation for Prophylaxis of VTE	Grade of Recommendation
General surgery Low risk (younger than 40 years, no CRFs, minor procedure)	Aspirin not recommended Early ambulation	C1
Moderate risk (older than 40 years, no CRFs, major procedure)	Either low-dose unfractionated heparin (LDUH), LMWH, intermittent pneumatic compression (IPC), or elastic stockings (ES)	A1
Higher risk (older than 40 years, CRFs, major procedure)	LDUH or higher-dose regimen of LMWH	A1
Higher risk and prone to wound infections or hematomas	IPC	A1
Very high risk (multiple CRFs)	LDUH or LMWH combined with IPC	B1
Selected very high risk	Perioperative warfarin (with warfarin therapy the international normalized ratio [INR] should be 2-3)	A2
Orthopedic procedures	Limit use of inferior vena cava (IVC) filter placement to high-risk patients when other prophylaxis is not feasible	C2
Elective total hip replacement (THR)	*Start either:* (1) LMWH 12-24 hr postoperatively (2) Warfarin therapy preoperatively or immediately after operation or (3) Adjusted-dose heparin preoperatively and ES or IPC	A1
Elective total knee replacement (TKR)	LMWH, warfarin or IPC	A1
Duration of prophylaxis for elective THR and TKR is uncertain	7-10 days' duration with LMWH or warfarin	A1
	Emerging data suggest benefits from 29-35 days duration of LMWH Routine duplex ultrasound screening not recommended for asymptomatic patients postoperatively	A2
Hip fracture surgical procedures	Either preoperative LMWH or preoperative or immediate postoperative warfarin therapy	A2
Elective neurosurgical procedures		
Intracranial procedures	IPC with or without ES; LMWH and LDUH may be acceptable alternatives	A1
	If high risk, a combination of pharmacologic and physical treatments may be more effective than either one alone	B1

Medical or Surgical Condition	Recommendation for Prophylaxis of VTE	Grade of Recommendation
Acute spinal cord injury	LMWH	B1
	IPC and ES may have benefit if used with LMWH or if anticoagulant agents are contraindicated	C1
	Rehabilitation phase: continuing LMWH or converting to full-dose oral anticoagulation may provide protection	C2
Trauma patients with CRF	Start LMWH as soon as safe and not contraindicated	A1
	If administration of LMWH is delayed, use IPC	C1
	If high risk or suboptimal prophylaxis, screen with duplex ultrasonography; if DVT is demonstrated and anticoagulation is contraindicated, insert IVC filter	C2
Medical conditions Myocardial infarction	LDUH Full anticoagulation	A1
	IPC and ES if heparin is contraindicated	C1
Ischemic stroke and lower extremity paralysis	LDUH and LMWH	A1
	IPC plus ES are probably effective	B1
General medical patients with CRFs and especially those with pulmonary infections and/or CHF	LDUH or LMWH	A1
Patients with long-term indwelling CVCs	Warfarin 1 mg/day or LMWH daily	A1
Patients with spinal puncture or epidural catheters for regional analgesia or anesthesia	Use LMWH with caution	C1

Adapted from Clagett G. P., et al. *(1998)*. Prevention of venous thromboembolism, *Chest* 114(5, Suppl.), 531S–561S.

13. **Describe nursing management during the acute phase of Mrs. Strange's PE event.**

Acute Phase
- Administer oxygen and elevate head of bed.
- Keep the patient in bed and avoid unnecessary movement.
- Attempt to relieve anxiety and remain with the patient and reassure/explain.
- Administer a narcotic analgesic and monitor the patient's status.
- Complete vital signs, differential tests (ABGs, ECG, and chest x-ray), and diagnostic tests as soon as possible.
- Monitor for subsequent PE events and be prepared to assist the patient in compensatory efforts.
- Have intubation and ventilatory equipment readily available.

- Monitor for pulmonary hypertension and right-sided ventricular failure (jugular vein distention, peripheral edema, arrhythmias, and tachypnea).
- Monitor cardiac output (tachycardia, hypotension, decreased cardiac output, and shock).
- Monitor PT (INR) and aPTT levels and assume that samples are drawn on time for accurate results. Assess for signs of bleeding.

14. Describe nursing management after the acute phase of Mrs. Strange's PE event.

After the Acute Phase

- Teaching after PE
- Need for lifestyle changes
- Signs and symptoms of DVT and the need for appropriate intervention
- Oral anticoagulation teaching regarding the medication, signs of hemorrhage, and control testing

15. What guidelines are available for Mrs. Strange's anticoagulation therapy in the treatment of PE?

Initial treatment for a DVT includes IV and subcutaneous administration of unfractionated heparin (UFH) or subcutaneous injection of LMWH followed by oral administration of warfarin. The UFH dosage is adjusted until the aPTT is prolonged one and one half to two times the control; the dose for LMWH is calculated by the patient's body weight, and the warfarin dosage is regulated to an INR of 2 (Graber, 1999). The UFH treatment for an uncomplicated DVT in the calf is found to be effective with a 5-day therapeutic dose, which reduces the risk of heparin-induced thrombocytopenia (HIT); whereas an extensive DVT in the ileofemoral vein still requires a 10-day UFH course of treatment (Hirsh et al, 1996a).

The potential for recurrence of DVT depends on the status of the individual's risk factors. If risk factors are reversed or decreased, recurrence within the first year is less than if risk factors remain the same. Most patients with reversible factors have normal noninvasive lower extremity studies after 3 months, and 90% have normal studies by 1 year, which indicates clot resolution but not necessarily a fully competent normal vein. If a patient develops postthrombotic syndrome, the rate of DVT recurrence is increased.

Anticoagulant Therapy

Heparin has been proven effective in the treatment of PE and should begin as soon as a PE is suspected unless heparin is contraindicated. The 1998 American Heart Medical/Scientific Statement on the Management of DVT and PE states that a bolus of heparin 5000 U should be followed by a subcutaneous injection of 17,500 U twice daily, an IV infusion of 1400 U/hr, or a weight-adjusted dosage regimen. Weight-adjusted heparin dosing includes a bolus of 80 U/kg, followed by an IV infusion of 18 U/kg/hr (Hirsh & Hoak, 1996).

Warfarin, an oral anticoagulant, should be started within 24 hours of the initiation of heparin therapy. PT is used to monitor the depression of factors II, VII, and X (three of the four vitamin K–dependent procoagulant clotting factors). The initial PT reflects the depression of factor VII, whereas the depression of factors II and X occurs later (Hirsh et al, 1998b). For this reason, heparin therapy is continued for about 5 days after the initiation of warfarin or when the warfarin dosage has kept the INR in the therapeutic range for 2 consecutive days.

Traditionally the PT has been stated as a ratio of the patient's time to the control time. Because response of thromboplastins varies depending on the source of the laboratory reagent used, confusion in determination of an appropriate therapeutic range has occurred and the recommended dosage of warfarin has been inadequate to maintain a therapeutic level. As a result of the differences in reagents and confusion in the therapeutic level for the PT, the INR is now recognized as a standardized means to report therapeutic levels and to monitor warfarin therapy. A therapeutic INR range of 2 to 3 is recommended for most uses of warfarin. Because the efficacy of the drug is reduced when the INR is less than

2, a target rate in the middle of the therapeutic range should be maintained. For example if the range is 2 to 3, a 2.5 target should be maintained and if the range is 2.5 to 3.5, a target of 3.5 should be maintained (Hirsh et al, 1998a).

Anticoagulant Therapy Guidelines

According to Hyers and associates (1998), grade A1 recommendations or guidelines for treatment of VTE or PE from the 1998 American College of Chest Physicians Consensus Conference on Antithrombotic Therapy include the following:

- IV heparin or an adjusted-dose subcutaneous heparin can be used to prolong the aPTT to a range corresponding to 0.3 to 0.6 IU/ml by an aminolytic anti-XA assay or a plasma heparin level of 0.2 to 0.4 IU/ml protamine sulfate.
- LMWH can be used in place of unfractionated heparin with PE when the patient is in a stable condition.
- If the PE is not massive, heparin or LMWH should be continued for at least 5 days, with oral anticoagulant therapy overlapping the heparin therapy for at least 4 to 5 days.
- If the PE is massive, a longer duration for heparin therapy may be used.
- Heparin therapy can be discontinued when the INR (used to monitor the warfarin therapy) is at a level of 2 for 2 consecutive days
- The duration of oral anticoagulants should prolong the PT to a target INR of 2.5 or a range of 2 to 3 and be continued for 3 months. If oral anticoagulants cannot be used, LMWH with or without unfractionated adjusted-dose heparin should be used so that the aPTT is prolonged to therapeutic plasma heparin level.

Other graded recommendations consist of the following:

- The duration for anticoagulant therapy should be 3 to 6 months in patients with time-limited or reversible risk factors and for at least 6 months in patients with a first-time idiopathic DVT event (Grade A2 recommendation).
- Patients with continued risk factors for VTE or recurrent venous thrombosis (RVT) events should receive therapy indefinitely (Grade C2 recommendation).
- Placement of an IVC shunt is recommended for patients who have complications with or contraindications for anticoagulant therapy, recurrent VTE with adequate anticoagulation therapy, concurrent surgical pulmonary embolectomy or endarterectomy, and chronic recurrent PE with pulmonary hypertension (no grade for recommendation) (Hyers et al, 1998).

16. Compare the action and monitoring of low-dose unfractionated heparin (LDUH) and low-molecular-weight heparin (LMWH). Identify advantages of LMWH.

UFH is a commercially isolated glycosaminoglycan heterogeneous mixture of bovine and porcine mucosa (Nutescu, 2002). Hirsh and associates (1998) identify UFH heterogeneous properties to be a broad range of molecular weights, anticoagulation effects in high and low affinity for antithrombin (AT)-III, and nonspecific protein binding. The short half-life of UFH and need for continuous infusion in high-risk patients are related to the fact that only one third of the UFH molecules are large enough to be drawn to the cofactor AT, which inactivates thrombin. The nonspecific protein binding of UFH requires frequent monitoring by aPTT and dosage adjustments (Hirsh et al, 1998b). Monitoring of UFH therapy consists of timely drawing of blood for aPTT assessment at 6 hours after bolus and initiation of the continuous IV infusion. Blood should be drawn at approximately the same time every morning for monitoring of aPTT levels during heparin therapy administration. The recommended therapeutic aPTT for PE is 1.5 to 2.5 times the control value (Erdman et al, 1997). Osteoporosis and venous and arterial thromboses resulting from HIT type II UFHs have been associated with the nonspecific protein binding property of UFH (Nutescu, 2002). HIT, an antibody-mediated reaction that occurs after 5 days of heparin therapy, is seen more often with UFH than with LMWH (Hirsh et al, 1998a).

Hirsh and coworkers (1998b) state that LMWH inactivates only factor Xa. LMWH requires no monitoring of the clotting status, and dosages are adjusted to the patient's weight as recommended by the product manufacturer. Monitoring of the LMWH clotting status is not required because it binds less to plasma protein, making the plasma concentration and dose independent of the plasma recovery and clearance. As a result the half-life of LMWH is two to four times longer than UFH. Nutescu (2002) states that LMWH can be administered effectively by the subcutaneous route and is believed to be safe for outpatient use. Advantages of LMWH are that it is less likely to produce HIT and thrombotic complications and that it is cost-effective. LMWH and UFH should not be given to patients with HIT (Nutescu, 2002).

Nutescu (2002) states the clinical efficiency and dosage of LMWHs vary. Dalteparin, enoxaparin, and tinzaparin are the three types of LMWH that have been studied. Enoxaparin and tinzaparin have compared equally with warfarin in lowering DVT incidence in patients with total knee replacements. The same results were not found in patients with total hip replacements (Nutescu, 2002).

17. Identify new anticoagulants available in addition to LDUH and LMWH.

Simmons (2002) states that new anticoagulants include direct and indirect thrombin inhibitors and defibrinating agents.

Direct thrombin inhibitors do not bind to antithrombin to produce anticoagulation. Instead recombinant hirudin (lepirudin), bivalirudin, and argatroban bind to thrombin. Recombinant hirudin and argatroban are approved for patients who develop HIT. A disadvantage of hirudin is that it has no natural antidote. Heparinoids or indirect thrombin inhibitors have a high affinity for antithrombin and are low-molecular-weight. The US Food and Drug Administration (FDA) has currently approved danaparoid, which is used for DVT. Ancrod, a defibrinating enzyme produces its anticoagulant effect by clinging to fibrinogen to decrease the amount of fibrinogen available in the blood. Ancrod is approved for use in HIT in Canada and compassionate use in the United States. An antivenin exists for ancrod (Simmons, 2002).

18. Explain the use of fibrinolytic therapy modalities in the management of PE.

Feied (2003) states that removal of a thrombus restores blood flow to maintain the structure and function of venous valves. Fibrinolysis can reduce the postphlebitic syndrome by 70% and recurrence of DVTs by 50%. Fibrinolytic therapy is used to dissolve PE in patients who are hemodynamically unstable and to prevent pulmonary hypertension and cor pulmonale. The mortality benefit from using early fibrinolytic therapy was realized in the last study conducted in the mid-1990s; the study was actually terminated before its completion because the test group (hemodynamically unstable patients treated with heparin) died and the trial group (hemodynamically unstable patients treated with fibinolysis) survived (Feied, 2003).

FDA-approved fibrinolytic agents for PE include alteplase (Activase), streptokinase, and urokinase. Alteplase is considered the fastest-acting safe infusion; streptokinase, the slowest-acting infusion, is no longer used for PE (Feied, 2003). Weaknesses of thrombolytic therapy include cost, increased risk of hemorrhage, and limited use when surgery may be indicated.

19. Describe management of PE.

Inferior Vena Cava Interruption and Filters

Ligation and clips can be used for IVC interruption, but the Greenfield filter is often preferred. The complication rate for IVC filters that is placed transvenously under fluoroscopy is low, but venous stasis can occur. IVC interruption and IVC filters prevent recurrences of major PE but not minor recurrent events or emboli that may generate from sites other than the lower extremities.

Pulmonary Embolectomy

According to Hyers and colleagues (1998), pulmonary embolectomy should be reserved for emergency treatment of PE by an experienced cardiac surgical team. Shock and cardiac arrest account for the high operative mortality rates that range from 10% to 75% with cardiopulmonary bypass standby and 50% to 94% in patients with cardiac arrest.

Candidates may have the following parameters: (1) massive PE (affects more than 50% of the pulmonary circulation), (2) shock and hemodynamically unstable condition despite resuscitative and anticoagulant therapy, and (3) a contraindication for, or failed, thrombolytic therapy. Postoperative complications include severe neurologic defects, acute respiratory distress syndrome, acute renal failure, and mediastinitis (Hyers et al, 1998).

PULMONARY EMBOLISM

References

Brashers, V. L. (2002). Alterations of pulmonary function. In K. L. McCance & S. E. Huether (Eds.), *Pathophysiology: The biologic basis for disease in adults and children* (4th ed., pp. 1105-1144). St Louis: Mosby.

Chestnutt, M. & Prendergast, T. (2002). Lung. In L. Tierney, S. McPhee, & M. Papadakis (Eds.), *Current medical diagnosis and treatment: Adult ambulatory and inpatient management* (pp. 332-341). New York, NY: McGraw-Hill.

Clagett, G. P., et al. (1998). Prevention of venous thromboembolism. *Chest, 114*(5, Suppl.), 531S-561S.

Erdman, S. M., Rodvold, K. A., & Friedenberg, W. R. (1997). Thromboembolic disorders. In J. T. DiPiro, R. L. Talbert, G. C. Yee, G. R. Matzke, B. G. Wells, & L. M. Posey (Eds.), *Pharmacotherapy: A pathophysiologic approach* (3rd ed., pp. 399-433). Stamford, CT: Appleton & Lange.

Fedullo, P. (2000). Pulmonary embolism and deep venous thrombosis. In W. Shoemaker, S. Ayers, A. Grenvik, & P. Holbrook (Eds.), *Textbook of critical care* (4th ed., pp. 1493-1508). Philadelphia: Saunders.

Feied, C. (2003).Venous thrombosis and pulmonary embolism. In J. Marx, et al (Eds.), *Rosen's emergency medicine: Concepts and clinical practice* (5th ed., pp. 1210-1234). St Louis: Mosby.

Ferri, F. (2003). *Ferri's clinical advisor: Instant diagnosis and treatment* (pp. 682-683, 800-801). St Louis: Mosby.

Gallus, A., Hirsch, J., Tuttle, R. (2001). Prevention of fatal post-operative pulmonary embolism by low doses of heparin. *Chest* 119(Suppl): 645-945.

Galvin, J. G. & Choi, B. S. (1999). Clinical presentation pulmonary embolus [WWW document]. www.vh.org/Providers/Tesxtbooks/ElectricPE/Text/ClinPresent.html.

Geerts, W., et al. (2001). Prevention of venous thromboembolism. *Chest 119*(Suppl): 132S-175S.

Gossage, J. (2003). Pulmonary embolism. In R. Rakel & E. Bope (Eds.), *Conn's current therapy 2003* (55th ed., pp. 262-265). Philadelphia: Saunders.

Graber, M. A. (1999). Pulmonary medicine: Pulmonary embolism and deep vein thrombosis [WWW document]. www.vh.org/Providers/ClinRef/FPHandbook/Chapter03/01-3.html.

Guyatt, G., et al. (2001). Grades of recommendation for antithrombotic agents. *Chest 119*(Suppl), 3S-7S.

Hirsh, J., et al. (1998a). Oral anticoagulants: Mechanism of action, clinical effectiveness, and optimal therapeutic range. *Chest, 114*(5, Suppl), 445S-469S.

Hirsh, J. & Hoak, J. (1996). Management of deep vein thrombosis and pulmonary embolism [WWW document]. www.americanheart.org/Scientific/statements/1996/069601.html.

Hirsh, J., et al. (1998b). Heparin and low-molecular-weight heparin. *Chest, 114*(5, Suppl), 489S-510S.

Hull, R., Pineo, G., & Raskob, G. (2000). In W. Shoemaker, S. Ayers, A. Grenvik, & P. Holbrook (Eds.), *Textbook of critical care* (4th ed., pp. 1744-1757). Philadelphia: Saunders.

Hyers, T. M., et al. (1998). Antithrombotic therapy for venous thromboembolic disease. *Chest, 114* (5, Suppl), 561S-578S.

Konstadt, S. (1999). Diagnostic dilemma [WWW document]. www.jcardioanesthesia.com/abs13_1/v13n1p105.html (visited March 17, 1999).

Langdale, L. (2002). In K. Bland, et al. (Eds.), *The practice of general surgery* (pp. 201-206). Philadelphia: W. B. Saunders.

Launius, B. K. & Graham, B. D. (1998). Understanding and preventing deep vein thrombosis and pulmonary embolism. *AACN Clinical Issues, 9*(1), 91-99.

Lipchik, R. J. & Presberg, K. W. (2001). Venous thromboembolism and pulmonary hypertensive diseases. In J. Noble, H. L. Green, W. Levinson, G. A. Modest, C.D. Mulrow, J. E. Scherger, & M. J. Young (Eds.), *Textbook of primary care medicine* (3rd ed., pp. 728-739). St Louis: Mosby.

Nutescu, E. (2002). Antithrombotic therapy for the prevention of venous thromboembolism. *U.S. pharmacist: The journal for pharmacists' education. Health Systems Edition, 27*(11), HS-65- HS-76.

Rodgers, M. L. (1999). Common respiratory problems: Pulmonary embolism, pneumothorax, and thoracic pulmonary surgery. In L. Bucher & S. Melander (Eds.), *Critical care nursing* (pp. 465-507). Philadelphia: W. B. Saunders.

Shorr, A.F. (2002). Pulmonary embolism: What have we learned since Virchow? *Chest, 122*, 1801-1817.

Simmons, E. (2002). Antithrombotic therapy. In Urden, L.D., Stacy, K.M., & Lough, M.E. *Thelan's critical care nursing: Diagnosis and management* (4th ed.). St. Louis: Mosby, (pp. 905-923).

Sue, D. & Vintch, J. (2002). Pulmonary disease. In F. Bongard & D. Sue (Eds.), *Current critical care: Diagnosis and treatment* (2nd ed., pp. 585-603). New York: McGraw-Hill.

Swearingen, P. & Keen, J. (2001). *Manual of critical care nursing: Nursing interventions and collaborative management* (4th ed., pp. 232-239). St Louis: Mosby.

Urden, L. D., Stacy, K. M, & Lough, M. E. (Eds.). (2002). *Thelan's critical care nursing: Diagnosis and management* (4th ed.). St Louis: Mosby.

10

Pulmonary Contusion

Judith A. Halstead, RN, MSN, DNS
Sheila Drake Melander, RN, DSN, ACNP-C, FCCM

Mr. Harrison, a 23-year-old, was involved in a late-night motor vehicle accident when he apparently fell asleep at the wheel. His car left the road, striking a tree head-on at approximately 35 miles per hour. He was not wearing a seatbelt. Mr. Harrison was arousable at the scene and slightly disoriented, but able to follow commands. He complained of chest and back pain. Oxygen at 2 L via nasal cannula and two peripheral intravenous (IV) lines were started before the patient was transported to the nearest hospital. On arrival at the emergency department, Mr. Harrison was alert and cooperative but anxious. He was able to communicate without difficulty and complained of right-sided chest pain, which he described as "rib pain," and some slight difficulty breathing. Marked ecchymosis in the right chest area with medial to lateral progression was noted. The following are his diagnostic data on admission:

BP	176/94 mm Hg	pH	7.43
HR	138 bpm, regular	Po_2	100 mm Hg
Respirations	32 breaths/min and	Pco_2	37 mm Hg
	slightly labored	K^+	3.1 mEq/L
Temperature	37.2° C (99° F)		

Arterial blood gas measurements with the patient receiving 2 L of oxygen by nasal cannula were the following:

Hgb	12 g/dl
Hct	36.3 g/dl
WBCs	10,500 mm^3

The chest x-ray film revealed four fractured ribs on the right side and two fractured ribs on the left side and was otherwise unremarkable. Findings from computed tomography (CT) scans of the head, chest, and abdomen were normal, and findings from the electrocardiogram were normal except for a sinus tachycardia. Physical examination revealed symmetric chest expansion, a midline trachea, bruising of the right chest and flank, and some facial bruising. Auscultation of the lungs revealed fine crackles in the right lung and clear breath sounds in the left lung field. Mr. Harrison was transferred to the telemetry unit for monitoring.

The physician ordered the following:

5% dextrose in 45% normal saline at 75 ml/hr
Clear liquids
Accurate intake and output
cefazolin 1 g IV q8h
Patient-controlled analgesia for pain: morphine sulfate 1 mg/1 ml, 1 mg every 10 minutes with lockout, not to exceed 20 mg in 4 hours
Repeat chest x-ray study in 12 hours

The repeat chest radiograph revealed patchy, irregular areas of density in the right lung indicative of a right pulmonary contusion. Mr. Harrison received education regarding the extent of his injuries and the potential dangers they may present. He was taught to use the incentive spirometer and instructed to use it hourly. Mr. Harrison progressed satisfactorily and was discharged from the hospital on the second day.

PULMONARY CONTUSION

QUESTIONS

1. Describe the mechanism of injury resulting in a pulmonary contusion.

2. Discuss the pathophysiology of a pulmonary contusion.

3. How is respiratory functioning affected by blunt chest trauma and the development of a pulmonary contusion?

4. What assessment findings may be indicative of a pulmonary contusion?

5. What laboratory and diagnostic methods are required for the diagnosis and monitoring of a pulmonary contusion?

6. What is the nurse's responsibility in the diagnosis of a pulmonary contusion?

7. What are the most common complications of a pulmonary contusion?

8. Describe the treatment for a patient who has a flail chest.

9. What nursing diagnoses might be appropriate for the care of a patient with a pulmonary contusion?

10. Identify the appropriate nursing interventions for a patient with a pulmonary contusion.

11. What discharge instructions would be appropriate for Mr. Harrison?

PULMONARY CONTUSION

QUESTIONS AND ANSWERS

1. Describe the mechanism of injury resulting in a pulmonary contusion.

Thoracic trauma leads to approximately 25% of the deaths resulting from trauma in the United States (Blank-Reid & Reid, 1999; Golden, 2000). Pulmonary contusions, which result from thoracic trauma, are usually the result of a blunt trauma and can be potentially life-threatening. The blunt forces causing pulmonary contusions are most commonly the result of motor vehicle accidents and falls (Johnson, 2000). Chest trauma rarely occurs in isolation, and the patient should be carefully assessed for associated injuries to other organs (Musto & Petersen, 1999; Yeo, 2001).

2. Discuss the pathophysiology of a pulmonary contusion.

Pulmonary contusions may be unilateral or bilateral depending upon the extent of the injury (Johnson, 2000). A pulmonary contusion usually develops as a result of a nonpenetrating, or blunt, chest injury. The rapid acceleration and deceleration that occur as the thorax comes into forcible contact with a blunt object or force (e.g., steering wheel, explosion) cause a disruption in the underlying pulmonary vasculature, tissue, and alveoli (Yeo, 2001). This disruption allows blood to enter the alveoli and interstitium, resulting in alveolar hemorrhage and interstitial edema. An inflammatory response develops at the level of the alveolar-capillary unit (Johnson, 2000; Yeo, 2001). The symptoms of a pulmonary contusion typically are insidious but progressive in nature. Evolution of symptoms may occur over a 24- to 48-hour period after an injury is sustained (Johnson, 2000). The nurse should suspect a pulmonary contusion in any patient who has experienced a blunt trauma, even in the absence of symptoms, and assess the patient accordingly. Interstitial edema can gradually develop, ultimately resulting in perfusion without ventilation, which leads to intrapulmonary shunting, hypoxemia, hypercapnia, and respiratory distress (Golden, 2000; Urden et al, 2002).

3. How is respiratory functioning affected by blunt chest trauma and the development of a pulmonary contusion?

Blunt chest trauma usually bruises the lung tissue; however, pulmonary tears or lacerations may be seen, especially if rib fractures are present. Rib fractures are the most frequent type of injury resulting from thoracic trauma, and can lead to hypoventilation (Lewis, 2000). Rib fractures have a mortality rate of 4% to 12% associated with them (Bansidhar, 2002), with certain rib fractures being more clinically significant. Fractures of the first, second, and third ribs are associated with a higher probability of injury to underlying pulmonary, vascular, and neurologic structures (Laskowski-Jones, 1999). Multiple rib fractures are also more significant than single rib fractures (Johnson, 2000). Multiple rib fractures can lead to the development of a flail chest, in which the fractured rib fragments are no longer attached to the rib cage and instead "float" independently from the rest of the chest wall (Golden, 2000; Johnson, 2000). In a pulmonary contusion the initial chest injury results in internal pulmonary hemorrhage, accompanied by alveolar and interstitial edema. Disruption of the alveolar-capillary unit leads to increased pulmonary vascular resistance and decreased pulmonary blood flow. Decreased lung compliance can also develop. A ventilation-perfusion mismatch occurs with hypoxia and hypercapnia developing (Johnson, 2000). If complications develop, ventilatory support may be required. Atelectasis can develop in the area of injury as a result of hypoventilation and fluid retention, leading to respiratory infection and potential respiratory failure (Laskowski-Jones, 1999; Johnson, 2000). Although pulmonary contusion typically is a secondary diagnosis, close monitoring, assessment of the patient, and identification of subtle changes in the patient's condition are extremely important. Other significant injuries associated with blunt chest trauma, which may be present along with a pulmonary contusion, include pneumothorax; hemothorax; cardiac contusion; trachea, bronchi, or diaphragm trauma; and great vessel trauma (Laskowski-Jones, 1999; Golden, 2000).

4. What assessment findings may be indicative of a pulmonary contusion?

Physical findings may include chest wall bruising and abrasions (Musto & Petersen, 1999). A cough and hemoptysis may be present, with moist crackles auscultated in the area of the contusion (Johnson, 2000). Other findings may include pain, dyspnea, tachypnea, with decreased chest excursion and breath sounds due to hypoventilation (Alspach, 1998). The extent of respiratory distress will depend upon the extent of the contusion; mechanical ventilation may be required if the contusions are extensive (Musto & Petersen, 1999; Urden et al, 2002). When a pulmonary contusion occurs with a flail chest, paradoxical chest movement occurs with the fractured segment moving inward during inspiration and outward upon expiration. In addition, the patient will exhibit pain upon inspiration, dyspnea, tachypnea, and crepitus at the point of fracture (Golden, 2000).

5. What laboratory and diagnostic methods are required for the diagnosis and monitoring of a pulmonary contusion?

The diagnosis of a pulmonary contusion is based on physical examination, tissue oxygenation measures, and radiologic findings. Arterial blood gases will be obtained and continuous pulse oximetry will be implemented in patients who have experienced blunt thoracic trauma to aid in the detection of injury and impaired lung function (Musto & Petersen, 1999). The presence of arterial hypoxemia indicates impaired lung functioning (Johnson, 2000). The definitive diagnosis of a pulmonary contusion is made by chest x-ray. Initial chest x-ray findings upon admission may be normal. Patches of pulmonary infiltration will be evident approximately 24 to 48 hours following injury, as the contusion continues to evolve (Musto & Petersen, 1999; Johnson, 2000). Large areas of contusion may produce the appearance of a "white-out" on the chest x-ray (Laskowski-Jones, 1999). Thoracic CT may be more accurate than the standard chest x-ray in diagnosing blunt chest trauma in general, and pulmonary contusions specifically, and may be ordered in conjunction with the chest x-ray (Omert, 2001). A pulmonary contusion usually resolves within about 2 weeks without complications (Yeo, 2001).

6. What is the nurse's responsibility in the diagnosis of a pulmonary contusion?

The assessment of patients who have experienced blunt thoracic trauma requires expert clinical skills to diagnose the potential and actual health problems that may develop. Initial symptoms of a pulmonary contusion may be subtle or absent. Nurses need to be familiar with the signs, symptoms, and management of thoracic trauma to prevent further injury or death (Golden, 2000). The diagnosis of a pulmonary contusion can be delayed or overlooked because of a lack of immediate radiographic changes and the presence of other traumatic injuries. Through a thorough physical assessment, history taking, and careful monitoring of laboratory and diagnostic data, the nurse can (1) identify acute respiratory problems, (2) anticipate potential changes in the patient's condition, (3) understand the underlying pathophysiology of the signs and symptoms, and (4) develop an appropriate plan of care (Brooks-Brunn, 1999). The nurse should gather information about the nature of the trauma and systematically assess the chest. The anterior and posterior chest should be inspected for the presence of bruising, abrasions, and traumatic marks from blunt objects (e.g., seatbelt or steering wheel imprints). The nurse should also inspect the chest wall for symmetrical excursion and note the quality of the patient's respirations. The trachea should be examined for any deviation from midline. Lung sounds should be auscultated to detect diminished, absent, or adventitious breath sounds. Percussion over normal lung tissue produces resonance. Dullness upon percussion of the lungs indicates the presence of fluid or consolidation. The presence of a pneumothorax will produce a hyperresonant sound. The nurse should also closely monitor the patient for developing hypoxemia, keeping in mind that initial changes in the patient's condition may be very subtle, such as restlessness or anxiety. With prompt diagnosis and treatment, the majority of pulmonary contusions resolve without complication.

7. What are the most common complications of a pulmonary contusion?

Because of chest pain or accompanying injuries such as rib fractures or a pneumothorax, patients with pulmonary contusions tend to breathe shallowly and have an impaired cough. This can lead to the development of atelectasis, infection, and pneumonia (Johnson, 2000; Urden et al, 2002). Adequate pain management, proper positioning, and use of incentive spirometry can help decrease the incidence of pneumonia.

Another potential complication of thoracic trauma is acute respiratory distress syndrome (ARDS) (Davies, 2002). Research studies have indicated that there is a direct relationship between pulmonary contusions and ARDS, with the risk increasing if the area of the contusion is larger than 20% of the lung tissue (Miller et al, 2002).

8. Describe the treatment for a patient who has a flail chest.

The major goal of treatment for the patient who has a flail chest is to promote and maintain optimal tissue oxygenation (Lewis, 2000). Specific treatment and nursing interventions for a patient who has a flail chest include:

1. Anticipating the need for endotracheal intubation and mechanical ventilation (Lewis, 2000)
2. Administering crystalloid IV fluids (Lewis, 2000) at a rate that maintains a urine output of 30 ml/hr, and normal hemodynamic values, being careful not to overhydrate the client (Harrahill, 1998)
3. Managing pain through the use of patient-controlled analgesia, an epidural catheter, or intercostal nerve block (Harrahill, 1998)
4. Implementing aggressive pulmonary physiotherapy through the use of incentive spirometry, turning, and postural drainage, suctioning, early ambulation, and "huff" coughing (Harrahill, 1998)

9. What nursing diagnoses might be appropriate for the care of a patient with a pulmonary contusion?

Nursing diagnoses appropriate for the care of the patient with pulmonary contusion include the following:

- Ineffective airway clearance related to decreased pulmonary compliance
- Impaired gas exchange related to interstitial hemorrhage
- Ineffective breathing pattern related to decreased pulmonary compliance
- Anxiety related to unusual muscular effort required for breathing
- Activity intolerance related to hypoxemia

10. Identify the appropriate nursing interventions for a patient with a pulmonary contusion.

The following nursing interventions are appropriate for the care of a patient with a pulmonary contusion (Urden & Stacy, 2000):

1. Maintaining the patient's arterial blood gases through supportive oxygen therapy, and when indicated, maintaining mechanical ventilation with positive end-expiratory pressure setting
2. Positioning the patient in a semi-Fowler's or high Fowler's position to decrease pressure on the diaphragm and increase inspiratory capacity
3. Assisting the patient with deep-breathing exercises and incentive spirometry hourly
4. Positioning the patient who has unilateral chest trauma with the injured side up to improve ventilation-perfusion; if chest trauma is bilateral, position the patient with the right lung down to improve perfusion to the largest area of lung tissue

5. Achieving adequate pain control to decrease hypoventilation and development of atelectasis
6. Monitoring the patient closely for complications, especially the development of ARDS and pneumonia

11. What discharge instructions would be appropriate for Mr. Harrison?

Discharge instructions for the patient with a pulmonary contusion must include information regarding potential changes in respiratory status. The patient should be instructed to report immediately to the physician any change in respiratory status such as tightness in the chest, increased sputum production, difficulty breathing deeply, or elevated temperature. Continued use of incentive spirometry, adequate fluid intake, and maintenance of mobility are other important self-care activities that the patient should implement at home to prevent the development of complications. It is crucial that patients understand that any change in respiratory status, as identified previously, may be indicative of developing respiratory complications.

PULMONARY CONTUSION

References

Alspach, J. G. (1998). *American Association of Critical-Care Nurses core curriculum for critical care nursing* (5th ed.). Philadelphia: Saunders.

Bansidhar, B. J. (2002). Clinical rib fractures: Are follow-up chest x-rays a waste of resources? *The American Surgeon Atlanta, 68*(5), 449-455.

Blank-Reid, C. & Reid, P. (1999). Taking the tension out of traumatic pneumothoraxes. *Nursing, 29*(4), 41-47.

Brooks-Brunn, J. (1999). Respiratory assessment. In L. Bucher & S. Melander (Eds.), *Critical care nursing* (pp. 369-388). Philadelphia: Saunders.

Davies, P. (2002). Guarding your patient against ARDS. *Nursing, 32*(3), 36-42.

Golden, P. A. (2000). Thoracic trauma. *Orthopedic Nursing, 19*(5), 37-47.

Harrahill, M. (1998). Flail chest: A nursing challenge. *Journal of Emergency Nursing, 24*(3), 288-289.

Johnson, K. (2000). Trauma. In L. Urden & K. Stacy (Eds.), *Priorities in critical care nursing* (pp. 396-413). St Louis: Mosby.

Laskowski-Jones, L. (1999). Trauma. In L. Bucher & S. Melander (Eds.), *Critical care nursing* (pp. 1094-1095). Philadelphia: Saunders.

Lewis, S. M. (2000). Nursing management: Lower respiratory problems. In S. Lewis, M. Heitkemper, & S. Dirksen (Eds.), *Medical-surgical nursing: Assessment and management of clinical problems* (pp. 611-659). St Louis: Mosby.

Miller, P., Croce, M., Kilgo, P., Scott, J., & Fabian, T. (2002). Acute respiratory distress syndrome in blunt trauma: Identification of independent risk factors. *The American Surgeon Atlanta 68*(10), 845-854.

Musto, J. & Petersen, J. (1999). Blunt chest trauma. *Australian Nursing Journal, 6*(8), CU1-CU4.

Omert, L. (2001). Efficacy of thoracic computerized tomography in blunt chest trauma. *The American Surgeon Atlanta, 67*(7), 660-664.

Urden, L. & Stacy, K. (2000). Nursing management plan of care: Ineffective airway clearance and ineffective breathing pattern. In L. Urden & K. Stacy (Eds.), *Priorities in critical care nursing* (pp. 472-474). St Louis: Mosby.

Urden, L. D., Stacy, K. M., & Lough, M. E. (Eds.). (2002). *Thelan's critical care nursing: Diagnosis and management* (4th ed.). St Louis: Mosby.

Yeo, T. P. (2001). Long-term sequelae following blunt thoracic trauma. *Orthopedic Nursing, 20*(5), 35-47.

11

Chronic Obstructive Pulmonary Disease with Pneumonia

Sheila Drake Melander, RN, DSN, ACNP-C, FCCM

CASE PRESENTATION

Mr. Bryant, a 62-year-old retired coal miner, has been experiencing a productive cough off and on for approximately 3 years. He decided to come to the emergency department because he has had difficulty in his breathing pattern on exertion. He states that he has had several bouts of chest colds during the past few years, but this time he says that he "can't seem to shake this round." His wife states that he is allergic to penicillin.

During his history Mr. Bryant stated that he has smoked two packs of cigarettes a day for 25 years. Crackles were noted in the lower bases of his lungs, with an occasional expiratory wheeze. He also said that he had been running a low-grade fever for approximately 2 to 3 days and had experienced chills and general weakness. A chest x-ray film disclosed some consolidation in the right lower lobe. Bronchography revealed nonuniform tapering of the airway. The following are additional diagnostic data:

BP	158/98 mm Hg	Pco_2	54 mm Hg
HR	107 bpm	HCO_3^-	30 mmol/L
Respirations	32 breaths/min	WBCs	20,000 mm^3
Temperature	38.9° C (102° F)	Hct	56%
pH	7.25	Gram Stain	Negative
Po_2	52 mm Hg (with room air)		

As a result of Mr. Bryant's arterial blood gas (ABG) levels, he was given 28% oxygen with a Venturi mask. His ABG levels 30 minutes after placement of the mask were as follows:

pH	7.42	Pco_2	48 mm Hg
Po_2	58 mm Hg	HCO_3^-	30 mmol/L

On the basis of these data, Mr. Bryant's diagnosis was chronic obstructive pulmonary disease (COPD) with an acute exacerbation of chronic bronchitis. Sputum cultures revealed a gram-positive organism, *Streptococcus pneumoniae*. Mr. Bryant received erythromycin after a secondary diagnosis of pneumonia was made. He also received theophylline at this time.

Mr. Bryant's condition improved in response to the antibiotic and bronchodilator therapy. He was discharged 3 days later.

CHRONIC OBSTRUCTIVE PULMONARY DISEASE WITH PNEUMONIA

QUESTIONS

1. Discuss the pathophysiology involved in the diagnosis of COPD.

2. Mr. Bryant's diagnosis was chronic bronchitis. This is one of the medical diagnoses associated with COPD. Discuss chronic bronchitis and the other two medical diagnoses that belong to the COPD group.

3. Were Mr. Bryant's presenting symptoms among the classic signs and symptoms exhibited by patients with COPD? Compare and contrast symptoms associated with bronchitis and emphysema.

4. Why is Mr. Bryant's temperature of concern?

5. Why was a Venturi mask chosen as the route of administration for oxygen therapy?

6. Is the organism found in Mr. Bryant's sputum cultures a common finding in patients with COPD?

7. Why was Mr. Bryant given erythromycin?

8. What are the contributing factors for the development of pneumonia in Mr. Bryant's case? List other contributing factors along with signs and symptoms associated with pneumonia not present in Mr. Bryant's case.

9. What diagnostic tests are significant in the determination of a diagnosis of pneumonia?

10. Discuss the medical management for a patient who has pneumonia.

11. What is the goal of therapy with theophylline, and what special considerations exist with this treatment for Mr. Bryant?

12. What is the clinical significance of the pH reading, and what is the appropriate range of partial pressure of oxygen (P_{O_2}) values in the patient with COPD?

13. Why were steroids not ordered for Mr. Bryant?

14. Were Mr. Bryant's laboratory results consistent with those expected for a patient with COPD and pneumonia?

15. What other pulmonary function tests would have assisted in the diagnosis of Mr. Bryant's COPD?

16. Had Mr. Bryant's condition deteriorated and not responded to the bronchodilator and antibiotic therapy, what considerations concerning ventilatory management would be important?

17. Discuss the occurrence of pneumonia in patients with COPD.

18. What teaching considerations are of special concern for Mr. Bryant before his discharge?

CHRONIC OBSTRUCTIVE PULMONARY DISEASE WITH PNEUMONIA

QUESTIONS AND ANSWERS

1. Discuss the pathophysiology involved in the diagnosis of COPD.

As stated by Bucher and Melander (1999), and Urden and associates (2002), COPD refers to a group of chronic diseases that obstruct airflow within the airways or the lung parenchyma. The description *chronic airflow limitation* may also be seen in the discussion of the patient with COPD. The disorders in the COPD group are as follows:

- Chronic bronchitis
- Emphysema
- Asthma

Asthma has been included in this listing, but it should be noted that with the increasing prevalence of asthma, some sources in the literature discuss asthma as a separate entity. COPD usually presents as a gradual decline in function, but an acute episode of respiratory failure can occur at any time because of the patient's lack of respiratory reserve. As described by Gawlinski and Hamwi (1999), dyspnea and hyperventilation are early signs of respiratory compromise in the patient with COPD.

Alspach (1998) and Urden and associates (2002) identified several factors in the pathogenesis of COPD:

- Tobacco use
- Air pollution
- Occupational exposure (coal miners; metal molders; workers handling stone, glass, or clay products; those who work with cotton or grain dust; firefighters; workers exposed to asbestos)
- Genetics

2. Mr. Bryant's diagnosis was chronic bronchitis. This is one of the medical diagnoses associated with COPD. Discuss chronic bronchitis and the other two medical diagnoses that belong to the COPD group.

Chronic Bronchitis

Chronic bronchitis is described as chronic cough and sputum production that is present for most days during at least 3 consecutive months for not less than 2 successive years (Heath & Mongia, 1998).

Pathophysiology

Production of mucus increases because of the enlargement of the bronchial mucus gland and an increase in the number of goblet cells. Other changes include inflammation of the bronchial and bronchiolar walls, loss of cilia, and the presence of mucus plugs. Physiologic changes are related to the narrowed airways. Chronic bronchitis is a disease of the central airways, and approximately 80% of the measurable airway resistance is in the central airways.

Bronchography shows the degree of tapering of the airway. The tapering is nonuniform, and the airway wall surfaces and outpouchings are irregular. It is believed that these changes account for the increased airway resistance seen in bronchitis. Functionally this resistance results in inspiratory and expiratory airflow obstruction, overinflation of the alveoli, and abnormal distribution of ventilation. The narrowed airway leads to overinflation of the alveoli with increased total lung capacity (TLC), increased residual volume (RV), and decreased vital capacity (VC) (Heath & Mongia, 1998; Madison & Irwin, 1998; Stein, 1998).

Emphysema

Emphysema is the abnormal enlargement of the air spaces distal to the terminal bronchioles, accompanied by nonuniformity in the pattern of respiratory airspace enlargement and destruction of the alveolar walls (Alspach, 1998; Stein, 1998; Urden et al, 2002).

Genetics

One cause of emphysema is a deficiency of a serum protein called α_1-protease inhibitor. Patients with decreased circulatory levels of this serum protein are predisposed to early development of emphysema. Two cells are seen in the inflammatory responses in the lungs: alveolar macrophages and polymorphonuclear leukocytes (PMNs). These cells manufacture elastase, the enzyme capable of breaking down elastin. PMNs are believed to be the major source of elastase in the lung. Most people also have an elastase *inhibitor* in the lung, which allows a balance between elastase and its inhibitor. When this balance is disturbed, either by an increase in elastase or a decrease in the inhibitor, damage to the alveolar walls occurs, resulting in emphysema (Alspach, 1998; Stein, 1998; Bucher & Melander, 1999).

Pathology

Emphysema destroys the alveolar walls and enlarges the air spaces distal to the terminal bronchioles. The portion of the lung distal to the terminal bronchioles—the acinus— comprises the functional units of the lung.

The loss of airway support contributes to airway narrowing because airways collapse on expiration. This loss of alveolar wall and reduction in elastic recoil also contribute to increased lung compliance, decreased driving pressure on expiration and subsequent hyperinflation, and increased RVs. Ultimately the surface area available for gas exchange decreases, causing alterations in diffusing capacities and ventilation-perfusion ($\dot{V}/\dot{Q}$) abnormalities. These abnormalities lead to the hypoxemia seen in emphysema.

Asthma

Asthma is a chronic disease of variable severity characterized by airway hyperactivity and airway narrowing of a reversible nature caused by bronchospasms. The bronchospasms cause air trapping, $\dot{V}/\dot{Q}$ mismatching, prolonged expiration acidosis, hypercapnia, and cough production of thick sputum. The lungs become stiff and overinflated and thus increase the workload of breathing. Intrathoracic pressure increases, thus decreasing venous return and cardiac output (Alspach, 1998; Niederman & Peters, 1998; Urden et al, 2002).

3. **Were Mr. Bryant's presenting symptoms among the classic signs and symptoms exhibited by patients with COPD? Compare and contrast symptoms associated with bronchitis and emphysema.**

Clinical Manifestations of Bronchitis

- Onset varies; symptoms are usually insidious.
- Cough and sputum production are present.
- Symptoms appear in patients in their 40s and 50s.
- Disability from the disease occurs in patients during their late 50s and early 60s.
- Patients have a history of frequent chest colds.
- Increased purulent sputum production is present.
- Dyspnea worsens as the disease progresses.
- Infections exacerbate the disease.
- Severe derangements in the $\dot{V}/\dot{Q}$ ratios may be seen later in the disease.
- Patients are characterized as a "blue bloaters."
- Low minute volumes are seen.
- Arterial hypoxemia and hypercapnia develop.
- Patients are usually stocky or obese.
- Central and peripheral cyanosis is seen.

- Wheezing may be present.
- Crackles (rales) may be present because of secretions.
- Pulmonary hypertension is present.
- Cor pulmonale is seen.
- Polycythemia is present.
- Hypoxemia and hypercapnia with compensated respiratory acidosis are seen.

Clinical Manifestations of Emphysema

- Signs and symptoms vary.
- Progressive expiratory flow obstruction and overinflation are seen.
- Dyspnea with exertion is seen at the beginning with dyspnea at rest as the disease progresses.
- Some patients have slow progression of disease; others rapidly become significantly disabled.
- Patients with advanced disease show enlargement of the anteroposterior diameter of the chest, dorsal kyphosis, elevated ribs, and wide costal angle (barrel chest).
- Patients have a thin physique with muscle wasting.
- Acyanotic unproductive minimal cough is seen.
- In later stages of disease, patients show signs and symptoms of right-sided ventricular failure (cor pulmonale).
- Accessory muscles are used for breathing.
- Patients may breathe through pursed lips with prolonged expiration ("pink puffers").
- Percussion shows increased resonance (hyperresonance) because of the increased lung volumes.
- Breath sounds are decreased and difficult to hear.
- Heart sounds are distant because of barrel chest.
- Expiratory wheezes may be present.
- Normal ABG values are seen in mild to moderate emphysema; in advanced emphysema, the P_{O_2} is commonly decreased and partial pressure of carbon dioxide (P_{CO_2}) is increased.
- Hypoxemia is greatest while patients are sleeping.

Often patients with emphysema are seen in the intensive care unit (ICU) as a result of infection, heart failure, pulmonary embolism, pneumothorax, bronchospastic episodes, gastrointestinal tract bleeding, or metabolic abnormalities. Some patients require medical attention because they changed the dosages of their medications without the physician's knowledge. Other patients are unable to maintain their medication regimens because of coughing, nausea, or vomiting. These patients sometimes require a change in their oxygen dosage, which may also trigger acute respiratory failure (Alspach, 1998; Stein, 1998; Gawlinski & Hamwi, 1999).

Common Findings in the ICU

- Cough and fatigue
- Mental confusion
- Irritability and lethargy
- Accessory muscle use
- Tachycardia
- Hypoxia
- Crackles, wheezes, or stridor or consolidation
- Cor pulmonale
- Oxygen saturation greater than 70% (acceptable if patient has adequate cardiac output)

Because of increased pulmonary vascular pressure, patients with COPD have increased pulmonary artery systolic, diastolic, and mean pressures (Alspach, 1998; Gawlinski & Hamwi, 1999; Urden et al, 2002).

The usual clinical findings for COPD are as follows:

- Significant and progressive reduction in expiration of airflow as measured by the forced expiratory volume (FEV_1)
- Varying degrees of exertional dyspnea
- Chronic cough and sputum production
- Decreased ABG values, hypoxemia, and hypercapnia with compensated respiratory acidosis
- Polycythemia

The bottom line becomes the following:

- The degree of airflow obstruction as measured by FEV_1
- The patient's age at the time of diagnosis
- The degree of reversibility
- The rate of change in the FEV over time

A higher prevalence of COPD is reported in men than in women, and mortality rates are related to socioeconomic status. It is estimated that as many as 35% of patients in the ICU have COPD (Eller et al, 1998; Madison & Irwin, 1998; Stein, 1998; Global Initiative for Chronic Obstructive Lung Disease [GOLD], 2001; Institute for Clinical Systems Improvement [ICSI], 2001; Snow et al, 2001).

4. Why is Mr. Bryant's temperature of concern?

Carbon dioxide and oxygen consumption increase as much as 10% for each degree Fahrenheit rise in temperature; thus treatment for an elevated temperature is recommended to prevent additional strain on the respiratory system (Stein, 1998; Bucher & Melander, 1999).

5. Why was a Venturi mask chosen as the route of administration for oxygen therapy?

The Venturi mask allows for precise delivery of oxygen. This is extremely important for the patient with COPD because of the "hypoxic drive." The goal of oxygen therapy is to keep the PaO_2 below 60 mm Hg and the $PaCO_2$ at a level to maintain pH within normal limits (Bucher & Melander, 1999).

6. Is the organism found in Mr. Bryant's sputum cultures a common finding in patients with COPD?

In discussing pneumonia, it is common to see it addressed as community-acquired pneumonia (CAP) and hospital-acquired pneumonia (HAP). Common causes of CAP include *S. pneumoniae, Haemophilus influenzae, Staphylococcus aureus,* anaerobic bacteria, *Moraxella catarrhalis, Klebsiella pneumoniae,* and *Legionella.* HAP is usually bacterial in origin and can include the following organisms: *Escherichia coli, K. pneumoniae,* Enterobacteriaceae, *Pseudomonas aeruginosa, S. aureus,* and *Serratia.* Pathogens may reach the lung in patients with CAP as a result of aspiration of gastric or oropharyngeal secretions into the lower respiratory tract.

One of the most common causes of bacterial pneumonia is *S. pneumoniae,* a gram-positive coccus. It is spread through droplets or airborne nuclei. The mortality rate is 50% for patients who are debilitated.

Nosocomial pneumonia is a concern for the hospitalized patient. Nosocomial pneumonia (gram-negative organisms) has been cited as one of the most commonly reported hospital-acquired infections (Gawlinski & Hamwi, 1999; Lucas et al, 1999; Grossman and Fein, 2000; Institute for Clinical Systems Improvement [ICSI], 2002).

7. Why was Mr. Bryant given erythromycin?

Mr. Bryant's respiratory status as evidenced by his chest radiograph and his arterial blood gas values made hospitalization necessary. However, many patients with CAP are treated as outpatients. This trend results from the growing necessity to contain medical costs and the increasing number of effective oral antibiotics. Because of the development of antibiotic-resistant strains of bacteria, the need for continued development of new agents is still important. As stated by Lucas and coworkers (1999), the increasing availability of effective antibiotics has caused controversy over first-line therapy. In its current guidelines, the Infectious Diseases Society of America (IDSA) as well as the Institute for Clinical Systems Improvement (2002) recommend a macrolide such as erythromycin, clarithromycin, or azithromycin. A newer fluoroquinolone and doxycycline were listed as the preferred agents for empiric outpatient therapy for CAP. Alternative first-line options include amoxicillin/clavulanate and some second- and third-generation cyclosporines, specifically cefuroxime. According to the IDSA, the choice for empiric therapy should be based on many patient variables, including the following:

- Severity of illness
- Antimicrobial intolerance
- Patient's age
- Comorbidities
- Concomitant medications
- Epidemiologic setting

The popularity of the macrolide erythromycin has grown because it is an excellent agent against atypical causes of CAP, which are increasingly being reported.

8. What are the contributing factors for the development of pneumonia in Mr. Bryant's case? List other contributing factors along with signs and symptoms associated with pneumonia not present in Mr. Bryant's case.

Contributing factors in Mr. Bryant's case were his frequent chest colds. Crackles were noted in the lower bases of the lung and an occasional expiratory wheeze. Mr. Bryant also had a low-grade fever for 2 to 3 days and an elevated white blood cell count, general weakness, and chills. The sputum culture showed *S. pneumoniae,* which confirmed the diagnosis of pneumonia. A chest x-ray study also revealed consolidation in the lower lung bases.

As noted by Bucher and Melander (1999), Bartlett and associates (2000), and Urden and colleagues (2002), the following have been identified as contributing factors for the development of pneumonia:

- Tracheal intubation
- Decreased level of consciousness (allowing for aspiration)
- Underlying chronic lung disorder
- Endotracheal intubation (bypasses upper airway and host defense mechanisms)
- Suctioning (creates mechanical irritation or injury to the mucosa, predisposing the lungs to inoculation and colonization of bacteria)

Signs and symptoms of bacterial pneumonia include the following:

- Sudden onset, including shaking, chills, and fever of 38.9° to 40.6° C (102° to 105° F)
- Cough initially dry, becoming productive and producing sputum that is rusty in color at first and then yellow-green (rusty color from a mixture of red blood cells and inflammatory cells in infected alveoli)
- Malaise, weakness
- Headache, myalgia
- Cyanosis (depending on the degree of respiratory compromise)
- Altered mental state in elderly patients
- Coarse inspiratory rales
- Friction rub may be present
- Pleuritic chest pain
- Either lobar consolidation or scattered interstitial infiltrates seen on the chest radiograph

9. **What diagnostic tests are significant in the determination of a diagnosis of pneumonia?**

The following tests are necessary for the diagnosis of pneumonia:

- Vital signs
- Blood cultures
- Sputum cultures (avoid collecting saliva; may have colonization)
- Chest radiographs
- ABG values
- Electrolyte values
- Electrocardiogram
- Hemoglobin and hematocrit
- Rales
- Respirations greater than 20

Therapy is based on results obtained from Gram stain and sputum cultures (Stein, 1998; Bucher & Melander, 1999; Bartlett et al, 2000; ICSI, 2002; Urden et al, 2002).

10. **Discuss the medical management for a patient who has pneumonia.**

All patients admitted to the hospital will be exposed to pathogens that make them candidates for acquiring pneumonia; prevention is the number one priority. The following criteria must be considered in the management of the patient with pneumonia (Stein, 1998; Bucher & Melander, 1999; Bartlett et al, 2000; Urden et al, 2002):

- Identification of risk factors and susceptible patient populations
- Aseptic technique, including hand washing and handling of respiratory equipment to prevent cross-contamination to susceptible patients
- Administration of antibiotic therapy
- Use of humidified oxygen
- Use of chest physical therapy
- Frequent turning, coughing, and deep breathing
- Assessment of airway protective mechanisms (cough, gag, and swallowing reflexes)
- Elevation of the head of the bed to decrease gastric reflux and facilitate swallowing and postural drainage
- Careful and frequent assessment of temperature, heart rate, respirations, chest sounds, respiratory effort, and use of accessory muscles with breathing; frequent chest x-ray studies
- Use of suctioning
- Assessment of patient's total volume fluid status
- Monitoring of fluid and electrolytes
- Use of bronchodilators

11. **What is the goal of therapy with theophylline, and what special considerations exist with this treatment for Mr. Bryant?**

Therapeutic blood levels of the theophylline compounds must be monitored closely in patients with COPD. Smokers tend to metabolize theophylline *faster* than nonsmokers, and patients with liver or cardiac disease metabolize theophylline *slower,* so dosages must be individualized.

The goal with theophylline therapy is to maintain a blood level of 10 to 20 µg/ml. Theophylline preparations have been used widely as bronchodilators for patients with COPD for more than 30 years. Theophylline treatment for patients with COPD has been analyzed by Van Andel and colleagues (1999). The consensus of a multicenter study of 3720 patients with COPD was that theophylline in selected patients continues to yield a beneficial respiratory effect especially if combined with an inhaled β-agonist. The study revealed that use of inhaled corticosteroids (CCSs) for the management of COPD has gained acceptance, although their role remains undetermined. Evidence from the 3720 patients revealed that the use of inhaled CCSs is widespread in patients with COPD and that the use of theophylline is declining.

12. What is the clinical significance of the pH reading, and what is the appropriate range of partial pressure of oxygen (Po_2) values in the patient with COPD?

Normal values for the patient with COPD are as follows:

Pao_2	<60 mm Hg
$Paco_2$	>50 mm Hg

As stated by Stein (1998), pH is the key to diagnosis. A severely acidotic range of 0.25 or less is often given as the marker for acute respiratory failure with increases in carbon dioxide and decreases in oxygen. The goal of oxygen therapy is to keep the Pao_2 between 55 and 65 mm Hg. In this range, saturation of hemoglobin is optimal without disruption of the "hypoxic drive" stimulus. Oxygen for the patient with COPD is delivered by Venturi mask, nasal cannula, rebreathing mask, and mechanical ventilation (Urden et al, 2002).

COPD increases pulmonary vascular pressures (pulmonary artery systolic and pulmonary artery diastolic), and the pulmonary artery pressure is 5 to 20 mm Hg higher than the pulmonary capillary wedge pressure. (Normally these two readings are within 1 to 2 mm Hg of each other.) Mechanical ventilators generate falsely elevated readings, and this is especially true when positive end-expiratory pressure (PEEP) is used.

13. Why were steroids not ordered for Mr. Bryant?

The use of steroids remains controversial. Practitioners use these agents more for the care of the patient with asthma than for the management of patients with chronic bronchitis. When steroids are used, patients should be monitored for side effects of short-term therapy, such as hyperglycemia, worsening hypertension, osteoporosis, cataracts, and opportunistic infections.

Steroids such as methylprednisolone (Solu-Medrol) are used intravenously for 1 to 2 days, followed by oral prednisone in increasingly lower dosages until a maintenance dosage is reached. Aerosol delivery of steroids has not proved effective. Because COPD is not primarily a disease of airway inflammation, it is less responsive to systemic steroids. The primary benefit of the use of steroids is their antiinflammatory effect (Hafner & Ferro, 1998).

14. Were Mr. Bryant's laboratory results consistent with those expected for a patient with COPD and pneumonia?

Usual Laboratory and Diagnostic Findings

Po_2	Decreased
Hct	Often elevated
Pco_2	Normal or elevated
Cor pulmonale	Increased neck vein distention, enlarged liver, and edema; common α_1-antiprotease phenotype
Recoil of lung	Normal

Chest X-Ray Films

Chest x-ray films usually are normal in patients who have chronic bronchitis and no complications. Classic findings seen in later stages are flattening of the diaphragm, hyperlucency, decreased vascular markings, widening of the rib spaces, and increased anteroposterior diameter (reflects hyperinflation).

ABG Levels

ABG levels may be normal in patients with mild to moderate emphysema. In advanced emphysema, the most common abnormality is decreased Po_2. Pco_2 levels may be normal or increased, especially when infection is present (Stein, 1998; Bucher & Melander, 1999; Urden et al, 2002).

15. What other pulmonary function tests would have assisted in the diagnosis of Mr. Bryant's COPD?

The following pulmonary function test results assist in diagnosing COPD:

- Increased RV and functional residual capacity
- Decreased VC
- Increased TLC
- Decreased diffusing capacity
- FEV_1 and ratio of FEV_1 to forced vital capacity decrease as the severity of COPD increases
- Flow-volume loop showing caved appearance

Pulmonary function tests with spirometry usually demonstrate normal findings. These may show an increased RV and a mild reduction in VC consistent with the degree of hyperinflation (Stein, 1998; Kamholz, 1999; Snow et al, 2001; Urden et al, 2002).

16. Had Mr. Bryant's condition deteriorated and not responded to the bronchodilator and antibiotic therapy, what considerations concerning ventilatory management would be important?

Ventilatory Management

Use of a ventilator allows the patient with COPD to rest and allows deep suctioning. The problem with ventilator use with this patient population is the difficulty of weaning patients from ventilator use.

Stein (1998), Bucher and Melander (1999), and Urden and colleagues (2002), state that when a patient is weaned from the ventilator, three areas must be monitored: oxygenation, carbon dioxide elimination, and mechanical efficiency. Some general guidelines for weaning that may be helpful to the clinician include the following:

- Oxygen concentration less than 50%
- PEEP less than 5 cm H_2O
- Respiratory rate less than 30 breaths/min
- Minute ventilation less than 10 L/min (volume of air patient breathes at rest)
- Low dynamic static pressures (compliance of at least 35 cm H_2O)
- Adequate ABG levels with the aforementioned guidelines

The current clinical practice for weaning is to use T-pieces or continuous positive airway pressure, alternating with full ventilator support such as synchronized intermittent mandatory ventilation or assist control. Pressure support is another mechanism for decreasing ventilator use while offering consistent internal alveoli support. The choice of weaning method will depend on the patient's underlying respiratory disorder and physical and psychologic responses to the weaning process. Patients who experience difficulty in weaning from the ventilator may benefit from techniques such as inspiratory resistance training, physical therapy, hypnosis, biofeedback, and pharmacologic support (Bucher & Melander, 1999).

17. Discuss the occurrence of pneumonia in patients with COPD.

Pneumonia occurs in 10% to 40% of intubated patients, requiring mechanical ventilation for more than 24 hours, and has a mortality rate of 30% to 70%. It should be noted that changes seen on the chest radiograph can be subtle and that establishing a specific cause may be difficult. Sputum cultures may be misleading, but gram-negative, antibiotic-resistant pathogens such as *P. aeruginosa* are the most prevalent, occurring in 20% to 30% of patients who have pneumonia and are being mechanically ventilated.

Although not all cases of pneumonia require combination antibiotic therapy, pneumonia caused by *Pseudomonas, Serratia, Acinetobacter,* or *Xanthomonas* does require this approach. In these patients, either an antipseudomonal penicillin or a third-generation cephalosporin and aminoglycoside are suggested.

Pneumococcal pneumonia may take some time to resolve, with consolidation in the lungs taking up to 6 weeks to clear. A chest radiograph of the patient with pneumococcal pneumonia will reveal consolidation manifested by dullness to percussion and increased fremitus (palpable vibrations transmitted through the bronchopulmonary system to the chest wall when the patient speaks). Mortality is related more often to concomitant host disease than to the type of gram-negative organism.

Staphylococcal pneumonia has an insidious onset in the chronically ill. High fever and chills may last up to 1 week in severe cases despite the use of antibiotics. Cough with blood-tinged sputum and tachypnea with cyanosis occur early in the course of the disease. Pneumonia caused by gram-negative bacteria has a highly variable course. It may progress slowly or rapidly over a few days. Patients will have a fever, a productive cough of purulent sputum, and pleuritic chest pain.

A vaccine is available for pneumococcal pneumonia. It is recommended prophylactically for high-risk groups, including elderly patients and those with COPD, congestive heart failure, renal failure, alcoholism, cirrhosis, splenic dysfunction or splenectomy, Hodgkin's disease, myeloma, or other immunocompromised states. The vaccine can be repeated in 6 years if needed. Influenza vaccines are also available and are recommended for high-risk patient populations (Hafner & Ferro, 1998; Gawlinski & Hamwi, 1999; Bartlett et al, 2000; Grossman & Fein, 2000).

18. What teaching considerations are of special concern for Mr. Bryant before his discharge?

As stated by Hafner and Ferro (1998), and Urden and associates (2002), pulmonary function deteriorates more rapidly in smokers than in nonsmokers, and because smokers are subject to more respiratory infections, health care personnel must be relentless in encouraging patients to stop smoking. It is common for the patient to have smoking cessation relapses. The clinician should discuss this with his or her patients and tell them that it is possible to achieve lifelong cessation, but it is common for this to take multiple attempts. Smoking cessation should be discussed at each visit, with new cessation dates set each time as necessary.

Patients with advanced pulmonary disease who stop smoking at age 65 years have an increased survival rate over those patients who continue to smoke. Other therapies that promote smoking cessation, including nicotine replacements such as gum and transdermal and intranasal formulations and bupropion (an antidepressant) should also be explored.

Other areas that need to be addressed with the patient before discharge include the following:

- Good hydration and sputum mobilization
- Prevention of and avoidance of exposure to infection
- Annual prophylactic multivalent influenza vaccines and an *S. pneumoniae* vaccine (which can be repeated after 6 years if an inadequate response is noted, such as a decline in the pneumococcal antibody titers)
- Avoidance of exposure to sudden temperature changes
- Understanding of bronchodilation therapy, normal blood levels, and diet management
- Referral to a support group

CHRONIC OBSTRUCTIVE PULMONARY DISEASE WITH PNEUMONIA

References

Alspach, J. G. (Ed.). (1998). *American Association of Critical-Care Nurses: Core curriculum for critical care nursing* (5th ed.). Philadelphia: Saunders.

Bartlett, J., et al. (2000). Practice guidelines for the management of community-acquired pneumonia. *Clinical Infectious Disease, 31*(2), 347-382.

Bucher, L. & Melander, S. (1999). *Critical care nursing.* Philadelphia: Saunders.

Eller, J., et al. (1998). Infective exacerbations of chronic bronchitis: Relation between bacteriologic etiology and lung function. *Chest, 113*(6), 1542-1547.

Gawlinski, A. & Hamwi, D. (1999). *Acute care nurse practitioner clinical curriculum and certification review.* Philadelphia: Saunders.

Global Initiative for Chronic Obstructive Lung Disease (GOLD), World Health Organization (WHO), National Heart, Lung, and Blood Institute (NHLBI). 2001. Global strategies for the diagnosis, management, and prevention of chronic obstructive pulmonary disease. Bethesda, MD: Global Initiative for Chronic Obstructive Lung Disease, World Health Organization, National Heart, Lung, and Blood Institute.

Grossman, R. & Fein, A. (2000). Evidence-based assessment of diagnostic tests for ventilator-associated pneumonia. *Chest, 117*(Suppl 2), 177s-181s.

Hafner, J. P. & Ferro, T. (1998). Recent developments in the management of COPD. *Hospital Medicine, 34*(1), 20-30, 32-38.

Heath, J. & Mongia, R. (1998). Chronic bronchitis: Primary care management. *American Family Physician, 57*(10), 2365-2368.

Institute for Clinical Systems Improvement (ICSI). Chronic obstructive pulmonary disease. Bloomington, MN: Institute for Clinical Systems Improvement (ICSI): 2001, December.

Institute for Clinical Systems Improvement (ICSI). Community-acquired pneumonia in adults. Bloomington, MN: Institute for Clinical Systems Improvement (ICSI): 2002, May.

Kamholz, S. (1999). Understanding pulmonary function tests. *The Clinical Advisor, 2*(9), 30-47.

Lucas, B., Armitage, B., Gross, P., & Yamauchi, T. (1999). Respiratory infections: Which antibiotics for empiric therapy? *Patient Care, 3*(1), 76-111.

Madison, J. & Irwin, R. (1998). Chronic obstructive pulmonary disease. *The Lancet, 352*(9126), 467-473.

Niederman, M. & Peters, S. (1998). Update in pulmonary medicine. *Annals of Internal Medicine, 128,* 208-215.

Snow, V., Lascher, S., & Motter-Pilson, C. (2001). Evidence base for management of acute exacerbations of chronic obstructive pulmonary disease. *Annals of Internal Medicine, 134*(7), 595-599.

Stein, J. (1998). *Internal medicine.* St Louis: Mosby.

Urden, L. D., Stacy, K. M., & Lough, M. E. (Eds.). (2002). *Thelan's critical care nursing: Diagnosis and management* (4th ed.). St Louis: Mosby.

Van Andel, A., Reisner, A., Menjoge, S., & Witek, T. (1999). Analysis of inhaled corticosteroid and oral theophylline use among patients with stable COPD from 1987 to 1995. *Chest, 15*(3), 703-707.

12

Acute Respiratory Distress Syndrome

Sharon West Angle, RN, BSN, MSN
Sheila Drake Melander, RN, DSN, ACNP-C, FCCM

CASE PRESENTATION

Postoperative Day 3

Mr. Gillian, a 62-year-old, 68 kg (150 lb) white man, had undergone an anterior colon resection for rectal polyps and had an uneventful postoperative course until the evening of the third postoperative day. He was monitored with telemetry and had no unusual complaints. At 10 PM on the third postoperative day, he began to complain of not feeling "right." Assessment of the patient revealed hypotension and shortness of breath. Within minutes he became confused and agitated. The shortness of breath worsened (he began gasping for air), and he experienced severe hypoxia. He was intubated and transferred to the intensive care unit (ICU). Initial assessment indicated the following:

BP	60/40 mm Hg	**pH**	7.3
HR	160 bpm	**Pco₂**	46 mm Hg
Respirations	12-35 breaths/min	**Po₂**	104 mm Hg
Temperature	38.8° C (101.8° F)	**HCO₃⁻**	22 mmol/L

On arrival in the ICU, mechanical ventilation in the synchronized intermittent mandatory ventilation (SIMV) mode was begun.

Fio₂	90%
SIMV Rate	6
Tidal Volume	800 ml

Mr. Gillian was given a 500 ml bolus of normal saline. He received dopamine (Intropin) 3 to 5 µg/kg/min for renal perfusion and was given vancomycin (Vancocin IV) 1 g intravenously (IV) every 12 hours for prophylaxis against staphylococcal infection. A pulmonary artery catheter (Swan-Ganz) was inserted, and the patient's pulmonary capillary wedge pressure was 12 mm Hg.

His fraction of inspired oxygen (Fio₂) increased from 90% to 100%, tidal volume (V_T) was 800 ml, and SIMV rate was 6 with total respiration of 16 breaths/min. At this time, a positive end-expiratory pressure (PEEP) of 5 cm H₂O was added, and he continued to receive pressure support of 7 cm H₂O. He was given several boluses of normal saline and continued to receive the dopamine infusion. The ventilator settings just outlined were

164

continued. The following arterial blood gas (ABG) values were obtained 2 hours after the ventilator settings were changed:

pH	7.42	Po_2	75.2 mm Hg
Pco_2	46 mm Hg	HCO_3^-	28.9 mmol/L

Postoperative Day 5

PEEP was increased to 10 cm H_2O, and V_T was increased to 1000 ml.

BP	130/60 mm Hg	pH	7.43
HR	120 bpm	Pco_2	46.2 mm Hg
Respirations	10 breaths/min	Po_2	86.8 mm Hg
Temperature	38.3° C (101° F)	HCO_3^-	30.5 mmol/L

After these changes, Mr. Gillian's oxygen levels gradually stabilized and he was weaned from ventilatory support. His urinary output also increased significantly after administration of the fluid boluses. Ten days after intubation, Mr. Gillian was extubated and received oxygen by nasal cannula.

ACUTE RESPIRATORY DISTRESS SYNDROME

QUESTIONS

1. What is ARDS?

2. Discuss the pathophysiologic changes associated with ARDS.

3. What are the pathophysiologic phases of ARDS?

4. How is ARDS diagnosed?

5. What are some medical complications seen with ARDS?

6. What laboratory findings are diagnostic for ARDS?

7. What radiologic changes are seen with ARDS?

8. What changes are seen in pulmonary function studies with ARDS?

9. Tissue hypoxia is a major finding in ARDS. Describe signs and symptoms found on assessment that would be seen with ARDS in the following systems: central nervous, pulmonary, cardiovascular, renal, and gastrointestinal/hepatic.

10. What is the goal of treatment for ARDS?

11. What are the principal treatments for ARDS? List and describe the types of ventilatory support available.

12. Describe nonventilatory means of pulmonary support.

13. What are some of the pharmacologic interventions used in ARDS?

14. What role does hemodynamic monitoring play in the management of ARDS?

15. Describe appropriate nursing diagnoses seen with ARDS.

16. What is the nurse's overall goal in caring for the patient with ARDS?

ACUTE RESPIRATORY DISTRESS SYNDROME

QUESTIONS AND ANSWERS

1. What is ARDS?

ARDS refers to acute respiratory distress syndrome, a set of manifestations presenting in the most extreme form of an acute lung injury (ALI) that is associated with a wide range of causes or associated conditions. ARDS was first described 30 years ago during the Vietnam War (Hudson & Steinberg, 1999). As stated by Bucher and Melander (1999) and Urden and colleagues (2002), the first widely used or standardized definition was published in 1994 by an American-European Consensus Conference. This definition describes ARDS as "a syndrome of inflammation and increased permeability associated with a constellation of clinical, radiologic, and physiologic abnormalities that could not be explained by left atrial hypertension." Based on definitions and criteria, ALI meets the same criteria as ARDS but with less severity of hypoxemia, allowing ARDS to be classified as a subset of ALI (Martin, 2002).

2. Discuss the pathophysiologic changes associated with ARDS?

There are four key criteria defining ARDS: acute onset, bilateral chest infiltrates, hypoxemia, and lack of left atrial hypertension (Martin, 2002). ARDS is a single pathologic process on a continuum of acute respiratory failure and only differ by their degree of severity. Pathophysiologic changes in ARDS as discussed by MacLaren and Jung (2002) are precipitated by either direct or indirect injury to the lungs, and arise from various sources. When the body is injured, a systemic inflammatory response syndrome (SIRS) is triggered. This takes the normal local inflammatory response that occurs with an injury and moves it from a local to a systemic response. There are many triggers for the SIRS response. The most common triggers found with ARDS are infection and trauma. Other events that may trigger SIRS include hypoxemia, major surgery, burns, and conditions with tissue necrosis. As stated by Urden and colleagues (2002), once SIRS is triggered, inflammatory mediators are released from the site of injury, resulting in an accumulation of neutrophils, macrophages, and platelets in the pulmonary capillaries. These cellular mediators then initiate the release of humoral mediators that cause damage to the alveolar capillary membrane. Damage of the epithelium of the alveolar capillary membrane causes an increase in permeability. This increase in permeability results in an accumulation of protein-rich fluid in the alveoli, causing edema.

The increase in alveolar fluid deactivates surfactant in the lungs. Without the surfactant, there is a decrease in alveolar tension, which causes the alveoli to collapse. The alveolar collapse creates a breakdown in the barrier and gas exchange functions in the lungs. The damage to the lung creates a further triggering of SIRS. As the process progresses, there is a fibroproliferation with deposits of collagen in the lungs, leading to lung remodeling. These deposits cause a further disruption of gas exchange, which leads to decreased elasticity of the lungs (Hudson & Steinberg, 1999).

As the alveoli collapse, there is a further disruption of gas exchange, and a ventilation-perfusion ($\dot{V}/\dot{Q}$) imbalance occurs because of an insufficient number of alveoli open to participate in gas exchange. As the process continues and additional alveoli become dysfunctional, the patient no longer responds to oxygen therapy. This hypoxemia leads to activation of the inflammatory process by the lungs.

3. What are the pathophysiologic phases of ARDS?

Bucher and Melander (1999) and Urden and associates (2002), describe three phases of ARDS. The first phase is called the exudative phase, and it is associated with alveolar edema caused by damage or injury to the pulmonary capillaries. Buildup of fibrin and leukocyte debris causes damage to the interstitium. Phase two is called the proliferative phase, which usually occurs after 7 to 10 days of the initial injury or insult. This phase is marked by persistent capillary and endothelial damage. There is a proliferation of type II cells and the beginning of squamous cell transformation. Injury to the alveolar epithelial cells and the loss of surfactant lead to alveoli collapse. Hypoxia then occurs as a result of intrapulmonary shunting and $\dot{V}/\dot{Q}$ mismatching. After 2 to 3 weeks the third phase, or the fibrotic phase, begins. This phase is more chronic in nature and is characterized by fibroproliferation with a thickening of the interstitium and an increase in type II cells and the development of pulmonary fibrosis. Structural remodeling occurs and the alveoli become enlarged and irregular in shape. Recovery occurs over several weeks with the resolution of fibrosis and restoration of the alveoli capillary membrane. Survival for these patients is dependant on not developing multiple organ dysfunction and sepsis.

4. How is ARDS diagnosed?

Understanding risk factors and identifying a history of a precipitating event that would trigger SIRS and the development of ARDS are key factors in identifying the onset of ARDS. Knowledge of a precipitating event, the presence of diffuse pulmonary infiltrates per chest x-ray, and refractory hypoxemia are characteristics that would lead to a diagnosis of ARDS (Wyncoll & Evans, 1999; Urden et al, 2002).

5. What are some medical complications seen with ARDS?

Mortality from ARDS is greater than 50%, although improvements have been seen in recent years, due to improved management protocols and ventilatory management. Nosocomial infections, especially pneumonia, and development of stress ulcers remain a threat. Prevention of these infections is an important goal in the treatment of patients with ARDS. Respiratory alkalosis and acidosis are problems at varying times during the course of ARDS. In addition, barotraumas, hypotension, volutrauma, sepsis, and multisystem organ failure are also complications associated with ARDS (Wyncoll & Evans, 1999; Urden et al, 2002).

6. What laboratory findings are diagnostic for ARDS?

Arterial blood gas measurements (ABG) are both diagnostic and treatment management tools in ARDS. They are used in the pulmonary treatment for ARDS through management of acid-base balance and arterial oxygenation in conjunction with assessment parameters and trends over time. ABG measurements are used to calculate a ratio of FiO_2 to the arterial partial pressure of oxygen (PaO_2) ($PaO_2 : FiO_2$ ratio). With ARDS, this ratio drops to less than 200 mm Hg regardless of the amount of PEEP used. The pH is high initially in many patients, but decreases as respiratory acidosis develops (Bucher & Melander, 1999; Urden et al, 2002).

7. What radiologic changes are seen with ARDS?

The hallmark of ARDS is the protein-rich fluid, which accumulates in the alveoli and interstitial spaces as a result of increased permeability. The alveoli become so filled with debris that they can no longer function and are no longer responsive to oxygen therapy. This is evident on the chest x-ray films as the characteristic finding of bilateral diffuse infiltrates or total whiteout (Bucher & Melander, 1999; Urden et al, 2002).

8. What changes are seen in pulmonary function studies with ARDS?

As a result of the many infiltrates, ARDS presents with changes in pulmonary function studies. The functional residual capacity decreases secondary to the microatelectasis and edema associated with the lung injury and the minute ventilation increases. The patient will begin to develop a right-to-left shunt, and then the alveolar to arterial gradient will begin to increase. Within 2 weeks of extubation, restorative impairments and abnormalities in diffusing capacity begin to subside and continued improvement is noted at 3 and 6 months with maximum improvement at 1 year (Hudson & Steinberg, 1999).

9. Tissue hypoxia is a major finding in ARDS. Describe signs and symptoms found on assessment that would be seen with ARDS in the following systems: central nervous, pulmonary, cardiovascular, renal, and gastrointestinal/hepatic.

Central Nervous System

Changes in oxygen leading to hypoxemia result in changes in the acid-base balance, which affect the level of consciousness, causing restlessness, fearfulness, agitation, confusion, and a sense of impending doom. As the disease progresses, the patient becomes increasingly lethargic and less responsive as decompensation continues (Bucher & Melander, 1999).

Pulmonary

Early in the disease process, there is an increase in respiration and dyspnea with crackles resulting from the fluid shifts occurring in the alveolar spaces. There is a cough with foamy, thick sputum production because of the protein, with hemoptysis from the inflammatory process. Initially the patient is alkalotic as a result of tachypnea. With increasing hypoxemia, responsiveness is decreased and the patient may develop cyanosis, pallor, and diaphoresis. As the disease progresses, crackles and wheezes are evident on physical examination. With further progression, the breath sounds become absent. Absence of breath sounds is an ominous sign because it signals the collapse of the alveoli. As the process continues, the patient may become acidotic (Bucher & Melander, 1999).

Cardiovascular

As hypoxia increases, there is evidence of tachycardia and arrhythmias. These are seen as a result of the increased cardiac output. The patient's cardiac output will be increased in an effort to compensate for the decreased oxygen saturation (Bucher & Melander, 1999).

Renal

As the body attempts to compensate for changes in cardiac output and decreased perfusion, the next system to be affected is the renal system. Because of the decreased cardiac output, blood flow through the kidneys will decrease, resulting in a reduction in urine output.

Gastrointestinal/hepatic

As other systems in the body begin to become affected, blood will be diverted from non-vital organs to assist in the compensatory mechanisms. The gastrointestinal (GI) tract is one system in which this will occur. As a result of decreased blood flow, the bowel can become ischemic and the patient could experience GI bleeding. An ischemic bowel is also an area where translocation of bacteria can occur. This would be an added risk factor for the development of infection, sepsis, or septic shock.

10. What is the goal of treatment for ARDS?

Because the damaged alveoli cannot be treated directly, the treatments are focused primarily on identifying the underlying cause, promoting gas exchange, supporting oxygenation, and preventing complications. Treatment efforts are focused on restoration of the alveolar capillary membrane integrity. The goal of the prevention of complications such as nosocomial infections, sepsis, and stress ulcers is imperative for a successful recovery. Additional goals are the maintenance of good nutritional status and fluid balance (Wyncoll & Evans, 1999; Urden et al, 2002).

11. What are the principal treatments for ARDS? List and describe the types of ventilatory support available.

The principal treatments for the patient with ARDS are ventilatory support and therapy for the underlying precipitating event. The major supportive therapy for ARDS is positive-pressure ventilation. Use of positive-pressure ventilation helps decrease workload and atelectasis. Collapsing alveoli and the increase in membrane permeability result in an impairment in gas exchange. This leads to decreased elasticity of lung tissue. Consequently, higher pressures are needed to distend the lung. High pressures and volume may lead to additional lung injury and/or barotrauma. Adjusting tidal volume and PEEP is key to the ventilatory management of ARDS patients. Recent clinical trials using lower tidal volumes have shown decreased mortality. One trial used a low tidal volume of 6 ml/kg and limiting pressure to 30 cm of H_2O with a reduction of mortality to 20%. A second study used higher PEEP levels without any significant improvement in mortality (Slutsky, 2002). To prevent additional lung injury, other methods of ventilation, including high-frequency jet ventilation, pressure-controlled inverse ratio ventilation, and pressure-controlled ventilation without the inverse ratio, have been tried. High-frequency jet ventilation has been used in the past 10 years to maintain gas exchange and decrease lung injury. High-frequency jet ventilation has been used effectively in the pediatric population, but results in adult patients have been conflicting. High-frequency jet ventilation allows the use of smaller volumes by creating constant airway pressure throughout the respiratory cycle (Velmahos et al, 1999).

Inverse ratio ventilation has become popular as a mode of ventilatory support to help provide improvement in gas exchange. This alternative prolongs the expiratory phase and shortens the inspiration time, which reverses the normal inspiratory/expiratory (I:E) ratio.

Pressure-controlled ventilation is used to deliver a preset pressure instead of volume. There is no reversal of the I:E ratio. Pressure-controlled ventilation without inverse ratio is used to support the patient's own breathing by delivering a preset volume with each patient-initiated breath (Efferen, 2001; Krieger, 2002; MacIntyre, 2002; Urden et al, 2002).

12. Describe nonventilatory means of pulmonary support.

Extracorporeal membrane oxygenation (ECMO) is a form of pulmonary support without the use of a ventilator. ECMO has been more widely used in the neonatal arena. ECMO has been used in nonneonatal acute respiratory failure. It is used most commonly when all other conventional therapies have failed and the patient has a recoverable pulmonary insufficiency. ECMO provides support when the supplemental oxygen, PEEP, and pressure ventilation limits reach the point at which continued use will cause irreversible damage and fibrosis of the lung (Meduri, 1999; Urden et al, 2002).

Surfactant therapy is one of the newer modalities being tested in adults with severe ARDS. There are different types of surfactant available, and the current thought is that there may be an advantage to the natural surfactant due to the associated surfactant proteins, which may provide better spreading of the drug and thus increased lung defense properties. Partial liquid ventilation and inhaled nitric oxide are also selectively being tried with severe ARDS patients.

It has also been demonstrated that providing supportive measures that provide optimal oxygenation are also important for the patient with ARDS. One supportive mechanism that has provided some improvement in oxygenation is prone positioning. Prone positioning seems to be more effective if initiated in the early phases of ARDS. The dependent areas of the lung are more heavily damaged, so turning the patient to the prone position improves perfusion to the less damaged areas, which improves $\dot{V}/\dot{Q}$ matching and decreases shunting (Reardon, 2002; Urden et al, 2002).

13. What are some of the pharmacologic interventions used in ARDS?

The pharmacologic agents used depend on the underlying processes being treated. Dopamine and dobutamine may be used to support cardiovascular dynamics by increasing cardiac output and hence blood pressure. Often, because sepsis is a significant precipitating event and because of the risk of nosocomial infections, antibiotic therapy is a key pharmacologic intervention. Neuromuscular blocking agents and sedatives are also widely used to aid with ventilatory support. Glucocorticoids may also be used because of their ability to inhibit the inflammatory response at all levels (Meduri, 1999).

14. What role does hemodynamic monitoring play in the management of ARDS?

Mechanical ventilation, which is a main component of therapy for the patient with ARDS, may have a great effect on cardiac output. The use of hemodynamic monitoring can help determine the effects of mechanical ventilation and PEEP on cardiac output as well as assist in the management of fluid volume. Hemodynamic monitoring also can help the health care professional differentiate between ARDS and congestive heart failure. Hemodynamic monitoring can be used to evaluate whether the current therapy modalities are effective.

15. Describe appropriate nursing diagnoses seen with ARDS.

Nursing diagnoses vary according to which body systems are affected and which complications occur with ARDS. The most common nursing diagnoses associated with ARDS include the following:

- Impaired tissue perfusion
- Alteration in cardiac output
- Ineffective breathing patterns
- Ineffective airway clearance
- Impaired gas exchange
- Alteration in nutrition
- Anxiety
- Alteration in communication
- High risk for infection
- High risk for impaired skin integrity

16. What is the nurse's overall goal in caring for the patient with ARDS?

The nurse has many roles in the care of the patient with ARDS. One of the first roles is to assist in finding the cause of the insult and stopping its progressive effects if possible. A second role is to ensure proper use of ventilation modalities to improve gas exchange and to monitor the patient's responses. A third very important role is for the nurse to continually assess for potential complications through the nursing assessment and to intervene to prevent the many complications associated with ARDS. A fourth role is to be supportive and provide palliative care for the patient while other treatment modalities are being used.

ACUTE RESPIRATORY DISTRESS SYNDROME

References

Bucher, L. & Melander, S. (Eds.). (1999). *Critical care nursing*. Philadelphia: Saunders.

Efferen, L. (2001). Mechanical ventilation in ARDS: Implementation of lung protective strategies, *Chest*: 67th Annual Scientific Assembly of the American College of Chest Physicians.

Hudson, L. D. & Steinberg, K. P. (1999). Epidemiology of acute lung injury and ARDS. *Chest, 116* (1 Suppl), 74S-82S.

Krieger, B. (2002). Top ten list in mechanical ventilation. *Chest, 122*(5), 1797-1800.

MacIntyre, N. (2002). Assessing the right strategies in lung recruitment for patients with ALI/ARDS. 32nd Critical Care Congress of Society of Critical Care Medicine—Mechanical Ventilation CME. Medscape. San Antanio Texas.

MacLaren, R. & Jung, R. (2002). Stress-dose cortocosteroid therapy for sepsis and acute lung injury or acute respiratory distress syndrome in critically ill adults. *Pharmacotherapy, 22*(9), 1140-1156.

Martin, G. (2002). Experts discuss ventilation strategies for improving outcomes in ALI/ARDSA. 98th International conference of the American Thoracic Society, May 17-22, Atlanta.

Meduri, G. U. (1999). Levels of evidence for the pharmacologic effectiveness of prolonged methylprednisolone treatment in unresolving acute respiratory distress syndrome. *Chest, 116*(1 Suppl), 116S-118S.

Reardon, C. (2002). Prone positioning in ARDS. *Medscape Critical Care, 3*(1).

Slutsky, A. (2002). Mechanical ventilation trials: How do they stand up over time? Conference coverage 15th Annual Congress of the European Society of Intensive Care Medicine. September 29-October 2, 2002, Barcelona, Spain.

Slutsky, A. (2002). New techniques in mechanical ventilation help keep patients more comfortable. Conference coverage 15th Annual Congress of the European Society of Intensive Care Medicine. September 29-October 2, 2002, Barcelona, Spain.

Urden, L. D., Stacy, K. M., & Lough, M. E. (Eds). (2002). *Thelan's critical care nursing: Diagnosis and management* (4th ed., pp. 947-963). St Louis: Mosby.

Velmahos, G. C., et al. (1999). High frequency percussive ventilation improves oxygenation in patients with ARDS. *Chest, 116*(2), 440-446.

Wyncoll, D. & Evans, T. (1999). Acute respiratory distress syndrome. *The Lancet, 354*(9177), 497-501.

NEUROLOGIC ALTERATIONS

13

Subarachnoid Hemorrhage with Aneurysm

Cinda Alexander, MSN, CCRN, CNRN, CNOR, CRNFA

CASE PRESENTATION

Sarah, a 42-year-old white woman, was seen in the emergency department with complaints of severe left temporal headaches after collapsing at work. Initially, while at work, Sarah was confused and incontinent of urine. After arrival in the emergency department, Sarah was cooperative, her pupils were equal and reactive, and she was mildly disoriented. She stated that the headaches were unlike any she had experienced before. According to Sarah's husband, Sarah had experienced these headaches for about 3 to 4 weeks. Additional symptoms included nausea, photophobia, and a mildly stiff neck. A computed tomographic (CT) scan of the head without contrast material revealed a subarachnoid hemorrhage in the area of the internal carotid artery. Her serum Na^+ level was 130 mmol/L, K^+ level was 3.6 mmol/L, and Cl^- level was 106 mmol/L.

Initial assessment data after admission to the emergency department were as follows:

BP	152/78 mm Hg
HR	102 bpm
Respirations	22 breaths/min
Temperature	37.2° C (99° F)
Sao$_2$	92% with room air

Neurologic signs were as follows:

- Lethargic, arouses to name
- Pupils equal and reactive
- Follows commands, moves all extremities equally
- Oriented to person only
- Glasgow Coma Scale score of 14

After admission and evaluation in the emergency department, Sarah's condition was stabilized and she was transferred to the critical care unit. She was scheduled for an arteriogram the next day. Treatment with aminocaproic acid (Amicar) and nimodipine

(Nimotop) was begun. Sarah continued to complain of a generalized headache and neck stiffness. Assessment data were as follows:

BP	142/80 mm Hg
HR	84 bpm
Respirations	24 breaths/min
Temperature	37.2° C (99° F)
Sao$_2$	98% with room air

Neurologic signs were as follows:

- Pupils equal and reactive
- Follows commands, moves all extremities equally, grasp equal
- Oriented to person and place
- Lethargic, arouses to name
- Glasgow Coma Scale score of 13

Sarah's condition was stable throughout the night. Her arteriogram the next morning revealed a left vertebral posterior inferior cerebellar aneurysm. Sarah and her family were present when the physician discussed the results of the arteriogram. Her treatment options were explored, and specific questions from the family were answered. Sarah's neurologic status remained stable, and the decision to proceed with "early surgery" was made.

SURGERY

At 10 AM the following day, Sarah underwent a craniotomy for a clip ligation of the left inferior cerebellar aneurysm.

POSTOPERATIVE COURSE

Immediately after surgery Sarah's vital signs were stable. She recovered from the general anesthesia, responded to her name, and moved all extremities to command during the initial hour of recovery in the intensive care unit. Sarah continued to show general recovery and recognized her family during the following hours. Several hours after surgery she developed a sudden headache, confusion, and gross weakness in her right hand. Her vital signs were as follows:

BP	162/94 mm Hg
HR	110 bpm
Respirations	32 breaths/min
Temperature	38.3° C (101° F)

Neurologic signs included the following:

- Pupils equal and reactive
- Follows command and moves all extremities, right grasp weak
- Disoriented, speech inappropriate
- Glasgow Coma Scale score of 11

An emergency CT scan of the head demonstrated postoperative changes associated with the surgery, an aneurysm clip artifact, minimal air, and no obvious collection of blood. The transcranial Doppler study demonstrated an increased velocity in the left middle cerebral artery, greater than 120 cm/sec. With no obvious postoperative hematoma, a decision was made to repeat the arteriogram, which demonstrated apparent narrowing of the arteries. The clinician concluded that Sarah was experiencing a vasospasm. Her Na$^+$ level was 145 mmol/L, K$^+$ level was 3.9 mmol/L, and Cl$^-$ level was 109 mmol/L.

After an arterial line and pulmonary artery (Swan-Ganz) catheter were inserted, hypervolemic/hyperfusion therapy was initiated and continued over the next 5 days. Sarah's neurologic status stabilized and improved with this therapy. Sarah was slowly weaned from this therapy, and her neurologic status remained stable for an additional 48 hours. Sarah was then transferred to a neurosurgical step-down unit. Neurologically, she was alert and oriented, although easily confused if given multiple instructions. She moved all extremities to command; however, she continued to demonstrate a mild weakness in her right hand and arm. She was discharged 8 days later to a rehabilitation unit with an anticipated discharge home after rehabilitation therapy.

SUBARACHNOID HEMORRHAGE WITH ANEURYSM

QUESTIONS

1. Discuss the clinical presentation of a subarachnoid hemorrhage.

2. Describe the incidence, risk factors, mortality, and morbidity associated with acute subarachnoid hemorrhage.

3. Discuss how a subarachnoid hemorrhage is diagnosed.

4. Describe the pathophysiology involved and consequences of blood in the subarachnoid space.

5. Give the rationale for Sarah's hyponatremia.

6. Describe how a subarachnoid hemorrhage is classified.

7. What therapeutic modalities should be anticipated for patients after subarachnoid hemorrhage? Give the rationale for each.

8. What parameters require close monitoring for patients after subarachnoid hemorrhage?

9. What are the general complications associated with aminocaproic acid (Amicar) and nimodipine (Nimotap)?

10. What are the general "aneurysm precautions" observed for patients with a subarachnoid hemorrhage who may have a cerebral aneurysm?

11. Describe the pathophysiology of cerebral aneurysm.

12. Define the different types of aneurysms.

13. Discuss the secondary cerebral injuries associated with a ruptured aneurysm and subsequent subarachnoid hemorrhage.

14. Discuss the advantages and disadvantages of early versus late surgical intervention.

15. Discuss why nursing care is of particular importance after a craniotomy.

16. Describe the pathophysiology and incidence of rebleeding. When is rebleeding likely to occur?

17. Discuss clinical changes that should be anticipated if a patient is experiencing rebleeding.

18. Describe how rebleeding would be diagnosed.

19. Discuss the treatment for rebleeding. What is the duration of treatment?

20. Describe the pathophysiology and incidence of vasospasm. When is vasospasm likely to occur?

21. Discuss the causes of vasospasm.

22. Identify how cerebral vasospasm is diagnosed. Include clinical symptoms that should be anticipated.

23. Discuss the mortality and morbidity of vasospasm and rebleeding.

24. Discuss current treatment for vasospasm. What additional approaches are discussed in the literature?

25. How long should the treatment of vasospasm be continued, and how long will Sarah remain at risk for vasospasm or rebleeding?

26. Discuss nonsurgical approaches available to patients unable to tolerate traditional surgical treatment.

SUBARACHNOID HEMORRHAGE WITH ANEURYSM

QUESTIONS AND ANSWERS

1. Discuss the clinical presentation of a subarachnoid hemorrhage.

Patients often report having sudden, severe, violent headaches, unlike any experienced before. Immediate loss of consciousness, nausea, vomiting, cranial nerve palsies, and focal neurologic deficits such as weakness of an extremity may also be present. Blood in the sub-arachnoid space produces signs and symptoms of meningeal irritation such as nuchal rigidity or stiff neck, photophobia, blurred vision, nausea and vomiting, headache, and fever. With the initial seepage of blood into the subarachnoid space, there may be a sudden onset of deep coma. As many as 40% of patients with subarachnoid hemorrhage have prodromal signs or warning symptoms, such as headache, that can indicate the occurrence of a small leakage of blood. However, these early symptoms are often ignored or attributed to other causes (Campbell & Edwards, 1997; Hickey, 1997; Becker, 1998; O'Sullivan & O'Sullivan, 2000; Urden et al, 2002).

2. Describe the incidence, risk factors, mortality, and morbidity associated with acute subarachnoid hemorrhage.

Subarachnoid hemorrhage occurs in 25,000 to 30,000 North Americans annually; of these, 50% to 60% die. One third of these deaths occur before the person enters the health care system. An additional 20% to 30% sustain permanent neurologic damage and disability. The average age of occurrence is 50 years, with patients ranging from 35 to 60 years (Campbell & Edwards, 1997; Hickey, 1997; Becker, 1998; Pfohman & Criddle, 2001; Urden et al, 2002). Johnston and colleagues (1998) reported that mortality decreased between 1994 and 1997 in the United States. Mortality is reported to be higher in women and African Americans. Risk factors include smoking, hypertension, and alcohol use (Becker, 1998; Pfohman & Criddle, 2001). The question of familial risk is gaining greater appreciation. According to Pfohman and Criddle (2001), there may be two- to seven-fold increase in risk in a first-degree relative. Recommendations for screening with MRI or CTI are gaining popularity. The major causes of death associated with aneurysmal subarachnoid hemorrhage are rebleeding and vasospasm (Lanzino & Kassell, 1998; O'Sullivan & O'Sullivan, 2000).

3. Discuss how a subarachnoid hemorrhage is diagnosed.

Diagnosis is based on history, clinical presentation, and a number of diagnostic procedures. Lumbar puncture may be used to confirm blood in the cerebrospinal fluid (CSF), which circulates in the subarachnoid space. The spinal fluid is bloody grossly and xanthochromic (a yellow discoloration of the CSF) after centrifugation. Lumbar puncture is avoided if intracranial hypertension is suspected because of the risk of brain herniation (Romeo, 1993; Wojner, 1999; O'Sullivan & O'Sullivan, 2000). A CT scan within 48 hours of the bleeding episode can demonstrate the blood in the subarachnoid space in 75% to 85% of all patients. Magnetic resonance imaging may be used to identify the subarachnoid blood and inner structures of the brain. Magnetic resonance angiography with intravenous gadolinium is a noninvasive approach to image cerebral vasculature and perhaps provide useful screening for suspected aneurysm or arteriovenous malformation. A four-vessel cerebral angiogram is the mainstay of diagnosis and usually is able to provide a definitive diagnosis of aneurysm or arteriovenous malformation. Cerebral angiography visualizes both intracranial and extracranial vessels. Contrast medium is injected, and a series of radiographic films is recorded (Hickey, 1997; Baxter et al, 1998; Van Tatenhove & Kelley, 1999; Urden et al, 2002).

4. Describe the pathophysiology involved and consequences of blood in the subarachnoid space.

The pathophysiology of subarachnoid hemorrhage is complex and not well understood but includes a number of events. *Subarachnoid hemorrhage* is arterial blood that has extravasated into the subarachnoid space, which normally contains CSF. Subarachnoid hemorrhage as a result of a ruptured aneurysm usually occurs around the circle of Willis at a point of bifurcation of the arterial vessels (Rusy, 1996). The amount of bleeding may range from small amounts to large amounts that extend beyond the site of leakage, flooding into cisterns and the ventricular system. Blood is an irritant to brain tissues that initiates an inflammatory response and cerebral edema. Studies suggest there is a rapid rise in intracranial pressure as well as a reduction of cerebral blood flow after a subarachnoid hemorrhage. There is often an abnormality in the cerebral vasculature response to partial pressure of carbon dioxide ($PaCO_2$), suggesting a disturbance in autoregulation. Patients with subarachnoid hemorrhage are often hypertensive after the initial bleeding episode, probably as a result of the release of catecholamines into the circulatory vasculature. This hypertension maintains or improves the cerebral perfusion pressure. Fibrin, platelets, and fluid around the point of arterial rupture, usually an aneurysm, seal off the tear (Macdonald, 1996; Hickey, 1997). After a subarachnoid hemorrhage, neurologic injury occurs immediately as a result of blood seeping into adjacent tissues or may be delayed as a result of a secondary event such as rebleeding or vasospasm. Estimates are that 45% of patients who survive the initial bleeding episode will have a transient loss of consciousness. This probably is caused by either intracranial hypertension and increased intracranial pressure or transient cardiac arrhythmias as a result of blood around the brainstem (Kirsch et al, 1989; Macdonald, 1996; McKhann & LeRoux 1998; Wojner, 1998; O'Sullivan & O'Sullivan, 2000; Sommargen, 2002).

5. Give the rationale for Sarah's hyponatremia.

According to Segatore (1993), hyponatremia is the most common electrolyte imbalance found in patients with subarachnoid hemorrhage. Hyponatremia is associated with a high incidence of brain ischemia and infarction. The pathogenesis of hyponatremia after subarachnoid hemorrhage remains unclear; it is probably caused by cerebral salt wasting or the syndrome of inappropriate secretion of antidiuretic hormone (ADH) (Segatore, 1993; Dorsch, 1996; McKhann & LeRoux, 1998).

6. Describe how a subarachnoid hemorrhage is classified.

The Hunt and Hess classification system is most commonly used to grade the severity of a subarachnoid bleeding episode in terms of clinical presentation and significance. The grades range from Grade I (asymptomatic or minimal headache) to Grade V (deep coma, extension abnormal, and moribund appearance). Timing of surgery may be judged by the presenting grade and clinical progression. The higher grades are associated with much higher mortality and morbidity (Campbell & Edwards, 1997; Hickey, 1997; Wojner, 1998, 1999; Cavanagh & Gordon, 2002).

7. What therapeutic modalities should be anticipated for patients after subarachnoid hemorrhage? Give the rationale for each.

After stabilization and control of systemic blood pressure, bed rest and aneurysm precautions are instituted. Elastic stockings or antithrombotic pumps may be used to counter the effects of bed rest and hemostasis. Normal hydration is supplemented with intravenous therapy. Drug therapy includes the following (Kirsch et al, 1989; Sikes & Nolan, 1993; Hickey, 1997; Feigin et al, 1998):

- *Anticonvulsants:* used prophylactically to prevent seizures because blood in the subarachnoid space is an irritant to the surrounding tissues
- *Steroids:* controversial but may be used if the patient shows signs of increased intracranial pressure, focal neurologic deficits, or cerebral edema

- *Calcium channel blocker:* used prophylactically to reduce or minimize the threat of vasospasm and subsequent secondary ischemia
- *Antifibrinolytic therapy:* controversial but used to prevent clot lysis at the point of rupture Agents such as aminocaproic acid or tranexamic acid reduce the risk of rebleeding during the first 2 weeks after rupture. The clot reinforces the wall of the aneurysm. If this therapy is used, it is initiated immediately upon diagnosis of a subarachnoid hemorrhage. Antifibrinolytic agents are discontinued upon ligation of the aneurysm.
- *Analgesics:* used to control the headaches and pain associated with meningeal irritation
- *Mild sedative:* possibly used if the patient is agitated and at risk for increased intracranial pressure because of combativeness
- *Stool softener:* used to prevent straining for bowel movements and initiation of Valsalva's maneuver, which may trigger increased intracranial pressure

8. What parameters require close monitoring for patients after subarachnoid hemorrhage?

Neurologic and vital signs are assessed for evidence of complications such as hydrocephalus, increased intracranial pressure, rebleeding, or vasospasm. The nurse also monitors for complications associated with prolonged bed rest. Detailed clinical assessment is paramount in the care of these patients to detect any early, subtle changes in neurologic status that may indicate secondary complications.

9. What are the general complications associated with aminocaproic acid (Amicar) and nimodipine (Nimotap)?

Aminocaproic acid (Amicar) has been associated with an increase in hydrocephalus and vasospasm. Calcium channel blockers are associated with hypotension, which can induce cerebral ischemia in the patient after subarachnoid hemorrhage. Calcium antagonists significantly limit the effectiveness of vasopressor drugs used to maintain systemic blood pressure (Kirsch et al, 1989; Feigin et al, 1998; LeRoux & Winn, 1998).

10. What are the general "aneurysm precautions" observed for patients with a subarachnoid hemorrhage who may have a cerebral aneurysm?

Aneurysm precautions include the following (Hickey, 1997):

- Place the patient in a quiet room.
- Control the room lighting to prevent strong, direct light.
- Allow reading and TV watching if these activities do not overstimulate the patient.
- Maintain good oxygen and carbon dioxide exchange; supplemental oxygen is usually ordered.
- Maintain head of bed elevation, generally 20 to 30 degrees to augment cerebral venous drainage.
- Maintain bed rest, possibly with bathroom privileges (avoid straining for bowel movements).
- Restrict visitors and discuss with visitors the importance of a calming, supportive environment.
- Schedule nursing care and diagnostic tests to avoid overstimulating the patient.

11. Describe the pathophysiology of cerebral aneurysm.

Cerebral aneurysms are saccular outpouchings of the walls of a cerebral artery. The causes of cerebral aneurysms are unclear. However, at least three theories have been identified in the literature. The congenital theory suggests that a congenital weakness exists in the wall of the artery's medial layer, allowing an outpouching. The degenerative theory suggests that a local weakness develops in the intima as a result of hemodynamically induced degenerative changes. In midlife, the vessel develops an outpouching of the intimal layer caused by hemodynamic stress on the weakened area (usually due to arteriosclerosis). Aneurysms often occur in the area of the circle of Willis at a point of bifurcation or a junction of the arteries. Rupture often occurs in association with physical activities or strain. Clinical studies suggest a seasonal variation for aneurysmal rupture in the spring and fall as well as a circadian cycle of increased episodes in the morning or evening. Also, there is a component of genetic predisposition (Dorsch, 1996; Rusy, 1996; Campbell & Edwards, 1997; Hickey, 1997; Becker, 1998; Connolly & Solomon, 1998).

12. Define the different types of aneurysms.

Types of aneurysms are best classified by their shapes. Common classification by shape is as follows (Rusy, 1996; Hickey, 1997; Wojner, 1998.)

- *Berry:* most common; berry shaped with a neck or stem
- *Saccular:* saccular outpouching
- *Fusiform:* outpouching without a neck or stem
- *Traumatic:* associated with head trauma
- *Mycotic:* caused by septic emboli
- *Charcot-Bouchard:* microscopic; associated with hypertension and often located in the brainstem and basal ganglia
- *Dissecting:* generally associated with atherosclerosis; blood is forced between the intimal layer and medial layer

13. Discuss the secondary cerebral injuries associated with a ruptured aneurysm and subsequent subarachnoid hemorrhage.

Rebleeding

Rebleeding occurs when an aneurysm releases additional blood into the subarachnoid space. With each additional rupture episode, patient mortality increases dramatically. Rarely do patients survive the third episode of a rupture and rebleeding (McKhann & LeRoux, 1998).

Hydrocephalus and increased intracranial pressure

Subarachnoid hemorrhage and subsequent clot(s) in the subarachnoid space may interfere with the flow and reabsorption of CSF via the arachnoid villi. Large clots may mechanically interfere with the flow of blood through the ventricular system, resulting in hydrocephalus, increased intracranial pressure, and reduced cerebral blood flow. The clinical presentation is generally a decrease or change in the level of consciousness (Kirsch et al, 1989; Hickey, 1997; LeRoux & Winn, 1998; McKhann & LeRoux, 1998).

Seizures

Seizures after a subarachnoid hemorrhage are more common in younger adults with a ruptured aneurysm and may occur in up to 25% of patients. Seizures associated with subarachnoid hemorrhage are divided into initial, early, and late. Initial seizures occur at the time of the rupture. Early seizures occur within 2 weeks, and late seizures usually occur more than 2 weeks after the initial hemorrhage. In the acute setting, seizures are often followed by rebleeding, probably because of the increased cerebral blood flow and perfusion pressure. Prophylactic anticonvulsant therapy is generally advocated but remains controversial, and often phenytoin (Dilantin) is the drug of choice (Kirsch et al, 1989; LeRoux & Winn, 1998; McKhann & LeRoux, 1998).

Vasospasm

Vasospasm is a narrowing of the vessels in the area of the subarachnoid hemorrhage. Vasospasm can lead to cerebral ischemia and a cerebral infarct (Kirsch et al, 1989; Bell & Kongable, 1996; Rusy, 1996; Mayberg, 1998; O'Sullivan & O'Sullivan, 2000).

Hypothalamic Dysfunction

Hypothalamic dysfunction may be exhibited as hyponatremia resulting from a disturbance in the regulation of ADH. Referred to as the syndrome of inappropriate secretion of ADH, this condition exists when the neurons of the supraoptic hypothalamic secrete ADH unrelated to true serum osmolarity or intravascular volume. Water is retained by the kidneys, and hyponatremia or hypervolemia results. Electrocardiogram changes may occur as a result of an overstimulated sympathetic system (Segatore, 1993; McKhann & LeRoux, 1998; Sommargen, 2002).

14. Discuss the advantages and disadvantages of early versus late surgical intervention.

Traditionally surgical repair of the aneurysm was delayed 7 to 14 days to allow cerebral edema to subside and to allow for medical stabilization of the patient. However, during the waiting period, the peak incidence of both rebleeding and vasospasm occurs. With improvements in microsurgical techniques and neuroanesthesia, the trend now is toward early surgery (i.e., within 1 to 3 days).

Early surgery enables the prevention of rebleeding and aggressive treatment with hypervolemia and hypertension for any vasospasm as necessary (Mendel & Carter, 1994). Early surgery consists of removal of the subarachnoid clot, which perhaps minimizes the vasospastic reaction to the clot (Lanzino & Kassell, 1998; Hosoda et al, 1999). Early surgery is associated with a higher risk probably because of the technically difficult nature of surgery on an edematous brain. Miyaoka and associates (1993) suggest in a retrospective analysis of 1622 cases that early surgery for patients with Grades I and II aneurysms was not a major factor in predicting outcome. However, early surgery for patients with Grades III and IV aneurysms does appear to provide additional benefits of preventing a rebleeding episode and allowing for aggressive treatment of vasospasm and clot removal at the time of surgery. The International Study on the Timing of Aneurysm Surgery (ISTAS) conducted during the 1980s indicated that good recovery was significantly higher in the early surgery group when the data collected by the North American Centers were analyzed separately. Early surgery allows for the concomitant removal of intraparenchymal hematoma. Delayed surgery may be considered based on the size and location of the aneurysm. Early surgery is not indicated for giant and technically difficult to approach aneurysms. Elderly patients and those with significant comorbidity may require a delayed approach (Lanzino & Kassell, 1998).

15. Discuss why nursing care is of particular importance after a craniotomy.

Overall and serial evaluation of neurologic status is critical to detect any changes associated with development of a postoperative intracranial blood clot. Airway maintenance is essential because these patients often have difficulty controlling their airway because of neurologic deficits. Evaluation of increased intracranial pressure related to cerebral edema is critical, particularly after suctioning or painful procedures. Electrolyte imbalances are also a concern postoperatively after a craniotomy because of the diuresis that occurs intraoperatively. As patients recover after a craniotomy, nutrition and complications of bed rest must be assessed carefully. Postoperative pain, particularly headache, requires attention with judicious use of pain medication (Romeo, 1993; Wojner, 1999).

16. Describe the pathophysiology and incidence of rebleeding. When is rebleeding likely to occur?

Rebleeding occurs when the fibrin-platelet clot is displaced by either hypertension or fibrinolysis. Women, patients in poor premorbid health, patients with elevated systolic blood pressures, and patients with a high clinical grade on the Hunt and Hess scale are more likely to have a rebleeding episode. Patients with aneurysms are at risk for rebleeding until the aneurysm is clipped or treated in some fashion. Peak incidence for rebleeding is 24 to 48 hours after the aneurysm (Kirsch et al, 1989; Rusy, 1996; Hickey, 1997; LeRoux & Winn, 1998; McKhann & LeRoux, 1998). Rebleeding occurs in as many as 30% of all patients with aneurysms, and the mortality is 45% (Lanzino & Kassell, 1998).

17. Discuss clinical changes that should be anticipated if a patient is experiencing rebleeding.

The clinical presentation of rebleeding is generally profound, with gradual or sudden deterioration in neurologic status. Patients may complain of increased pain associated with a headache. Often there may be a sudden onset of nausea and vomiting and a rise in systolic blood pressure and intracranial pressure (Dorsch, 1996; McKhann & LeRoux, 1998).

18. Describe how rebleeding would be diagnosed.

The definitive diagnosis of rebleeding is made by a second CT scan. The results of the second scan are compared with the initial CT scan. The second CT scan can also reveal evidence of increasing subarachnoid hemorrhage, which is indicative of a rebleeding episode.

19. Discuss the treatment for rebleeding. What is the duration of treatment?

Ideally, treatment consists of prevention. The definitive prevention is surgical clip ligation of the aneurysm. The efficacy of prophylactic treatment while waiting for surgical intervention is controversial. Antifibrinolytic agents such as aminocaproic acid (Amicar) may be administered with the initial diagnosis of subarachnoid hemorrhage to prevent clot lysis. Aminocaproic acid is discontinued intraoperatively once the clip is in place. The placement of Guglielmi detachable coils provides some protection against rebleeding during the acute phase (Martin, 1998; McKhann & LeRoux 1998; Nelson, 1998).

20. Describe the pathophysiology and incidence of vasospasm. When is vasospasm likely to occur?

Vasospasm is a narrowing of the arteries in the area of the aneurysm and subarachnoid hemorrhage. The specific cause of vasospasm is debated in the literature. A correlation is suggested between the incidence of vasospasm and the amount of blood released into the subarachnoid space. The extent of the clot (when located in the basal cisterns and cerebral fissures) should be considered when evaluating the probability of spasm. Subarachnoid clots larger than 3 by 5 mm in the basal cisterns or layers of blood 1 mm or thicker in the area of the cisterns have a high correlation with spasm (Bell & Kongable, 1996; Hickey, 1997; O'Sullivan & O'Sullivan, 2000). The following have a high incidence of vasospasm: patients with a high clinical grade on the Hunt and Hess scale and patients with hyponatremia, hypovolemia, electroencephalogram abnormalities, increased cerebral blood flow velocity, decreased regional cerebral blood flow, or fibrinogen degradation products greater than 80 µg/ml in the CSF (Sikes & Nolan, 1993). Vasospasm is also associated with a loss of autoregulation, tissue ischemia, and ultimately, tissue infarction. The onset of vasospasm is usually 3 to 14 days after the initial subarachnoid hemorrhage, with a peak around day 7. The threat of vasospasm persists for up to 3 weeks (Kirsch et al, 1989; Bell & Kongable, 1996; Dorsch, 1996; Rusy, 1996; Campbell & Edwards, 1997; Hickey, 1997).

21. Discuss the causes of vasospasm.

The cause of vasospasm is still unknown; however, a dominant theory exists. Once the clot in the subarachnoid space begins to break down, spasmodic agents are released, resulting in vasospasm. Theories of etiology include the following:

- Biochemical process resulting in contraction of arterial muscle cells
- Release of spasmodic substances during the breakdown of erythrocytes and platelets in the subarachnoid blood
- Release of mitogenic substances from platelets, resulting in structural vessel changes
- An inflammatory process resulting in vasculopathy

There is also much interest in the role that oxygen-free radicals may play in the development of vasospasm (Campbell & Edwards, 1997; Mayberg, 1998; O'Sullivan & O'Sullivan, 2000).

22. Identify how cerebral vasospasm is diagnosed. Include clinical symptoms that should be anticipated.

Sequential neurologic assessment is crucial to identify the clinical symptoms of vasospasm. The clinician must carefully observe for lethargy, confusion, restlessness, disorientation, new headaches, hemiparesis, seizures, labile blood pressure, change in speech, elevated fever, or slight leukocytosis, all of which are indicative of the onset of vasospasm. Transcranial Doppler study may detect vessel narrowing with elevated velocities. The demonstrated increase in velocity may often precede clinical symptoms. With deterioration of neurologic function and no radiographic evidence of rebleeding, a second angiogram provides definitive diagnosis of vasospasm. Other causes of a change in condition (e.g., electrolyte imbalance, development of hydrocephalus) must be considered as well (Bell & Kongable, 1996; Campbell & Edwards, 1997; Manno, 1997; Mayberg, 1998; O'Sullivan & O'Sullivan, 2000).

23. Discuss the mortality and morbidity of vasospasm and rebleeding.

Mortality and morbidity related to vasospasm is high, approaching 50%. Among those who survive the initial subarachnoid hemorrhage, 40% will develop clinical symptoms of vasospasm, resulting in delayed cerebral ischemia. Morbidity is associated with the degree of cerebral ischemia, infarction, and permanent neurologic injury. Mortality associated with rebleeding is as high as 70% and increases with each episode of rebleeding. Patients rarely survive a third rebleeding event. Morbidity is associated with the location and degree of cerebral tissue injury with each event and can be quite severe (Kirsch et al, 1989; Rusy, 1996; Campbell & Edwards, 1997; Hickey, 1997; McKhann & LeRoux, 1998).

24. Discuss current treatment for vasospasm. What additional approaches are discussed in the literature?

Current modalities of treatment are focused on increasing cerebral perfusion pressure using hypervolemic/hypertensive therapy and pharmacologic agents to dilate cerebral arteries, improve rheologic findings, and maximize cardiac performance (Sikes & Nolan, 1993; Campbell & Edwards, 1997; Hickey, 1997; O'Sullivan & O'Sullivan, 2000).

Hypervolemic/hypertensive therapy is also referred to as *hyperdynamic therapy* or *triple-H therapy.* This consists of induced hypervolemia, hemodilution, and hypertension. The goal is to increase cerebral blood flow, cerebral perfusion pressure, and cerebral microcirculation. Much of the improvement in mortality associated with subarachnoid hemorrhage has been attributed to aggressive treatment of vasospasm after the clip ligation of the aneurysm. Vasopressor agents such as dopamine or phenylephrine (Neo-Synephrine) may be useful to elevate systolic blood pressure. Hypervolemia is induced with combined use of colloids (albumin) or crystalloids (5% dextrose in lactated Ringer's solution [D5LR] or in normal saline). Intravenous solutions such as D5LR may be given at high rates (125 to 300 ml/hr). Triple-H therapy is not without risk and hazards. The patient must be monitored carefully for complications such as pulmonary edema, congestive heart failure, cerebral edema, increased intracranial pressure, myocardial infarction, intracerebral hemorrhage, and systemic complications of prolonged vasopressor administration. Guidelines for hypervolemic/hypertensive therapy are as follows (Mendel & Carter, 1994; Rusy, 1996; Campbell & Edwards, 1997; Hickey, 1997; Mayberg, 1998; O'Sullivan & O'Sullivan, 2000):

- Central venous pressure >10 mm Hg
- Pulmonary capillary wedge pressure 14 to 20 mm Hg
- Hematocrit 33% to 38%
- Heart rate >70 bpm
- 30% rise in mean arterial blood pressure (130 to 150 mm Hg)
- Systolic blood pressure 160 to 200 mm Hg

Despite the interest in a variety of drugs to prevent the narrowing of arteriole walls, the results have not been promising. The greatest interest is currently in the use of calcium antagonists. Of the calcium channel blockers available, nimodipine is currently the drug of choice. Nimodipine is more potent than nifedipine (Procardia), is lipid soluble, readily crosses the blood-brain barrier, and perhaps has fewer systemic effects from hypotension.

Nimodipine promotes collateral circulation, reduces platelet aggregation, and blocks calcium influx into single nerve cells, thus promoting an antispasmodic effect. Nimodipine enhances the cardiac function by reducing afterload. Treatment is continued for 21 days. The typical dosage is 60 mg every 4 hours orally. Although other calcium channel blockers (e.g., nicardipine, AT877) are available, the drug of choice remains nimodipine (Feigin et al, 1998).

Rheology is the study of blood's ability to flow. Patients with a subarachnoid hemorrhage often have increased blood volume within the brain tissue, suggesting microstagnation. Increased hematocrit, erythrocyte aggregation, platelet aggregation, plasma viscosity, and shear rate affect blood viscosity. The hematocrit is the easiest to manipulate and is done so by hemodilution. Crystalloids and colloids are used in conjunction to provide hemodilution and hypervolemic therapy to increase the cerebral perfusion to the tissues deprived by vasospasm. Plasma protein fraction (Plasmanate), 5% albumin, hetastarch (Hespan), or dextran may also be used (Sikes & Nolan, 1993).

Additional drugs may be used to maximize cardiac performance and promote supported hypervolemic/hypertensive therapy. The mean arterial blood pressure is elevated to the point at which the clinical condition of the patient improves and is then titrated down to the point at which neurologic status is maintained. Therapy can be much more aggressive in patients who have clipped or surgically secured aneurysms once the threat of rebleeding has been removed.

Inotropic and vasoconstrictive therapy may be necessary to support the desired elevation in blood pressure. Dopamine (Intropin) (3 to 10 µg/kg/min), dobutamine (Dobutrex) (2.5 to 10 µg/kg/min), and phenylephrine hydrochloride (Neo-Synephrine) (10 to 100 µg/min) are commonly used. Atropine sulfate may be necessary to block vagal bradycardia induced by hypervolemia. Vasopressin (Pitressin) may be used to keep urine output at less than 200 ml/hr and to prevent diuresis as a response to hypervolemia. Cardiac pharmacologic management such as digitalis (Digoxin) may be necessary for the patient at risk for pulmonary compromise and cardiac failure with the added stress of hypervolemia therapy (Sikes & Nolan, 1993; McKhann & LeRoux, 1998).

Cerebral angioplasty is indicated for patients who do not improve with conventional therapy. This investigative therapy involves temporary balloon dilation of the affected arterial segment(s). Arterial dilation is immediate and permanent. Complete recovery has been reported using this technique. Possible use of oxygen-free radical scavengers (lazaroids) is being considered to prevent cellular damage. Intracisternal injection of the drug recombinant tissue plasminogen activator is also under evaluation (Sikes & Nolan, 1993; Mendel & Carter, 1994). This may reduce vasospasm by improving the process of clot lysis and clearance, thus preventing prolonged exposure to perivascular blood and the release of oxyhemoglobin (Bell & Kongable, 1996; Rusy, 1996; Mayberg, 1998; McKhann & LeRoux, 1998).

25. How long should the treatment of vasospasm be continued, and how long will Sarah remain at risk for vasospasm or rebleeding?

Hypervolemic therapy is maintained until stabilization of the patient's condition and resolution of the acute phase. Calcium antagonists are usually continued for 21 days.

The risk for rebleeding is present until the aneurysm is surgically treated by clip ligation or clamp of the main feeder artery. In patients with untreated aneurysms after the first year, the risk of rebleeding is cumulative at 3% for each year. The risk for vasospasm is present for approximately 21 days, then the incidence drops off dramatically (LeRoux & Winn, 1998).

26. Discuss nonsurgical approaches available to patients unable to tolerate traditional surgical treatment.

Endovascular occlusion is an option for patients unable to undergo traditional surgical treatment. Coil embolization has been advocated for poor-grade patients (Hunt and Hess scale), advanced age, medical instability, difficult location of the aneurysm, and so on. One approach is the placement of platinum Guglielmi detachable coils within the aneurysmal sac. Thrombosis around the coil promotes occlusion of the aneurysm. There are many questions regarding long-term stability and recurrence after coil treatment. Another option includes treatment with stereotactic radiosurgery (LeRoux & Winn, 1998; Martin, 1998; Nelson, 1998).

SUBARACHNOID HEMORRHAGE WITH ANEURYSM

References

Baxter, A., Cohen, W. A., & Maravilla, R. (1998). Imaging of intracranial aneurysms and subarachnoid hemorrhage. *Neurosurgery Clinics of North America, 9*(3), 445-462.

Becker, K. J. (1998). Epidemiology and clinical presentation of aneurysmal subarachnoid hemorrhage. *Neurosurgery Clinics of North America, 9*(3), 435-444.

Bell, T. & Kongable, G. (1996). Innovations in aneurysmal subarachnoid hemorrhage: Intracisternal t-PA for the prevention of vasospasm. *Journal of Neuroscience Nursing, 25*(2), 107-110.

Campbell, P. & Edwards, S. (1997). Hyperdynamic therapy: The nurse's role in the treatment of cerebral vasospasm. *Journal of Neuroscience Nursing, 29*(5), 318-326.

Cavanagh, S. J. & Gordon, V. L. (2002). Grading scales used in the management of aneurysmal subarachnoid hemorrhage: A critical review. *Journal of Neuroscience Nursing, 34*(6), 288-295.

Connolly, E. & Solomon, R. (1998). Management of symptomatic and unsymptomatic unruptured aneurysms. *Neurosurgery Clinics of North America, 9*(3), 509-524.

Dorsch, N. (1996). Special problems associated with subarachnoid hemorrhage. In J. R. Youmans (Ed.), *Neurological surgery* (pp. 1438-1448). Philadelphia: Saunders.

Feigin, V., Rinkel, G., Algra, A., Vermeulen, M., & Van Gijn, J. (1998). Calcium antagonist in patients with aneurysmal subarachnoid hemorrhage. *Neurology, 50*(4), 876-881.

Hickey, J. (1997). *Neurological and neurosurgical nursing.* Philadelphia: JB Lippincott.

Hosoda, K., et al. (1999). Effects of clot removal and surgical manipulation on regional cerebral blood flow and delayed vasospasm in early aneurysm surgery for subarachnoid hemorrhage. *Surgical Neurology, 51*(1), 81-88.

Johnston, S., Selvin, S., & Gress, D. (1998) The burden, trends, and demographics of mortality from subarachnoid hemorrhage. *Neurology, 50*(5), 1413-1418.

Kirsch, J., Diringer, M., Borel, C., & Hanley, D. (1989). Cerebral aneurysms: Mechanisms of injury and critical care interventions. *Critical Care Clinics, 5*(4), 755-772.

Lanzino, G. & Kassell, N. (1998). Surgical treatment of the ruptured aneurysm. *Neurosurgery Clinics of North America, 9*(3), 541-547.

LeRoux, P. & Winn, H. (1998). Management of the ruptured aneurysm. *Neurosurgery Clinics of North America, 9*(3), 525-540.

Macdonald, R. (1996). Pathophysiology and clinical evaluation of subarachnoid hemorrhage. In J. R. Youmans (Ed.), *Neurological surgery* (pp. 1224-1242). Philadelphia: Saunders.

Manno, E. (1997). Transcranial Doppler ultrasonography in the neurocritical care unit. In M. N. Diringer (Ed.), *Critical care clinics* (pp. 79-104). Philadelphia: Saunders.

Martin, N. (1998). The combination of endovascular and surgical techniques for the treatment of intracranial aneurysms. *Neurosurgery Clinics of North America, 9*(4), 897-916.

Mayberg, M. (1998). Cerebral vasospasm. *Neurosurgery Clinics of North America, 9*(3), 615-628.

McKhann, G. & LeRoux, P. (1998). Perioperative and intensive care unit care of patients with aneurysmal subarachnoid hemorrhage. *Neurosurgery Clinics of North America, 9*(3), 595-610.

Mendel, R. & Carter, L. (1994). Evaluation and treatment of clinical vasospasm following subarachnoid hemorrhage. *Contemporary Neurosurgery, 16*(6), 1-6.

Miyaoka, M., Sato, K., & Ishii, S. (1993). A clinical study of the relationship of timing to outcome of surgery for ruptured cerebral aneurysms. *Journal of Neurosurgery, 79*, 373-378.

Nelson, P. (1998). Neurointerventional management of intracranial aneurysms. *Neurosurgery Clinics of North America, 9*(4), 879-896.

O'Sullivan, M. M. & O'Sullivan, J. C. (2000). Hyperperfusion therapy for cerebral vasospasm following ruptured cerebral aneurysm. www.aacn.org/aacn/conteduc.nsf, 9.

Pfohman, M. & Criddle, L. (2001). Epidemiology of intracranial aneurysmal and subarachnoid hemorrhage. *Journal of Neuroscience Nurses, 33*(1), 39-41.

Romeo, J. (1993). Patients with craniotomies. In J. M. Clochesy, C. Breu, S. Cardin, E. B. Rudy, & A. A. Whittaker (Eds.), *Critical care nursing* (pp. 788-793). Philadelphia: Saunders.

Rusy, K. (1996). Rebleeding and vasospasm after subarachnoid hemorrhage: A critical care challenge. *Critical Care Nurse, 16*(1), 41-47.

Segatore, M. (1993). Hyponatremia after aneurysmal subarachnoid hemorrhage. *Journal of Neuroscience Nurses, 25*(2), 92-99.

Sikes, P. & Nolan, S. (1993). Pharmacologic management of cerebral vasospasm. *Critical Care Nurse Quarterly, 15*(4), 78-88.

Sommargen, C. E. (2002). Electrocardigraphic abnormalities in patients with subarachnoid hemorrhage. *American Journal of Critical Care, 11*(1), 48-56.

Urden, L. D., Stacy, K. M., & Lough, M. E. (Eds.). (2002). *Thelan's critical care nursing: Diagnosis and management* (4th ed.). St Louis: Mosby.

Van Tatenhove, J. & Kelley, C. (1999). Neurodiagnostic tests. In L. Bucher & S. Melander (Eds.), *Critical care nursing* (pp. 824-842). Philadelphia: Saunders.

Wojner, A. (1998). Neurovascular disease. In M. R. Kinney, S. B. Dunbar, J. A. Brooks-Brunn, N. Molter, & J. M. Vitello-Cicciu (Eds.), *AACN clinical reference for critical care nursing* (pp. 733-768). St Louis: Mosby.

Wojner, A. (1999). Neurovascular disorders. In L. Bucher & S. Melander (Eds.), *Critical care nursing* (pp. 913-939). Philadelphia: Saunders.

14

Head Trauma and Subdural Hematoma

Cinda Alexander, MSN, CCRN, CNRN, CNOR, CRNFA

CASE PRESENTATION

Joyce, a 27-year-old right-handed patient, was involved in a motor vehicle accident. Joyce was an unrestrained passenger in a car that swerved off the road and struck a tree. She was ejected from the car and was found unconscious by the emergency medical service personnel.

After being placed on a spinal board and in a Philadelphia collar, Joyce was transported by helicopter to the nearest emergency department trauma center. Joyce was somewhat combative and unresponsive to commands at arrival. Her pupils were reactive bilaterally (left > right). Her respiratory rate was 40 breaths/min and labored. Subsequently, an endotracheal tube was placed, and mechanical ventilation was started. Additional treatment included placement of a subclavian intravenous (IV) line, arterial catheter, and Foley catheter. Initial evaluation of her cervical spine revealed no abnormal findings, and the long spine board and Philadelphia collar were removed. Joyce's diagnostic data were as follows:

BP	90/40 mm Hg
HR	100 bpm
Respirations	40 breaths/min
Temperature	36.7° C (98° F)
Pupils Reactive	left > right
Glasgow Coma Scale score	9

Joyce's initial computed tomography (CT) scan of the head revealed a left temporal cerebral contusion with a midline shift of brain structures. The CT scan also revealed a left temporal parietal subdural hematoma (SDH).

After surgical removal of the hematoma, Joyce was transferred to the critical care unit. Intubation and mechanical ventilation were continued. An intracranial pressure (ICP) monitoring device was placed. The following were her diagnostic data after surgery:

ICP	25 mm Hg
BP	130/88 mm Hg
HR	100 bpm
Respirations	12 breaths/min
Temperature	37.8° C (100° F)
pH	7.48

P_{CO_2}	40 mm Hg
P_{O_2}	434 mm Hg
HCO_3^-	20.4 mmol/L

Ventilator settings were as follows:

V_T	700 ml
Rate	12/min
FiO_2	100%

As Joyce recovered from the general anesthesia, she opened her eyes to speech, verbalized incomprehensible sounds, and exhibited abnormal general flexion to obtain a Glasgow Coma Scale score of 8. Over the next 2 hours, Joyce's body temperature increased to 38.3° C (101° F). Despite hyperventilation, Joyce's ICP remained elevated. Her serum osmolality was 282 mOsm/L, K^+ level was 3.9 mmol/L, and Na^+ level was 139 mmol/L. Postoperative orders included the following:

- Fluid restriction to maintain patient's osmolality between 305 and 315 mOsm/L
- Furosemide (Lasix) 20 mg q6h, IV
- Mannitol (Osmitrol) 25 to 50 g periodic bolus
- Phenytoin (Dilantin) 100 mg IV q6h

Joyce's ICP remained elevated for more than 72 hours, then gradually her pressure stabilized. After 2 weeks in the intensive care unit, Joyce was transferred to a neurologic step-down unit and then to a head injury rehabilitation unit.

HEAD TRAUMA AND SUBDURAL HEMATOMA

QUESTIONS

1. Where does head trauma rank as a cause of death in the United States? What are the statistics associated with head trauma? Include morbidity and mortality information.

2. Identify the leading causes of head injury.

3. What is the rationale for Joyce being placed on a long spine board with a Philadelphia collar?

4. What is the Glasgow Coma Scale? How is this scale helpful?

5. Differentiate the types of skull fractures associated with head trauma. What clinical presentations and pathophysiology are pertinent in these types of trauma?

6. Identify special considerations that are necessary for patients with basilar skull fractures for placement of an endotracheal or nasogastric tube.

7. List and describe the focal injuries associated with traumatic head injury. Include the mechanism of injury and clinical presentation associated with each.

8. List and describe the diffuse injuries associated with traumatic head injury.

9. Discuss the significance of a midline shift.

10. Identify the types of SDHs. Include the pathology and clinical presentation of SDH.

11. What surgical intervention is indicated for patients with SDH?

12. Define ICP. What methods are available for monitoring ICP? Describe the potential complications of ICP monitoring.

13. What factors determine when an ICP monitoring device is placed?

14. List and describe possible secondary injuries with head injury.

15. Based on Joyce's arterial blood gas results, what ventilator changes should be anticipated? What is the desirable arterial carbon dioxide pressure ($PaCO_2$) range in the presence of increased ICP?

16. Discuss the effect hyperventilation has on cerebral blood flow and increased ICP.

17. Describe the pathophysiology of intracranial hypertension. What is the general cause of increased ICP in patients with acute head injury?

18. What is autoregulation and how does it affect cerebral blood flow and ICP?

19. Given an ICP of 25 mm Hg and blood pressure of 120/72 mm Hg, calculate Joyce's cerebral perfusion pressure (CPP). Is the CPP an acceptable value? Discuss the drawbacks of using CPP values.

20. Discuss the medical management that should be anticipated for patients with head injuries. Include the rationale and identify at least one potential complication associated with each.

21. Define and discuss the clinical significance of posturing such as abnormal flexion and abnormal extension.

22. Describe the relevance of controlling hyperthermia in the management of patients with head injuries.

23. What nursing management actions are essential to prevent or minimize the effects of secondary injury in patients with head injuries?

24. What are the potential extracranial effects of increased ICP?

25. Which cranial nerves must be intact before the patient eats or drinks?

HEAD TRAUMA AND SUBDURAL HEMATOMA

QUESTIONS AND ANSWERS

1. **Where does head trauma rank as a cause of death in the United States? What are the statistics associated with head trauma? Include morbidity and mortality information.**

   Head trauma is the third leading cause of death in the United States. It is estimated that more than 1.5 million head injuries occur each year. Approximately 373,000 hospitalizations and 75,000 deaths are associated with head injury (Zink & Lanter, 2001). Of all trauma-related deaths, 70% involve a head injury. Mortality from head injury alone is estimated to be approximately 50%. Most of these deaths occur before the person enters the health care system. The incidence of head injury is two to three times greater in males than in females, peak incidence is at age 15 to 24 years, and the most common cause of death for people younger than the age of 45 (Walleck, 1993; Sullivan et al, 1994; Guidelines for the Management of Severe Head Injury, 1995; McNair, 1999; Littlejohns & Bader, 2001; Lovasik et al, 2001).

2. **Identify the leading causes of head injury.**

   Motor vehicle accidents are the leading cause of head injury with alcohol or drug consumption often associated as a contributing factor. Other causes include shootings, falls, assaults, and sporting accidents (Mansfield, 1997; March, 1999; Littlejohns & Bader, 2001).

3. **What is the rationale for Joyce being placed on a long spine board with a Philadelphia collar?**

   It is known that Joyce was traveling in a vehicle and was not wearing a seatbelt. It is also known that after the automobile she was riding in hit a tree, Joyce was ejected from the vehicle. It is well documented that there is a strong correlation between spinal cord trauma and head trauma or general trauma. Therefore if head or spinal trauma is suspected, it is always recommended that victims at the site of an accident be placed on a spinal board and in a Philadelphia collar to prevent any secondary trauma to either the spine or the head and neck area. Motor vehicle accidents account for 47.7% of all spinal cord injuries (Hickey, 1997). There is a higher incidence of spinal cord injury associated with victims who are ejected from the vehicle as in Joyce's case.

4. **What is the Glasgow Coma Scale? How is this scale helpful?**

   The Glasgow Coma Scale is a standardized scale used to evaluate neurologic response. The scale is divided into three sections designed to assess consciousness, verbal abilities, and motor response. The scores range from 3 to 15, with 15 representing normal function. It is generally accepted that a score of 8 or less constitutes coma. The scale is a useful tool to communicate the patient's neurologic condition after a rapid assessment (Nikas, 1998; March, 1999; McNair, 1999; Fischer & Mathieson, 2001; Hartshorn & Gauthier, 2001; Cavanagh & Gordon, 2002; Urden et al, 2002).

5. **Differentiate the types of skull fractures associated with head trauma. What clinical presentations and pathophysiology are pertinent in these types of trauma?**

   Skull fractures are categorized as linear, depressed, or basilar and may be simple, comminuted, or compound in nature. The presence of a skull fracture does not delineate the degree of injury to the brain structures within the skull (Davis & Briones, 1998; Zink & Lanter, 2001).

Linear Skull Fracture

Linear skull fractures are nondisplaced fractures of the skull. Most linear skull fractures are not displaced and do not require intervention unless they extend into a major sinus or across a major vascular channel (Nikas, 1998; March, 1999). If there is a fracture across a major vascular channel, such as the middle meningeal artery in the temporal parietal area, the patient should be evaluated carefully for acute epidural bleeding.

Depressed Skull Fracture

A depressed skull fracture is characterized by an inward depression of the outer table of the skull. Patients will have an open laceration in the area of the depression and varying degrees of neurologic alterations based on the degree of brain tissue involvement. Surgical intervention may be necessary to remove bone fragment from the meninges or brain tissue. The area of tissue and compression by the bony fragments can become a source of irritability and seizure focus (Hartshorn & Gauthier, 2001). If the fracture is severe, clinical presentation may extend to seepage of cerebrospinal fluid (CSF) and brain tissue from the fracture site.

Basilar Skull Fracture

A basilar skull fracture is located at the base of the skull. If the fracture is significant, the underlying dura may be torn, which allows direct communication with the subarachnoid space and brain tissue. Infection and meningitis are of major concern with this type of fracture. Clinical presentation may include the following (Walleck, 1993; Davis & Briones, 1998; March, 1999):

- Seepage of CSF from the nose (rhinorrhea)
- Bilateral periorbital ecchymosis (raccoon eyes) if the anterior fossa is involved
- Leakage of CSF from the ears (otorrhea) if the middle fossa is involved
- Ecchymosis of the mastoid sinus (Battle's sign) if the posterior fossa is involved

6. **Identify special considerations that are necessary for patients with basilar skull fractures for placement of an endotracheal or nasogastric tube.**

The inherent risk associated with endotracheal intubation and passage of a nasogastric tube is penetration through the fracture site and passage into the brain itself. Precautions include the use of the oral route for intubation and nasogastric tubes to minimize this risk. In addition, the nose should never be suctioned for removal of drainage in patients with basilar skull fractures (Walleck, 1993).

7. **List and describe the focal injuries associated with traumatic head injury. Include the mechanism of injury and clinical presentation associated with each.**

The most common focal injuries associated with head injury are laceration, contusion, and intracranial hematomas (Butterworth & DeWitt, 1989; Hickey, 1997; Mansfield, 1997; March, 1999; Zink & Lanter, 2001).

Contusions and Lacerations

A *contusion* is bruising of the brain. Contusions can be mild, involving a small portion of the brain tissue with minimal clinical symptoms, or they can be large, usually in the case of impact injuries, where the size increases as a result of edema and may produce significant increases in ICP. Injury to the brain usually results from accelerations and decelerations of the brain within the cranial vault. Contusions and lacerations tend to occur in the frontal and temporal areas and are commonly associated with skull fractures. A laceration is the tearing of brain parenchyma and is often associated with a depressed skull fracture. The significance of contusions and lacerations and severity of the neurologic injury are related to the degree of secondary insults such as edema, hemorrhage, and ischemia (Butterworth & DeWitt, 1989; March, 1999).

Hematomas

Intracranial hematomas are classified as extradural or intradural. Extradural hematomas are referred to as *epidural* and generally are arterial in nature, usually occurring from a laceration of the middle meningeal artery. The clot forms between the inner table of the skull and the outer dura. Clinical symptoms develop quickly and are manifested as a sudden deterioration of consciousness, a fixed and dilated ipsilateral pupil, and hemiplegia or paresis. SDHs *(intradural)* form when there is bleeding between the dura and arachnoid layers. SDHs are generally venous in nature and often result from tears of cortical bridging veins but can result from bruising of the cortical tissue as well. The bleeding creates direct pressure and irritation of the cortical tissue. Clinical presentation includes a significantly depressed level of consciousness, pupillary changes (unequal to dilated and fixed), headache, agitation, confusion, and motor deficits. The degree of symptoms usually depends on the location and size of the clot formation (Walleck, 1993; March, 1999).

8. List and describe the diffuse injuries associated with traumatic head injury.

Concussion

A *concussion* is a transient, temporary condition of the brain without any structural damage. The clinical symptoms usually include a brief (generally seconds) loss of consciousness, confusion, and some amnesia. However, concussion can be severe enough to induce brief respiratory arrest, pronounced confusion, and severe amnesia. Concussions can be graded I through IV, with IV being the most severe. Clinical presentation and the lack of adequate supervision at home may necessitate hospitalization (March, 1999; Zink & Lanter, 2001).

Diffuse axonal injury

Diffuse axonal injury (DAI) is a shear injury to the white matter with stretching and tearing of the reticular activating fibers. Microscopic focal lesions in the white matter include axon contraction balls throughout white matter, gathering of microglial cells, followed by degradation of long tracts. Microhemorrhagic or necrotic lesions appear in the corpus callosum and in the dorsolateral part of the upper brainstem (Sahuquillo-Barris et al, 1988; Liau et al, 1996; McNair, 1999). Clinical presentation includes deep and profound coma, abnormal posturing, increased ICP, hypertension, and hyperthermia. The hallmark of DAI is immediate and prolonged coma without radiographic identification of a specific cause (Butterworth & DeWitt, 1989; Crow, 1991; Walleck, 1993; Mansfield, 1997; Davis & Briones, 1998; March, 1999).

9. Discuss the significance of a midline shift.

A midline shift on a CT or magnetic resonance imaging scan indicates that the delicate structures of the central portion of the brain, such as the ventricles and brainstem, have been displaced laterally. Brain tissue displacement is poorly tolerated and leads to areas of ischemia, diffuse edema, and shearing of structures (Walleck, 1993; Liau et al, 1996; McNair, 1999; Zink & Lanter, 2001).

10. Identify the types of SDHs. Include the pathology and clinical presentation of SDH.

SDHs are classified as acute, subacute, and chronic, with mortality ranging from 52% to 90% (Wilberger et al, 1991; Walleck, 1993; March, 1999; Urden et al, 2002). Acute SDH generally occurs within 48 hours of the initial injury. Clinical presentation is usually progressive, with possible headache, symptoms of increased ICP, pupillary and motor changes, and marked coma.

Subacute SDH develops 2 to 24 days after the initial injury. SDHs are often difficult to diagnose and are strongly indicated by failure to regain consciousness after head trauma.

Chronic SDH can develop from minor head trauma. Often, chronic SDH is associated with the elderly population because of cerebral atrophy, which can result from a minor fall or bump of the head. In the chronic state the blood clot becomes encased within a membrane. Clinical symptoms generally are subtle and vague, with progressive confusion, drowsiness, headache, seizures, and hemiparesis. Symptoms associated with chronic SDH may not become apparent until several weeks to months after the initial injury. Persons with alcoholism are prone to chronic SDH formation as a result of frequent falls and changes in clotting factors associated with alcoholism (Walleck, 1993; Hickey, 1997; March, 1999; McNair, 1999).

11. What surgical intervention is indicated for patients with SDH?

Small SDHs can be treated medically because they can be reabsorbed if there is no evidence of significant increased ICP or shifting of brain structures. Acute SDH is surgically treated by craniotomy and removal of the clot. The greater the thickness of the clot and the greater the midline shift, the higher the morbidity and mortality (Zumkeller et al, 1996; Baldisseri, 2003). Subacute SDH may require a craniotomy flap or may be treated by burr holes if the clot has degenerated into a thick viscous liquid. Chronic SDH is treated with burr holes and placement of a temporary drain. Persistent chronic SDH may require a craniotomy flap to remove the membrane flap (Walleck, 1993).

12. Define ICP. What methods are available for monitoring ICP? Describe the potential complications of ICP monitoring.

ICP is a dynamic state of equilibrium that exists among the three components within the cranial vault: blood, brain, and CSF. Any increase in one component necessitates a decrease in another component for the dynamic equilibrium to remain constant; otherwise, an increase in ICP occurs (Monro-Kellie doctrine) (Hickey, 1997).

Various methods are available to measure ICP, including catheters and transducer setups that measure pressure from the epidural area, subdural area, subarachnoid space, tissue, and intraventricular spaces. The major complication associated with ICP monitoring is infection. Generally, the more invasive the method, the greater the risk of serious consequences of infection. Other complications associated with ICP monitoring include hematoma and migration of the catheter or device (Davis & Briones, 1998; Nikas, 1998; Van Tatenhove & Kelley, 1999; Michael, 2003).

13. What factors determine when an ICP monitoring device is placed?

Indications for an ICP monitor are somewhat controversial. General guidelines for placement include the following (Butterworth & DeWitt, 1989; Andrews, 1998; Van Tatenhove & Kelley, 1999; Michael, 2003):

- A Glasgow Coma Scale score of ≤8
- Intradural hematomas or contusions
- Demonstrated cerebral edema on CT scan
- Midline shifts

The Guidelines for the Management of Severe Head Injury (1995) indicate that ICP monitoring is appropriate if the CT scan is abnormal. In addition, if the CT scan is normal, ICP monitoring is appropriate if two or more of the following are noted:

- Age older than 40
- Motor posturing
- Systolic blood pressure <90 mm Hg

Other parameter(s) may be available for monitoring cerebral oxygenation. There is a growing interest in the use of venous jugular bulb saturation to estimate cerebral ischemia. An oximeter catheter can be placed in the jugular bulb to measure cerebral venous oxygen saturation (SaO_2). This parameter allows the calculation of tissue oxygen delivery and consumption. In addition to ICP monitoring devices, other monitoring may include transcranial Doppler, end-tidal CO_2, cerebral lactate levels, as well as other investigative approaches under evaluation (Kidd & Criddle, 2001).

14. List and describe possible secondary injuries with head injury.

Secondary insults precipitated by brain trauma may include hypoxia, hypercapnia, hypotension, and cerebral edema or intracranial hypertension. Secondary processes may be immediate or delayed and are mediated by biochemical and cellular responses to the initial insult (Mansfield, 1997; Davis & Briones, 1998; March, 1999; McNair, 1999; Wright, 1999; Lovasik et al, 2001).

Hypoxia

Brain injury often leads to irregular and inadequate respiratory efforts. Early management of the airway at the scene of injury and aggressive respiratory support are critical. Hypoxemia contributes to neurologic damage because the brain compensates for a deceased oxygen supply by increased cerebral blood flow. This offers a luxury perfusion to the uninjured tissue and contributes to increased cerebral blood volume, thus increasing ICP (March, 1999; McNair, 1999). The Guidelines for the Management of Severe Head Injury (1995) recommend that hypotension (systolic blood pressure <90 mm Hg) or hypoxia (arterial oxygen pressure [PaO_2] <60 mm Hg) must be avoided and corrected immediately.

Hypercapnia

Carbon dioxide is a potent cerebrovasodilator that will increase cerebral blood flow and contribute to increased intracranial hypertension.

Hypotension

Hypotension is often the result of multisystem injury and overall blood loss. The mean arterial pressure (MAP) must be sufficient to maintain cerebral perfusion. Systemic hypotension contributes to general cerebral hypoperfusion (March, 1999).

Intracranial Hypertension

Cerebral edema associated with head trauma may be local or diffuse. Cerebral edema exaggerates the amount and severity of neurologic injury and leads to increased ICP. Intracranial hypertension is a major complication and is the most common cause of death associated with brain injury. Most of the care of patients with head injuries is focused on control of ICP (Bouma et al, 1992; Hickey, 1997; Marion & Letarte, 1997; Andrews, 1998). Wilberger and associates (1991) found that control of increased ICP after removal of an SDH was a variable more critical to the patient's outcome than timing of surgery for removal of the clot.

15. Based on Joyce's arterial blood gas results, what ventilator changes should be anticipated? What is the desirable arterial carbon dioxide pressure ($Paco_2$) range in the presence of increased ICP?

Ventilator changes to reduce the $Paco_2$ include increasing the rate (frequency) or tidal volume. Decreasing the fraction of inspired oxygen (Fio_2) to minimize the effect of oxygen toxicity is also indicated.

16. Discuss the effect hyperventilation has on cerebral blood flow and increased ICP.

Hyperventilation, a cornerstone in the management of traumatic brain injury, assists with the reduction of carbon dioxide, a potent cerebrovasodilator. With a reduction of $Paco_2$ there is vasoconstriction of the cerebral blood vessels, decreased cerebral blood volume, and thus decreased ICP. Severely lowered $Paco_2$ levels have a potential for causing ischemia and infarction (Walleck, 1993; Littlejohns & Bader, 2001; Urden et al, 2002; Michael, 2003). Because traumatic brain injury is associated with a reduction of cerebral blood flow in the initial 24 hours after injury, hyperventilation is not without risk. Chronic use of hyperventilation of less than $PaCO_2$ of 25 mm Hg should be avoided because it may contribute to cerebral ischemia in an already compromised brain (Guidelines for the Management of Severe Head Injury, 1995; Littlejohns & Bader, 2001; Mansfield, 1997; Walleck, 1993; Wright, 1999; Yundt & Diringer, 1997).

Guidelines for the Management of Severe Head Injury (1995) include the following:

- Chronic, prolonged hyperventilation ($PaCO_2$ = 25 mm Hg) should be avoided
- Prophylactic hyperventilation ($PaCO_2$ = 35 mm Hg) should be avoided the first 24 hours after injury

17. Describe the pathophysiology of intracranial hypertension. What is the general cause of increased ICP in patients with acute head injury?

The Monro-Kellie doctrine describes the skull encasing a closed system with three components: blood, CSF, and brain tissue. If the volume of any of these three components increases without a concurrent decrease in one of the other, increased ICP will result. Normal ICP is 0 to 15 mm Hg. Some variations may be associated with the type of monitoring device used. *Intracranial hypertension* is a sustained increase in ICP greater than 15 mm Hg caused by the following conditions:

- Conditions that increase brain volume such as hematomas or cerebral edema
- Conditions that increase cerebral blood flow, including hyperemia and hypercapnia
- Conditions that increase CSF volume such as increased production of CSF, decreased absorption, and obstruction hydrocephalus

Cerebral edema is a common complication of moderate to severe brain injury that can result in intracranial hypertension and reduction of cerebral blood flow. Eisenhart (1994) describes three major causes of cerebral edema: increased cerebral blood flow, biochemical changes at the cellular level, and brain ischemia.

Initially, after acute head injury, cerebral blood flow increases, with an associated increase in ICP or intracranial hypertension, because there is engorgement of the brain tissue. As the ICP elevates, there is an associated tissue ischemia. Cerebral edema is also triggered at the cellular level via chemical changes and the release of excitatory amino acids. The state of increased pressure is further complicated by hypotension, resulting in decreased oxygenation to the tissues, and hypercapnia, resulting in cerebrovasodilation (Hickey, 1997; Nikas, 1998). Treatment now focuses on management of brain tissue perfusion and promotion of cerebral perfusion (Mansfield, 1997; Davis & Briones, 1998; March, 1999; McNair, 1999; Littlejohns & Bader, 2001; Michael, 2003). However, according to the Guidelines for the Management of Severe Head Injury (1995), ICP treatment should be initiated at an upper threshold of 20 to 25 mm Hg. In addition, interpretation and treatment of ICP should be correlated by frequent clinical review of the CPP data. Cerebral blood flow must be maintained at a minimal level to ensure adequate tissue perfusion. Because cerebral blood flow is difficult to measure in the clinical setting, the CPP can be estimated and used as an index (see question 19).

18. What is autoregulation and how does it affect cerebral blood flow and ICP?

Autoregulation is the automatic change in cerebral blood vessels in response to varying systemic pressures to maintain a continuous perfusion pressure gradient to the tissues without wide fluctuation of flow. The reflex maintains constant perfusion despite wide variations in systemic MAP. When autoregulation is disrupted, as may be the case in traumatized brain tissue, that area of tissue is dependent on systemic pressure for perfusion (Walleck, 1993; Rosner, 1995; Hickey, 1997; March, 1999; McNair, 1999; Michael, 2003).

19. **Given an ICP of 25 mm Hg and blood pressure of 120/72 mm Hg, calculate Joyce's cerebral perfusion pressure (CPP). Is the CPP an acceptable value? Discuss the drawbacks of using CPP values.**

To calculate MAP:

$$\frac{\text{Systolic} + (2 \times \text{Diastolic})}{3} = \text{MAP}$$

To calculate CPP: MAP – ICP = CPP

$$\frac{120 + (2 \times 72)}{3} = 88 \text{ mm Hg (MAP)}$$

$$88 - 25 = 63 \text{ mm Hg (CPP)}$$

The focus has shifted from the single measurement of ICP to management of cerebral perfusion. Controversy exists over the "minimal" acceptable CPP value. Generally, 60 mm Hg is considered the lowest acceptable value. Once ICP rises and CPP begins to fall, cerebral tissue is deprived of sufficient blood flow, and ischemia and infarction occur. If the ICP rises too high, the brain tissue herniates, followed by ischemia and infarction. If the herniation process continues without intervention, death caused by brainstem compression is usually the result (Kirsch et al, 1989; Walleck, 1993; Liau et al, 1996; March, 1999; Littlejohns & Bader, 2001; Urden et al, 2002). The recommendation of the Guidelines for the Management of Severe Head Injury (1995) is to maintain a CPP of 70 mm Hg.

20. **Discuss the medical management that should be anticipated for patients with head injuries. Include the rationale and identify at least one potential complication associated with each.**

CSF drainage

A ventriculostomy will allow the drainage of CSF as well as ICP monitoring. Generally the drainage point, or the point at which the CSF should drain via the ventriculostomy, is set for 20 mm Hg. The drainage point may be lowered to 15 mm Hg to promote additional CSF drainage if there is an increase in ICP (Hickey, 1997; Marion & Letarte, 1997). A serious complication of a ventriculostomy is infection or ventriculitis. Generally a ventriculostomy in place longer than 7 to 10 days is associated with a significantly higher incidence of infection. Care should be taken to not allow "overdrainage" of the CSF and subsequent collapse of the ventricles.

Hyperventilation

Hyperventilation is induced to decrease the $Paco_2$ and promote vasoconstriction of cerebrovasculature, thereby decreasing cerebral blood flow and ICP. However, severe reduction of $Paco_2$, below 20 mm Hg, can cause hypoxia and tissue ischemia or infarction (Nikas, 1998; Littlejohns & Bader, 2001). Hyperventilation should be used judiciously only if uncontrolled ICP is present (Eisenhart, 1994; Fischer & Mathieson, 2001).

Osmotic diuretics

Osmotic diuretics decrease brain edema by creating a vascular gradient promoting movement of water from brain tissue into the vascular compartment. Hyperosmolarity and renal failure are potential complications of this treatment. Mannitol is the drug of choice because of its rapid onset of action (Guidelines for the Management of Severe Head Injury, 1995; Hickey, 1997; March, 1999; Marion & Letarte, 1997; Yanko & Mitcho, 2001). Serum osmolarity should be maintained below 320 mOsm. The Guidelines for the Management of Severe Head Injury (1995) suggest that an intermittent bolus may be more effective than a continuous IV infusion.

Loop diuretics

Loop diuretics, such as furosemide (Lasix), are often used in combination with osmotic diuretics. The benefits probably relate to the ability of loop diuretics to reduce total body fluid and shifting of extravascular space, preventing acute pulmonary edema and congestive heart failure that can be a complication of osmotic therapy (March, 1999; Yanko & Mitcho, 2001). Joyce's hydration status must be evaluated carefully because the overuse of loop diuretics can lead to severe dehydration.

Fluid management

Fluid restriction remains controversial in the care of patients with head injuries. Too much fluid restriction may result in severe dehydration. The patient's osmolality is the best guide for fluid therapy with a goal of 305 to 315 mOsm/L (normal 280 to 300 mOsm/L) with the goal of euvolemia (Hickey, 1997; Yanko & Mitcho, 2001).

Glucocorticosteroids

The Guidelines for the Management of Severe Head Injury (1995) state that use of glucocorticosteroids is not recommended for improving outcome or reducing ICP in patients with severe brain injury. Steroids are still widely used in the treatment of brain tumors. Side effects associated with large doses of steroids include decreased resistance to infection and gastrointestinal hemorrhage (Hickey, 1997; March, 1999; Littlejohns & Bader, 2001).

Barbiturate therapy

Barbiturate therapy for coma is still considered for patients with uncontrolled ICP associated with cerebral edema. Barbiturates lower ICP; however, the mechanism is not well understood. Barbiturates are associated with numerous complications, including hypotension and decreased cardiac output (Kirsch et al, 1989; Walleck, 1993; Kelly et al, 1996). An ICP monitoring device must be used during barbiturate therapy so that the nurse can evaluate the patient's neurologic status because the patient is in a drug-induced coma (Guidelines for the Management of Severe Head Injury, 1995; March, 1999; Littlejohns & Bader, 2001; Lovasik et al, 2001).

Seizure control

Posttraumatic epilepsy occurs in 5% to 20% of patients with head injuries. The more severe the injury, the greater the likelihood of seizure activity. Seizures may occur early, within the first 7 days, or late after brain injury. Late posttraumatic seizures should not be treated prophylactically with anticonvulsants (Guidelines for the Management of Severe Head Injury, 1995; March, 1999; Littlejohns & Bader, 2001). Risk factors to assess include intracranial hematoma, focal neurologic deficits, posttraumatic amnesia lasting more than 24 hours, depressed skull fracture, and age younger than 5 years. The treatment of early posttraumatic seizures may reduce secondary injury and ischemia. Seizure activity in the presence of brain injury can lead to a severe elevation in ICP and place increased metabolic demands on a compromised brain. Phenytoin (Dilantin) is the drug of choice for seizure control. Potential adverse effects of IV phenytoin are hypotension and cardiac arrhythmias.

Sedation, analgesics, and neuromuscular blockade

Benzodiazepines are the most commonly used sedatives. Propofol is the most popular. Because sedatives do not provide analgesia, consideration must be given for pain control. Parenteral narcotics, such as small doses of morphine or fentanyl, may be used. Short-acting neuromuscular blockade (e.g., with vecuronium) may be used to counteract the ICP response to stimulation associated with activities such as personal care or suctioning (Fowler et al, 1995; Hickey, 1997; Marion & Letarte, 1997; March, 1999; Fischer & Mathieson, 2001; Yanko & Mitcho, 2001). Potential complications of these agents include hypotension and respiratory depression.

Neuroprotectants

There is much interest in investigational drugs called *neuroprotectants*. These drugs are thought to treat or control the pathologic response to the secondary insult of ischemia (March, 1999). As ischemia occurs in an injured brain, it is believed that there are biochemical processes that trigger a "neurotoxic cascade" of reactions. These biochemical changes may include the release of excitatory amino acids as well as the generation of oxygen-free radicals. The eventual result is cellular damage and destruction, which may not be restricted to the initially injured cells. Pharmacologic agents such as oxygen-free radical scavengers, glutamate antagonists, calcium channel blockers, nonglucocorticosteroids, and excitatory amino acid antagonists are now being studied in various trial phases (Eisenhart, 1994; Guidelines for the Management of Severe Head Injury, 1995; March, 1999; McNair, 1999; Littlejohns & Bader, 2001).

21. Define and discuss the clinical significance of posturing such as abnormal flexion and abnormal extension.

Noxious stimuli can initiate abnormal stereotypic motor responses referred to as *posturing*. Posturing, such as abnormal extension and abnormal flexion, is often associated with abnormal brainstem function and damage to the cerebral hemisphere.

Decortication is the hyperflexion of the upper extremities and the hyperextension of the lower extremities. Decortication, also referred to as *flexion abnormal,* may indicate damage to the cerebral hemispheres and internal capsule. Decerebration is the hyperextension of both the upper and lower extremities and internal rotation of the upper extremities. Decerebration, also referred to as *extension abnormal,* can indicate brainstem dysfunction. The presence of abnormal posturing does not clearly predict the outcome after acute head injury. However, it emphasizes the need for close neurologic monitoring because the brain has been severely compromised (Hartshorn & Gauthier, 2001).

22. Describe the relevance of controlling hyperthermia in the management of patients with head injuries.

Hyperthermia increases metabolic activity in the brain tissue, resulting in a greater oxygen demand. This leads to an increase in cerebral blood flow and production of carbon dioxide in a brain already compromised by cerebral edema and increased ICP (Walleck, 1993; March, 1999; Fischer & Mathieson, 2001). There is increased interest in the use of hypothermia with the core temperature 34° to 35° C, to help decrease ICP. Hypothermia is believed to stabilize cell membranes. The risks of complications include infection, cardiac arrest, cardiac arrhythmia, rewarming shock, renal failure, and rebound ICP (Fischer & Mathieson, 2001).

23. What nursing management actions are essential to prevent or minimize the effects of secondary injury in patients with head injuries?

Walleck (1993) outlines the following guidelines for patient care:

- *Patient positioning:* The patient's position should always promote venous drainage from the brain. The head, neck, and chest are maintained in alignment to prevent obstruction of the jugular veins and twisting of the neck. The head of the bed is usually elevated. According to Feldman and colleagues (1992), elevation of the head at 30 degrees significantly reduces ICP without compromising cerebral blood flow and CPP.
- *Ventilation:* Airway management and pulmonary toilet are important protocols to manage patients with head injuries and prevent pulmonary complications.
- *Hyperventilation and oxygenation:* Hyperventilation and oxygenation before and after pulmonary suctioning can minimize the negative effects of suctioning. Caution must be observed to prevent overhyperventilation, which may lead to $PaCO_2$ values less than 25 mm Hg.
- *Maintenance of blood pressure:* Hemodynamic stability is critical in the patient with a head injury to prevent wide fluctuations in MAP. Appropriate treatment of hypotension with IV fluids and pharmacologic agents and ongoing assessment of the MAP are indicated.

- *Normothermia:* Monitoring and maintenance of normal body temperature are necessary to prevent the effects of a hypermetabolic state on ICP.
- *Neurologic assessment:* Ongoing assessment of the patient's neurologic function is paramount to detect subtle changes that may indicate deterioration of the patient's condition. Serial evaluation and collaboration among caregivers are critical to ensure that any changes in status are noted.
- *Physical care*: There has been much interest in the literature as to the effects of personal care such as bathing, oral hygiene, and range of motion on ICP. Individualization based on patient response is necessary to determine which activities are well tolerated and which should be avoided. Generally it is accepted that physical activities should be spaced to allow the patient recovery time and to prevent compounded effects on the ICP.

24. What are the potential extracranial effects of increased ICP?

The following are major extracerebral effects of traumatic brain injury (March, 1999; Fischer & Mathieson, 2001).

Pulmonary Effects

- *Hypoxia:* Hypoxia occurs as a result of ventilation-perfusion mismatch or pulmonary shunt.
- *Noncardiogenic pulmonary edema:* Cerebral ischemia triggers a response of sympathetic discharge that alters capillary permeability in the lungs and creates an increase in atrial pressure.
- *Acute respiratory distress syndrome (ARDS):* ARDS is a common complication of patients with head injuries, resulting in an increase in dead space, a decrease in pulmonary compliance, and formation of hyaline membrane.
- *Aspiration pneumonitis:* In patients with head injuries, the airway is often not guarded because of a depressed level of consciousness, leaving them at risk for aspiration.
- *Fat emboli:* Fat emboli are often associated with long bone fractures seen in patients with multiple trauma.
- *Pulmonary contusion:* Pulmonary contusion often accompanies head injury caused by multiple trauma.

Cardiovascular Effects

- *Hyperdynamic cardiovascular response:* Hyperdynamic cardiovascular response is a cardiovascular effect associated with head trauma, a state of elevated cardiac output, increased heart rate, and increased blood pressure.
- *Posttraumatic hypertension:* Posttraumatic hypertension is precipitated by increased sympathetic activity, resulting in increased systolic blood pressure associated with Cushing's phenomenon.

Gastrointestinal Effects

- *Pancreatitis:* Pancreatitis is a gastrointestinal effect caused by blunt trauma to the abdomen that may be difficult to diagnose because of the patient's decreased level of consciousness.
- *Stress ulceration:* Stress ulceration may be present as erosive gastritis or gastrointestinal bleeding resulting from increased acidity.

Electrolyte and Metabolic Derangements

- *Hyponatremia:* Hyponatremia is associated with diarrhea, vomiting, gastric suction, and syndrome of inappropriate secretion of antidiuretic hormone.
- *Hypernatremia:* Hypernatremia usually represents water loss and may also be the result of diabetes insipidus.
- *Potassium deficits:* Deficiencies may be related to inadequate potassium replacement, diuretics, or alkalemia.
- *Thyroid and adrenal malfunction:* Trauma to the hypothalamus and pituitary glands results in thyroid and adrenal malfunction.

Nutrition

- *Autocatabolic state:* Autocatabolic state is an effect of increased ICP caused by stress-related hypermetabolism and gluconeogenesis.
- *Coagulation abnormalities:* Disseminated intravascular coagulation (DIC) is the most common coagulopathy associated with severe head trauma, especially with acute SDH and contusions. The cause of DIC is high thromboplastic activity of brain tissue.

25. **Which cranial nerves must be intact before the patient eats or drinks?**

It is essential that the nurse evaluate the following cranial nerves before the patient eats or drinks:

- Cranial nerve V (trigeminal): chewing
- Cranial nerve VII (facial): facial muscles
- Cranial nerves IX and X (glossopharyngeal and vagus): gag and swallowing
- Cranial nerve XII (hypoglossal): tongue

Only if these cranial nerves are intact bilaterally can the patient take nourishment by mouth (Walleck, 1993).

HEAD TRAUMA AND SUBDURAL HEMATOMA

References

Andrews, B. T. (1998). Intensive care for the neurosurgical patient. *Contemporary Neurosurgery, 20*(3), 1-6.

Baldisseri, M. R. (2003). Subdural hematoma. In J. A. Kruse, M. P. Fink, & R. W. Carlson (Eds.), *Saunders' manual of critical care* (pp. 291-292). Philadelphia: Saunders.

Bouma, G. J., Muizelaar, J. P., Bandoh, K., & Marmarou, A. (1992). Blood pressure and intracranial pressure-volume dynamics in severe head injury: Relationship with cerebral blood flow. *Journal of Neurosurgery, 77*, 15-19.

Butterworth, J. F. & DeWitt, D. S. (1989). Severe head trauma: Pathophysiology and management. *Critical Care Clinics, 5*(4), 807-819.

Cavanagh, S. J. & Gordon, V. L. (2002). Grading scales used in the management of aneurysmal subarachnoid hemorrhage: A critical review. *Journal of Neuroscience Nursing, 34*(6), 288-295.

Crow, W. (1991). Aspects of neuroradiology of head injury. *Neurosurgery Clinics of North America, 2*(2), 321-340.

Davis, A. E. & Briones, T. L. (1998). Intracranial disorders. In M. R. Kinney, S. B. Dunbar, J. A. Brooks-Brunn, N. Molter, & J. M. Vitello-Cicciu (Eds.), *AACN clinical reference for critical care nursing* (pp. 685-710). St Louis: Mosby.

Eisenhart, K. (1994). New perspectives in the management of adults with severe head injury. *Critical Care Nurse Quarterly, 17*(2), 1-12.

Feldman, Z., et al. (1992). Effect of head elevation on intracranial pressure, cerebral perfusion pressure, and cerebral blood flow in head-injured patients. *Journal of Neurosurgery, 76*, 207-211.

Fischer, J. & Mathieson, C. (2001). The history of the Glasgow Coma Scale: Implications for practice. *Critical Care Nursing Quarterly, 23*(4), 52-58.

Fowler, S. B., Hertzog, J., & Wagner, B. (1995). Pharmacological interventions for agitation in head-injured patients in the acute care setting. *Journal of Neuroscience Nursing, 27*(2), 119-123.

Guidelines for the Management of Severe Head Injury: A joint initiative of The Brain Trauma Foundation, The American Association of Neurological Surgeons, The Joint Section on Neurotrauma and Critical Care. (1995). www.braintrauma.org/guidelines.nsf.

Hartshorn, J. C. & Gauthier D. M. (2001). Nervous system alterations. In M. L. Sole, M. I. Lamborn, & J. C. Hartshorn (Eds.), *Introduction to critical care nursing* (3rd ed., pp. 283-344). Philadelphia: Saunders.

Hickey, J. V. (1997). *Neurological and neurosurgical nursing.* Philadelphia: JB Lippincott.

Kelly, D. F., Nikas, D. L., & Becker, D. P. (1996). Diagnosis and treatment of moderate and severe head injuries in adults. In J. R. Youmans (Ed.), *Neurological surgery* (pp. 1618-1718). Philadelphia: Saunders.

Kidd, K. C. & Criddle, L. (2001). Using jugular venous catheters in patients with traumatic brain injury. *Critical Care Nurse, 21*(6), 16-24.

Kirsch, J. R., Diringer, M. N., Borel, C. O., Hart, G. K., & Hanley, D. F. (1989). Medical management and innovations. In K. A. Gould (Ed.), *Critical care nursing clinics of North America* (pp. 143-151). Philadelphia: Saunders.

Liau, L. M., Bergsneider, M., & Becker, D. P. (1996). Pathology and pathophysiology of head injury. In J. R. Youmans (Ed.), *Neurological surgery* (pp. 1549-1594). Philadelphia: Saunders.

Littlejohns, L. R. & Bader, M. K. (2001). Guidelines for the management of severe head injury: Clinical application and changes in practice. *Critical Care Nurse, 21*(6), 48-65.

Lovasik, D., Kerr, M. E., & Alexander, S. (2001). Traumatic brain injury research: A review of clinical studies. *Critical Care Nursing Quarterly, 23*(4), 24-41.

Mansfield, R. T. (1997). Head injuries in children and adults. In M. M. Parker (Ed.), *Critical care clinics* (pp. 611-625). Philadelphia: Saunders.

March, K. (1999). Acute head injury. In L. Bucher & S. Melander (Eds.), *Critical care nursing* (pp. 843-868). Philadelphia: Saunders.

Marion, D. W. & Letarte, P. B. (1997). Management of intracranial hypertension. *Contemporary Neurosurgery, 19*(3), 1-6.

McNair, N. D. (1999). Traumatic brain injury. *Nursing Clinics of North America, 34*(3), 637-659.

Michael, D. B. (2003). Intracranial hypertension. In J. A. Kruse, M. P. Fink, & R. W. Carlson (Eds.), *Saunders' manual of critical care* (pp. 293-297). Philadelphia: Saunders.

Nikas, D. L. (1998).The neurologic system. In J. G. Alspach (Ed.), *American Association of Critical-Care Nurses: Core curriculum for critical care nursing* (pp. 339-463). Philadelphia: Saunders.

Rosner, M. J. (1995). Introduction to cerebral perfusion pressure management. *Neurosurgery Clinics of North America, 6*(4), 761-774.

Sahuquillo-Barris, J., Lamarca-Ciuro, J., Vilata-Castan, J., Rubio-Garcia, E., & Rodriguez-Pazos, M. (1988). Acute subdural hematoma and diffuse axonal injury after severe head trauma. *Journal of Neurosurgery, 68*, 894-900.

Sullivan, T. E., Schefft, B. K., Warm, J. S., & Dember, W. N. (1994). Closed head injury assessment and research methodology. *Journal of Neuroscience Nursing, 26*(1), 27-29.

Urden, L. D., Stacy, K. M. & Lough, M. E. (Eds.). (2002). *Thelan's critical care nursing: Diagnosis and management* (4th ed.). St Louis: Mosby.

Van Tatenhove, J. C. & Kelley, C. B. (1999). Neurodiagnostic tests. In L. Bucher & S. Melander (Eds.), *Critical care nursing* (pp. 824-842). Philadelphia: Saunders.

Walleck, C. A. (1993). *Patients with head injury and brain dysfunction* (pp. 677-706). Philadelphia: Saunders.

Wilberger, J. E., Harris, M., & Diamond, D. L. (1991). Acute subdural hematoma: Morbidity, mortality, and operative timing. *Journal of Neurosurgery, 74,* 212-218.

Wright, M. M. (1999). Resuscitation of the multitrauma patient with head injury. *AACN Clinical Issues, 10*(1), 32-43.

Yanko, J. R. & Mitcho, K. (2001). Acute care management of severe traumatic brain injuries. *Critical Care Nursing Quarterly, 23*(4), 1-23.

Yundt, K. D. & Diringer, M. N. (1997). The use of hyperventilation and its impact on cerebral ischemia in the treatment of traumatic brain injury. In M. N. Diringer (Ed.), *Critical care clinics* (pp.163-184). Philadelphia: Saunders.

Zink, B. J. & Lanter, P. L. (2001). Traumatic brain injury. In P. C. Ferrera, S. A. Colucciello, J. A. Marx, V. P. Verdile, & M. A. Gibbs (Eds.), *Trauma management* (pp. 127-135). St Louis: Mosby.

Zumkeller, M., Behrmann, R., Heissler, H. E., & Dietz, H. (1996). Computed tomographic criteria and survival rate for patients with acute subdural hematoma. *Neurosurgery, 39*(4), 708-712.

15

Epidural Hematoma

Cinda Alexander, MSN, CCRN, CNRN, CNOR, CRNFA

CASE PRESENTATION

Steven, age 24 years, was driving home from a party late at night when he lost control of his car and hit a tree. On impact his head hit the windshield. A witness to the accident stated that Steven was unconscious for at least 5 minutes but was awake when the paramedics arrived on the scene at 3 AM.

On arrival at the emergency department (ED), Steven was awake and restless with little memory of the accident. He was slightly combative with the ED staff, and his breath was reported to smell of alcohol. A small laceration was observed on his left temple. Skull x-ray films identified a left-sided temporal fracture. Vital signs were as follows:

BP	128/80 mm Hg
HR	88 bpm
Respirations	22 breaths/min
Temperature	36.6° C (97.8° F)

Steven was admitted to the neurologic critical care unit for observation. He remained alert and oriented throughout the night, with no changes noted in his neurologic status. However, at 9 AM, the assessment revealed that Steven was very irritable and did not know the date or time. He became drowsy and was mumbling incoherently. The physician on call was notified, and an immediate computed tomography (CT) scan was ordered, which revealed a left-sided epidural hematoma (EDH).

EMERGENCY SURGERY

Steven was immediately taken to the operating room, where a craniotomy was performed to remove the clot. He tolerated the procedure well and was returned to the neurologic critical care unit after surgery.

POSTOPERATIVE COURSE

After surgery Steven was drowsy but arousable to voice. His pupils were equal and reactive. A large head dressing was in place with no signs of drainage noted. An arterial line was placed, and a peripheral intravenous line of 5% dextrose in lactated Ringer's solution was infusing at 100 ml/hr. Steven was also receiving oxygen at 3 L/min via nasal cannula.

Diagnostic data were as follows:

BP	90/60 mm Hg (arterial line)
HR	92 bpm
Respirations	24 breaths/min
Temperature	37.7° C (99.7° F)
HCO₃⁻	28 mmol/L
pH	7.35
Pao₂	82 mm Hg
Paco₂	35 mm Hg
Sao₂	95%

Two days later Steven was awake and alert with no neurologic deficits noted. Vital signs remained stable. The arterial line was discontinued, and he was tolerating a regular diet. He was transferred to the neurologic unit and discharged 1 day later.

EPIDURAL HEMATOMA

QUESTIONS

1. Describe the pathophysiology of epidural hematoma (EDH).

2. What is the classic clinical picture of EDH?

3. What diagnostic modalities are used to identify an EDH?

4. Discuss the options for surgical intervention in patients with EDH.

5. Discuss the incidence of and mortality associated with EDH. What prognostic indicators may be assessed to predict outcome?

6. Discuss the nursing responsibilities for monitoring and assessment of the patient with EDH.

EPIDURAL HEMATOMA

QUESTIONS AND ANSWERS

1. Describe the pathophysiology of epidural hematoma (EDH).

EDH is a collection of blood between the inner periosteum of the skull and the dura mater. Most EDHs result from arterial bleeding; however, venous bleeding from damage to the meningeal vein or dura sinus is also a potential source. The most common location for an EDH is the temporal fossa. Other sites may include the subfrontal region or occipital-suboccipital area. A temporal fracture may lead to a laceration of the meningeal artery because the temporal region is the thinnest portion of the skull. An epidural hemorrhage occurs as a result of the bleeding meningeal artery. An EDH may lead to cerebral displacement and uncal herniation rather than direct brain injury. The hematoma can push the temporal lobe medially, causing herniation of the uncus and hippocampal gyrus over and through the tentorial notch. The result is a compromised blood supply that suppresses brainstem functions (Hickey, 1997; Nikas, 1998; March, 1999; McNair, 1999; Zink & Lanter, 2001; Urden et al, 2002).

2. What is the classic clinical picture of EDH?

The classic picture of EDH consists of a brief loss of consciousness as a direct result of the injury, followed by a lucid interval. An estimated 30% to 50% of patients will experience the lucid period (Nikas, 1998; Urden et al, 2002). The lucid interval can last anywhere from a few minutes to hours and is followed by a depression in the level of consciousness. Additional symptoms may include ipsilateral pupillary changes progressing to fixed and dilated pupils with simultaneous contralateral motor weakness or paresis. As the mass effect continues, the patient's level of consciousness will rapidly deteriorate (Hickey, 1997; March, 1999; McNair, 1999; Valadka, 2000; Zink & Lanter, 2001; Shpeitz, 2002).

3. What diagnostic modalities are used to identify an EDH?

In the patient with an EDH, a CT scan will reveal an area of density that indicates the location and extent of the hematoma. As the clot expansion strips the dura away from the inner table of the skull, it takes on a biconvexity appearance with sharp margins on CT imaging (Crow, 1991). The CT scan allows rapid identification of the hematoma so treatment can be initiated quickly with a resulting reduction in mortality and morbidity for these patients. After the initial evaluation there is a need for clinical vigilance and subsequent examinations, even though the initial CT scan may be normal, because the EDH may not have yet developed in the patient. Because most patients with EDH have a skull fracture, typically in the thin squamous portion of the temporal area, an x-ray film of the head and neck is diagnostically beneficial (Hickey, 1997, March, 1999; McNair, 1999; Valadka, 2000; Zink & Lanter, 2001).

4. Discuss the options for surgical intervention in patients with EDH.

According to Lee and associates (1998), a delay in evacuation of a hematoma increases the morbidity and mortality of patients with EDH after clinical symptoms of herniation develop. Surgical removal of the clot is necessary to minimize any neurologic deficit by preventing herniation or a shift in brain tissue. A craniotomy consists of incising through the scalp and muscle and creating a bone flap to expose the dura mater. At this time the clot can be removed and the damaged vessel repaired. A small, thin EDH may not require surgical intervention and can be treated with observation (Hickey, 1997; McNair, 1999; Valadka, 2000).

5. **Discuss the incidence of and mortality associated with EDH. What prognostic indicators may be assessed to predict outcome?**

   The overall mortality for EDH is reported to be between 9.4% and 33%. With increased access to CT imaging, mortality of less than 10% can be expected. Traumatic EDH accounts for 0.2% to 6% of all head injuries. Lee and coworkers (1998) identified the following prognostic indicators for unfavorable functional outcome:

   - A longer period of herniation until operative decompression
   - Associated brain injury such as diffuse axonal injury
   - Greater clot density (>50 ml) and degree of midline shift (>10 mm)
   - Total obliteration of the basal cisterns
   - Reoperative motor response of abnormal posturing

6. **Discuss the nursing responsibilities for monitoring and assessment of the patient with EDH.**

   It is beneficial to obtain a thorough patient history, including the type of injury involved, level of consciousness at time of injury, baseline vital signs, behavior, and motor function, to identify any significant changes in assessment from the baseline. The most reliable indicator of neurologic function is level of consciousness. The Glasgow Coma Scale is the most reliable scale for assessing the level of consciousness by assessing the patient's best eye opening and verbal and motor responses. Scale scores range from 3 to 15. The lower the score, the more severe the head injury. Pupil size and reaction to light should be assessed frequently for changes. Ipsilateral pupil dilation is an indication of herniation from a hematoma, lesion, or edema and is often a late sign.

   Blood pressure and heart rate must be assessed frequently to ensure that brain tissues are adequately perfused. Bradycardia, systolic hypertension, and bradypnea are the set of clinical manifestations known as *Cushing's triad;* however, these are late signs of increased ICP. Bradycardia, junctional escape rhythms, and idioventricular rhythms can occur in patients with cerebral hemorrhage and increased ICP. Therefore continuous cardiac monitoring is required. Respiratory patterns must be assessed frequently to identify possible herniation.

   Urine output, serum sodium, and osmolarity levels must be monitored to rule out the syndrome of inappropriate secretion of antidiuretic hormone, which may be a secondary effect of head injury (Hickey, 1997; Nikas, 1998; March, 1999; McNair, 1999).

   Patients may sustain traumatic brain injury at the time of the initial trauma. Additional treatment may be required for head trauma. The reader is referred to Chapter 14 for information regarding traumatic brain injury.

EPIDURAL HEMATOMA

References

Crow, W. (1991). Aspects of neuroradiology of head injury. *Neurosurgery Clinics of North America, 2*(2), 321-340.

Hickey, J. V. (1997). *Neurological and neurosurgical nursing.* Philadelphia: JB Lippincott.

Lee, E., Hung, Y., Wang, L., Chung, K., & Chen, H. (1998). Factors influencing the functional outcome of patients with acute epidural hematomas: Analysis of 200 patients undergoing surgery. *The Journal of Trauma: Injury, Infection, and Critical Care, 45*(5), 946-952.

March, K. (1999). Acute head injury. In L. Bucher & S. Melander (Eds.), *Critical care nursing* (pp. 843-868). Philadelphia: Saunders.

McNair, N. D. (1999). Traumatic brain injury. *Nursing Clinics of North America, 34*(3), 1206-1216.

Nikas, D. L. (1998). The neurologic system. In J. G. Alspach (Ed.), *American Association of Critical-Care Nurses: Core curriculum for critical care nursing* (5th ed., pp. 339-463). Philadelphia: Saunders.

Shpeitz, D. W. (2002). Interventions for critically ill clients with neurologic problems. In. D. D. Ignatavicius & L. M. Workman (Eds.), *Medical surgical nursing* (pp. 989-995). Philadelphia: Saunders.

Urden, L. D., Stacy, K. M., & Lough, M. E. (Eds.). (2002). *Thelan's critical care nursing: Diagnosis and management* (4th ed.). St Louis: Mosby.

Valadka, A. B. (2000). Injury to the cranium. In K. L. Mattox, D. V. Feliciano, & E. E. Moore (Eds.), *Trauma* (4th ed., pp. 378-387). New York: McGraw-Hill.

Zink, B. J. & Lanter, P.L. (2001). Traumatic brain injury. In P. C. Ferrera, S. A. Colucciello, J. A. Marx, V. P. Verdile, & M. A. Gibbs (Eds.), *Trauma management* (pp. 127-135). St Louis: Mosby.

U N I T

IV

RENAL
ALTERATIONS

16

Acute Renal Failure

Amy Reese Ramirez, RN, BSN, MSW, MSN, FNP-C
Sheila Drake Melander, RN, DSN, ACNP-C, FCCM

CASE PRESENTATION

Ann Hayes, age 68, initially was admitted to the hospital for elective surgical repair of an abdominal aortic aneurysm. Her surgery was documented as uneventful. However, complications developed during her fifth postoperative day as a result of a small bowel perforation.

Postoperative Day 5

Vital signs and laboratory results were as follows:

BP	170/94 mm Hg
HR	110 bpm
Respirations	30 breaths/min
Temperature	38.6° C (101.4 ° F) (rectal)
Hgb	10.1 g/dl
Hct	30%
RBCs	$3.5 \times 10^6/mm^3$
WBCs	$20,000/mm^3$

Urine tests showed the following:

Creatinine	0.6 g/24 hr
Osmolarity	460 mOsm/kg
Specific Gravity	1.01
pH	9.0
Na^+	45 mmol/L
K^+	15 mmol/L
Cl^-	48 mmol/L

Results of serum measurements were the following:

Na^+	135 mmol/L
K^+	4.8 mmol/L
Cl^-	88 mmol/L
Ca^{++}	6 mg/dl
BUN	27 mg/dl
Creatinine	1.4 mg/dl
Uric Acid	9 mg/dl

| Phosphorus | 5.2 mg/dl |
| Alkaline Phosphatase | 14.8 King-Armstrong units/dl |

Laboratory results and vital signs were telephoned to her physician. Her physician's orders included the following:

- Hydralazine (Apresoline) at 10 mg qid
- Gentamicin sulfate (Garamycin) IV at 5 mg/kg tid in divided doses
- Piperacillin sodium (Pipracil) 3 g q12h

Gastrointestinal Fistula Repair

As a result of an abnormal abdominal x-ray film, Mrs. Hayes was returned to surgery for repair of a small bowel perforation. Four days after Mrs. Hayes's bowel surgery, she developed a gastrointestinal fistula. She was again taken to surgery for repair of the fistula. Postoperatively her blood pressure dropped to 80/52 mm Hg and her urine output was 20 ml/hr, requiring invasive monitoring. Mrs. Hayes's oxygen saturations and arterial blood gas values dropped significantly. She required intubation and was transferred to the intensive care unit (ICU).

Intensive Care Unit Admission

After Mrs. Hayes's admission to the ICU, the staff took a complete history that revealed her congestive heart failure. Mrs. Hayes weighed 76.5 kg (170 lb) (preoperative weight was 71 kg [158 lb]) and had 2+ pitting edema in her lower extremities. Her skin was pale, shiny, and dry. She complained of nausea and stated that she "felt as if she had no energy left." Fluid intake for the past 24 hours was 1400 ml, and her output was 510 ml. Jugular vein distention was noted, and crackles were auscultated bilaterally in the lung bases. The initial cardiac rhythm was tachycardia with a rate of 110 bpm, a PR interval of 0.18 second, QRS complex of 0.14 second, and peaked T waves.

A fluid challenge was administered unsuccessfully. Despite volume replacement and diuretics, Mrs. Hayes's renal status deteriorated further, and acute renal failure (ARF) was diagnosed. Dopamine (Intropin) was started at 2 µg/kg/min and dobutamine (Dobutrex) at 3 µg/kg/min, and continuous arteriovenous hemofiltration dialysis (CAVHD) was begun. Diagnostic data at this time were the following:

Weight	82 kg (182 lb)
BP	90-110 mm Hg (systolic)
HR	124 bpm
Urine Output	15 ml/hr
Na$^+$	146 mmol/L
K$^+$	5.8 mmol/L
Cl$^-$	98 mmol/L
Ca^{++}	7 mg/dl
BUN	36 mg/dl
Creatinine	3.9 mg/dl
PAP	36/16 mm Hg
PAWP	15 mm Hg

After 4 days of CAVHD, blood urea nitrogen (BUN) and creatinine levels began falling, and blood pressure stabilized with a decrease in weight and edema. Electrolyte and laboratory values returned to normal limits. Total parenteral nutrition (TPN) was begun, and renal function continued to improve until CAVHD was discontinued 5 days later.

ACUTE RENAL FAILURE

QUESTIONS

1. Discuss the pathophysiology involved in acute renal failure (ARF).

2. Describe the four phases in the clinical course of ARF.

3. Compare and contrast oliguric and nonoliguric renal failure.

4. What clinical assessment data support the diagnosis of ARF for Mrs. Hayes? What other information may be useful in the diagnosis of ARF?

5. What is the significance of the use of gentamicin sulfate (Garamycin) and piperacillin sodium (Pipracil) in Mrs. Hayes's treatment regimen?

6. Discuss the major nephrotoxic drug classifications, including risk factors and prevention of nephrotoxicity.

7. What is the rationale for including dopamine (Intropin) in Mrs. Hayes's treatment plan?

8. Identify other pharmacologic agents used in the treatment of ARF and the rationale for their use.

9. Discuss the dietary management of the patient with ARF.

10. Discuss the three different forms of dialysis used in the treatment of ARF, including the indications and contraindications for each. Why was CAVHD indicated for Mrs. Hayes?

11. List nursing diagnoses appropriate for care of the patient with ARF.

12. What are the nursing responsibilities and potential complications related to continuous renal replacement therapy (CRRT)?

ACUTE RENAL FAILURE

QUESTIONS AND ANSWERS

1. Discuss the pathophysiology involved in acute renal failure (ARF).

Definition

Acute renal failure (ARF) occurs when there is an abrupt decrease in renal function sufficient to result in retention of nitrogenous waste (e.g., BUN and creatinine) in the body. According to Rakel (2002), the frequency of ARF varies greatly depending on the clinical setting. The frequency among hospitalized patients is about 5% but can be as high as 15% after cardiopulmonary bypass. Despite major advances in dialysis and intensive care, the mortality rate among patients with severe ARF requiring dialysis has not decreased significantly over the past 50 years. This may be explained in part by the fact that increased age and coexisting serious illnesses are increasingly more common among these patients. These facts reinforce the need for focusing on prevention strategies (Rakel, 2002).

Etiology

ARF can be classified as prerenal, postrenal, or intrarenal (Rakel, 2002). Prerenal failure results from decreased renal perfusion caused by hemorrhage, dehydration, decreased cardiac output, or fluid shifts. Postrenal failure is caused by an obstruction in the flow of urine from conditions such as benign prostatic hypertrophy, tumor, and bladder, renal, or ureteral calculi. Intrarenal failure is accompanied by tubular, interstitial, glomerular, or vascular renal tissue damage, such as that occurring in acute tubular necrosis (ATN), glomerulonephritis, renal vascular disease, and interstitial nephritis. According to Rakel (2002) the most common form of ARF in hospitalized patients is ATN resulting from ischemic or toxic damage to the nephrons. Patients at risk for developing ATN include those who have suffered a decrease in blood flow to peripheral organs, usually accompanied by hypotension and shock.

Pathophysiology

The pathophysiology of ARF involves changes in renal hemodynamics, cellular metabolism, and nephron structure and function. Filtration ceases when tubular hydrostatic pressure equals that of glomerular filtration pressure. Urine formation decreases because of the lack of filtrate to process (Urden et al, 2002). A reduction in renal blood flow (RBF) is the common cause of a decreased glomerular filtration rate (GFR). This decreased RBF eventually leads to ischemia and cell death. Oxygen-free radicals and enzymes are produced, which continue to cause cell injury even after renal blood flow is restored. The cell damage disrupts the tight junctions between cells, permitting a backleak of glomerular filtrate. Dying cells slough off into the tubules, which further decreases GFR and leads to oliguria (Sinert & Peacock, 2002).

      The amount of renal cell damage depends on the ischemic time period. Earlier normalization of RBF predicts better prognosis for recovery of renal function. Recovery involves the restoration of circulating blood volume in prerenal failure, and the relief of urinary obstruction in postrenal failure. The removal of tubular toxins and the treatment of the causative glomerular disease lead to recovery in intrinsic renal failure (Sinert & Peacock, 2002).

2. Describe the four phases in the clinical course of ARF.

The four phases of ARF include the (1) onset phase, (2) oliguric-anuric phase, (3) diuretic phase, and (4) convalescent or recovery phase.

Onset Phase

The onset phase represents the time from when an insult occurs until cell injury. This phase can last from hours to days and is characterized by renal blood flow and oxygen consumption at 25% of normal, urine output at 30 ml or less per hour, and urinary sodium excretion greater than 40 mEq/L (Bucher & Melander, 1999). Only 50% of patients are oliguric, with the remainder excreting greater than 600 ml/8 hr (Urden et al, 2002). According to Urden and colleagues (2002), irreversible damage can be alleviated if treatment is initiated during this phase.

Oliguric-Anuric Phase

The oliguric-anuric phase lasts about 8 to 14 days and is characterized by further damage to the tubular wall and basement membranes. The GFR is greatly reduced, leading to increased levels of BUN and creatinine, electrolyte abnormalities (hyperkalemia, hyperphosphatemia, hypocalcemia), and metabolic acidosis. The nonoliguric phase is reflective of decreased tubular damage, as well as a better prognosis. The mortality of patients with nonoliguric ATN is 25%, whereas it rises to 66% in the presence of oliguria (Urden et al, 2002).

Diuretic Phase

The diuretic phase appears when the sources of obstruction have passed, but scarring and edema remain. This phase, which lasts 7 to 14 days, is characterized by an increase in GFR with a urine output as high as 2 to 4 L/day (Urden et al, 2002). The urine is able to flow through the tubular space, but the cells cannot concentrate the urine. The high glomerular flow rate can contribute to a passive loss of electrolytes. Intravenous (IV) administration of crystalloids is necessary to maintain hydration during this phase (Bucher & Melander, 1999).

Convalescent or Recovery Phase

The convalescent or recovery phase begins with stabilization of laboratory values and can range from several months to 1 year (Bucher & Melander, 1999). During this phase edema diminishes and the tubular cells begin to slowly resume normal functioning, with a GFR 70% to 80% of normal within 1 to 2 years (Urden et al, 2002). If significant renal damage has occurred, BUN and creatinine may never return to normal levels.

3. **Compare and contrast oliguric and nonoliguric renal failure.**

Oliguric ATN

Oliguria is defined as a urine output between 100 and 400 ml/day (Sinert & Peacock, 2002). Oliguric ATN, the classic presenting form of ATN, involves tubular damage, resulting in a tubular backleak of filtrate and tubular obstruction. During oliguria the kidney is unable to concentrate urine, resulting in excretion of urine that is rich in sodium but lacking in excess volume, electrolytes, and waste. The patient exhibits fluid overload, electrolyte and acid-base imbalances, azotemia, anemia, and increased risk of infection. The recovery time of oliguric ATN ranges from a minimum of 12 to 16 days to a maximum of 3 to 12 months; however, the mortality rate ranges between 50% and 70% in critically ill patients (Bucher & Melander, 1999).

Nonoliguric ATN

Nonoliguria is defined as a urine output of greater than 400 ml/day (Sinert & Peacock, 2002). In contrast to oliguric ATN, tubular damage in the nonoliguric kidney is less severe. The presence of nonoliguria signals only epithelial damage to the tubules. There is no basement membrane damage, no cracks in the tubular wall, and no sloughing of cells obstructing the tubular space. The urine can pass freely in large volumes but cannot be concentrated. Urine output varies from normal to as large as 2 L per hour. The passive loss of waste products and electrolytes, due to the increased flowd of the glomerular filtrate, contributes to the decreased need for dialysis. As compared with oliguric ATN, the time for recovery is greatly decreased to a minimum of 5 to 8 days (Bucher & Melander, 1999).

4. What clinical assessment data support the diagnosis of ARF for Mrs. Hayes? What other information may be useful in the diagnosis of ARF?

Assessment Data

Mrs. Hayes's assessment data support the diagnosis of ARF (Bucher & Melander, 1999). Mrs. Hayes's assessment information included jugular vein distention, pulmonary congestion, tachypnea, tachycardia, hypotension, and intake and output imbalances. Hypotension and tachycardia are apparent clues to Mrs. Hayes's decreased renal perfusion. Other evaluation measures for hypovolemia include orthostatic hypotension, mucosal membrane moisture, and tissue turgor (Sinert & Peacock, 2002). Mrs. Hayes's complaint of nausea and vomiting was probably caused by her uremic state. Anemia is the main hematologic effect of ARF, which may have contributed to her lethargy as well as her increased heart rate (Campbell, 2003).

Patient History

Aspects of the patient's history that are important in diagnosing ARF include renal symptoms, systemic diseases, laboratory results, and medication history. Mrs. Hayes had a history of cardiovascular disease and had experienced a hypotensive episode postoperatively along with sepsis. These findings in addition to the presence of other systemic diseases, such as hematopoietic or immunologic diseases, have a direct impact on the renal system. Also, Mrs. Hayes was being treated with two nephrotoxic agents: gentamicin sulfate (Garamycin) and piperacillin sodium (Pipracil) (Mitchell & Coburn, 2002).

Laboratory Data

Laboratory studies for the evaluation of ARF include routine blood chemistry and complete blood count and differential white blood cell count; urinalysis including specific gravity, dipstick, sulfosalicylic acid, microscopy; and, urine chemistry, eosinophils, and/or immunoelectrophoresis (Brenner & Rector, 2000). Mrs. Hayes's creatinine and BUN levels were both elevated, indicating reduced GFR. A creatinine level of 4 mg/dl reflects a 70% to 85% reduction in GFR (Sinert & Peacock, 2002). BUN levels are the less helpful of the two measures because many processes increase BUN, including internal bleeding, protein metabolism, and infection (Campbell, 2003). Mrs. Hayes had elevations in sodium, potassium, chloride, phosphorus, uric acid, and alkaline phosphatase levels that support the diagnosis of ARF.

As in Mrs. Hayes's case, the key renal effect of ARF is decreased urine output that leads to fluid retention and edema; however, urine volume is not always a good measure of renal function because some patients may exhibit nonoliguric renal failure. Patterns of urine output must be monitored to identify renal perfusion status. Analysis of the sediment and supernatant of a centrifuged urine specimen is valuable for distinguishing between prerenal, intrinsic, and postrenal causes of ARF (Brenner & Rector, 2000). Urine sediment should be inspected for the presence of cells, casts, and crystals. Urine laboratory values supporting ARF include the following:

- Decreased creatinine level and osmolality
- Increased sodium, potassium, and chloride levels
- Increased pH
- Fixed specific gravity and normal glucose and protein levels

It should be noted, however, that urinary laboratory values vary depending on the etiology of the ARF and the pathophysiologic changes involved (Brenner & Rector, 2000).

Diagnostic Information

Noninvasive diagnostic procedures that should be performed for Mrs. Hayes and other patients with ARF include fluid intake and output, daily weighing, and x-ray examinations of the kidney, ureters, and bladder. Invasive procedures that may be used include intravenous pyelography, computed tomography, renal angiography, nephrosonography, and renal biopsy (Bucher & Melander, 1999). An electrocardiogram may demonstrate changes associated with hyperkalemia, including a flattened P wave, prolonged QRS complex, and tall, tented T waves (Campbell, 2003).

5. **What is the significance of the use of gentamicin sulfate (Garamycin) and piperacillin sodium (Pipracil) in Mrs. Hayes's treatment regimen?**

Gentamicin sulfate (Garamycin) and piperacillin sodium (Pipracil) are both nephrotoxic agents (Mitchell & Coburn, 2002). Piperacillin sodium, a penicillin, may lead to interstitial nephritis with ARF owing to a hypersensitive reaction. Gentamicin sulfate, an aminoglycoside, may lead to renal dysfunction with ATN. Aminoglycosides are major culprits in the development of nephrotoxic ATN.

6. **Discuss the major nephrotoxic drug classifications, including risk factors and prevention of nephrotoxicity.**

Nephrotoxic Drug Classifications

Medications are primary causes of ARF. Angiotensin-converting enzyme (ACE) inhibitors and nonsteroidal antiinflammatory drugs (NSAIDs) are the primary drug classifications causing prerenal ARF due to their impairment of renal blood flow (Agrawal & Swartz, 2002. To reduce the risk of antibiotic-induced drug toxicity, the patient should be given the shortest course with once-daily dosing; in addition, serum concentrations must be monitored carefully. Radiocontrast media and aminoglycosides are the agents most likely to cause ATN. The potential for renal damage is increased in patients with congestive heart failure, diabetes, or poor renal perfusion (Agrawal & Swartz, 2000).

Prevention of Nephrotoxicity

Due to its mortality rate of 50% to 80%, the best intervention is prevention of ARF (Bucher & Melander, 1999). Identifying patients at risk, avoiding potentially nephrotoxic agents, and using strategies to prevent renal injury may prevent nephrotoxicity. Patients at risk are the elderly, those with preexisting renal disease, and those who are volume depleted. Compelling evidence exists that aggressive restoration of intravascular volume dramatically reduces the incidence of ATN after major surgery, trauma, and burns. When the use of potentially nephrotoxic agents cannot be avoided, steps should be taken to reduce the risk of ARF. Hydration and high urine flow rates are protective against the toxicity of sulfonamides and chemotherapeutic agents, including methotrexate and cisplatin (Rakel, 2002).

7. **What is the rationale for including dopamine (Intropin) in Mrs. Hayes's treatment plan?**

Dopamine has been widely used to prevent and treat renal dysfunction (Kellum & Decker, 2001). However, debate exists regarding dopamine's benefit in the prevention, development, and course of ARF. Dopamine dilates renal arterioles and increases renal blood flow and GFR. However, as stated by Kellum and Decker (2001), it is not known whether ATN is always a result of a decrease in renal blood flow or whether increasing renal blood flow will reverse or prevent renal injury. Low-dose dopamine can also cause tachycardia, tachyarrhythmias, myocardial ischemia, and intestinal ischemia (Al-Khafaji & Corwin, 2001). Kellum and Decker (2001) conclude that on the basis of available evidence, low-dose dopamine cannot be justified for the treatment or prevention of ARF.

8. Identify other pharmacologic agents used in the treatment of ARF and the rationale for their use.

Pharmacologic Management

In addition to dopamine (Intropin), loop diuretics such as furosemide (Lasix) and osmotic diuretics such as mannitol are used in the treatment of ARF when fluid overload is present (Agrawal & Swartz, 2000). Diuretics are used in ARF to increase urinary flow with the intent of flushing out the cellular debris causing tubular obstruction and possibly creating a non-oliguric ATN. Osmotic diuretics and loop diuretics dilate renal arteries by increasing the synthesis of prostaglandins, resulting in restoration of renal blood flow. Because the impact of a decrease in renal perfusion is greatest in the initial stages of ARF, it is crucial to use diuretics as an early intervention. If administered early in the course of the ARF, both mannitol and furosemide can convert an oliguric state to a nonoliguric state (Mitchell & Coburn, 2002).

The main electrolyte abnormalities seen in ARF are hyperkalemia and acidosis. Intravenous administered calcium is cardioprotective and temporarily reverses the neuromuscular effect of hyperkalemia. Potassium can also be shifted into the intracellular space using insulin and glucose, inhaled β-agonists, or sodium bicarbonate. Potassium can be excreted using polystyrene sulfonate (Kayexalate) and/or diuretics. Acidosis can be treated with sodium bicarbonate (Agrawal & Swartz, 2000).

9. Discuss the dietary management of the patient with ARF.

Nutritional support is critical in the patient with ARF. Reasons include increased energy expenditure, extensive catabolic state, and the negative nitrogen balance. Tissue catabolism commonly develops in patients with ARF, which leads to increases in BUN levels, metabolic acidosis, and hyperkalemia. To prevent even greater stress on the kidneys, nutrition should provide adequate calories without increasing protein load. A diet low in protein and sodium but higher in fats and carbohydrates is recommended. Restricted sodium intake of 2 to 4 g/day to prevent further fluid retention, reduced potassium intake to decrease cardiac arrhythmia potential, and limited phosphorus intake to prevent reductions in blood calcium levels are all recommended dietary restrictions (Campbell, 2003).

10. Discuss the three different forms of dialysis used in the treatment of ARF, including the indications and contraindications for each. Why was CAVHD indicated for Mrs. Hayes?

Between 20% and 60% of ARF patients require short-term dialysis. Dialysis is indicated when acidosis or electrolyte disturbances cannot be corrected using pharmacologic therapy or when fluid overload does not respond to diuretics (Agrawal & Swartz, 2000). The three dialysis options in the critically ill patient are peritoneal dialysis, hemodialysis, and continuous renal replacement therapy (CRRT).

Peritoneal Dialysis

Peritoneal dialysis has become less utilized as a form of dialysis in the ICU over the past decade. Peritoneal dialysis is a slow, efficient form of dialysis that involves an exchange of fluid and solutes between the peritoneal cavity and peritoneal capillaries. Peritoneal dialysis does provide for hemodynamic stability; however, its clearance is less efficient than with other forms of dialysis (Al-Khafaji & Corwin, 2001).

Hemodialysis

Until recently, hemodialysis was the primary method of renal replacement therapy in patients with ARF (Al-Khafaji & Corwin, 2001). According to Schiffl (2002), alternate day hemodialysis continues to remain the most commonly used method of renal replacement in North America. Hemodialysis provides ultrafiltration for rapid water removal and diffusion for solute removal. It is indicated for uremia, electrolyte imbalances, fluid overload, and severe metabolic acidosis. Hemodialysis is the preferred method when quick removal of water or toxins is needed. However, because this process requires moving large amounts of fluid from the intravascular system, hypotension is a risk factor from hypovolemia (Campbell, 2003).

CRRT

CRRT is an ongoing therapy that may be used for days or months by allowing slow volume removal while maintaining hemodynamic stability. Continuous replacement therapies are the most common methods used for the treatment of ARF in Australia and Europe (Schiffl, 2002). The arteriovenous forms, such as continuous arteriovenous hemofiltration (CAVH) and CAVHD, are gradually being replaced by venovenous forms, including continuous venovenous hemofiltration (CVVH) and continuous venovenous hemodialysis (CVVHD) (Vanholder et al, 2001).

The theoretic benefits of CRRT include hemodynamic stability, correction of metabolic acidosis, shorter recovery time of renal function, correction of malnutrition, and solute removal (Vanholder et al, 2001). However, despite the theoretical advantages of continuous renal replacement therapy in patients with ARF, there are no controlled studies that show superiority of this technique compared with intermittent hemodialysis (Vanholder et al, 2001; Schiffl, 2002). The disadvantages of CRRT include the potential problems associated with the continuous need for anticoagulation therapy, the need for immobilization of the patient, and the greater expense than intermittent hemodialysis (IHD) (Vanholder et al, 2001). The choice of using CRRT over IHD is largely based on the availability of CRRT and care provider preferences, rather than on evidence-based indications of its superiority (Schiffl, 2002).

CRRT rather than traditional hemodialysis was an appropriate dialysis option for Mrs. Hayes because of her hemodynamically unstable condition. Mrs. Hayes also had a large daily fluid requirement that included TPN. Mrs. Hayes's unresponsiveness to diuretic therapy also supported the need for CRRT.

11. List nursing diagnoses appropriate for care of the patient with ARF.

As cited by Bucher and Melander (1999), the following nursing diagnoses should be considered in the care of the patients with ARF:

- Alteration in urinary elimination
- Fluid volume deficit
- Fluid volume excess
- Altered nutrition: less than body requirements
- Risk for impaired skin integrity
- Knowledge deficit
- Decreased cardiac output
- Anxiety or fear
- Activity intolerance
- Body image disturbance
- Altered thought processes
- Risk for infection, ineffective patient or family coping

12. What are the nursing responsibilities and potential complications related to continuous renal replacement therapy (CRRT)?

Nursing Responsibilities

Before CRRT is begun, patient and family teaching concerning the procedure should be completed. Once the therapy has started, it is crucial to monitor the patient's hemodynamic status frequently to observe the patient's response to fluid removal. Continuous assessment of heart rate, blood pressure, and cardiac rhythm along with assessment of fluid status, including central venous pressure and pulmonary artery pressure, provide important clinical data. Nursing responsibilities also include monitoring changes in mental status, breath sounds, and skin turgor and for the presence of cardiac arrhythmias, edema, signs of bleeding, and signs of infection. Hypotension in response to hypovolemia requires aggressive management with rapid administration of crystalloid solution and adjustment of the ultrafiltration rate (Kaplow & Barry, 2002). Fluid volume overload can also occur, requiring the nurse to decrease or temporarily discontinue fluid replacement. The nurse must ensure that all connections are secure due to the significant risk of hemorrhage caused by the accidental disconnection of the lines from the body; and in some instances sedation may be indicated to avoid disconnection (Kapow & Barry, 2002). Electrolyte and acid-base imbalances can be significant, indicating the need for close monitoring of electrolyte imbalances.

Prevention of Complications

Prevention of complications related to CRRT requires early intervention by the nursing staff. Restrictions on patient activity may lead to complications related to skin integrity, requiring a turning schedule via logrolling. As previously discussed, dislodgment of the catheter lines may lead to hemorrhage. Therefore patients receiving CRRT may require restraints or sedation (Kaplow & Barry, 2002). Thrombosis is another potential complication that requires close monitoring of distal extremity pulses and perfusion. Monitoring for signs of infection, including fever and white blood cell count elevations, is critical along with assessing the catheter insertion sites and changing sterile dressings according to hospital policy (Kapow & Barry, 2002).

ACUTE RENAL FAILURE

References

Agrawal, M. & Swartz, R. (2000). Acute renal failure. *American Family Physician, 61,* 2077-2088.

Al-Khafaji, A. & Corwin, H. L. (2001). Acute renal failure and dialysis in the chronically critically ill patient. *Clinics in Chest Medicine, 22,* 165-174.

Brenner, B. M. & Rector, F. C. (Eds.). (2000). *The kidney* (6th ed.). Philadelphia: W. B. Saunders.

Bucher, L. & Melander, S. (Eds.). (1999). *Critical care nursing.* Philadelphia: W. B. Saunders.

Campbell, D. (2003). How acute renal failure puts brakes on kidney function. *Nursing2003, 33,* 59-63.

Kaplow, R. & Barry, R. (2002). Continuous renal replacement therapies. *American Journal of Nursing, 102,* 26-33.

Kellum, J. A. & Decker, J. M. (2001). Use of dopamine in acute renal failure: A meta-analysis. *Critical Care Medicine, 29(8),* 1526-1531.

Mitchell, S. A. & Coburn, S. (2002). Acute renal failure: Early detection and prompt intervention can improve outcomes. *Oncology Nursing Update, 102,* 6-12.

Rakel, R. E. (Ed.). (2002). *Conn's current therapy.* Philadelphia: W. B. Saunders.

Schiffl, H. (2002). Intermittent hemodialysis and/or continuous renal replacement therapy: Are they complementary or alternative therapies? *American Journal of Kidney Diseases, 40,* 1097-1099.

Sinert, R. & Peacock, P. R. (2002). Renal failure, acute. *eMedicine* [On-line]. Available: emedicine.com/emerg/topic500.

Urden, L. D., Stacy, K. M., & Lough, M. E. (Eds.). (2002). *Thelan's critical care nursing: Diagnosis and management* (4th ed.). St Louis: Mosby.

Vanholder, R., Van Biesen, W. I. M., & Lameire, N. (2001). What is the renal replacement method of first choice for intensive care patients? *Journal of the American Society of Nephrology, 12,* S40-S43.

17

Chronic Renal Failure and Renal Transplantation

Phyllis Ann Egbert, MSN, RN, ACNP-C, CNN

CASE PRESENTATION

Michael Miller, age 67, has end-stage renal disease (ESRD) caused by chronic pyelonephritis. He receives hemodialysis at an outpatient chronic renal failure and renal transplantation clinic three times a week. He travels with his wife approximately 75 miles to reach the clinic. A short experience with home dialysis was unsuccessful, and Mr. Miller had begun to miss one, and sometimes, two clinic appointments each week. Mr. Miller has no active malignancy or infectious process. He has a strong support system with siblings willing to donate a living donor kidney. He is financially secure through income and health insurance coverage.

Mr. Miller arrived at the emergency department with a 2-day history of not feeling well, accompanied by nausea and vomiting. He was agitated and slightly confused. He was complaining of moderate to severe chest pain diffused over the precordium. Initial assessment revealed jugular vein distention, scattered crackles bilaterally throughout the lung bases, and pitting peripheral edema bilaterally in the lower extremities. Cardiac monitoring demonstrated sinus tachycardia with a rate of 116 bpm. A pericardial friction rub and an S_3 gallop were auscultated. His wife informed the nurse that Mr. Miller had missed his previous appointment for dialysis. He was 8 kg (18 lb) heavier than his estimated dry weight of 74 kg (164 lb). Current vital signs and laboratory results were as follows:

BP	180/110 mm Hg
HR	116 bpm
Respirations	36 breaths/min
Temperature	38.7° C (101.6° F) (rectal)
Height	175 cm (5 ft 10 in)
Weight	82 kg (182 lb)
RBCs	$3.1 \times 10^6/mm^3$
WBCs	13,500/mm³
Platelets	226,000/mm³
Hgb	8.5 g/dl
Hct	26%
Na⁺	136 mmol/L
K⁺	7.3 mmol/L

Cl⁻	110 mmol/L

Cl⁻   110 mmol/L
CO_2 10 mmol/L
Mg^{++} 1.3 mEq/L
PO_4^- 12 mg/dl
Creatinine   26.9 mg/dl
BUN   127 mg/dl
Glucose   95 mg/dl
pH   7.2
$Paco_2$ 53 mm Hg
Sao_2 85%
HCO_3^- 10 mmol/L

Note: These values were in room air (21% oxygen).

The physician ordered admission to the medical intensive care unit for immediate hemodialysis. Oxygen was administered by a 40% face mask, and hemodialysis was initiated via a permanent arteriovenous (AV) fistula in the right forearm. An initial 4-hour dialysis treatment reduced Mr. Miller's body weight to 76.5 kg (170 lb). After dialysis Mr. Miller was alert and oriented to place and person. Postdialysis assessment revealed the following: blood pressure 160/90 mm Hg, heart rate 94 bpm, and respirations 26 breaths/min. Mr. Miller was given a diet restricted to 20 g of protein and 1000 ml of fluid per day. His medication orders included the following:

- Sevelamer hydrochloride (Renagel) 800 mg, 6 tablets po tid with meals
- Vitamin B complex with C, one tablet po daily (after dialysis on dialysis days)
- Losartan (Cozaar) 50 mg po bid

Hemodialysis was continued on a daily schedule of 4-hour sessions, and Mr. Miller was transferred to the step-down unit. Mr. Miller's condition progressively improved. He was able to resume his regular 4-hour dialysis regimen three times per week and he was scheduled for discharge. Discharge assessment revealed the following:

BP   160/95 mm Hg
HR   92 bpm
Respirations   20 breaths/min
Temperature   36.8° C (98.2° F)
Weight   76.5 kg (170 lb)
RBCs $4.1 \times 10^6/mm^3$
WBCs $12,000/mm^3$
Platelets $226,000/mm^3$
Hgb   9.1 g/dl
Hct   28.1%
Na⁺   136 mmol/L
K⁺   5.8 mmol/L
Cl⁻   98 mmol/L
CO_2 15 mmol/L
Ca^{++} 8.4 mg/dl
Mg^{++} 2.3 mEq/L
PO_4^- 6.2 mg/dl
Creatinine   12.6 mg/dl
BUN   80 mg/dl
Glucose   125 mg/dl
pH   7.48
HCO_3^- 25 mmol/L
Sao_2 95%

Paco$_2$	30 mm Hg
Pao$_2$	135 mm Hg

Note: These values were in room air (21% oxygen).

Mr. Miller told his physician that he was unwilling to accept the limitations and restrictions in his life imposed by this illness and requested to have a kidney transplant. He informed the physician that he had discussed this at length with his three brothers and three sisters, and each is prepared to undergo testing to determine whether a transplant match is possible. Mr. Miller was informed that he would have to prove to the transplant team that he could be compliant with his dialysis and medicine regimen for 6 months before he would be considered for a living-related kidney transplant. Mr. Miller agreed not to miss any more dialysis treatments and to take his medications as ordered.

6 MONTHS LATER

The testing of Mr. Miller's siblings resulted in a suitable donor for his kidney transplant. Six months after discharge, Mr. Miller was admitted to the transplant unit. Clinical and laboratory assessment revealed the following data:

BP	150/85 mm/Hg
HR	92 bpm
Respirations	20 breaths/min
Temperature	36.8° C (98.2° F)
RBCs	$4.3 \times 10^6/mm^3$
WBCs	9000/mm^3
Cl$^-$	98 mmol/L
CO$_2$	15 mmol/L
Ca^{++}	8.6 mg/dl
Mg^{++}	2.0 mEq/L
PO$_4^-$	6.5 mg/dl
Platelets	230,000/mm^3
Hgb	10.8 g/dl
Hct	32.4%
Na$^+$	136 mmol/L
K$^+$	5.8 mmol/L
Creatinine	10.1 mg/dl
BUN	90 mg/dl
Glucose	125 mg/dl
HCO$_3^-$	25 mmol/L
pH	7.48
Sao$_2$	95%
Paco$_2$	30 mm Hg
Pao$_2$	135 mm Hg

Note: These values were in room air (21% oxygen).

Preoperatively Mr. Miller was given methylprednisolone (Solu-Medrol), antithymocyte globulin (ATG), and sirolimus (Rapamune). A right kidney was transplanted during an uneventful operation. Estimated blood loss was 200 ml. During the procedure Mr. Miller received 1400 ml of crystalloid intravenous solution and 2 U of packed red blood cells. He was transferred from the postanesthesia recovery room to the surgical intensive care unit. He received oxygen via a 40% face mask and dopamine at 2 µg/kg/min for renal perfusion. He had a Jackson-Pratt drain in the right flank and a Foley catheter to straight drainage.

The initial postoperative assessment revealed the following clinical data:

BP	138/92 mm Hg
HR	92 bpm
Respirations	22 breaths/min
Temperature	36.9° C (98.4° F)
CVP	5 mm Hg
RBCs	$4.6 \times 10^6/mm^3$
WBCs	12,500/mm^3
Platelets	235,000/mm^3
Hgb	11.1 g/dl
Hct	33.5%
Na^+	131 mmol/L
K^+	4.8 mmol/L
Cl^-	92 mmol/L
CO_2	18 mmol/L
PO_4^-	4.3 mg/dl
Creatinine	9.3 mg/dl
BUN	71 mg/dl
pH	7.36
HCO_3^-	25 mmol/L
Sao_2	99%
$Paco_2$	35 mm Hg
Pao_2	138 mm Hg

Over the next 4 postoperative days, Mr. Miller continued to improve. Blood urea nitrogen (BUN) and creatinine levels continued to drop, urine output averaged more than 100 ml/hr, and his condition was hemodynamically stable. Immunosuppression therapy included methylprednisolone 30 mg a day, mycophenolate mofetil 1000 mg every 12 hours, cyclosporine 300 mg every 12 hours, and ATG 1000 mg IV daily for 7 days. On the seventh postoperative day, the relevant laboratory data were the following:

BP	138/92 mm Hg
HR	92 bpm
Respirations	22 breaths/min
Temperature	36.9° C (98.4° F)
RBCs	$4.6 \times 10^6/mm^3$
WBCs	13,800/mm^3
Platelets	296,000/mm^3
Hgb	12.9 g/dl
Hct	36.7%
Na^+	135 mmol/L
K^+	4.4 mmol/L
Cl^-	92 mmol/L
CO_2	22 mmol/L
Ca^{++}	8.5 mg/dl
PO_4^-	3.3 mg/dl
Creatinine	1.9 mg/dl
BUN	32 mg/dl
Intake	2250 ml
Output (Urine)	2050 ml
Output (JP Drain)	5 ml
Weight	75.0 kg (165 lb)
Sao_2	99%

The Jackson-Pratt drain was removed. On the eighth postoperative day, Mr. Miller began to complain of not feeling well; he had minimal abdominal tenderness on palpation and complained of nausea. His temperature fluctuated between 38.4° and 38.8° C (101.2° and 101.8° F). Urinary output dropped to an average of 25 ml/hr. Furosemide (Lasix) boluses did not improve his urinary output. Mr. Miller had a renal ultrasound, which showed no evidence of hydronephrosis, obstruction, or other abnormalities. An emergency renal biopsy was performed which was consistent with acute rejection. On postoperative day 9, his weight was up to 78 kg (172 lb), creatinine level was 4.3 mg/dl, and BUN was 63 mg/dl. Mr. Miller was given pulse-dose of methylprednisolone (Solu-Medrol) and muromonab-CD3 (Orthoclone OKT3) was started. His renal function showed progressive improvement over the next week and he did not have to receive hemodialysis to support his renal function. Tacrolimus (Prograf) was added to his immunosuppression therapy regimen and cyclosporine was discontinued. Mr. Miller's laboratory data 1 week after his acute rejection episode were as follows:

BP	142/88 mm Hg
HR	82 bpm
Respirations	18 breaths/min
Temperature	36.9° C (98.4° F)
RBCs	$4.6 \times 10^6/mm^3$
WBCs	$7800/mm^3$
Platelets	$320,000/mm^3$
Hgb	9.5 g/dl
Hct	28.7%
Na⁺	137 mmol/L
K⁺	4.6 mmol/L
Cl⁻	92 mmol/L
Ca⁺⁺	8.9 mg/dl
CO₂	24 mmol/L
PO₄⁻	3.3 mg/dl
Creatinine	2.1 mg/dl
BUN	31 mg/dl
Intake	2750
Output (Urine)	2625
Weight	76.4 kg (168 lb)

On the eighteenth postoperative day, Mr. Miller was discharged home with the following regimen:

- Mycophenolate mofetil (CellCept) 1000 mg bid
- Tacrolimus (Prograf) 400 mg every 12 hours
- Prednisone 30 mg qd
- Ranitidine (Zantac) 150 mg po q̄d
- Metoclopramide 10 mg HS
- Diltiazem 240 mg qd
- Nystatin 100,000 U/ml, 5 ml swish and swallow qid
- Bactrim DS 1 tablet every day × 4 weeks
- Ganciclovir 900 mg qd × 4 weeks

CHRONIC RENAL FAILURE AND RENAL TRANSPLANTATION

QUESTIONS

1. Discuss the pathophysiology involved in chronic renal failure.

2. Discuss the typical laboratory findings seen with chronic renal failure.

3. Describe the symptoms of uremia that might be manifested by Mr. Miller.

4. Describe how the relationship between calcium and phosphorus is altered in chronic renal failure.

5. Discuss the pathophysiology of aluminum toxicity in chronic renal failure.

6. Discuss the pathophysiology of pericarditis in chronic renal failure. Why was Mr. Miller particularly prone to this complication?

7. Discuss the different forms of dialysis used in the treatment of renal failure, including the indications and contraindications for each. Support the decision to use hemodialysis in treating Mr. Miller.

8. Identify pharmacologic agents used to treat chronic renal failure and the rationale for their use.

9. Discuss the dietary management of the patient with chronic renal failure.

10. Identify clinical complications arising from noncompliance that were manifested by Mr. Miller.

11. List nursing diagnoses appropriate for the care of the patient with chronic renal failure. Include nursing diagnoses appropriate for the care of the patient with a permanent AV fistula for dialysis access.

12. List the components of the teaching plan for the patient with chronic renal failure.

13. List the criteria used in the selection of patients for kidney transplantation.

14. Discuss hemodialysis and renal transplantation as alternative treatment modalities for Mr. Miller. Support Mr. Miller's decision to select renal transplantation rather than hemodialysis.

15. List the advantages and disadvantages of a living donor versus a cadaver donor. Why was it imperative that Mr. Miller receive a living donor kidney?

16. Describe the cadaver kidney preservation process.

17. Briefly describe the surgical process of renal transplantation.

18. Discuss possible postoperative complications of renal transplantation.

19. List the nursing diagnoses appropriate for the care of the patient undergoing renal transplantation during the recovery period.

20. Discuss the pathophysiology of acute rejection. Describe the clinical manifestations of acute rejection in Mr. Miller.

21. Discuss the immunosuppressive pharmacologic agents methylprednisolone, muromonab-CD3 (Orthoclone OKT3), cyclosporine, mycophenolate mofetil (CellCept), and tacrolimus (Prograf). Why did the physician add muromonab-CD3 and change cyclosporine to tacrolimus?

22. List the components of the teaching plan for Mr. Miller.

CHRONIC RENAL FAILURE AND RENAL TRANSPLANTATION

QUESTIONS AND ANSWERS

1. **Discuss the pathophysiology involved in chronic renal failure.**

   The kidneys are paired organs located in the dorsal abdominal cavity in the retroperitoneal space in front of and on both sides of the spinal column between the twelfth thoracic and third lumbar vertebrae. The right kidney is slightly lower than the left because the liver lies above it. The main function of the kidneys is to maintain proper fluid and electrolyte balance and remove metabolic wastes from the body. Fluid balance is achieved by the kidneys' ability to concentrate or dilute urine. Electrolyte balance is achieved by the appropriate absorption and secretion of electrolytes within the tubular system of the nephron. Chronic renal failure may develop slowly over months or years or rapidly over weeks. Irreversible kidney damage occurs when 85% to 90% of renal function is lost. The hallmark of renal failure is an increase in urea and other nonprotein nitrogens, which is termed *uremia* or *azotemia* (Pisoni & Remuzzi, 2001). All body systems are affected by metabolic waste accumulation, fluid overload, and electrolyte imbalances. Initially, as the glomerular filtration rate (GFR) begins to fall, medication, diet, and fluid restrictions are used to maintain and support system function. However, with the loss of 90% of nephrons, GFR will decrease to 5 ml/min (normal is 125 ml/min), and symptoms of uremia (anorexia, nausea, vomiting, angina, dyspnea, insomnia, and loss of libido) will be seen. At this point, hemodialysis, peritoneal dialysis, or kidney transplantation is necessary to maintain the integrity of the body's internal environment (Amerling & Levin, 2001; Greenberg & Palevsky, 2001; Pisoni & Remuzzi, 2001; Urden et al, 2002).

2. **Discuss the typical laboratory findings seen with chronic renal failure.**

   Normal values are the following:

Hct	40%-54% men; 37%-47% women
BUN	10-26 mg/dl
Creatinine	0.6-1.2 mg/dl
Na^+	136-148 mmol/L
K^+	3.5-5.0 mmol/L
Cl^-	96-106 mmol/L
CO_2 (HCO_3^-)	24-30 mmol/L
Ca^{++}	8.4-10.2 mg/dl
Phosphate	2.7-4.5 mg/dl

   Pertinent laboratory tests include a blood chemistry analysis, with particular attention to the complete blood count (CBC) and electrolyte, serum creatinine, BUN, calcium, and phosphorus levels to establish baseline data. Anemia is common with chronic renal failure because of the decrease in production of erythropoietin (a protein hormone produced by the kidneys to stimulate the bone marrow to produce red blood cells). It is not unusual to find hematocrit values of 20% to 25%. In addition, it is common to find serum potassium and phosphorus levels elevated and serum sodium and calcium levels decreased. BUN and serum creatinine levels are significantly elevated in patients with chronic renal failure. These patients demonstrate some degree of metabolic acidosis and decreased carbon dioxide (HCO_3^-) levels because nonfunctioning kidneys can no longer produce new bicarbonate (Parker, 1998; Amerling & Levin, 2001; Greenberg & Palevsky, 2001; Pisoni & Remuzzi, 2001; Urden et al, 2002).

3. Describe the symptoms of uremia that might be manifested by Mr. Miller.

Uremia refers to the constellation of signs and symptoms associated with the deterioration of biochemical and physiologic functions that occur with renal failure. It results from the retention of substances that are ordinarily removed by healthy kidneys (urea, creatinine, and other organic and inorganic compounds) and derangements of hormonal and enzymatic homeostasis. Body systems affected by renal failure and possible clinical manifestations are as follows (Parker, 1998; Vanholder, 1998; Amerling & Levin, 2001; Pisoni & Remuzzi, 2001):

- *Genitourinary system*: decreased urine volume, increased serum urea nitrogen level, and increased serum creatinine level
- *Cardiovascular system*: volume overload, pulmonary edema, hypertension, pericarditis, cardiomyopathy
- *Neurologic system*: encephalopathy, convulsions, altered mental state, memory loss, decreased muscle strength, psychosis, insomnia, neuropathy
- *Hematologic system*: anemia, thrombocytopenia
- *Gastrointestinal system*: anorexia, nausea, vomiting, gastritis, ulcers, uremic fetor (urine breath), constipation
- *Integumentary system*: yellow, gray-tinged skin, dryness, itching
- *Skeletal system*: bone demineralization, osteodystrophy, metastatic calcification

4. Describe how the relationship between calcium and phosphorus is altered in chronic renal failure.

Normal values are the following:

Serum Phosphorus	2.7-4.5 mg/dl
Serum Calcium	8.4-10.2 mg/dl
Calcium-Phosphorus Product	30-40 mg/dl

Approximately 98% of the total body calcium can be found within the bone, with the remaining 2% found in the plasma. It is the ionized plasma calcium level that controls the absorption of calcium from the gastrointestinal tract. Vitamin D must be metabolized by the kidney into its active form, 1,25-dihydroxycholecalciferol, to facilitate calcium absorption from the gastrointestinal tract. Plasma calcium and phosphorus exist in a reciprocal relationship so that when the phosphorus level decreases, the calcium level increases. The amount of phosphorus excreted by the kidney is directly proportional to the level of phosphorus in the plasma. Thus, if the serum phosphorus level is elevated, the kidneys increase the excretion of phosphorus to maintain the plasma level between 2.7 and 4.5 mg/dl. The parathyroid hormone plays a significant role in maintaining the calcium-phosphorus balance. When the serum calcium level decreases, parathyroid hormone is released by the parathyroid gland, which causes calcium to be released by the bone and phosphorus to be excreted by the kidney. With irreversible damage to the kidney, the complex relationship between calcium and phosphorus is severely altered. The kidney can no longer excrete the majority of phosphorus necessary to maintain balance; thus an elevated plasma phosphorus level occurs. The reciprocal relationship results in a decrease in plasma calcium. The state of hypocalcemia worsens because the kidney cannot metabolize the active form of vitamin D, which reduces calcium absorption from the gastrointestinal tract and impairs calcium mobilization from the bone. The parathyroid glands respond to the decreased plasma calcium levels and release parathyroid hormone to stimulate the reabsorption of calcium by the bone, which in turn increases the plasma calcium level. With both the serum calcium and phosphorus levels elevated, the calcium-phosphorus level is significantly elevated. If the calcium-phosphorus product exceeds 70 mg/dl, calcium phosphate crystals may precipitate in the brain, eyes, myocardium, lungs, skin, and bone. The increased production of parathormone may lead to further bone demineralization (Parker, 1998; Ahmad, 2000; Massry & Smogorzewski, 2001).

5. **Discuss the pathophysiology of aluminum toxicity in chronic renal failure.**

Aluminum is a cation found in certain medications, such as aluminum-based phosphate binders (e.g., Amphojel, ALternaGEL, Basaljel), untreated tap water, fruits and vegetables grown in soil with high aluminum levels, food cooked in aluminum vessels, and unprocessed water used to prepare hemodialysis solution. Aluminum is absorbed from the gastrointestinal tract and partially excreted by the kidneys. About 80% of aluminum is protein bound, so it does not readily diffuse across the glomerular membrane for renal excretion. Patients undergoing dialysis are particularly prone to developing toxicity that results in bone disease, myopathy, encephalopathy, seizures, microcytic anemia, and myocardiomyopathy (Delmez, 1998; D'Haese & DeBroe, 2001; Kovalik, 2001; Ritz et al, 2001).

6. **Discuss the pathophysiology of pericarditis in chronic renal failure. Why was Mr. Miller particularly prone to this complication?**

Pericarditis is inflammation of the visceral and parietal pericardial layers of the pericardium that develops as a result of toxic metabolic wastes found with renal failure. Toxins inflame and irritate the layers of the pericardium, causing a "rub" instead of gliding smoothly across each other during systole and diastole. Uremic pericarditis is commonly seen in patients who have not yet started dialysis. It is also seen during the first few months of dialysis therapy and in those whose dialysis is inadequate. The classic triad of symptoms for pericarditis is chest pain, fever, and pericardial friction rub. The chest pain is usually sharp and typically radiates over the left shoulder, neck, and left arm. The pain increases when the patient is supine, intensifies with deep breathing, and is relieved by sitting forward. The pericardial friction rub can be heard upon auscultation by placing the stethoscope's diaphragm over the left midsternal to lower sternal border; the amplitude may increase or decrease with inspiration or expiration. The most life-threatening complication of pericarditis is cardiac tamponade (Lancaster, 2001).

7. **Discuss the different forms of dialysis used in the treatment of renal failure, including the indications and contraindications for each. Support the decision to use hemodialysis in treating Mr. Miller.**

Two major forms of dialysis are available for treatment of chronic renal failure: peritoneal dialysis and hemodialysis. Both techniques use diffusion, osmosis, and filtration via a semipermeable membrane to remove excess metabolic waste and excess fluid and electrolytes. Peritoneal dialysis uses the body's own peritoneal membrane in the abdominal cavity and requires placement of a catheter into the peritoneal cavity. The principle of osmosis is used to promote fluid shifts from the peritoneal vasculature into the dialysis solution. The osmotic gradient is created by the concentration of glucose in the peritoneal dialysis solution.

Hemodialysis is a process using an extracorporeal circuit and an artificial membrane (dialyzer) to mimic the functions of the glomerulus of the human kidney. It requires access to the central circulation, dialysis solution, treated water, dialyzer, and a dialysis machine (Salai, 1998; Daugirdas & Van Stone, 2001; Palmer, 2001; Urden et al, 2002). Either modality can be used in the treatment of acute or chronic renal failure. The patient should be given the choice after the risks and benefits of both have been explained. Mr. Miller already had an AV fistula in his right forearm, which was created as a permanent access to his central circulation for hemodialysis.

8. **Identify pharmacologic agents used to treat chronic renal failure and the rationale for their use.**

Antianemics are drugs used to treat the anemia associated with decreased erythropoietin production by renal tissue; decreased red blood cell survival; chronic blood loss through blood sampling, dialysis, or gastrointestinal losses; and iron and vitamin B_{12} and folate deficiencies. Common antianemics include the following:

- Epoetin alfa (Epogen): glycoprotein that is biologically and immunologically identical to endogenous erythropoietin and functions by acting on erythroid tissues within the bone marrow to stimulate the differentiation of erythroid progenitor and early precursor cells
- Iron preparations: ferrous sulfate (Iberet, Feosol); iron dextran (InFeD) injection; sodium ferric gluconate complex in sucrose (Ferrlecit) injection; polysaccharide-iron complex (Niferex)
- Folic acid (Folvite)
- Pyridoxine (pyridoxine hydrochloride)

Phosphate-binding agents are used to bind phosphates in the gastrointestinal tract to facilitate their excretion via feces. Phosphate-binding agents used include the following:

- Calcium acetate (PhosLo)
- Calcium carbonate (Os-Cal, Tums)
- Aluminum hydroxide (Amphojel, ALternaGEL, Alucaps)
- Sevelamer hydrochloride (Renagel): the first calcium-free, aluminum-free phosphate binder

Vitamins are also used as supplements because of dietary restrictions, dialysis therapy, and metabolic imbalances. Important vitamins to replace are the following:

- All B with C
- Vitamin B complex with C
- Nephrocaps
- Nephro-Vite

Vitamin D supplementation and analogs are used to help normalize serum calcium and alkaline phosphatase levels and may lower elevated parathyroid hormone levels. Patients with chronic renal failure can no longer convert vitamin D into the active form, contributing to the development of hypocalcemia and secondary hyperparathyroidism. Medications used to maintain homeostasis are the following:

- Ergocalciferol (Calciferol), least active
- Dihydrotachysterol
- 1,25-Dihydroxycholecalciferol/calcitriol (Rocaltrol), most active
- Calcitriol (Calcijex) injection
- Paricalcitol (Zemplar) injection

9. Discuss the dietary management of the patient with chronic renal failure.

A diet controlled for protein, phosphorus, or both may retard the progression of renal insufficiency to chronic renal failure. Kimmel (1998) and Pisoni and Remuzzi (2001) report that a low-protein diet reduces intraglomerular pressure and capillary blood flow and decreases urinary protein loss, thus slowing the progression to chronic renal failure. The current recommendation for protein intake in patients with GFRs between 25 and 60 ml/min is 0.6 g/kg/day with two thirds provided as high biologic value protein to meet the essential amino acid requirements, and the recommendation for calorie intake is 35 to 50 kcal/kg. Patients with renal insufficiency are monitored for volume depletion or fluid overload. A minimum urinary volume of approximately 600 ml is required for the excretion of the average load of solids. Peripheral edema, hypertension, and congestive heart failure are potential complications that must be watched for. The diet for dialysis compensates for lack of kidney function, dialysate losses, and current nutritional status. The recommendations for the patient with renal failure is sodium intake of 1000 to 3000 mg/day, potassium intake of 2000 to 3000 mg/day, fluid intake to limit weight gains between dialysis treatments to 0.5 to 1 kg/day, and phosphorus intake of 600 to 1200 mg/day (McCann, 2002). Calorie and protein intake for patients receiving dialysis needs to be higher because the process of dialysis is catabolic. During hemodialysis, amino acid losses may exceed 10 to 12 g per treatment; with peritoneal dialysis, 5 to 15 g of amino acids and albumin are lost daily and 50% to 80% is as albumin. Recommendations for protein intake in patients receiving hemodialysis is ≥1.2 g/kg of body weight (Louden & Goodship, 2002) and 1.2 to 1.3 g/kg of body weight for patients receiving peritoneal dialysis (Vychytil & Hörl, 2002).

10. Identify clinical complications arising from noncompliance that were manifested by Mr. Miller.

Mr. Miller had an accumulation of uremic toxins resulting from noncompliance with his medical regimen. Mr. Miller experienced nausea and vomiting, agitation, and confusion. In addition he had chest pain, described as moderate to severe in intensity and diffusely located over the precordium. Pulmonary overload was revealed through neck vein distention, crackles scattered bilaterally throughout the lung bases, and pitting peripheral edema bilaterally in the lower extremities. He had a weight gain of 8 kg (17.6 lb). Cardiac monitoring demonstrated sinus tachycardia with a rate of 116 bpm. A pericardial friction rub and an S_3 gallop were auscultated. These symptoms are consistent with pericarditis. Laboratory values revealed metabolic acidosis, hyperkalemia, hyponatremia, hyperphosphatemia, hypocalcemia, and anemia.

11. List nursing diagnoses appropriate for the care of the patient with chronic renal failure. Include nursing diagnoses appropriate for the care of the patient with a permanent AV fistula for dialysis access.

- Fluid volume excess related to noncompliance with prescribed medical regimen
- Noncompliance with medical regimen related to limitations of disease
- Alteration in self-image related to skin changes and changes in lifestyle
- Impaired gas exchange related to pulmonary edema
- Alteration in nutrition: less than body requirements related to nausea and vomiting
- High risk for infection related to impaired defense barriers
- Alteration in self-image related to skin changes
- High risk for alteration in cardiac output related to uremic pericarditis and patency of the access (Molzahan, 1998)

12. List the components of the teaching plan for the patient with chronic renal failure.

- Compliance with components of medical regimen such as dialysis schedule, medications and diet and fluid restriction
- Prevention of infection
- Regular exercise
- Maintenance of dialysis access: teaching about how to check for patency of the access, and signs and symptoms of infection
- Prevention of complications (Bucher & Melander, 1999)

13. List the criteria used in the selection of patients for kidney transplantation.

Renal transplantation is considered a viable alternative for treatment of ESRD when the patient does not have other medical problems that could increase the risks associated with the procedure. The usual age range of candidates for renal transplantation is 2 to 65 years. Patients at either end of the transplantation age continuum have an increased risk for complications. A thorough body systems assessment is performed before the person is considered for organ transplantation (Mudge et al, 1998; Kendrick, 2001).

The number of patients awaiting organ transplantation has increased dramatically from 1997 to 2003 because of the advances made in transplantation procedures. As of March 2003, 86,157 patients were awaiting vital organs for transplantation in the United States, with 56,895 of these awaiting cadaver kidney transplantation (United Network for Organ Sharing [UNOS], 2003). All potential organ recipients are entered into the national computer system through the United Network for Organ Sharing (UNOS). A point system has been instituted to allow equitable distribution of this scarce resource. Blood type compatibility between donor and recipient is mandatory.

Specific criteria have been established for potential kidney recipients. First, priority is given to the potential recipient with the best antigen match. Second, priority is also given to potential recipients who have preformed antibodies to major histocompatibility complex antigens because the presence of these antibodies can limit the number of kidneys for which the potential recipient would be eligible. Priority is also given to potential recipients who are considered "medical emergencies." The most common circumstance that qualifies a patient as needing an emergency kidney transplantation is the inability to maintain AV access for hemodialysis. The final criterion has to do with logistic factors based on the ease and rapidity with which the transplantation can be performed (Alspach, 1998; Katznelson et al, 2001).

Organs from living-related donors provide the highest rates of renal graft survival. General physical criteria for donors include the absence of systemic disease and infection, no history of cancer, absence of hypertension and renal disease, and adequate renal function as evidenced by diagnostic studies. In addition, living-related donors must express a clear understanding of the associated surgery and a willingness to donate a kidney. Some transplant centers also require a psychiatric evaluation to determine the motivation of the donor.

14. Discuss hemodialysis and renal transplantation as alternative treatment modalities for Mr. Miller. Support Mr. Miller's decision to select renal transplantation rather than hemodialysis.

Hemodialysis and renal transplantation are alternative treatment modalities for Mr. Miller. It is most often the patient's preference that determines the type of therapy instituted. Patients should consider which modality would best be suited to their physical condition and lifestyle. Mr. Miller has no active malignancy or infectious process. He has a strong support system, with siblings willing to donate a living donor kidney. He is financially secure through income and health insurance coverage. Although Mr. Miller has had difficulty complying with the medical regimen of hemodialysis because of transportation difficulties and distance to the health care facility, he stated that he is now willing to comply with the medical regimen after transplantation because these transportation issues will be eliminated.

Conservative medical management of ESRD with dialysis is costly. Although transplantation procedures are expensive, current success rates have made transplantation a cost-effective treatment option compared with traditional medical management. For example, a patient undergoing hemodialysis costs the federal government, through Medicare, about $56,000 per year. The cost of a kidney transplant is approximately $90,000 for the first year and $18,000 yearly for follow-up care. If the transplant functions for 5 years, the cost is approximately $90,000 as opposed to $280,000 for 5 years of hemodialysis (U.S. Renal Data System [USRDS], 2002). Because Mr. Miller was employed full-time before beginning dialysis and plans to return to work after the transplantation, other financial considerations are his potential earning power and the discontinuation of any disability benefits previously required.

One of the major obstacles to a successful renal transplant is finding a suitable donor. Blood relatives make the most compatible donors and result in an approximate 95% success rate at 1 year for the patient (Katznelson et al, 2001). Mr. Miller had three brothers and three sisters consenting to be a donor if a transplant match was possible. It is imperative that Mr. Miller receive a living donor kidney because the more similar the tissue antigens of the donor are to those of the recipient, the more likely it is that the transplant will be successful and immunologic rejection will be avoided.

Renal transplantation could also eliminate the lifestyle restrictions for the patient. Mr. Miller was required to report to a community-based hemodialysis clinic 75 miles from his home three times a week. Approximately 24 hours each week were required for travel and treatment time. By choosing renal transplantation, Mr. Miller hopes to alleviate the inconvenience and discomfort of the frequent dialysis treatments.

15. List the advantages and disadvantages of a living donor versus a cadaver donor. Why was it imperative that Mr. Miller receive a living donor kidney?

Cadaver organ donors are those from previously healthy individuals who have suffered irreversible brain injury of a known cause. The most common causes of injury are cerebral trauma from motor vehicle accidents, gunshot wounds, intracerebral or subarachnoid hemorrhage, primary brain tumor, and anoxic brain damage resulting from drug overdose or cardiac arrest. The brain-dead donor must have effective cardiovascular function and must be supported on a ventilator to preserve organ viability. The donor must be free of extracranial malignancies, sepsis, and communicable diseases, including hepatitis, syphilis, tuberculosis, and human immunodeficiency virus infection. The age range of most suitable donors is between 6 and 65 years. Age is generally less important than the quality of organ function; however, kidneys from children younger than 6 years pose significant technical challenges and increase the risk of delayed graft function (Alspach, 1998; Bucher & Melander, 1999; Gritsch et al, 2001; Young & Gaston, 2001).

Cadaver Donor Kidney

1. Advantages
   - Success rate of transplantation has improved to 85% to 90%.
   - Cadaver kidneys can maintain viability for as long as 72 hours after removal from the donor.
   - The average cost of transplant is $90,000 (same as that for living donor transplants).

2. Disadvantages
   - The potential organ recipient is placed on a national registry (UNOS) to allow equitable distribution of scarce organ supply.
   - The organ recipient may die while waiting for a kidney because of limited supply and great demand.
   - Few kidneys are available for transplantation, and surgery must be done as kidneys become available.
   - Recipient's physical and psychologic health may not be optimal.

Living-Related Donor Kidney

1. Advantages
   - The recipient is not placed on the national registry to wait for a kidney.
   - A living-related donor provides the highest rate of renal graft survival (95%).
   - The average cost is $90,000 and it is more cost-effective over the long term than hemodialysis.
   - Current research favors donor-specific blood transfusion, in which blood from the kidney donor is transfused into the recipient. This has improved graft survival, especially of organs from living donors.
   - Surgery can be scheduled electively to optimize the patient's state of health. The organ suffers less ischemia because it is not transported.

2. Disadvantages
   - Kidney removal from a living donor requires greater surgical care and is a delicate procedure that lasts 3 to 4 hours.
   - Donors experience more pain than recipients.
   - There is a small risk of complication or death for the donor.
   - The donor must have annual physical examinations for life to assess the function of the remaining kidney.
   - There is a psychologic impact for both the donor and the recipient.

At 67 years of age, if Mr. Miller were to receive a living donor kidney, it would enhance his chances for a successful transplantation. The procedure could be scheduled electively, which would allow for an optimal state of health at the time of surgery. The living donor transplantation also would allow decreased ischemic time for the kidney by eliminating transport time.

16. Describe the cadaver kidney preservation process.

The cadaver donor nephrectomy is conducted as a sterile autopsy in the operating room. All arterial and venous vessels are carefully preserved (Bucher & Melander, 1999). The aorta and vena cava are cannulated from below and ligated above the renal arteries and veins. The cadaver kidneys are flushed with cold Ringer's lactate solution containing heparin 10,000 U/L. Once the transplantable kidney has been surgically removed, it is preserved in a sterile, iced electrolyte solution and transported to a transplant center. Kidneys can maintain viability for as long as 72 hours before they must be transplanted (Bucher & Melander, 1999; Gritsch et al, 2001).

Preservation by Perfusion

The kidneys are perfused with a cold (6° to 10° C) solution at low flow, low pressure to provide nutrients and oxygen and to remove products of metabolism. The kidneys can be preserved in this process for up to 72 hours (Gritsch et al, 2001).

Preservation by Cold Storage

A high-potassium, low-sodium solution that resembles the electrolyte balance inside kidney cells is used to flush the kidney, and then the kidneys are stored in this solution in sterile plastic bags at temperatures of 6° C or less. The kidneys can be preserved in this process for up to 30 hours (Gritsch et al, 2001).

17. Briefly describe the surgical process of renal transplantation.

After induction of anesthesia, the genitalia and abdominal skin are prepared and a Foley catheter is placed in the urinary bladder. The bladder is rinsed with a broad-spectrum antibiotic solution and gravity filled to capacity, and the catheter is clamped until the urinary tract reconstruction portion of the operation begins. Usually the kidney graft is placed in the extraperitoneal area in the contralateral iliac fossa through a Gibson incision on the same side from which it was removed from the donor. The renal artery is attached to the hypogastric or internal iliac artery, and the renal vein is anastomosed to the external iliac vein. Mannitol (0.5 to 1 g/kg) is infused during and immediately after renal revascularization to act as an osmotic diuretic. The urinary tract reconstruction is by transvesical or extravesical ureteroneocystostomy. The recipient's own nonfunctioning kidney is usually not removed unless it is infected, greatly enlarged, or causing medically uncontrollable hypertension (Kendrick, 2001).

18. Discuss possible postoperative complications of renal transplantation.

Numerous potential complications are associated with renal transplantation. Vascular complications nearly always require surgical intervention. Stenosis of the renal artery may occur, which is evident by the presence of hypertension, auscultation of a bruit over the artery anastomoses site, and decreased renal function. To correct stenosis of the renal artery, the clinician must surgically resect the involved artery and anastomose the kidney to another artery. Other vascular problems include vascular leakage and thrombosis, both of which require an emergency nephrectomy.

   Wound complications include hematomas, abscesses, and lymphoceles. Genitourinary tract complications such as ureteral leakage, ureteral fistulas, ureteral obstruction, calculus formation, bladder neck contractures, scrotal swelling, and graft rupture may also necessitate surgical intervention (Mudge et al, 1998; Gritsch & Rosenthal, 2001). The most common and most life-threatening complication of renal transplantation is rejection. In tissue rejection, a reaction occurs between the antigens in the transplanted kidney and the antibodies and cytotoxic T cells in the recipient's blood. These immunologic substances treat the transplanted kidney as a foreign invader and cause tissue destruction, thrombosis, and eventual necrosis of the tissue (Mudge et al, 1998; Bucher & Melander, 1999).

19. List the nursing diagnoses appropriate to the care of the patient undergoing renal transplantation during the recovery period.

- Altered tissue perfusion related to rejection or acute tubular necrosis
- Potential for fluid volume excess related to intraoperative and postoperative fluid administration and/or inadequate urinary elimination
- Potential for fluid volume deficit related to excessive output, diuretic therapy, inadequate fluid administration, vomiting/diarrhea, and/or bleeding
- Altered patterns of urinary elimination related to bladder spasms, anatomic size, or obstruction due to clots, bladder leak, infection, or diabetic neurogenic bladder
- Potential for electrolyte imbalance related to level of renal function after transplantation, intraoperative blood transfusions, metabolic disorders associated with acidosis and hyperglycemia, or side effects of medications (e.g., cyclosporine, steroids)
- Potential for infection related to alterations in the immune system secondary to immunosuppressive therapy, presence of invasive lines and Foley catheter
- Potential for constipation or gastroparesis related to anesthesia, immobility, pain medication, fear of straining on defecation, presence of Foley catheter, inadequate dietary intake
- Altered comfort related to incisional pain and bladder spasms
- Alteration in nutrition: less than body requirements related to nausea and vomiting and postoperative pain
- Alteration in body image related to medication side effects and transplantation
- Alteration in self-image related to changes in lifestyle
- Potential for knowledge deficit related to the short/long posttransplant course, unfamiliar tests and procedures, home management, medications, rejection, and risk of infection
- Noncompliance with medical regimen related to limitations of disease and physical changes secondary to medication

20. Discuss the pathophysiology of acute rejection. Describe the clinical manifestations of acute rejection in Mr. Miller.

The types of rejection are hyperacute, acute, and chronic. Hyperacute rejection occurs within 48 hours after transplant surgery. No treatment exists for this type of rejection, and after recognition of the problem, the rejected kidney is removed quickly to prevent further complications. Clinical manifestations include elevated temperature, elevated blood pressure, and pain at the transplant site (Bucher & Melander, 1999; Amend et al, 2001). Acute rejection usually occurs between 7 and 14 days after surgery but may occur up to 2 years after transplantation. The most common manifestations of acute rejection include oliguria or anuria, temperature greater than 37.8° C (100° F), enlarged and tender kidney, fluid retention, increased blood pressure, chronic fatigue, and changes in urinalysis and blood chemistry laboratory values. Acute rejection can be halted with early recognition and immediate administration of increased dosages of immunosuppressive drugs. Chronic rejection occurs gradually over months to years. The clinical manifestations include gradually increasing BUN and creatinine levels and changes in serum electrolyte levels. No treatment exists for chronic rejection, and the patient is conservatively managed until renal function deteriorates and dialysis is required (Bucher & Melander, 1999; Nast & Cohen, 2001).

     On the eighth postoperative day, Mr. Miller began to demonstrate signs and symptoms of acute rejection. He complained of not feeling well, of minimal abdominal tenderness on palpation, and of nausea. His temperature fluctuated between 38.4° and 38.8° C (101.2° and 101.8° F). Urinary output dropped to an average of 55 ml/hr and did not improve with furosemide (Lasix) boluses. On the ninth postoperative day, laboratory data revealed that his weight had increased to 78 kg (172 lb). His creatinine level was 4.3 mg/dl, and his BUN level was 63 mg/dl.

21. Discuss the immunosuppressive pharmacologic agents methylprednisolone, muromonab-CD3 (Orthoclone OKT3), cyclosporine, mycophenolate mofetil (CellCept), and tacrolimus (Prograf). Why did the physician add muromonab-CD3 and change cyclosporine to tacrolimus?

Methylprednisolone (Solu-Medrol)

Methylprednisolone, a corticosteroid, acts as an antiinflammatory agent to prevent movement of leukocytes into tissue during resection. In addition, methylprednisolone limits antibody production and blocks the antigen-antibody complex formation. Numerous side effects of corticosteroids include infections, gastrointestinal tract bleeding, ulcers, pancreatitis, delayed wound healing, diabetes mellitus, psychosis, cataracts, fluid and electrolyte imbalances, and hypertension (*Physicians' Desk Reference,* 2003).

Muromonab-CD3 (Orthoclone OKT3)

Muromonab-CD3 is a monoclonal anti–T-cell antibody that reacts with and blocks the function of all T cells, thereby reversing acute renal allograft rejection. The usual dosage of muromonab-CD3 is 5 mg/day. The drug is administered by intravenous bolus only. Muromonab-CD3 may not be given with any other drug. Side effects include respiratory complications such as acute pulmonary edema. This drug requires meticulous nursing assessment because it is given intravenously and reactions frequently occur with the first administration. Clinical manifestations of a reaction include fever, chills, dyspnea, and chest pain (Danovitch, 2001; *Physicians' Desk Reference,* 2003).

Cyclosporine

Cyclosporine is a calcineurin inhibitor medication used to prevent and treat rejection of organ transplants. Cyclosporine works by interfering with T-cell growth and can be given orally or intravenously. If administered orally, the drug may be diluted in various liquids but should be taken 1 to 2 hours after meals at the same time each day to maintain a consistent absorption rate and thereby maintain a consistent blood level. The usual dosage of cyclosporine is 6 mg/kg in divided doses every 12 hours. Mr. Miller's creatinine level had dropped to 1.9 mg/dl, so cyclosporine was added to the regimen. Cyclosporine is added to the medical regimen when the creatinine level is 2.5 mg/dl or less. Cyclosporine increases the risk of renal failure and hepatotoxicity.

Nursing responsibilities require observing for nephrotoxicity, hepatotoxicity, and potential malignancy, especially lymphoma. The nurse should monitor blood levels of the drug to ensure they are therapeutic but not toxic. Therapeutic trough levels range between 250 and 350 mg/ml. Six to 8 weeks after renal transplantation, the dosage is usually decreased to 4 to 5 mg/kg (*Physicians' Desk Reference,* 2003).

Mycophenolate mofetil (CellCept)

Mycophenolate mofetil (MMF) is a more selective antimetabolite. It does not affect cytokine production or the more proximal events following antigen recognition. MMF blocks the proliferation of T and B cells, inhibits antibody formation, and inhibits the generation of cytotoxic T cells. It also down-regulates the expression of adhesion molecules on lymphocytes, thereby impairing their binding to vascular endothelial cells. MMF is available in 250 mg and 500 mg capsules. The standard dose is 1 g twice daily. It is rapidly absorbed and well tolerated. Gastrointestinal side effects usually occur with doses greater than 1 g twice daily. Leukopenia, anemia, and thrombocytopenia also are side effects (Danovitch, 2001; Gourishankar & Halloran, 2001).

Tacrolimus (Prograf)

Tacrolimus is a calcineurin inhibitor. Although biochemically distinct from cyclosporine, it is remarkably similar in its mechanism of action, clinical efficacy, and side effect profile. Tacrolimus is available in intravenous formulation and as capsules. Its gastrointestinal absorption is independent of bile salts and it is absorbed primarily from the small intestines. A potential benefit of tacrolimus is rapidity of gastric emptying, which may be beneficial for patients with gastric motility disorders (Danovitch, 2001). An additional cardiovascular benefit to taking tacrolimus over cyclosporine is a reduction in serum cholesterol (Miller, 2001).

Muromonab-CD3 was added to Mr. Miller's medical regimen on the ninth postoperative day, when his laboratory values indicated worsening signs of acute rejection. Muromonab-CD3 drug therapy was added to block cytotoxic human T cells and the generation of other T-cell functions. The symptoms of renal allograft rejection, such as those noted in Mr. Miller's condition, are subtle and difficult to differentiate from similar symptoms of drug-induced nephrotoxicity.

Mycophenolate mofetil was added to Mr. Miller's immunosuppressive regimen as a primary prevention of renal allograft rejection. MMF inhibits the recruitment of mononuclear cells into rejection sites and the ensuing interaction of these cells with target cells. MMF has a preventive effect on the development and progression of proliferative arteriolopathy, which is a pathologic lesion in rejection (Danovitch, 2001; Gourishankar & Halloran, 2001).

Tacrolimus replaced cyclosporine because it has been shown to be a potent agent for rescue therapy for patients with acute cellular rejection on cyclosporine-based immunosuppression (Miller, 2001).

22. List the components of the teaching plan for Mr. Miller.

- Teach the patient the routine after a kidney transplant (e.g., what the patient will feel and see when he or she awakes from surgery, how often vital signs will be needed, and what type of a hospital unit he or she will be in after surgery).
- Inform the patient of the importance of all medications prescribed after transplantation, including purpose, side effects, dosage schedule, and frequency.
- Educate the patient about the laboratory values that will be monitored (e.g., BUN, creatinine, electrolytes, drug levels, CBC, platelets, and liver function studies) and discuss their importance.
- Teach the patient and family members the signs and symptoms of rejection (decreased urine output, pain over the kidney, a general feeling of illness, and weight gain) and the appropriate actions to take if any of these are seen.
- Teach the patient and the family members the signs and symptoms of infection, the importance of monitoring clinical manifestations, and the appropriate action to take if infection is suspected.
- Inform the patient and family members about dietary and fluid changes and/or restrictions.
- Arrange a consultation for nutritional support when convenient for the patient and family members.
- Educate the patient about the importance of skin care, use of sunscreen, and acne prophylaxis to prevent complications.
- Provide information stressing the importance of routine dental care, brushing, flossing, and gum care.
- Educate the patient and family members about family planning, use of contraceptives, and risks of pregnancy.
- Inform the patient of the importance of exercise and encourage the patient to establish a regular exercise routine.

- Teach health maintenance skills needed for monitoring the patient's health status and have the patient validate learning through return demonstrations (e.g., temperature, weight, blood pressure, pulse, glucose monitoring, incision care).
- Reinforce the importance of keeping all follow-up appointments with the physician or for diagnostic procedures.
- Provide information about kidney transplantation and local organizations and support groups.
- Provide information regarding the financial, psychologic, and rehabilitative resources available.
- Emphasize to the patient the importance of carrying medical alert information at all times.

CHRONIC RENAL FAILURE AND RENAL TRANSPLANTATION

References

Ahmad, S. (2000). Renal osteodystrophy. In S. Ahmad (Ed.), *Manual of clinical dialysis* (pp. 130-138). London: Science Press.

Alspach, J. G. (Ed.). (1998). *American Association of Critical-Care Nurses: Core curriculum for critical care nursing* (5th ed.). Philadelphia: W. B. Saunders.

Amend, J. C., Jr., Vincenti, F., & Tomlanovich, S. J. (2001). The first two post-transplant months. In G. Danovitch (Ed.), *Handbook of kidney transplantation* (3rd ed., pp. 163-181). Baltimore: Lippincott Williams & Wilkins.

Amerling, R. & Levin, N. W. (2001). Uremia. In S. Massry & R. Glassock (Eds.), *Textbook of nephrology* (4th ed., pp. 555-561). Philadelphia: Lippincott Williams & Wilkins.

Bucher, L. & Melander, S. (Eds). (1999). *Critical care nursing*. Philadelphia: W. B. Saunders.

Danovitch, G. M. (2001). Immunosuppressive medications and protocols for kidney transplantation. In G. Danovitch (Ed.), *Handbook of kidney transplantation* (3rd ed., pp. 62-110). Baltimore: Lippincott Williams & Wilkins.

Daugirdas, J. T. & Van Stone, J. C. (2001). Physiologic principles and urea kinetic modeling. In J. Daugirdas, P. Blake, & T. Ing (Eds.), *Handbook of dialysis* (3rd ed., pp. 15-45). Philadelphia: Lippincott Williams & Wilkins.

Delmez, J. A. (1998). Renal osteodystrophy and other musculoskeletal complications of chronic renal failure. In A. Greenburg (Ed.), *Primer on kidney diseases* (2nd ed., pp.448-455). San Diego: Academic Press.

D'Haese, P. C. & DeBroe, M. E. (2001). Aluminum toxicity. In J. Daugirdas, P. Blake, & T. Ing (Eds.), *Handbook of dialysis* (3rd ed., pp. 548-561). Philadelphia: Lippincott Williams & Wilkins.

Gourishankar, S. & Halloran, P. F. (2001). Action, efficacy, and toxicities: Mycophenolate mofetil. In D. Norman & L. Turka (Eds.), *Primer on transplantation* (2nd ed., pp.138-143). Mt. Laurel: American Society of Transplantation.

Greenberg, A. & Palevsky, P. M. (2001). Disturbances in fluid, electrolyte, and acid-base balance. In S. Massry & R. Glassock (Eds.), *Textbook of nephrology* (4th ed., pp. 1381-1387). Philadelphia: Lippincott Williams & Wilkins.

Gritsch, H. A. & Rosenthal, J. T. (2001). The transplant operation and its surgical complications. In G. Danovitch (Ed.), *Handbook of kidney transplantation* (3rd ed., pp. 146-162). Baltimore: Lippincott Williams & Wilkins.

Gritsch, H. A., Rosenthal, J. T., & Danovitch, G. M. (2001). Living and cadaveric kidney donation. In G. Danovitch (Ed.), *Handbook of kidney transplantation* (3rd ed., pp. 111-129). Baltimore: Lippincott Williams & Wilkins.

Katznelson, S., Terasaki, P. I., & Danovitch, G. M. (2001). Histocompatibility testing, crossmatching, and allocation of cadaveric kidney transplants. In G. Danovitch (Ed.), *Handbook of kidney transplantation* (3rd ed., pp. 39-61). Baltimore: Lippincott Williams & Wilkins.

Kendrick, E. (2001). Evaluation of the transplant recipient. In G. Danovitch (Ed.), *Handbook of kidney transplantation* (3rd ed., pp. 130-145). Philadelphia: Lippincott Williams & Wilkins.

Kimmel, P. L. (1998). Management of the patient with chronic renal disease. In A. Greenberg (Ed.), *Primer on kidney diseases* (2nd ed., pp. 433-440). San Diego: Academic Press.

Kovalik, E. (2001). Endocrine and neurological manifestations of renal failure. In A. Greenberg (Ed.), *Primer on kidney diseases* (3rd ed., pp. 446-454). San Diego: Academic Press.

Lancaster, L. E. (2001). Systemic manifestations of renal failure. In L. E. Lancaster (Ed.), *Core curriculum for nephrology nursing* (4th ed., pp. 117-158). Pitman, NJ: Jannetti.

Louden, J. D. & Goodship, T. H. J. (2002). Nutritional requirements of hemodialysis patients. In W. Mitch & S. Klahr (Eds.), *Handbook of nutrition and the kidney* (4th ed., pp. 118-125). Philadelphia: Lippincott Williams & Wilkins.

Massry, S. & Smogorzewski, M. (2001). Divalent ion metabolism and renal osteodystrophy. In S. Massry & R. Glassock (Eds.), *Textbook of nephrology* (4th ed., pp. 1394-1425). Philadelphia: Lippincott Williams & Wilkins.

McCann, L. (2002). Pocket guide to nutrition assessment of the renal patient (3rd ed.). New York: National Kidney Foundation.

Miller, L. W. (2001). Action, efficacy, and toxicities: Tacrolimus. In D. Norman & L. Turka (Eds.), *Primer on transplantation* (2nd ed., pp. 130-137). Mt. Laurel: American Society of Transplantation. Philadelphia, PA.

Molzahn, A. C. (1998). Psychosocial impact of renal disease. In J. Parker (Ed.), *Contemporary nephrology nursing* (pp. 269-284). Pitman, NJ: Jannetti.

Mudge, C., Carlson, L., & Brennan, P. (1998). Transplantation. In J. Parker (Ed.), *Contemporary nephrology nursing* (pp. 693-778). Pitman, NJ: Jannetti.

Nast, C. C. & Cohen, A. H. (2001). Pathology of kidney transplantation. In G. Danovitch (Ed.), *Handbook of kidney transplantation* (3rd ed., pp. 290-312). Baltimore: Lippincott Williams & Wilkins.

Palmer, B. (2001). Dialyzers, dialysates, and delivery systems. In S. Massry & R. Glassock (Eds.), *Textbook of nephrology* (4th ed., pp. 1488-1494). Philadelphia: Lippincott Williams & Wilkins.

Parker, K. P. (1998). Acute and chronic renal failure. In J. Parker (Ed.), *Contemporary nephrology nursing* (pp. 199-265). Pitman, NJ: Jannetti.

Physicians' desk reference. (2003). Montvale, NJ: Medical Economics Co.

Pisoni, R. & Remuzzi, G. (2001). Progression of renal disease. In A. Greenburg (Ed.), *Primer on kidney diseases* (3rd ed., pp. 385-395). San Diego: Academic Press.

Ritz, E., Schoemig, M., & Massry, S. (2001). Uremic myopathy. In S. Massry & R. Glassock (Eds.), *Textbook of nephrology* (4th ed., pp. 1426-1429). Philadelphia: Lippincott Williams & Wilkins.

Salai, P. B. (1998). Hemodialysis. In J. Parker (Ed.), *Contemporary nephrology nursing* (pp. 527-576). Pitman, NJ: Jannetti.

United Network for Organ Sharing (UNOS). (2003). Update. [Homepage]. www.unos.org.

Urden, L. D., Stacy, K. M., & Lough, M. E. (2002*). Thelan's critical care nursing: Diagnosis and management* (4th ed.). Philadelphia: Mosby.

U.S. Renal Data System [USRDS]. (2002). The 2002 annual data report [WWW document]. www.usrds.org.

Vanholder, R. (1998). The uremic syndrome. In A. Greenburg (Ed.), *Primer on kidney diseases* (2nd ed., pp. 403-407). San Diego: Academic Press.

Vychytil, A. & Hörl, W. H. (2002). Nutrition and peritoneal dialysis. In W. Mitch & S. Klahr (Eds.), *Handbook of nutrition and the kidney* (4th ed., pp. 253-271). Philadelphia: Lippincott Williams & Wilkins.

Young, C. J. & Gaston, R. S. (2001). Cadaver kidney donor selection. In D. Norman & L. Turka (Eds.), *Primer on transplantation* (2nd ed., pp. 425-427). Mt. Laurel: American Society of Transplantation. Philadelphia, PA.

GASTROINTESTINAL ALTERATIONS

18

Gastrointestinal Tract Bleeding

Judi Kuric, PhD, MSN, RN, APRN, BC, CRRN-A, CNRN

CASE PRESENTATION

Scott Mitchell, age 44 years, was transferred from the emergency department (ED) to the intensive care unit (ICU) with a diagnosis of probable gastrointestinal (GI) tract bleeding. The ED history states that he had been seen as an outpatient 1 week ago because of epigastric pain after heavy alcohol consumption at a New Year's party. He stated he had been "hungover and nauseated" for 48 hours and has had severe epigastric pain since the party. Gastritis was diagnosed, and he was sent home with antiemetic and antacid medications and advised to stop smoking. Although he returned to his job as a commodities trader, he has not felt well since the party. He has been taking two buffered aspirin two or three times daily for epigastric pain in addition to his prescribed medications. He returned to the ED because of nausea, two episodes of vomiting large amounts of "dark brown" liquid, and complaints of extreme weakness. He also experienced dizziness when he stood or sat up abruptly.

Vital signs at admission and laboratory data at 6 PM were as follows:

BP	96/60 mm Hg lying; 84/50 mm Hg standing
HR	102 bpm
Respirations	20 breaths/min
Temperature	tympanic 37.9° C (100.2° F)
Hgb	12.5 g/dl
Hct	40%
WBCs	1200/mm^3

EMERGENCY DEPARTMENT RECORD

A 14-gauge nasogastric tube (NGT) was placed, and 350 ml of dark-brown, guaiac-positive "coffee ground" liquid returned. His stomach was lavaged with 500 ml of normal saline (NS), and the drainage subsequently became clear.

Mr. Mitchell's ICU admission orders were as follows:

1. Monitor electrocardiogram, vital signs, and intake and output every hour.
2. Maintain bed rest.

The editor would like to thank Cynthia S. Goodwin for her contribution to this chapter in the second edition of *Case Studies in Critical Care Nursing.*

3. Suction NGT at low intermittent setting; for active bleeding, notify physician and irrigate with 30 ml of NS q2h and prn until drainage becomes clear.
4. Give nothing by mouth (NPO) except for sips of water with oral medications.
5. Give medications orally (po); clamp NGT for 30 minutes after administration of medication.
6. Give magnesium hydroxide (Mylanta) 30 ml q4h po.
7. Give cimetidine (Tagamet) 300 mg q6h po.
8. Give promethazine (Phenergan) 25 mg IV q6h prn for nausea.
9. Start intravenous (IV) infusion of 5% dextrose in lactated Ringer's solution (D5LR) at 100 ml/hr.
10. Schedule for esophagogastroduodenoscopy (EGD) at 7 AM in GI laboratory.
11. Measure hemoglobin (Hgb) and hematocrit (Hct) at 9 PM.
12. Perform complete blood count and platelet count, prothrombin time (PT), partial thromboplastin time (PTT), complete metabolic profile electrolytes, and urinalysis in the morning.

Mr. Mitchell had an uneventful evening. His medical record reflected the data shown in Table 18-1.

At midnight his NGT was clamped to administer medication. When the NGT was unclamped at 12:30 AM, 300 ml of bloody drainage returned. He became restless and anxious. His skin was pale and moist. Oxygen was started by nasal cannula at 4 L/min. Vital signs at 12:30 AM were as follows:

BP	84/50 mm Hg lying
HR	126 bpm
Respirations	28 breaths/min

The physician was called, and the following orders were received:

1. Lavage the NGT with saline until clear.
2. Immediately measure Hgb and Hct and call results.
3. Type and crossmatch for two units of packed red blood cells (PRBCs); type and screen for an additional four units of PRBCs.
4. Place a triple-lumen subclavian IV line.
5. Measure central venous pressure (CVP) hourly; if it is less than 10 mm Hg, give 500 ml of NS IV fluid challenge and repeat the fluid challenge once if needed.
6. Anchor an indwelling urinary catheter and measure urine amount hourly.
7. Notify the gastroenterologist and surgeon.

Table 18-1	*Vital Signs and Flow Sheet Data*			
Time	**HR (bpm)**	**Respirations (breaths/min)**	**BP (mm Hg)**	**Other Client Data**
7 PM	112	16	104/64	
8 PM	115	18	100/60	Temperature 37.9° C (100.2° F)
9 PM	120	20	98/60	
10 PM	120	20	100/60	Hgb 12.3 g/dl Hct 36%
11 PM	120	20	96/54	Sleeping
Midnight	112	20	92/50	Temperature 36.7° C (98° F) (tympanic) Voided 120 ml amber urine

Table 18-2 *Vital Signs and Flow Sheet Data*

Time	HR (bpm)	Respirations (breaths/min)	BP (mm Hg)	CVP (mm Hg)	Urine Output	Other Client Data
2 AM	120	26	84/50	10	30	
3 AM	116	24	90/58	12	75	
4 AM	112	20	94/62	12	90	
5 AM	110	18	96/64	12	94	
6 AM	110	18	98/62	13	80	
7 AM	104	18	98/64	12	68	Hgb 10.1 g/dl Hct 28%

The interventions were carried out. No urine was obtained when the catheter was inserted. Assessment and laboratory data at 1 AM were as follows:

CVP	8 mm Hg
Hgb	9.8 g/dl
Hct	24%

At 1:30 AM after two 500 ml fluid challenges, Mr. Mitchell's CVP was 12 mm Hg and he had urine output of 30 ml/hr. D5LR was infusing at 50 ml/hr in a peripheral line and NS at 150 ml/hr in a central line. The physician ordered two units of PRBCs, which Mr. Mitchell received at 2 AM. His chart reflected the data shown in Table 18-2.

At 7:10 AM, Mr. Mitchell was transported to the GI laboratory for the EGD. The gastroenterologist found diffuse gastritis with a 2 cm duodenal ulcer. No clots were visible, and the ulcer was not actively bleeding. A biopsy specimen taken from the gastric wall tested positive for *Helicobacter pylori,* and a culture and sensitivity test were then performed.

Pharmacologic treatment for *H. pylori* was instituted, along with histamine-receptor antagonists and supplemental antacids. Mr. Mitchell's physicians chose to treat him conservatively with medication, and he progressed well. He was released from the ICU to the step-down unit in 24 hours and discharged home after 3 days.

GASTROINTESTINAL TRACT BLEEDING

QUESTIONS

1. What is the incidence of and mortality associated with acute GI tract bleeding?

2. Identify common causes of GI tract bleeding and list predisposing factors specific to Mr. Mitchell.

3. Discriminate between the characteristics of upper and lower GI tract bleeding.

4. What complication did Mr. Mitchell experience?

5. Which factors determine whether blood products will be administered to a patient with GI tract bleeding?

6. Mr. Mitchell's Hgb and Hct values dropped dramatically from admission to 7 AM. Discuss the drop in Hgb and Hct values in relation to Mr. Mitchell's blood loss.

7. If a patient continues to have active bleeding from the GI tract despite conservative management, what other medical procedures might be implemented?

8. Identify pharmacologic therapy commonly used in the treatment of GI tract bleeding.

9. What are the indications and types of surgical procedures for upper GI tract bleeding?

10. Identify six nursing diagnoses appropriate for Mr. Mitchell.

11. What is the incidence of *H. pylori* infection in gastritis and duodenal ulcers?

12. What is the treatment of choice for *H. pylori* infection?

GASTROINTESTINAL TRACT BLEEDING

QUESTIONS AND ANSWERS

1. What is the incidence of and mortality associated with acute GI tract bleeding?

More than 300,000 Americans with acute GI tract bleeding are admitted to hospitals each year, with an overall mortality of 10% (Savides & Jensen, 2000). Half the episodes are caused by peptic ulcers, and esophageal varices are the second leading cause. Mortality from bleeding esophageal varices ranges from 40% to 70% (Urden et al, 2002). For all causes of GI tract bleeding, mortality is greater in those who are older than age 60, who are in shock upon admission, who have a rebleeding episode within 72 hours, or whose red nasogastric aspirate fails to clear (Zuckerman, 2003).

2. Identify common causes of GI tract bleeding and list predisposing factors specific to Mr. Mitchell.

Causes of acute upper GI tract bleeding include gastric and duodenal ulcers, esophageal varices, erosive gastritis or esophagitis, Mallory-Weiss tears, angiomas of the stomach or small bowel, and aortoenteric fistulas. Common causes of acute lower GI tract bleeding include colonic angiomas (angiodysplasia), diverticula, and internal hemorrhoids.

Less common causes of GI tract bleeding include gastrointestinal cancer, inflammatory bowel disease, bowel infarction with perforation, and stress ulcers. Contributing factors may include liver disease, bleeding disorders, a history of abdominal aortic aneurysm repair, and nonsteroidal antiinflammatory drug or anticoagulation therapy. Mr. Mitchell's predisposing factors included alcohol ingestion, smoking, aspirin intake, and a stressful job.

3. Discriminate between the characteristics of upper and lower GI tract bleeding.

Bleeding above the duodenojejunal junction is defined as upper GI bleeding. Upper GI tract bleeding is characterized by *hematemesis* (vomiting bright or dark red blood) or vomiting old digested blood, a dark material that looks like coffee grounds. Bleeding from the stomach and esophageal sources is common, and in 90% of bleeding duodenal ulcers, blood also refluxes into the stomach (Alspach, 1998). Bleeding below the ligament of Treitz seldom results in vomiting of blood.

Lower GI bleeding from the colon, rectum, or anus is characterized by *hematochezia* (rectal passage of red blood or mahogany-colored stool) (Cello, 2000). *Melena*, the passage of black or tarry stools, occurs from digestion of blood from an upper GI hemorrhage and may take several days to clear after the bleeding stops (Beejay, 2000). In massive rapid upper GI tract bleeding, the patient may have both hematemesis and hematochezia.

4. What complication did Mr. Mitchell experience?

Mr. Mitchell experienced hypovolemia as a result of acute blood loss. His tachypnea, tachycardia, low CVP, orthostatic hypotension, low urine output, skin color changes, and restlessness indicated a class III hemorrhage, with a 30% to 40% loss of blood volume and moderately severe hemorrhagic shock (Urden, 2002, p. 810).

5. Which factors determine whether blood products will be administered to a patient with GI tract bleeding?

Blood administration is based on the level of shock, the response to IV fluid replacement, and changes in Hgb and Hct levels. Unstable vital signs after infusion of 2 L of crystalloid fluid replacement indicate the need for blood replacement. A Hgb value less than 10 mg/dl and an Hct less than 25% are also indicators for blood replacement. The amount of bloody drainage and the presence of active bleeding are also considered. PRBCs are commonly used because they decrease exposure to plasma antibodies and the risk of fluid volume overload (Bucher & Melander, 1999).

6. Mr. Mitchell's Hgb and Hct values dropped dramatically from admission to 7 AM. Discuss the drop in Hgb and Hct values in relation to Mr. Mitchell's blood loss.

Hgb and Hct values are poor indicators of the severity or rapidity of blood loss (Urden et al, 2002, p. 810). Initial Hgb and Hct values will not match the degree of blood loss because it takes 48 to 72 hours for intravascular and extravascular equilibration to occur (Urden et al, 2002). In Mr. Mitchell's case, the drop in Hgb and Hct values probably reflected some actual blood loss. However, part of the decrease, which occurred despite his receiving two units of PRBCs, was caused by hemodilution from fluid replacement therapy.

7. If a patient continues to have active bleeding from the GI tract despite conservative medical management, what other medical procedures might be implemented?

Therapies that may be used to treat acute GI bleeding include the following:

- Iced saline NGT lavage is sometimes used. However, evidence suggests that iced saline actually prolongs bleeding and increases clotting time compared with no lavage and that saline lavage resolves clots but does not halt bleeding (Zuckerman, 2003).
- Endoscopic hemostasis can be achieved via coagulation by cautery or injection of sclerosing agents. Electrocoagulation is achieved with heater probes, photocoagulation, or laser therapy, which is more expensive than traditional electrocoagulation. Sclerosing agents such as ethanolamine, sodium tetradecyl sulfate, or other solutions can also be injected into bleeding sites.
- Band ligation can be used during endoscopy to treat esophageal varices. This method is as effective as sclerotherapy in achieving initial hemostasis and reducing rebleeding rates. Small elastic "O" rings are placed around the varices, causing strangulation, sloughing, and fibrosis (Zuckerman, 2003).
- Octreotide, a long-acting analog of somatostatin, causes selective splanchnic vasoconstriction without cardiac complications when given by IV infusion and is currently the drug of choice as an adjunct to endoscopy (Savides & Jensen, 2000).
- Vasopressin infusion acts to constrict arteries and contract the bowel, thus reducing blood flow and stimulating the formation of thrombus. Vasopressin is associated with a high rate of cardiac complications and is no longer the drug of choice for pharmacologic hemostasis (Ferri, 2001).
- Transcatheter embolization using angiography to identify and embolize a bleeding artery may also be used. Substances such as coils, Gelfoam, cyanoacrylate glue, clots, and polyvinyl alcohol may be used. Ischemia or infarction may occur if collateral circulation is inadequate.
- Mechanical tamponade with the use of Ewald, Cantor, Minnesota, Sengstaken-Blakemore, or Linton-Nachlas tubes to apply direct pressure to bleeding sites may be used as a last-resort measure. Although balloon therapy provides initial tamponade 85% to 98% of the time, there is a 30% rate of serious complications and up to a 60% rate of rebleeding after deflation (Savides & Jensen, 2000).

8. Identify pharmacologic therapy commonly used in the treatment of GI tract bleeding.

Pharmacologic therapy is used to treat underlying conditions that cause GI tract bleeding and as an adjunct to management of bleeding. IV histamine-receptor antagonists are commonly used, but there is no evidence that they stop or prevent rebleeding. However, oral omeprazole (Prilosec), a proton pump inhibitor, significantly decreases recurrent bleeding for peptic ulcers that are not actively bleeding (Zuckerman, 2003). Stress ulcers are treated with a combination of sucralfate, histamine-receptor antagonists, and antacids. Metoclopramide (Reglan) may be used to decrease nausea, vomiting, and gastric stasis (Savides & Jensen, 2000).

Histamine-receptor antagonists inhibit the action of histamine on the receptor sites of the parietal cells by competing for the sites. They reduce the amount and concentration of gastric secretions. Examples include ranitidine (Zantac), cimetidine (Tagamet), nizatidine, and famotidine (Pepcid). Common side effects include headache, dizziness, diarrhea, and constipation (Bucher & Melander, 1999).

Antacids work by chemical neutralization of hydrochloric acid. By increasing the stomach's pH, antacids decrease the erosion of the stomach and duodenum by gastric acid. Long-term use of antacids may lead to metabolic alkalosis, increased serum sodium levels (sodium bicarbonate antacids), hypercalcemia and renal impairment (calcium carbonate antacids), constipation, phosphate depletion (aluminum-containing antacids), diarrhea, and hypermagnesemia (magnesium-containing antacids). Administration of antacids and histamine blockers should be staggered to allow for maximum absorption of both drugs.

9. What are the indications and types of surgical procedures for upper GI tract bleeding?

Indications for surgery are persistent bleeding after medical treatment, presence of neoplasm or malignancy, perforation of obstruction, and recurrence of ulcers.

Surgical interventions range from oversewing the ulcer site to gastric resection. Billroth I or II procedures involve partial resection of the stomach. Intractable ulcer disease and bleeding may be treated with a total gastrectomy. Vagotomy may be done in conjunction with or separate from these operations. Vagotomy reduces gastric secretions by eliminating vagal stimulation to the stomach.

Several surgical options exist to create portosystemic shunts. Placement of a transjugular intrahepatic portosystemic shunt device can also be used to reduce portal hypertension seen with esophageal varices.

10. Identify six nursing diagnoses appropriate for Mr. Mitchell.

- Fluid volume deficit related to vomiting, active bleeding, and decreased circulatory volume
- Altered tissue perfusion related to hypotension, decreased oxygen transport, increased oxygen demand, and metabolic acidosis
- Pain (acute abdominal) related to disruption of the mucosal barrier of GI tract (Alspach, 1998)
- Anxiety related to fear of death, hemorrhage, and unfamiliar procedures
- Altered nutrition: less than body requirements related to prolonged NPO status and NGT suction
- Knowledge deficit related to risk factor control (smoking, alcohol, stress management, and acetylsalicylic acid intake), medications, and treatments

11. What is the incidence of *H. pylori* infection in gastritis and duodenal ulcers?

H. pylori, first identified in 1984, is found in 90% to 100% of duodenal ulcers and 70% to 90% of gastric ulcers. It is recognized as the major cause of environmental (nonautoimmune) gastritis and peptic ulcer (Cello, 2000).

12. What is the treatment of choice for *H. pylori* infection?

H. pylori eradication therapy usually consists of an antisecretory agent and two antibiotics. The U.S. Food and Drug Administration (FDA)–approved therapy consists of omeprazole 20 mg, amoxicillin 1 g, and clarithromycin 500 mg twice a day for 2 weeks (Wynne et al, 2002). Current therapy may substitute bismuth subsalicylate, metronidazole, tetracyclines or lansoprazole for the previously mentioned antibiotics (Ferri, 2001). Recurrence of ulcers after healing is less than 10%, and reinfection rates are 1% to 2% per year after treatment (Cello, 2000).

GASTROINTESTINAL TRACT BLEEDING

References

Alspach, G. (1998). *Core curriculum for critical care nurses* (5th ed). W.B. Saunders, Philadelphia.

Beejay, U. & Wolfe, M. M. (2000). Acute gastrointestinal bleeding in the intensive care unit: The gastroenterologist's perspective. *Gastroenterology Clinics of North America, 29*, 309.

Bucher, L. & Melander, S. (1999). *Critical care nursing*. Philadelphia: W. B. Saunders.

Cello, J. P. (2000). Gastrointestinal hemorrhage and occult GI bleeding. In J. G. Bennett & L. Goldman (Eds.), *Cecil textbook of medicine* (21st ed.). Philadelphia: W. B. Saunders.

Ferri, F. F. (2001). *Practical guide to the care of the medical patient* (5th ed.). St Louis: Mosby.

Savides, T. K. & Jensen, D. M. (2000). Severe gastrointestinal hemorrhage. In W. C. Shoemaker, S. M. Ayres, A. Grenvik, & P. R. Holbrook (Eds.), *Textbook of critical care* (4th ed.). Philadelphia: W. B. Saunders.

Urden, L. D., Stacey, K. M., & Lough, M. E. (Eds.). (2002). *Thelan's* critical *care nursing: Diagnosis and management* (4th ed.). St Louis: Mosby.

Wynne, A. L., Woo, T. M., & Millard, M. (2002). *Pharmacotherapeutics for nurse practitioner prescribers*. Philadelphia: F. A. Davis.

Zuckerman, G. R. (2003). GI bleeding: Principles of diagnosis and management. In R. S. Irwin, J. M. Rippe, & H. P. Goodheart (Eds.), *Irwin & Rippe's intensive care medicine* (5th ed.). Philadelphia: Lippincott Williams & Wilkins.

19

Acute Pancreatitis

Ann H. White, RN, PhD, MBA, CNA

Carol, a 43-year-old, came to the emergency department (ED) with acute abdominal pain. This pain had been present for approximately 2 days but had increased in severity over the last 6 hours. The pain was localized to the upper-left abdominal quadrant with some radiation to the back. She had vomited three times in the last 6 hours with no relief of pain. Carol's brother, who accompanied her to the ED, reported that Carol drinks heavily and has a history of intravenous (IV) drug use. Her brother reported that she no longer uses IV drugs but has continued to drink at least a fifth of hard liquor a day. Carol admitted to having a past problem with alcohol and drug use but stated she is now "clean." Carol agreed to have blood drawn for analysis and gave permission to have blood alcohol and drug screening tests done.

Vital signs and laboratory results obtained in the ED were as follows:

BP	134/76 mm Hg
HR	68 bpm
Respirations	24 breaths/min
Temperature	38.6° C (101.4° F) (tympanic)

Complete bloodwork revealed the following:

WBCs	$11 \times 10^3/mm^3$
RBCs	$11 \times 10^6/mm^3$
Hgb	12.3 g/dl
Hct	52%
Na⁺	141 mmol/L
K⁺	3 mmol/L
Mg⁺⁺	1.3 mg/dl
Ca⁺⁺	7.3 mg/dl
Glucose	266 ml/dl
Total Protein	4.9 g/dl
Albumin	2.4 g/dl
Amylase	505 U/L
Lipase	519 U/L
Alkaline Phosphatase	120 U/L
AST (SGOT)	307 U/L
LDH	891 U/L
Blood Alcohol	205 mg/dl

Drug screening results are pending.

Arterial blood gas (ABG) measurements were as follows:

pH	7.35
P_{CO_2}	33 mm Hg
P_{O_2}	90 mm Hg
HCO_3^-	25 mmol/L
Base Excess	+1
Sa_{O_2}	91%

After a 2-hour stay in the ED, Carol reported increased pain in the upper-left abdominal quadrant. She vomited 100 ml of brown liquid with no relief of pain. Her vital signs were as follows:

BP	90/60 mm Hg
HR	100 bpm
Respirations	28 breaths/min
Temperature	39.4° C (103° F) (tympanic)

On physical examination, her abdomen was tender with guarding in all abdominal quadrants and bowel sounds were hypoactive. A nasogastric tube (NGT) was inserted and an IV line was started in the ED. Carol was transferred to the intensive care unit (ICU) with a preliminary diagnosis of acute pancreatitis. The following orders accompanied Carol to the ICU:

1. IV infusion of 0.45% normal saline (NS) solution with 20 mEq of potassium/bag to run at 150 ml/hr
2. Daily CBC, amylase and lipase levels, and basic metabolic profile
3. ABGs in the morning
4. Morphine sulfate 3 mg IV push q2h prn for severe pain
5. Nothing by mouth (NPO); includes no ice chips
6. NGT to intermittent suction
7. Two sets of blood cultures if not done in the ED
8. Gentamicin (Garamycin) 80 mg IV piggyback q8h after blood for cultures is drawn
9. Famotidine (Pepcid) 20 mg IV every 6 hours

Carol's laboratory results after the first 24 hours in the ICU were as follows:

WBCs	$14.6 \times 10^3/mm^3$
RBCs	$3.82 \times 10^6/mm^3$
Hgb	10.3 g/dl
Hct	42%
Na^+	139 mmol/L
K^+	3.2 mmol/L
Mg^{++}	1.3 mg/dl
Ca^{++}	7.8 mg/dl
Glucose	203 ml/dl
Total Protein	4.6 g/dl
Albumin	2.2 g/dl
Amylase	575 U/L
Lipase	789 U/L
Alkaline Phosphatase	139 U/L
AST (SGOT)	436 U/L
LDH	798 U/L

Drug screening results were negative.
ABG results were the following:

pH	7.22
Pco$_2$	26 mm Hg
Po$_2$	84 mm Hg
HCO$_3^-$	10 mmol/L
Base excess	+6
Sao$_2$	80%

Additional orders received included the following:

1. Change IV infusion to 0.45% saline with 30 mEq of potassium and 9 mEq of magnesium/IV bag to run at 125 ml/hr.
2. Administer oxygen at 2 L via nasal cannula.
3. Repeat basic metabolic profile 20 and ABG measurements in the morning.

Carol's heart monitor revealed a normal sinus rhythm with a prolonged QT interval. Carol's pain subsided after 72 hours, bowel sounds were heard, and she was started on ice chips and progressed to a clear liquid diet. After 24 hours without pain, Carol was transferred to a medical-surgical unit.

ACUTE PANCREATITIS

QUESTIONS

1. Discuss the pathophysiology of acute pancreatitis.

2. Describe the classic assessment findings that support a diagnosis of acute pancreatitis. Relate Carol's history and physical assessment findings to this description.

3. Compare and contrast mild (edematous) and severe (necrotizing) acute pancreatitis.

4. Discuss significant diagnostic studies that assist in confirming or in monitoring the progress of acute pancreatitis. Relate the diagnostic studies completed on Carol to this discussion.

5. Carol requested pain medication. What should be the initial nursing actions?

6. Discuss the appropriateness of administering gentamicin (Garamycin) to patients with acute pancreatitis.

7. Discuss the reason(s) for ordering famotidine (Pepcid).

8. Discuss the dietary management of a patient with acute pancreatitis. What is the purpose of the nasogastric tube (NGT) and the NPO status?

9. List the nursing diagnoses, outcomes, and interventions appropriate for a patient with acute pancreatitis.

10. Identify complications of acute pancreatitis. Based on the change in vital signs, laboratory data, and history, which complication has most likely occurred in this case study?

11. Discuss the prognosis for a patient with acute pancreatitis.

12. Discuss the psychosocial aspects of caring for a patient with acute pancreatitis.

ACUTE PANCREATITIS

QUESTIONS AND ANSWERS

1. Discuss the pathophysiology of acute pancreatitis.

The pancreas is a large gland with two distinct roles. As an exocrine gland, the acinar cells of the pancreas produce the inactive enzymes (trypsinogen, chymotrypsin, carboxy-polypepticlase, pancreatic lipase, and pancreatic amylase) that are activated in the intestinal track. The pancreas also produces trypsin inhibitor, which normally prevents the enzymes from being activated. Because trypsin is the initiator of activating the other enzymes, preventing its release results in no other enzymes being activated (McArdle, 2000). As an endocrine gland, the α- and β-cells of the pancreas produce insulin, glucagons, and somatostatin (McArdle, 2000). Pancreatitis typically is initiated in the exocrine portion of the pancreas but may alter both the exocrine and endocrine functions.

Acute pancreatitis is an acute inflammatory process of the pancreas that is believed to result from the premature activation of pancreatic enzymes as listed above that cause autodigestion and major cellular destruction (edema, vascular damage, hemorrhage, and necrosis) of the pancreas and surrounding gastrointestinal structures (Huether, 2002). The tissue damage that occurs in the pancreas initiates the inflammation response system, resulting in release of mediators (cytokines), movement of serum albumin, third-spacing, and pancreatic edema (Cole, 2002).

Most experts believe the initial injury is in the acinar cells. As a result of this cellular injury, pancreatic enzymes are released into the surrounding tissues. These enzymes become activated, thus initiating the autodigestion process, which results in damage to the surrounding tissue and injury to additional acinar cells (Huether, 2002). Trypsin is believed to be the enzyme that is initially activated and begins the autodigestion process by releasing phospholipase A, elastase, and kallikrein. With the release of these enzymes, pancreatic tissue and fat cell necrosis occurs with the release of free fatty acids. Kallikrein initiates the release of bradykinin and kallidin that causes a decrease in peripheral vascular resistance, vasodilation, and increased vascular permeability.

Several theories have been proposed to explain the destruction of the pancreatic tissue, none of which are conclusive. The following discussions summarizes these theories:

- Certain substances act as cell toxins, which are believed to alter the metabolic processes of the acinar cells. The acinar cells are responsible for the production and release of pancreatic juice, which contains digestive enzymes. Normally these enzymes are not activated until they reach the intestines. The hormone cholecystokinin (pancreozymin) stimulates the release of the enzymes through the pancreatic duct system to reach the intestine. Once in the intestine, trypsinogen is converted to trypsin, which activates the other pancreatic enzymes (Giuliano & Scott, 1999).
- Alcohol consumption has been closely associated with pancreatitis. Although the exact mechanism is unclear, alcohol is a known irritant to pancreatic tissue, which may cause protein that may obstruct the ductules (Hale et al, 2002). Alcohol may also induce ischemia to the pancreatic tissues due to secondary hypertriglyceridemia (Giuliano & Scott, 1999). Another possible explanation for the high incidence of acute pancreatitis with alcohol ingestion is the edema or destruction of the ampulla of Vater. This allows the release/reflux of duodenal contents or bile, which seems to activate the process (Steer, 2000).
- Pancreatic duct obstruction is another theory. This theory focuses on the obstruction in the release of pancreatic juices as a result of distal obstruction of the biliary ductal system, in particular the sphincter of Oddi. The distal obstruction is commonly caused by gallstones actually blocking the duct or by the resulting edema that forms as a gallstone passes. The resulting ductal hypertension may lead to the rupture of small ducts and the release of the enzymes (Steer, 2000).

- The bile reflux theory is that gallstone(s) may obstruct the flow of bile. As a result, the bile takes the path of least resistance, which is to back up into the pancreatic duct, leading to the activation of the enzymes. This is also referred to as the *common channel theory*. This theory is being challenged as an increasing number of patients who have pancreatitis but do not have this common channel are found (Steer, 2000).
- The duodenal reflux theory proposes that the duodenal contents back up into the pancreas as a result of potential damage to the system during the passage of a gallstone. Because of activation of the pancreatic enzymes when they reach the intestines, autodigestion and cell damage begin.

Other factors that can lead to acute pancreatitis include the use of certain drugs such as thiazides, acetaminophen, tetracyclines, estrogen-containing contraceptives, pentamidine, valproic acid, sulfonamides, and possibly steroids (Friedman, 2003). Surgical procedures including exploration of the common bile duct, pancreatic biopsy, and endoscopic retrograde cholangiopancreatography (ERCP), may also predispose the patient to the development of acute pancreatitis. Recent research has indicated that infectious agents and toxins may also cause acute pancreatitis (Laws & Kent, 2000). Whatever the cause, the result is autodigestion and cellular damage in the pancreas and surrounding tissues. Once the cycle is begun, it is perpetuated by the cellular damage that causes cell destruction and death. This results in further release of pancreatic enzymes and destruction of more pancreatic cells as a result of autodigestion. The cycle continues until medical intervention is sought.

2. Describe the classic assessment findings that support a diagnosis of acute pancreatitis. Relate Carol's history and physical assessment findings to this description.

History taking should include gathering detailed information with particular focus on gallbladder disease, recent abdominal surgical procedures, alcohol use, and any type of medication use. Specific medications to inquire about include thiazides, acetaminophen, tetracyclines, and oral contraceptives containing estrogen as well as those listed earlier. The patient should be asked about recent consumption of alcohol or a large meal with high levels of fat.

Classic assessment findings include abdominal pain that is almost always severe, persistent, and penetrating (Giuliano & Scott, 1999). The pain usually begins abruptly and may precede nausea (Steer, 2000). The patient may describe the pain as knifelike or twisting (Cole, 2002). The pain typically is located in the upper-left abdominal quadrant or may be in the midepigastric area and may radiate to the back or flank areas. The onset of pain may be directly associated with consumption of alcohol or a large meal with fatty foods. Patients experiencing pain associated with acute pancreatitis may prefer to sit up or lie in a fetal position to decrease the intensity.

Physical assessment of the abdomen may include decreased or absent bowel sounds. The abdomen may be somewhat distended, guarded, and tender to palpation. This tenderness is noted more in the upper quadrants but may be present in all four abdominal quadrants. Ecchymotic areas may be noted in the flank and umbilical areas. Cullen's sign is an irregular hemorrhagic area around the umbilicus. Grey Turner's sign is a bluish discoloration of the abdominal flank or lower back area (Westfall, 1999a).

In addition, nausea and vomiting may occur. Vomiting without a decrease in pain is considered a hallmark symptom of acute pancreatitis (Cole, 2002). Vomiting, along with the extensive third spacing, may lead to dehydration. As a result, the patient may have poor skin turgor and dry mucous membranes. With extensive loss of fluid through vomiting and third spacing, symptoms of hypovolemic shock may be seen. Plasma volume may also be lost due to release of enzymes and kinins, which cause vasodilatation and increased cell permeability (Huether, 2002). Immediate resuscitation with fluids is critical to prevent death (Braganza, 2001).

Because the respiratory system may be seriously compromised by the development of acute pancreatitis, respirations and lung sounds must be monitored carefully. Assessment findings may include dyspnea, tachypnea, hypoxemia, diminished or absent breath sounds, and referred pain to the shoulder. Careful assessment of the respiratory status is required to prevent acute respiratory distress syndrome (ARDS), the most serious respiratory problem associated with acute pancreatitis (Friedman, 2003).

An elevated temperature may also be indicative of acute pancreatitis. The elevated temperature, if present, is typically less than 39° C (102.2° F). Persistent temperature elevation may indicate complications, including infection or abscess formation (Giuliano & Scott, 1999).

Carol had several assessment findings that supported the diagnosis of acute pancreatitis. Her history of alcohol abuse is definitely a factor. Although alcohol abuse and acute pancreatitis are more commonly associated with men in their 50s, this does not preclude other patients from exhibiting this clinical picture. Carol also had the abdominal pain radiation associated with acute pancreatitis. She vomited without relief of pain, which further supports the diagnosis of acute pancreatitis. Carol's temperature was elevated.

3. Compare and contrast mild (edematous) and severe (necrotizing) acute pancreatitis.

With mild or acute edematous (interstitial) pancreatitis, there is edema in the surrounding tissues with minimal necrotizing of the fat tissue. Activated enzymes are released, causing cellular damage. Typical symptoms have been described in the previous answer. Severe (necrotizing) acute pancreatitis is considered the more serious form and is characterized by necrosis of the pancreatic tissue with bleeding into the surrounding tissue. The patient may have all the symptoms of interstitial pancreatitis as well as Grey Turner's sign and Cullen's sign as described earlier. The bleeding into the tissue is thought to be the result of damage caused by circulating trypsin to the intravascular structures (Giuliano & Scott, 1999). Both signs are grave indications of the progression of the disease. The mortality rate with necrotizing acute pancreatitis is high, with the latest figures estimating a 50% mortality rate (Hale et al, 2002).

4. Discuss significant diagnostic studies that assist in confirming or in monitoring the progress of acute pancreatitis. Relate the diagnostic studies completed on Carol to this discussion.

Specific laboratory studies to assist in confirming the diagnosis of acute pancreatitis include serum and urine amylase levels, isoamylase levels, serum lipase levels, CBC, basic metabolic profile 20 (electrolytes, blood glucose, liver enzymes, blood urea nitrogen [BUN]), ABGs, and culture and sensitivity tests of blood and any drainage.

Serum and urine levels of amylase are usually elevated. The serum amylase level is elevated within the first 12 to 72 hours after the onset of symptoms and returns to normal in 1 week (Munoz & Katerndahl, 2000). However, many other disease processes and drugs can also cause an elevation, and this elevation may not reflect the extent of the disease process. Common drugs that have been associated with amylase elevations include meperidine, morphine, and codeine (Westfall, 1999b).

Isoamylase levels are more specific but have not proven useful (Steer, 2000). In addition, many laboratories are unable to perform these types of tests because they do not have the equipment required. Friedman (2003) reported that a serum amylase level three times the normal level (25-125 Somogyi U/dl) and a serum lipase level three times the normal (10-140 Somogyi U/L) in a patient with symptoms associated with acute pancreatitis confirms the diagnosis. Serum lipase levels are also elevated during the first 24 hours of the onset of symptoms and remain elevated for 8 to 14 days. Lipase is found predominantly in the pancreas; however, other disease processes can cause this elevation. The lipase levels are considered a better indicator than amylase levels especially in identifying acute pancreatitis related to alcohol consumption (Munoz & Katerndahl, 2000).

Nonspecific abnormal laboratory findings include an elevated white blood cell count with a left shift that may be caused by an infection (Steer, 2000). The hematocrit may be elevated initially because of third-space fluid losses but later may decrease because of hemorrhaging. Sodium, potassium, calcium, and magnesium levels may be decreased because of vomiting, fluid shifts, and the saponification of fats. Calcium levels may also be decreased as a result of low levels of albumin. The calcium level may appear to be low because of the close association with albumin. Once the albumin level is corrected, the calcium level may return to normal (Giuliano & Scott, 1999). However, in severe cases of acute pancreatitis, the calcium level may be decreased and must be monitored carefully. The blood glucose level may be elevated if the islets of Langerhans are affected by the disease process and are unable to produce insulin. The BUN level may be elevated because of dehydration. Liver enzyme levels will also be elevated, and prothrombin time may be prolonged with concurrent biliary tract disease and liver involvement.

ABG determinations are imperative because of the respiratory compromise associated with acute pancreatitis. Blood for serial ABG measurements should be drawn to monitor development of metabolic acidosis and hypoxemia. Culture and sensitivity tests of the blood and any other drainage should be performed to gather information about the infectious process. The sensitivity will identify any antimicrobial therapy that must be started.

Radiologic testing that may be useful in the diagnosis of acute pancreatitis includes flat plates of the abdomen, contrast-enhanced computed tomography (CE-CT) scan, or magnetic resonance imaging (MRI) with specific detail to the pancreas. CE-CT scanning is commonly used today. Specific detail of the pancreas and surrounding structures involved may be well defined with the use of this radiologic test (Steer, 2000).

The final diagnostic tool to consider is an electrocardiogram or telemetry. If the patient with acute pancreatitis has a low calcium level, the cardiac rhythms must be monitored carefully. A low calcium level may lead to a prolonged QT interval, with the potential for R on T phenomenon and torsades de pointes or ventricular tachycardia. Correction of the calcium level should prevent the occurrence of arrhythmias (Giuliano & Scott, 1999).

Carol has many of the above identified lab abnormalities with elevated amylase and lipase levels, abnormal blood gas levels, abnormal electrolyte levels, and lab values consistent with third spacing. Carol did not have a CE-CT done, and this might need to be ordered if there is any concern about another diagnosis.

5. Carol requested pain medication. What should be the initial nursing actions?

After carefully assessing her pain, a call to the physician is the appropriate action to ensure that the most effective pain medication is given. Opiate analgesics (morphine) are widely used for the relief of acute pain. However, in this case, morphine may not be the drug of choice to manage pancreatic pain. Because morphine may cause biliary colic and spasms of the sphincter of Oddi, meperidine (Demerol) usually is ordered for a patient with acute pancreatitis. Experts in the care of patients with acute pancreatitis have reported in recent studies with morphine that patients achieve significant pain relief with minimal effect on the sphincter of Oddi (Cole, 2002). Reported use of oral forms of morphine (elixir) appears to provide pain relief with minimal effect on the pancreatic tissue (Hale et al, 2002).

Pain management is an important component of treating patients with the diagnosis of acute pancreatitis. Not only does the patient experience a great deal of discomfort but also severe pain increases the metabolic activity in the body. This increase in metabolic activity further increases the release of pancreatic enzymes, which is detrimental because of the pathology occurring in the pancreas (Cole, 2002).

6. Discuss the appropriateness of administering gentamicin (Garamycin) to patients with acute pancreatitis.

The use of antimicrobials in the treatment of mild to moderate forms of acute pancreatitis has not been supported by research findings or clinical trials. Antimicrobials are sometimes ordered if an infection is suspected or in severe cases of necrotizing acute pancreatitis (Laws

& Kent, 2000). Typically antimicrobials are ordered only once an infection has been confirmed through culture and sensitivity tests, when a CE-CT scan has confirmed necrotizing pancreatitis, or when additional clinical symptoms (e.g., an elevation in temperature) are present. Infection is more common 14 to 21 days after the initial attack (Laws & Kent, 2000). The initial antimicrobials of choice are imipenem-cilastatin (Primaxin), cefuroxime (Zinacef), and ceftazidime (Ceptaz) (Munoz & Katerndahl, 2000).

7. Discuss the reason(s) for ordering famotidine (Pepcid).

Patients with acute pancreatitis have high stress levels due to hospitalization and disease process. In addition, the NPO status and possible NGT increase the risk of stress ulcers. The famotidine is ordered to prevent the development of stress ulcers in this type of patient.

8. Discuss the dietary management of a patient with acute pancreatitis. What is the purpose of the nasogastric tube (NGT) and the NPO status?

The initial strategy of diet management is to minimize pancreatic secretions. It was believed that placing an NGT connected to suction should indirectly decrease the release of pancreatic secretions by preventing the release of secretin, which requires an acid environment to be released. With the nasogastric suction removing gastric secretions, it was thought that the acid environment would not be created. However, recent clinical studies have not demonstrated this to be true. Today nasogastric suction should be used only for patients with vomiting, gastric distention, ileus, or an altered mental status (Munoz & Katerndahl, 2000).

The patient will be assigned NPO (including no ice chips) status for a period of time until the pain subsides, bowel sounds are clearly present, and the serum amylase levels are normal. Diet intake should begin gradually, starting with clear liquids and progressing to more solid food based on patient tolerance. As the diet is advanced, fat, cholesterol, and triglycerides should be kept to a minimum. If an increase in pain develops, the patient should return to NPO status. An increase in pain indicates that enzymes have been released into the tissue and the resulting autodigestion has begun again. Returning to NPO status is an attempt to rest the pancreas and decrease or minimize pancreatic secretions.

Nutritional support is imperative during this time. The patient with acute pancreatitis requires aggressive therapy to meet metabolic and healing needs without stimulation of the pancreas. Total parenteral nutrition (TPN) should be considered for patients with moderate to severe pancreatitis. Composition of the TPN depends on the patient's clinical picture and laboratory values. Typically an amino acid and glucose base is used with essential minerals and vitamins. Electrolyte replacement depends on the laboratory values. The inclusion of insulin in the TPN solution depends on the production of insulin by the pancreas and the blood glucose levels. Lipid preparations are not typically used for the patient with pancreatitis because their use will lead to an increase in the release of pancreatic enzymes (Cole, 2002).

9. List the nursing diagnoses, outcomes, and interventions appropriate for a patient with acute pancreatitis.

Table 19-1 is a compilation of nursing care plans developed by Smolen (2001) and Giuliano and Scott (1999) for the patient with acute pancreatitis. Although specific nursing diagnoses must be identified based on the patient's clinical picture, this plan provides the basis for care. See Table 19-1 for nursing diagnoses, outcomes, and interventions.

Table 19-1	*Nursing Diagnoses, Outcomes, and Interventions for Acute Pancreatitis*	
Nursing Diagnoses	**Outcome Criteria**	**Nursing Interventions**
Fluid volume deficit related to fluid, plasma, albumin, and blood losses into peritoneum and retroperitoneal space, nausea and vomiting	Hemodynamic stability (blood pressure, pulse, central venous pressure; pulmonary arterial pressure, adequate peripheral circulation, urine output within normal limits)	1. Monitor and record intake and output every hour. 2. Monitor and record central venous pressure and pulmonary arterial pressure. 3. Weigh patient daily. 4. Monitor vital signs every 1-2 hr. Assess peripheral circulation and level of consciousness. 5. Monitor laboratory values for abnormal hemoglobin and hematocrit, electrolyte imbalance (calcium, magnesium, potassium), and blood urea nitrogen and creatinine. 6. Monitor for signs of bleeding (hemorrhagic pancreatitis: Cullen's sign, Grey Turner's sign, increased abdominal girth). 7. Monitor for signs of hypocalcemia: Chvostek's sign, Trousseau's sign. 8. Monitor for signs of cardiac failure such as dyspnea, chest pain, edema. 9. Provide IV fluids; monitor for signs of fluid overload, such as shortness of breath, edema, abnormal breath sounds (crackles).
Altered comfort; pain related to inflammation of pancreas or obstruction of pancreatic duct	Pain at tolerable level Vital signs stable	1. Assess patient's pain using a pain-rating scale; use pain rating to evaluate response to pain management interventions. 2. Provide analgesics as ordered and before activity or diagnostic procedures; remember to draw blood to determine amylase levels before giving first dose of analgesic to avoid false elevation in amylase. 3. Assist patient to assume a comfortable position to decrease pain. 4. Maintain bed rest and limit activities to reduce metabolic stress. 5. Eliminate oral intake and maintain nasogastric suction, if ordered, to decrease nausea and vomiting and rest the pancreas

Continued

Table 19-1   *Nursing Diagnoses, Outcomes, and Interventions for Acute Pancreatitis—cont'd*

Nursing Diagnoses	Outcome Criteria	Nursing Interventions
		6. Provide alternative methods of pain control (i.e., back massage, guided imagery, and relaxation techniques).
High risk for ineffective breathing patterns related to abdominal distention and pain	Maintains an effective breathing pattern	1. Assess respiratory status every 2 hr. 2. Maintain aggressive pulmonary hygiene. 3. Monitor fluid volume. 4. Place patient in semi-Fowler's position. 5. Maintain effective pain management.
Impaired gas exchange related to inflammatory process and aggressive fluid therapy, respiratory distress syndrome, atelectasis, microemboli, pain, pleural effusion	Effective breathing patterns with adequate ventilation and oxygenation (PaO_2 and $PaCO_2$ within normal limits) Absence of atelectasis Absence of reduction of pleural effusion, pulmonary edema, microemboli	1. Administer analgesics to relieve pain and allow adequate ventilation. 2. Provide chest physiotherapy and reposition every 1-2 hr to prevent atelectasis. 3. Provide oxygen therapy as ordered to prevent hypoxemia. 4. Monitor chest x-ray films for presence of atelectasis, effusion, or edema. 5. Perform respiratory assessments every 1-2 hr and note presence of tachypnea, dyspnea, or wheezing; identify presence of adventitious breath sounds and absence of normal breath sounds. 6. Monitor arterial blood gas results for hypoxemia, hypercapnia, or acidosis.
High risk for tissue injury related to pancreatic inflammation, peritonitis, formation of pseudocyst, formation of abscesses, bleeding, formation of fistulas	Absence or resolution of peritonitis Absence of fever, pseudocyst, abscesses	1. Administer antibiotics as ordered if causative organism(s) has been identified. 2. Monitor vital signs, especially increases in temperature, and monitor for increase in white blood cell count. 3. Observe for signs of pseudocyst: upper abdominal pain, mass, tenderness, fever, deterioration, or no improvement in condition. 4. Observe for signs of abscess: abdominal pain, distention tenderness, fever, leukocytosis, tachycardia, and hypotension. 5. Assess for paralytic ileus and fluid accumulation; auscultate bowel sounds every shift.

Table 19-1	*Nursing Diagnoses, Outcomes, and Interventions for Acute Pancreatitis—cont'd*	
Nursing Diagnoses	**Outcome Criteria**	**Nursing Interventions**
		6. Observe for respiratory distress resulting from ascites or abdominal mass; check breath sounds, presence of cough, sputum production, shallow breathing, elevated diaphragm, and fluid accumulation.
		7. Provide skin care for draining fistulas; use skin barrier to protect skin from pancreatic enzymes; monitor fistula output.

Alteration in nutrition and metabolic status related to pancreatic dysfunction with altered production of digestive enzymes, insulin, and glucagon; decrease or absence of oral intake; alcoholism; abnormal metabolism	Normal nutritional status
	Weight gain or maintenance
	Positive nitrogen balance
		1. Eliminate oral intake during acute phase of illness.
		2. Assess nutritional status and general appearance for the following:
		  a. Poor skin turgor
		  b. Lethargy
		  c. Anorexia
		  d. Dry, flaky, discolored skin
		  e. Sunken eyeballs
		  f. Decreased muscle mass and decreased muscular control
		  g. Tremors, twitching
		3. Monitor the following:
		  a. Serum amylase
		  b. Urine amylase
		  c. Lipase
		  d. Glucose
		4. Provide nutritional support as ordered.
		5. Monitor laboratory results to prevent complications of nutritional support.
		6. Provide oral care every 4-8 hr.
		7. Monitor nasogastric output.
		8. Maintain ongoing assessment of nutritional status and therapy, including the following:
		  a. Daily weights
		  b. Intake and output
		  c. Nutritional laboratory data (albumin, transferrin, total lymphocyte count)
		  d. Nitrogen balance
		  e. Altered mental status
		  f. Skin turgor
		  g. Muscle atrophy or weakness
		9. Monitor fistula drainage and record output every shift.

Continued

Table **19-1**   *Nursing Diagnoses, Outcomes, and Interventions for Acute Pancreatitis—cont'd*

Nursing Diagnoses	Outcome Criteria	Nursing Interventions
Anxiety (patient or family) related to insufficitnt knowledge of disease process, treatment, and diagnostic procedures	Reduction in patient's or family's anxiety with information about disease process, treatment, and diagnostic procedures Patient and family participate in care planning process	1. Assess patient's or family's reason for and level of anxiety. 2. Provide information to patient and family about disease process, treatment(s), and diagnostic procedures. 3. Include patient and family in care planning process. 4. Evaluate reduction in patient's or family's anxiety.
Knowledge deficit related to change in lifestyle, care, and diet needs	Increased patient knowledge of disease and thus better compliance with treatment regimen	1. Develop client teaching plan. 2. Include significant others in plan. 3. Allow verbalization of concerns regarding care and change in lifestyle. 4. Return demonstration of information understood. 5. Encourage group support such as Alcoholics Anonymous.

10. **Identify complications of acute pancreatitis. Based on the change in vital signs, laboratory data, and history, which complication has most likely occurred in this case study?**

A common complication associated with acute pancreatitis is hypovolemic shock. If this complication occurs, it carries with it the potential to cause renal failure, pulmonary insult, electrolyte imbalances, pancreatic pseudocyst, and pancreatic abscess (Friedman, 2003). All of these complications should be treated immediately.

Hypovolemic shock commonly occurs as a result of third spacing. Fluid shifts from the vascular system to the intraperitoneal and retroperitoneal spaces as a result of the injury to the abdominal structures from the activated enzymes. Cole (2002) also reported the release of kinins as a result of the inflammation. With the release of these kinins, there is vasodilation and increased capillary permeability. As a result, large amounts of plasma and protein leave the vascular system, adding to the potential for hypovolemic shock. Hypovolemia can be extensive, with as much as 4 to 6 L of fluid shifting into the abdomen with severe pancreatitis. Further loss of fluid in the vascular system results from decreased dietary intake of protein, thus affecting the oncotic pressure. Patients usually do not take anything by mouth and may experience vomiting, which also add to the loss of fluid in the vascular system. Without aggressive replacement therapy, renal failure and death may result because of hypoperfusion of the kidneys and other major organs (Braganza, 2001).

The inflammatory response in the pancreatic and surrounding tissues also leads to the release of agents such as myocardial depressant factor, histamine, and prostaglandin, that depress the myocardial tissue, cause vasodilation, and increase capillary permeability. With the release of these agents and the subsequent response, the body is unable to compensate for the decreased fluid volume, thus increasing the potential for hypovolemic shock (Giuliano & Scott, 1999).

Pulmonary complications are common with acute pancreatitis, including the development of atelectasis, acute lung injury, and pleural effusion. The most serious pulmonary complication is adult respiratory distress syndrome (ARDS). ARDS usually occurs within the first 3 to 7 days after the initial attack and is seen more often in patients who required a large volume of plasma and fluids due to hypovolemia (Friedman, 2003)

Factors that have an impact on the development of respiratory complications include splinting, minimal movement, and decreased coughing during episodes of severe pain. In addition, abdominal distention related to fluid shifting that leads to decreased diaphragmatic effort can also depress respirations (Giuliano & Scott, 1999). The development of pancreatic fluid can also result in the development of pleural effusions and direct injury to the lungs (Cole, 2002). Assessment findings indicating pulmonary complications include adventitious breath sounds, tachypnea, diminished breath sounds, and dyspnea.

Electrolyte imbalances include losses of sodium, potassium, calcium, and magnesium. Sodium and potassium loss is the result of third spacing and gastrointestinal losses with the NGT or vomiting. Hypocalcemia is a common electrolyte imbalance seen with acute pancreatitis. Calcium deficits may result from hypoalbuminemia. Careful review of the calcium and albumin laboratory values is necessary. Careful monitoring for neuromuscular irritability and prolonged QT intervals is required with hypocalcemia. Another concern is the development of hyperglycemia, which occurs when the pancreatic cells are no longer able to produce insulin.

A pancreatic pseudocyst is the development of necrotic pancreatic tissue, fluid, debris, enzymes, and blood encapsulated in a fibrous tissue (Friedman 2003). A pseudocyst usually resolves by itself but must be monitored through the use of a CT scan or MRI. The cyst may begin to obstruct abdominal structures, or it may rupture, leading to hemorrhagic shock. Assessment findings indicating the development of a pseudocyst include abdominal pain, nausea and vomiting, weight loss, and anorexia after the acute episode of pancreatitis has subsided.

Pancreatic abscesses may form in patients with acute pancreatitis. An abscess will usually develop 4 weeks after an episode and are the result of necrosis of tissue and translocation of gastrointestinal bacteria such as *Escherichia coli, Pseudomonas, Staphylococcus,* and *Klebsiella* (Munoz & Katerndahl, 2000). Assessment findings that indicate the formation of an abscess include an elevated temperature, abdominal pain, vomiting, and possibly a palpable mass in the abdomen. A pancreatic abscess typically requires a surgical procedure for incision and drainage. Antibiotic therapy may also be ordered.

Hematologic complications may result from altered levels of fibrinogen and factor VIII. These alterations are thought to be a result of the activation of trypsin in the pancreas (Cole, 2002). Based on Carol's clinical picture, her most likely complication is hypovolemic shock. However, with the elevation in temperature a possible source of infection must be considered.

11. Discuss the prognosis for a patient with acute pancreatitis.

One method to predict the outcome of an episode of acute pancreatitis is to use the guidelines established by Ranson in 1974 (Friedman, 2003). Eleven criteria were identified by Ranson to help predict the prognosis for patients with pancreatitis. Five of the criteria are evaluated in the ED. The remaining six are evaluated during the first 48 hours after treatment is begun. (See Box 19-1 for Ranson criteria [Giuliano & Scott, 1999]). Patients with three or more of the criteria listed in Box 19-1 require supportive care. Patients with seven or more of the criteria are considered a medical challenge with an estimated 90% to 100% mortality (Giuliano & Scott, 1999). Recent studies conducted to test the validity of using Ranson's criteria have established that the scoring remains a valid tool for predicting prognosis in patients with acute pancreatitis (Eachempati et al, 2002).

Another method to establish severity of the disease and the prognosis is use of the Acute Physiology and Chronic Health Evaluation (APACHE II) system (Fig. 19-1). A patient with eight or more points from Figure 19-1 requires supportive care. The APACHE II system has the added advantage of being able to monitor the patient after the first 48 hours (Munoz & Katerndahl, 2000).

Text Continued on p. 283.

HIGH ABNORMAL RANGE

PHYSIOLOGIC VARIABLE	+4	+3	+2	+1
1. TEMPERATURE—rectal (°C)	≥41°	39°–40.9°		38.5°–38.9°
2. MEAN ARTERIAL PRESSURE (mm Hg)	≥160	130–159	110–129	
3. HEART RATE (ventricular response)	≥180	140–179	110–139	
4. RESPIRATORY RATE (nonventilated or ventilated)	≥50	35–49		25–34
5. OXYGENATION: A-aDO$_2$ or PaO$_2$ (mm Hg) a. FiO$_2$ ≥ 0.5: record A-aDO$_2$	≥500	350–499	200–349	
b. FiO$_2$ < 0.5: record only PaO$_2$	--------	--------	--------	--------
6. ARTERIAL pH	≥7.7	7.6–7.69		7.5–7.59
7. SERUM SODIUM (mmol/L)	≥180	160–179	155–159	150–154
8. SERUM POTASSIUM (mmol/L)	≥7	6–6.9		5.5–5.9
9. SERUM CREATININE (mg/100 mL) (Double point score for acute renal failure)	≥3.5	2–3.4	1.5–1.9	
10. HEMATOCRIT (%)	≥60		50–59.9	46–49.9
11. WHITE BLOOD CELL COUNT (total/mm^3) (in 1000 sec)	≥40		20–39.9	15–19.9
12. GLASGOW COMA SCALE (GCS): Score = 15 minus actual GCS				
A Total ACUTE PHYSIOLOGY SCORE (APS) Sum of the 12 individual variable points				
Serum HCO$_2$ (venous: mmol/L) (Not preferred, use if no ABGs)	≥52	41–51.9		32–40.9

B AGE POINTS

Assign points to age as follows:

AGE (years)	POINTS
≤44	0
45–54	2
55–64	3
65–74	5
≥75	6

C CHRONIC HEALTH POINTS

If the patient has a history of severe organ system insufficiency or is immunocompromised, assign points as follows:

a. For nonoperative or emergency postoperative patients: 5 points

or

b. For elective postoperative patients: 2 points

DEFINITIONS: Organ insufficiency or immunocompromised state must have been evident prior to this hospital admission and conforms to the following criteria:

LIVER: Biopsy-proven cirrhosis and documented portal hypertension, episodes of past upper GI bleeding attributed to portal hypertension; or prior episodes of hepatic failure/encephalopathy/coma.

CARDIOVASCULAR: NY Heart Association Class IV.

RESPIRATORY: Chronic restrictive, obstructive, or vascular disease resulting in severe exercise restriction (e.g., unable to climb stairs or perform household duties); or documented chronic hypoxia, hypercapnia, secondary polycythemia, severe pulmonary hypertension (>40 mm Hg), or respirator dependency.

RENAL: Recurring chronic dialysis.

Figure **19-1** APACHE II Severity of Disease Classification System. (*Reprinted from Sleisenger, B. & Fordtran, M. (1998). Gastrointestinal and liver disease: Pathophysiology/diagnosis/management [6th ed.]. Philadelphia: W. B. Saunders.*)

Continued

LOW ABNORMAL RANGE

0	+1	+2	+3	+4
36°–38.4°	34°–35.9°	32°–33.9°	30°–31.9°	≤29.9°
70–109		50–69		≤49
70–109		55–69	40–54	≤39
12–24	10–11	6–9		≤5
<200 -------- PO_2 >70	-------- PO_2 61–70	--------	-------- PO_2 55–60	-------- PO_2 <55
7.33–7.49		7.25–7.32	7.15–7.24	<7.15
130–149		120–129	111–119	<110
3.5–5.4	3–3.4	2.5–2.9		<2.5
0.6–1.4		<0.6		
30–45.9		20–29.9		<20
3–14.9		1–2.9		<1
22–31.9		18–21.9	15–17.9	<15

IMMUNOCOMPROMISED: The patient has received therapy that suppresses resistance to infection (e.g., immunosuppression, chemotherapy, radiation, long-term or recent high-dose steroids) or has a disease that is sufficiently advanced to suppress resistance to infection (e.g., leukemia, lymphoma, AIDS).

APACHE-II SCORE
Sum of **A** + **B** + **C**

A APS points _____

B Age points _____

C Chronic health points _____

Total APACHE-II SCORE _____

Figure **19-1,** cont'd.

Score	Date		
(Enter one score for each of the following categories listed below)	month	day	year
	Time		24-hr clock

	Verbal	Oriented	5	
		Confused	4	
		Inappropriate words	3	
		Incomprehensible sounds	2	
		None	1	
	Motor	Obeys commands	6	
		Localizes pain	5	
		Flexion to pain	4	
		Decorticate movement	3	
		Extension to pain	2	
		None	1	
	Eye	Spontaneous	4	
		To speech	3	
		To pain	2	
		None	1	
	GCS total score			

Completed by _____

Date | month | day | year

Figure **19-1**, cont'd.

Box 19-1   Ranson Criteria

Use in the Emergency Department
1. Age >55 yr
2. White blood cell count >16 × 10^3/mm^3
3. Blood glucose >200 mg/dl
4. Lactate dehydrogenase >350 U/L
5. AST (SGOT) >250 U/L

During the First 48 Hours
1. Hematocrit decreases >10%
2. Blood urea nitrogen >5 mg/dl above baseline
3. Calcium levels <8 mg/dl
4. Arterial P$_{O_2}$ <60 mm Hg
5. Base deficit increases >4 mmol/L
6. Estimated fluid sequestration >6000 ml

Based on the Ranson guidelines, Carol has 6 of the 11 criteria, including a blood glucose level of more than 200 mg/dl, lactate dehydrogenase (LDH) level more than 350 U/L, and AST level more than 250 U/L in the ED. After 24 hours her calcium levels dropped below 8 mg/dl, hematocrit dropped more than 10 percentage points, and base deficit increased more than 4 mmol/L. Based on the APACHE II system, Carol received a score of 11 points with an acute pancreatitis scale (APS) score of 6 (elevated temperature, low potassium, high hematocrit, and heart rate); no age points, and 5 points for chronic health problems. Both ratings indicate that Carol requires treatment in the ICU and must be monitored closely.

Recent use of drug therapy including pancreatic secretion inhibitors (somatostatin and octreotide) may improve patient outcomes. Further research is necessary to confirm use of these drugs as part of the treatment protocol for acute pancreatitis. Both medications modulate the immune response through neurologic and endocrine pathways. Somatostatin inhibits the release of "cytokines, tumor necrosis factor, and interferon-gamma while octreotide increases the phagocytosis activity of monocytes" (Hale et al, 2002, p. 16). Both mechanisms serve to protect pancreatic tissue.

12. Discuss the psychosocial aspects of caring for a patient with acute pancreatitis.

Once a patient has experienced the pain of acute pancreatitis, that patient never wants to experience it again. If the acute pancreatitis is caused by consumption of alcohol, the patient must stop drinking alcohol to decrease the episodes of acute pancreatitis. Counseling of the patient and significant others must be encouraged and supported by the nursing staff.

With other causes of acute pancreatitis, such as biliary obstruction resulting from gallstones, patients usually have surgery to decrease the possibility of further episodes of acute pancreatitis. However, they must realize the need to be cautious regarding consumption of high-fat diets and alcohol.

ACUTE PANCREATITIS

References

Braganza, J. (2001). Towards a novel treatment strategy for acute pancreatitis: 2. Principles and potential practice. [Electronic version]. *Digestion 63*(3), 143-162.

Cole, L. (2002). Unraveling the mystery of acute pancreatitis. [Electronic version]. *Dimensions of Critical Care Nursing 21*(3), 86-90.

Eachempati, S., Hydo, L., & Barie, P. (2002). Severity scoring for prognostication in patients with severe acute pancreatitis: Comparative analysis of the Ranson score and the APACHE III score. [Electronic version]. *Archives of Surgery, 137*(8), 730-736.

Friedman, L. (2003). Liver, biliary tract, and pancreas. In L. Tierney, S. McPhee, & M. Papadakis (Eds.), *Current medical diagnosis and treatment* (pp. 666-669). New York: Lange Medical Books.

Giuliano, K. & Scott, S. (1999). Acute pancreatitis. In L. Bucher & S. Melander (Eds.), *Critical care nursing* (pp. 764-778). Philadelphia: W. B. Saunders.

Hale, A., Moseley, M., & Warner, S. (2002). Treating pancreatitis in the acute care setting. [Electronic version]. *Dimensions of Critical Care Nursing 19*(4), 15-21.

Huether, S. (2002). Alterations of digestive functions. In K. McCance & S. Huether (Eds.), *Pathophysiology: The biologic basis for disease in adults and children* (4th ed., pp. 1298-1299). St Louis: Mosby.

Laws, H. & Kent, R. (2000). Acute pancreatitis: Management of complicating infection. [Electronic version]. *The American Surgeon, 66*(2), 145-152.

McArdle, J. (2000). The biological and nursing implications of pancreatitis. [Electronic version]. *Nursing Standard 14*(48), 46-53.

Munoz, A. & Katerndahl, D. (2000). Diagnosis and management of acute pancreatitis. *American Family Physician 62*(1), 164-174.

Smolen D. (2001). Management of clients with exocrine pancreatic and biliary disorders. In J. Black, J. Hawks, & A. Keene (Eds.), *Medical-surgical nursing* (6th ed., pp. 1194-1299). Philadelphia: W. B. Saunders.

Steer, M. (2000). Acute Pancreatitis. In A. Grenvik (Ed.), *Textbook of critical care* (4th ed., pp. 1621-1624). Philadelphia: W. B. Saunders.

Westfall, U. (1999a). Gastrointestinal assessment. In L. Bucher & S. Melander (Eds.), *Critical care nursing* (pp. 692-704). Philadelphia: W. B. Saunders.

Westfall, U. (1999b). Gastrointestinal laboratory and diagnostic tests. In L. Bucher & S. Melander (Eds.), *Critical care nursing* (pp. 705-725). Philadelphia: W. B. Saunders.

20

Peritonitis

M. Lynn Rodgers, RNC, MSN, CCRN, CNRN, ACNP-BC

CASE PRESENTATION

Jane Harold, age 40 years, came to the emergency department (ED) with severe lower-left abdominal pain. The day before her admission she felt nauseated and had abdominal distention, which she attributed to having had no bowel movement for 4 days. Mrs. Harold has diverticulosis and stated that she only has a bowel movement twice a week. She often takes a laxative, which she had done the day before her ED visit. She had no results from the laxative, was still quite nauseated, and had vomited one time. Her last menstrual period was 3 weeks ago. She is 165 cm (5 feet 6 inches) tall and weighs 74 kg (165 lb).

PHYSICAL ASSESSMENT

Mrs. Harold was lying on her back with her knees flexed. Her face was flushed, and she was quietly crying, obviously in great distress. Bowel sounds were absent. Her abdomen was slightly distended, firm, and rigid. Rebound tenderness existed over the lower-left abdominal quadrant, although her entire abdomen was painful to light palpation. Breath sounds were clear, but respirations were shallow. Mrs. Harold's diagnostic data were as follows:

BP	96/50 mm Hg lying; 84/46 mm Hg standing
HR	112 bpm lying; 128 bpm standing
Respirations	28 breaths/min
Temperature	38.7° C (101.6° F)
RBCs	$3.8 \times 10^6/mm^3$
WBCs	$19,000/mm^3$
Hgb	12.6 g/dl
Hct	48%
Na⁺	148 mmol/L
K⁺	3.6 mmol/L
Cl⁻	107 mmol/L
Creatinine	1.6 mg/dl
BUN	50 mg/dl
Amylase	60 U/L
HCG	Negative
Urinalysis	Normal findings

Immediate treatment included the following:

- Lactated Ringer's solution (LR) was started at 150 ml/hr via an 18-gauge intravenous (IV) catheter.
- Green fluid was aspirated from the nasogastric tube (NGT), which was connected to low continuous suction.
- Immediately after a Foley catheter was anchored, 100 ml of clear, dark urine was returned. Hourly urine specimens were obtained.
- A right subclavian triple-lumen central line was inserted. Initial central venous pressure (CVP) and right atrial pressure (RAP) were 1 mm Hg.
- Kidneys, ureters, and bladder x-ray (KUB) and upright chest x-ray examination showed free air under the diaphragm and good location of the CVP line. No pneumothorax was evident. Large distended intestinal loops were obvious.

Further treatment included the following:

- Morphine sulfate 1 to 2 mg IV push was given every 10 to 15 minutes, with a total of 14 mg given in the first 2 hours.
- Over the next 2 hours, 2000 ml of LR was infused. Breath sounds and orthostatic blood pressure (BP) changes were reevaluated every 15 to 30 minutes. Breath sounds remained clear, and orthostatic changes in BP were less than 6 mm Hg. Urine output was 45 to 50 ml/hr. CVP and RAP increased to 4 mm Hg.
- Clavulanic acid/ticarcillin 3.1 g IV partial fill was initiated immediately and then ordered every 6 hours.
- A consultation with the enterostomal therapist was held to assess and mark the patient's abdomen for stoma placement, to implement preoperative teaching, and to provide further emotional support to the patient and family.
- An exploratory laparotomy was performed, and the suspected ruptured diverticulum was confirmed. A temporary colostomy was created.

SURGICAL INTENSIVE CARE UNIT

After an uneventful recovery room stay, Mrs. Harold was transferred to the surgical intensive care unit (SICU). She received LR at 125 ml/hr, oxygen 28% via Venturi mask, and morphine sulfate by a patient-controlled anesthesia pump. Her CVP readings were 6 to 8 mm Hg, and her urine output was 50 to 70 ml/hr. Her NGT remained at low suction. Her lower abdominal incision was well approximated without drainage. Her colostomy was brick red with only a small amount of serosanguineous fluid in the ostomy bag. She had no bowel sounds. Her blood urea nitrogen (BUN) and creatinine levels dropped to normal by the second postoperative day. Her white blood cell (WBC) count peaked at 21,000/mm³ but also started to drop by the second postoperative day. She was transferred out of the SICU during the afternoon of her second postoperative day in stable condition.

PERITONITIS

QUESTIONS

1. What is the function of the peritoneum?

2. Discuss the pathophysiology and potential causes of peritonitis.

3. What are the clinical signs and symptoms of peritonitis?

4. Explain the abnormalities in Mrs. Harold's admission laboratory results.

5. What are the significant findings of the KUB and chest x-ray examinations?

6. What is the rationale for checking Mrs. Harold's BP in the lying and sitting positions?

7. Discuss the reason for initiating fluid resuscitation in the ED.

8. Discuss the rationale for the IV antibiotic chosen for Mrs. Harold.

9. Identify other possible diagnoses that were considered and ruled out for Mrs. Harold.

10. What interventions helped relieve Mrs. Harold's pain? Why?

11. Give the rationale for withholding pain medication immediately after Mrs. Harold's admission to the ED.

12. What is the prognosis for patients with peritonitis?

13. What are the primary nursing diagnoses for Mrs. Harold?

14. Do the signs and symptoms of peritonitis differ in elderly patients?

15. What other specific abdominal diagnostic tests could be done to confirm or rule out this or other diagnoses for abdominal pain?

PERITONITIS

QUESTIONS AND ANSWERS

1. What is the function of the peritoneum?

The peritoneum is the largest semipermeable serous membrane in the body. It is made up of the visceral peritoneum, which envelops the viscera, and the parietal peritoneum, which lines the outer walls of the abdominal cavity. As described by Markey (1999), the large folds of these peritoneal layers bind the abdominal contents together and contain the nerve, blood, and lymph supplies to these organs. Exchange of fluids and electrolytes occurs between the visceral and parietal peritoneal layers via these blood and lymph vessels. The peritoneal cavity is the potential space between these two membranes. It contains less than 50 ml of serous fluid secreted by the cells of the serosa that keep the two surfaces moist. This lubrication allows the organs within the abdominal cavity to slide freely against one another during peristalsis. In addition, the peritoneum will react to the presence of chemical or bacterial contaminants with a localized inflammatory reaction (Hirsch & Caswell, 1999).

2. Discuss the pathophysiology and potential causes of peritonitis.

According to Zaleznick and Kasper (2001b), *peritonitis* is an inflammation of the peritoneum, resulting from bacterial or chemical invasion of the peritoneal cavity. Peritonitis may be classified as primary or secondary and as localized or diffuse, depending on the cause and the severity of the condition. Primary peritonitis is an acute bacterial infection that is not associated with a perforated viscus or organ. A bacterial infection originating in another area of the body and then transported to the peritoneum by the vascular system is typically the causative agent. Tuberculosis elsewhere in the body or alcoholic cirrhosis and ascites are examples of potential sources of primary peritonitis (Rimola et al, 2000).

Another source of primary peritonitis is through peritoneal dialysis, especially patient-administered continuous ambulatory peritoneal dialysis (CAPD). Of those receiving CAPD, 60% to 70% will develop peritonitis in the first year of therapy. Between 60% and 70% of cases are caused by gram-positive organisms such as *Staphylococcus aureus* and *S. epidermidis,* 15% to 30% are caused by gram-negative organisms such as *Escherichia coli,* and only 5% to 10% are caused by fungi such as *Candida albicans* and are most common in immunosuppressed patients (Zaleznik & Kasper, 2001a). Sclerosing peritonitis and sclerosing encapsulating peritonitis are extremely serious complications of CAPD with multifactorial causes.

Secondary peritonitis can occur with a perforation or rupture of the abdominal viscus, as in Mrs. Harold's case. Any abdominal organ, including any part of the gastrointestinal tract, gallbladder, pancreas, liver, ovary, or fallopian tube, may be involved (Isselbacher & Epstein, 2001). Bacteria from the ruptured organ and severe chemical reactions resulting from the released pancreatic enzymes, digestive fluids, and bile instigate the inflammatory insult. Initially, when the peritoneum is contaminated, macrophages, mast cells, eosinophils, and basophils are released from the visceral peritoneal mesentery. These inflammatory cells release prostaglandins and histamine, which results in a localized vascular dilation and increased capillary permeability. This allows movement into the peritoneal space of inflammatory serous fluid that is high in immunoglobulins, fibrin, complement, clotting factors, and chemotaxins such as leukotriene C_{5a} and B_4. This inflammatory exudate attracts phagocytic WBCs into the peritoneal cavity to begin destruction of bacteria. Fibroblastic inflammatory exudate coats the peritoneum and essentially isolates the inflammatory process by sealing off the abdominal contents from the contaminant (Zaleznik & Kasper, 2001a).

If effective, these polymorphonuclear neutrophil leukocytes ingest or wall off the offending substances, resulting in a contained or localized peritonitis. If these attempts fail or if the contamination is continuous or massive, generalized peritonitis develops (Hirsch & Caswell, 1999). Generalized or diffuse peritonitis is a result of bacterial invasion into a large majority of the peritoneum. The tissues begin to swell, fibrous exudate develops, and adhesions may form. When the irritant is eliminated, these adhesions may or may not shrink and disappear. Diffuse peritoneal infection can affect the entire body and eventually can result in bacteremia or septic shock (Lucey, 2000).

Infectious peritonitis can be caused by several different organisms; however, in Mrs. Harold's case, *E. coli* was the causative agent. Such organisms can also be the culprits if peritonitis results from a rupture of the appendix or from perforation caused by colonic obstruction, toxic megacolon, or traumatic intestinal injury (Zaleznik & Kasper, 2001b). Pneumococcal peritonitis is a common occurrence in patients with pneumococcal pneumonia and should be suspected, especially during the winter months. Tuberculous peritonitis is slow to develop and slow to heal, causing little or no pain. It should be suspected in patients at high risk for tuberculosis such as those who are infected with human immunodeficiency virus. Gonococcal peritonitis can occur occasionally after massive gonococcemia. A vaginal swab for gonorrhea will help in establishing this diagnosis (Rockey, 2000).

Chemical peritonitis occurs when the inflammation of the peritoneum results primarily from the caustic effects of some substance rather than from infection by an organism. Offending substances are gastric acid, pancreatic fluid, bile, or starch. There are also reports in the literature of peritoneal contamination resulting from peritoneal leakage of gastric nutritional feedings after percutaneous endoscopic gastrostomy. Although this complication is rare, occurring only in 1% of cases, this can develop in the first 2 weeks after gastrostomy tube placement until a permanent fibrous tract between the skin and the gastric wall has formed (Zaleznik & Kasper, 2001b).

3. What are the clinical signs and symptoms of peritonitis?

The most common symptom reported in acute peritonitis is abdominal pain and fever, being present in one half to two thirds of patients (McQuaid, 2003). Pain may be localized or diffuse, but the most intense pain has been reported in the area of the patient's primary gastrointestinal disorder. Referred pain to either the shoulder or thoracic area is common. Movement often aggravates this pain. Rebound tenderness, muscular rigidity and spasm, and guarding of the abdomen are other major signs of irritation of the peritoneum. Often the patient assumes a side-lying position with knees and hips flexed to decrease the peritoneal irritation. A history of low-grade fever is also common. Pain usually is followed by spikes of fever (39.4° C [103° F]), chills, extreme weakness, and absolute exhaustion (McQuaid, 2003). A complete and thorough history and physical examination of the patient with abdominal pain should include type, onset, character, and distribution of pain; chronologic appearance of symptoms; and exact time, mode and acuteness of symptom onset (Rockey, 2000).

Accumulation of serous fluid and inflammatory exudate in the peritoneal cavity results in ascites and abdominal distention. As more intravascular fluid enters the peritoneal cavity, the patient becomes volume depleted and dehydrated as evidenced by dry mucous membranes, poor skin turgor, thirst, tachycardia, orthostatic BP changes, and decreased urinary output. A shallow and rapid breathing pattern develops, decreasing diaphragm excursion and thereby lessening peritoneal irritation and pain. Paralytic ileus commonly occurs in the patient with acute peritonitis. Nausea, vomiting, inability to pass feces and flatus, and absence of bowel sounds are common findings. If a pelvic abscess does develop, diarrhea and urinary urgency may be present. Malaise, vomiting, and a generalized "toxic" ill appearance are usually seen in proportion to the severity of the peritonitis. Complications associated with peritonitis are hypovolemic shock, septicemia, organ failure, and mental confusion. Multisystem organ failure is the ultimate result of extensive peritonitis.

4. Explain the abnormalities in Mrs. Harold's admission laboratory results.

Mrs. Harold's complete blood count revealed some important information. Her red blood cell (RBC) count was 3.8×10^6/mm³, which could indicate some blood loss. Her WBC count was elevated at 19,000/mm³, with the normal range being 5000 to 10,000/mm³. Her particular laboratory values are important in determining the severity of the infectious process (McQuaid, 2003). The hemoglobin level is important for determining the oxygen-carrying capacity of the blood. The normal range for women is between 12 and 16 g/dl. Mrs. Harold's hemoglobin result was 12.6 g/dl, which is within the lower limits of the normal range. The normal hematocrit for women is 40% to 48%. Mrs. Harold's result was 48%, which could indicate hemoconcentration resulting from a shift of fluid out of the intravascular space into the peritoneal cavity (Hirsch & Caswell, 1999).

Normal levels for serum creatinine are between 0.6 and 1.2 mg/dl for women. Mrs. Harold's level was elevated at 1.6 mg/dl. Initial vital signs indicated tachycardia and orthostatic hypotension, which are commonly seen in situations in which blood or volume loss occurs. Elevated creatinine levels could be caused by the resulting decrease in kidney function. Her urine output of 100 ml of clear, dark urine upon catheterization further indicates a decrease in her kidney perfusion. The BUN level is normally 7 to 18 mg/dl. Mrs. Harold's result of 50 mg/dl may indicate a serious condition. Several possible factors causing this condition could be gastrointestinal hemorrhage, shock, dehydration, and impaired renal function (Urden et al, 2002). Normal sodium levels are 135 to 148 mmol/L. Mrs. Harold's sodium level was 148 mmol/L, which may be increased because of dehydration, insufficient fluid intake, and a shift of intravascular fluid to the interstitial areas. Her potassium level was within the normal limits of 3.5 to 5 mmol/L but should be monitored closely for a decrease resulting from fluid loss and sodium conservation efforts by the kidney. Normal blood values for chloride are 98 to 106 mmol/L. Mrs. Harold's slightly elevated level of 107 mmol/L could possibly be caused by dehydration.

5. What are the significant findings of the KUB and chest x-ray examinations?

The significant radiographic findings that apply to acute abdominal pain are free intraperitoneal air and dilated loops of the intestine (Isselbacher & Epstein, 2001). Free intraperitoneal air can indicate perforation of a hollow viscus. In Mrs. Harold's case, a ruptured diverticulum was suspected. Dilated loops of the intestine can indicate a paralytic ileus, also commonly seen with a ruptured colon. A chest x-ray film was obtained after central line placement to rule out accidental pneumothorax, chest problems that could contribute to abdominal pain, and pneumonia, which can develop with peritonitis as a result of decreased lung excursion and possible bacteremia. The patient should be kept in an upright position long enough for free air to collect beneath the diaphragm so it will show on the x-ray film (McQuaid, 2003).

6. What is the rationale for checking Mrs. Harold's BP in the lying and sitting positions?

Mrs. Harold's BP was checked in the lying and sitting positions to determine whether she had postural or orthostatic hypotension. According to Jones and Bucher (1999), when a person experiences blood or fluid loss that significantly affects total blood volume, BP will decrease as the patient sits and then stands. With a decrease in BP, there is also a compensatory increase in the heart rate to maintain a consistent cardiac output. A decrease in BP of 10 to 20 mm Hg or more and an increase in heart rate of 10 to 20 bpm or more with position changes is called a postural drop. Mrs. Harold's BP and heart rate did change significantly enough to warrant this diagnosis. Further monitoring of orthostatic hypotension would be indicated if blood and fluid losses increased or if the sitting position is contraindicated. Other significant measurements from the subclavian line were the initial CVP and RAP, which measure the pressure on the right side of the heart. Normal values are 0 to 8 mm Hg. Mrs. Harold's low reading of 1 mm Hg could indicate a decrease in blood volume and a "dry" condition intravascularly (Urden et al, 2002).

7. Discuss the reason for initiating fluid resuscitation in the ED.

Mrs. Harold was obviously volume depleted, as evidenced by the assessment changes discussed. The CVP and RAP were initially 1 mm Hg, were 4 mm Hg after 2000 ml of IV fluids, and were 6 to 8 mm Hg while she was in the SICU. Mrs. Harold's hypotensive state needed to be corrected as soon as possible to prevent hypovolemic shock. The treatment of choice for hypotension resulting from a volume deficit is to correct the volume problem rather than constrict the vasculature (Gawlinski et al, 1999; Urden et al, 2002).

8. Discuss the rationale for the IV antibiotic chosen for Mrs. Harold.

IV antibiotics should be administered as soon as possible preoperatively once the diagnosis of peritonitis is established because the time that antibiotics are started is the biggest determinant of successful treatment (McQuaid, 2003). Selection of antibiotics for peritonitis is based on severity, etiology, and practitioner preference, but the antibiotic chosen must be effective for colonic aerobes and anaerobes. For mild to moderate peritonitis, second-generation cephalosporins such as cefuroxime or third-generation penicillins such as ampicillin/sulbactam are suggested. For severe peritonitis, broad-spectrum penicillins such as piperacillin or ticarcillin or aminoglycosides such as gentamicin with metronidazole for anaerobic bacteria are recommended (Hirsch & Caswell, 1999). A single antibiotic with effectiveness against both aerobes and anaerobes was selected for Mrs. Harold. Thus clavulanic acid/ticarcillin (Timentin) was administered. Antibiotics should be continued throughout the preoperative, operative, and postoperative periods. If the patient is afebrile, has a normal leukocyte count, and has a band count of less than 3%, the chance of recurrent sepsis after discontinuation of antibiotic therapy is virtually zero (McQuaid, 2003). With these criteria, antibiotics may be discontinued as early as the fourth postoperative day. If the patient does not meet these criteria, postoperative antibiotics are continued for a minimum of 7 to 10 days.

9. Identify other possible diagnoses that were considered and ruled out for Mrs. Harold.

A brief review of Mrs. Harold's laboratory work and symptoms in the ED indicated that other possible diagnoses needed to be ruled out. These included bowel obstruction, appendicitis, pancreatitis, peptic ulcer, urinary tract stones, ectopic pregnancy, and ovarian cyst (Ferri, 2001).

Mrs. Harold had severe lower-left abdominal pain, nausea, vomiting, and abdominal distention. She had a history of diverticulosis and frequent laxative use. Assessment revealed that she was doubled over in acute pain, her face was flushed, and she was crying. Bowel sounds were absent, and the abdomen was slightly distended, firm, and rigid. Rebound tenderness was noted over her lower-left abdominal quadrant with her entire abdomen painful to light touch. Her respirations were shallow.

All of the aforementioned signs and symptoms, including a WBC count greater than 15,000/mm^3, seemed to indicate appendicitis or possible bowel obstruction. The only symptom that possibly negated a diagnosis of appendicitis was that the severe pain and rebound tenderness were on the side opposite to the appendix.

Acute pancreatitis is another possible cause for her symptoms. Certainly the symptoms of nausea, vomiting, elevated temperature, tachycardia, hypovolemia, and hypotension are similar in both diseases, but the location of pain is a key difference. Pancreatic pain is usually felt in the epigastric region or the upper-left abdominal quadrant. Abdominal rigidity usually indicates a late sign of pancreatitis, which does not correspond to Mrs. Harold's history. Mrs. Harold's serum amylase level was 60 U/L, which is normal and thus ruled out pancreatitis. Amylase levels are significantly increased in patients with pancreatitis within 3 to 6 hours after the onset of pain (Ferri, 2001).

Peptic ulcer could also be another consideration because of the sudden onset of constant intense pain. The pain with peptic ulcer is more generalized and has a tendency to be affected by food intake. Signs of hemorrhagic shock that occur with bleeding peptic ulcers were also present. However, lack of blood in the NGT drainage and the lack of history ruled out this diagnosis (Ferri, 2001).

The last diagnosis to be considered is a genitourinary complication, such as an ectopic pregnancy, ovarian cyst, or urinary tract stone. The human chorionic gonadotropin test in this case was negative, which rules out a possible pregnancy; the urinalysis was normal, which rules out urinary tract stones. Ultrasonography or an abdominal computed tomography (CT) scan could have diagnosed an ovarian cyst, but ovarian cysts generally do not result in absent bowel sounds (Ferri, 2001).

10. What interventions helped relieve Mrs. Harold's pain? Why?

Initially an NGT was inserted, and green drainage was aspirated. This drainage could be irritating to a ruptured diverticulum and even more irritating to the peritoneum. Decompressing the stomach may also decrease intraabdominal pressure and thus decrease pain. Insertion of a Foley catheter can also relieve intraabdominal pressure. Morphine sulfate 1 to 2 mg IV push was given at 10- to 15-minute intervals for a total of 14 mg within the first 2 hours of appearance of symptoms. The position of comfort Mrs. Harold assumed also helped decrease intraabdominal pressure (Hirsch & Caswell, 1999).

11. Give the rationale for withholding pain medication immediately after Mrs. Harold's admission to the ED.

Obtaining an accurate assessment of Mrs. Harold's pain required that all pain medications be withheld. The identification of the exact location of the most severe pain is very important in diagnosing her condition. Pain medication would have masked the signs and symptoms of pain, wasted valuable time, and possibly led to an erroneous diagnosis (McQuaid, 2003). When the diagnosis was confirmed, pain medication was given, and other steps were taken to reduce Mrs. Harold's pain.

12. What is the prognosis for patients with peritonitis?

Intraabdominal infections are associated with significant mortality and morbidity despite the powerful antibiotics made available over the past 35 years. Survival is most strongly associated with the body's response to the peritoneal contamination rather than the medical interventions performed. Mortality of 30% to 50% has been reported (Lucey, 2000; McQuaid, 2003). The risk of death is increased in patients whose peritonitis develops after surgery or trauma compared with patients with peritoneal infection at admission. Mortality is also increased in patients requiring more than one surgical intervention or when intervention is delayed more than 24 hours after presentation. The type of surgical procedure performed does not influence the mortality rate, nor does better drainage of the peritoneal cavity. Prognosis depends on the cause of peritoneal inflammation, the amount of time the infection has been present, the body's immunologic response to the infection, the extent of surgical intervention, and body systems involved. Fluid and electrolyte resuscitation, antibiotic therapy, and surgical repair of any perforated viscus are still the most important interventions to prevent death (Hirsch & Caswell, 1999).

13. What are the primary nursing diagnoses for Mrs. Harold?

The following nursing diagnoses are most applicable in Mrs. Harold's situation:

- Alteration in comfort, pain, and anxiety
- High risk for infection
- Fluid volume deficit: actual
- Alteration in tissue perfusion
- Anxiety
- Body image disturbance
- Ineffective patient and family coping

14. Do the signs and symptoms of peritonitis differ in elderly patients?

Patients who are 65 years of age or older are three times more likely to have generalized peritonitis than younger patients (Lucey, 2000; Urden et al, 2002). These findings are consistent with the hypothesis that the biologic features of peritonitis differ in elderly patients. Impaired local peritoneal responses can result in less localized and less severe abdominal pain, leading to the development of generalized peritonitis by the time treatment is pursued. Because pain is not intense, older patients may delay in seeking medical assistance. Such delays may be attributed to difficulties leaving home, fear of hospitalization, alterations in usual symptoms, diminished perception of symptoms, or diminished ability to express them effectively. In addition, elderly patients do not always develop a significant febrile response to peritonitis. To further complicate the diagnosis, WBC counts do not always rise in elderly patients in response to infection, although an elevation in immature leukocyte numbers or a shift to the left does occur (Isselbacher & Epstein, 2001).

15. What other specific abdominal diagnostic tests could be done to confirm or rule out this or other diagnoses for abdominal pain?

Hirsch and Caswell (1999) and McQuaid (2003) concluded that the following diagnostic tests can be useful for the diagnoses listed when developing differential diagnoses for abdominal pain:

- *Chest x-ray film:* can indicate the presence of free air, pleural effusion, pneumonia, or bibasilar atelectasis that may infer inflammatory disease
- *Abdominal ultrasound:* can indicate abdominal masses such as abscesses or tumors, gallbladder disease, pancreatitis, abdominal fluid or free air, ectopic pregnancy, or uterine and ovarian disease
- *Abdominal series:* can indicate free air under the diaphragm, bowel obstruction or ileus, organ displacement, a space-occupying lesion, or air within the colon
- *CT scan with contrast:* can indicate with great specificity most diagnoses although it is expensive and requires exposure to radiation
- *Radionuclide scan:* can isolate difficult-to-locate abdominal abscesses

PERITONITIS

References

Ferri, F. (2001). *Practical guide to the care of the medical patient*, ed 5. St Louis: Mosby.

Gawlinski, A., McCloy, K., Caswell, D., & Quinones-Baldrich, W. J. (1999). Cardiovascular disorders. In A. Gawlinski & D. Hamwi (Eds.), *Acute care nurse practitioner: Clinical curriculum and certification review*. Philadelphia: W. B. Saunders.

Hirsch, C. G. & Caswell, D. (1999). Gastrointestinal disorders. In A. Gawlinski & D. Hamwi (Eds.), *Acute care nurse practitioner: Clinical curriculum and certification review*. Philadelphia: W. B. Saunders.

Isselbacher, K. J. & Epstein, A. (2001). Diverticular, vascular, and other diseases of the intestine and peritoneum. In Brauwald (Ed.), *Harrison's principles of internal medicine* (15th ed.). New York: McGraw-Hill.

Jones, K. M. & Bucher, L. (1999). Shock. In L. Bucher & S. Melander (Eds.), *Critical care nursing*. Philadelphia: W. B. Saunders.

Lucey, M. R. (2000). Diseases of the peritoneum, mesentery, and omentum. In E. Goldman, L. Bennett, & J. Claude (Eds.), *Textbook of internal medicine* (21st ed.). Philadelphia: W. B. Saunders.

Markey, D. W. (1999). Gastrointestinal anatomy and physiology. In L. Bucher & S. Melander (Eds.), *Critical care nursing*. Philadelphia: W. B. Saunders.

McQuaid, K. R. (2003). Peritonitis. In L. M. Tierney, S. J. McPhee, & M. A. Papadaki (Eds.), *Conn's 2003 current therapy*. Philadelphia: W. B. Saunders.

Rimola, A. et al. Diagnosis, treatment, and prophylaxis of spontaneous bacterial peritonitis: A consensus document. *Journal of Hepatology,* 2000, 32(1),142-153.

Rockey, D. C. (2000). Peritonitis. In R. W. Wachter, L. Goldman, & H. Hollander (Eds.), *Hospital medicine*. Philadelphia: Lippincott Williams & Wilkins.

Urden, L. D., Stacy, K. M. & Lough, M. E. (Eds). (2002). *Thelan's critical care nursing: Diagnosis and management* (4th ed.). St Louis: Mosby.

Zaleznik, D. F. & Kasper, D. L. (2001a). Intraabdominal infections and abscesses. In Brauwald (Ed.), *Harrison's principles of internal medicine* (15th ed.). New York: McGraw-Hill.

Zaleznik, D. F. & Kasper, D. L. (2001b). Peritonitis. In Brauwald E. (Ed.), *Harrison's principles of internal medicine* (15th ed.). New York: McGraw-Hill.

21

Esophageal Varices

Linda K. Evinger, RN, MSN, C-OGNP

Bruce Eggert, age 59 years, was brought to the emergency department (ED) with complaints of dizziness, dyspnea, restlessness, and anxiety. Mr. Eggert currently works as an accountant for a large firm. He is married and has two children living at home. He reported a 2-day history of hematemesis with some bright red blood and large amounts of "coffee ground" emesis. Mr. Eggert denied any recent or chronic illnesses and was unable to remember if anyone in his family had ever had problems with gastrointestinal (GI) tract bleeding. He did admit to drinking six to eight alcoholic beverages almost every day for the past 7 years. Initial assessment revealed cool and clammy skin, a distended abdomen with hyperactive bowel sounds, and tachycardia.

Current vital signs and laboratory results are as follows:

BP	92/60 mm Hg
HR	120 bpm
Respirations	28 breaths/min
Temperature	36.9° C (98.3° F) (oral)
Ammonia	60 µg/dl
Glucose	87 mg/dl
LDH	500 U/L
AST (SGOT)	950 U/L
ALT (SGPT)	1000 U/L
Alkaline Phosphatase	165 U/L
Total Bilirubin	2.5 mg/dl
Albumin	2.3 g/dl
PT	26 sec
PTT	85 sec

Three hours after arriving in the ED, Mr. Eggert was admitted to the intensive care unit (ICU) with an intravenous infusion of normal saline. Two units of packed red blood cells were administered. Twenty units of vasopressin (Pitressin) in 100 ml of 5% dextrose in water (D5W) were given intravenously over 20 minutes. A continuous infusion of vasopressin 0.4 U/min was then initiated. Sublingual nitroglycerin was added to the medication regimen. Diagnostic fiberoptic endoscopy, immediately preceded by a saline lavage, was scheduled for the following day. Endoscopy revealed a large esophageal varix (1.5 cm) above the gastroesophageal junction. Only a small amount of bright red blood was observed, so sclerotherapy was performed. A solution of 5% ethanolamine oleate was given by intravariceal injection. Mr. Eggert's condition remained stable after sclerotherapy and he was transferred to a medical floor. Subsequent sclerotherapy sessions were scheduled on a weekly basis for 4 weeks.

ESOPHAGEAL VARICES

QUESTIONS

1. Define and discuss the pathophysiology of esophageal varices and portal hypertension.

2. What do Mr. Eggert's laboratory tests indicate about his current health status?

3. Explain how Mr. Eggert's history and laboratory results relate to portal hypertension.

4. Discuss the clinical manifestations of esophageal varices.

5. Identify the diagnostic procedures and nursing implications for esophageal varices.

6. Compare and contrast the treatment options and nursing implications for esophageal varices.

7. Discuss the rationale for Mr. Eggert's vasopressin therapy, management of side effects, and nursing concerns.

8. Identify the relevant nursing diagnoses for Mr. Eggert while he is in the ICU.

9. Discuss the patient/family teaching indicated for Mr. Eggert.

10. What special nursing considerations are prompted by Mr. Eggert's past drinking pattern?

11. Discuss the psychosocial aspects of the care of Mr. Eggert and his family.

ESOPHAGEAL VARICES

QUESTIONS AND ANSWERS

1. **Define and discuss the pathophysiology of esophageal varices and portal hypertension.**

    Esophageal varices are defined as "large dilated veins in the submucosa of the stomach and lower esophagus" (Driscoll, 1999, p. 725). *Portal hypertension* is described as an increase in portal venous pressure in the liver (Urden et al, 2002). Blood enters the liver through the hepatic artery and the portal vein. The liver is a highly vascular organ that normally offers little resistance to splanchnic blood flow.

    Alcohol is oxidized to aldehyde by the liver. This change results in permanent hepatocellular damage. Excessive and chronic consumption of alcohol causes an increase of smooth endoplasmic reticulum in the cells of the liver. This stimulates an increased production of cholesterol that accumulates in the liver. Mitochondria swell, which leads to increased inflammation, fibrosis, and necrosis of the liver's cells (Altman, 1999).

    This chronic injury to the liver leads to irreversible scarring. The scarring and regeneration nodules that develop result in a distortion of the vascular bed, which leads to portal hypertension (Altman, 1999). In an attempt to compensate, the liver develops collateral circulation connecting the portal veins to other organs. This effort is inefficient and results in venous backflow into the spleen, esophagus, stomach, and intestines. Because the veins in the esophagus and upper stomach are thin walled, they dilate and become engorged, forming varices (Urden et al, 2002). This occurs with an increase in portal venous pressure greater than 10 mm Hg. Bleeding typically occurs when the pressure exceeds 12 mm Hg. The development of esophageal varices occurs annually in 5% to 15% of individuals with cirrhosis (Hegab & Luketic, 2001). Variceal bleeding occurs more often in patients who have more severe liver dysfunction and in those who have large varices or have varices with red signs, which are considered to be varices on varices (Burroughs & Patch, 1999).

2. **What do Mr. Eggert's laboratory tests indicate about his current health status?**

    Mr. Eggert has advanced liver disease. He experienced blood loss resulting in hypovolemia, which decreased the hemoglobin level and hematocrit and elevated the white blood cell (WBC) count, platelet count, and blood urea nitrogen (BUN) level. His sodium and potassium levels were decreased because of the vomiting. His ammonia level was elevated because the diseased liver was unable to convert ammonia to urea for excretion. Lactate dehydrogenase (LDH), aspartate aminotransferase (AST), and alanine aminotransferase (ALT) levels were elevated because enzymes and end products are released into the blood with the destruction of liver cells. The alkaline phosphatase level was increased because of biliary obstruction. The albumin level was low because of impaired liver synthesis. The bilirubin level was elevated because of the liver's inability to conjugate bilirubin, and the prothrombin time (PT) was longer because of diminished synthesis of prothrombin by the liver.

3. **Explain how Mr. Eggert's history and laboratory results relate to portal hypertension.**

    Portal hypertension is the primary cause of esophageal varices. The esophageal varices caused the symptoms experienced by Mr. Eggert. Hematemesis is bloody emesis that is either bright red, indicating fresh bleeding, or a dark "coffee ground" color, indicating that blood has been in the stomach where gastric juices have had a chance to act on it. The blood loss accounts for his dizziness, dyspnea, restlessness, tachycardia, and anxiety. Mr. Eggert's admission of long-term heavy alcohol intake implies cirrhosis as a cause for the portal hypertension. It also suggests liver disease as a cause for the abnormal laboratory test results indicated in question 2. Abdominal distention may be explained by ascites from liver disease. The cool and clammy skin is a sign of shock.

Portal hypertension is the cause of esophageal varices. The varices, by rupturing, then cause hypovolemia, resulting in a decreased hemoglobin level and hematocrit and an increased BUN level, WBC count, and platelet count. The vomiting contributes to the decreased sodium and potassium levels. Increased ammonia, LDH, alkaline phosphatase, AST, ALT, and total bilirubin levels; increased PT; and a decreased albumin level also are common in advanced liver disease. The calcium level is low because of the decreased albumin level and because 50% of the total calcium is protein bound.

4. Discuss the clinical manifestations of esophageal varices.

A common symptom of ruptured esophageal varices is hematemesis, which may be a bright red or "coffee ground" color. Patients may also report hematochezia, blood in the feces, when the upper GI bleeding is rapid and excessive (Urden et al, 2002). Sometimes patients report signs and symptoms of blood loss, which include dizziness, dyspnea, restlessness, and anxiety. Hypotension, tachycardia, decreased level of consciousness, decreased urinary output, and shock may also be seen.

5. Identify the diagnostic procedures and nursing implications for esophageal varices.

Endoscopy is used in the diagnosis of esophageal varices. Once the patient's condition is hemodynamically stable, gastric lavage may be performed to improve visualization before endoscopy. The patient should be reassured that the endoscopy procedure is safe and informed that gagging may occur but that medication will be given to minimize the gagging response. Usually about 5 minutes before endoscopy is begun, the patient is given a medication such as lorazepam, meperidine, or midazolam for sedation. An endoscope is used because it has a fiberoptic light source that enables a clear view of the upper GI tract. The patient is instructed to lie on the left side. A rubber mouthpiece is inserted to protect the patient's teeth. The endoscope is inserted into the esophagus and then into the stomach and duodenum. Complications of endoscopy include aspiration, perforation of the esophagus, and rupture of the varices (Ross, 2001, p. 658).

6. Compare and contrast the treatment options and nursing implications for esophageal varices.

Endoscopic Injection Sclerotherapy

Injection therapy is used to treat active bleeding. "The most commonly used agent is epinephrine, which results in localized vasoconstriction and enhanced platelet aggregation" (Urden et al, 2002, p. 822). Sclerotherapy is considered by some as the treatment of choice for an acute episode of bleeding from esophageal varices (Hegab & Luketic, 2001). Sclerosing agents include alcohol, polidocanol, and ethanolamine. An intravariceal injection, which delivers the agent directly into the lumen of the varix, causes a thrombus to form in the vein and this in turn stops the bleeding. The number of injections is based on the patient, extension of the bleeding area, and effect of the sclerosing agent on the varices (Urden et al, 2002). During sclerotherapy the patient is kept lying on the left side with the head of the bed elevated 30 degrees to reduce the risk of aspiration. General anesthesia may not be recommended because of the liver disease and the resulting inability to metabolize the anesthetic agents. The nurse must closely monitor the patient's respiratory status during and after the procedure. Complications include ulceration of the esophagus, mucosal sloughing, esophageal perforation, stenosis of the esophagus, variceal bleeding, venous embolism, esophageal spasm resulting in substernal chest pain, fever, aspiration pneumonia, and an allergic reaction to the sclerosant (Driscoll, 1999, pp. 738-739).

Endoscopic Band Ligation

Another treatment option is ligation of the varices using the endoscope. Results are favorable, and the procedure may produce fewer complications and therefore better survival rates (Krige et al, 2000). Bands or clips are used to prevent or control bleeding. Application of the tight bands or clips causes obstruction of the veins, which controls bleeding. Necrosis results in scar formation (Urden et al, 2002). Ulceration of the mucosa and bleeding caused by the bands or clips are the most common complications (Ziegler, 2000). Endoscopic variceal ligation has a success rate of 86% in controlling bleeding (Urden et al, 2002).

Intravenous Vasopressin (Pitressin)

Vasopressin, somatostatin, and octreotide have all been used to reduce blood flow to the gut and decrease portal flow and pressure. Although vasopressin is more commonly seen, there is discussion about whether octreotide might be preferable due to the reduced incidence of cardiac effects (Hegab & Luketic, 2001). When vasopressin is used, there is often a loading dose of 20 U in 50 ml of D5W given for 30 minutes; then a maintenance dose ranging from 0.1 to 0.5 U/min is begun. No more than 0.9 U/min is considered safe. The vasopressin dosage must be tapered over at least 24 hours when discontinuation is chosen (Altman, 1999). The critical care nurse must continuously monitor the patient's electrocardiogram and blood pressure. Side effects include myocardial infarction, arrhythmias, bradycardia, hypertension, decreased cardiac output, abdominal cramps, and coronary artery vasoconstriction. Concurrent administration of nitroglycerin may help decrease the side effects of vasopressin therapy (Savides & Jensen, 2000).

Balloon Tamponade

Balloon tamponade is another method infrequently used to control the bleeding. Several types of tubes may be used for balloon tamponade therapy. The Sengstaken-Blakemore tube is a triple-lumen tube in which one lumen is for gastric aspiration, one is for inflating the esophageal balloon, and one is for inflating the gastric balloon. Another type is the Minnesota tube, which has one additional lumen for aspiration of the esophagus. A third type is the Linton tube, a triple-lumen tube in which one lumen is for gastric aspiration, one is for esophageal aspiration, and the other is for inflation of a large gastric balloon. Balloon inflation puts pressure on the varices, which will stop the blood flow. The Minnesota tube may be preferred due to the dual balloons and suction access, enabling suction to be utilized in both the esophagus and the stomach (Urden et al, 2002). Initially the tip of the balloon is inserted into the stomach and inflated and clamped. The tube is then withdrawn until resistance is felt, causing pressure to be exerted at the gastroesophageal junction. An external traction source may be used via a helmet or the foot of the bed. Traction must be monitored carefully and is believed to be uncomfortable for the patient. If bleeding still is not controlled, the esophageal balloon is inflated with pressure from 25 to 40 mm Hg. Tissue damage can occur in only a few hours. The esophageal balloon should not be left inflated for more than 72 hours. Confirmation of the gastric balloon port below the gastroesophageal junction is done by x-ray examination. The nurse must monitor the balloon tamponade patient for more bleeding or tube complications, including pulmonary aspiration. Emptying the stomach and then anchoring an endotracheal tube prior to inserting the balloon tamponade tube helps to decrease the occurrence of pulmonary aspiration (Urden et al, 2002). Evaluation of the bleeding status of the varices should be done during the deflation time, and the nurse must be prepared for rebleeding and hematemesis. For deflation, the esophageal balloon is deflated first to prevent airway occlusion by displacement of the tube upward. Scissors should be kept at the bedside to facilitate immediate removal of the tube by cutting the lumens if airway obstruction occurs. Suction may be applied above the most proximately located balloon to reduce the possibility of aspiration. Symptoms of esophageal rupture include sudden onset of upper abdominal or back pain, which is accompanied by a sudden drop in blood pressure. The naris used for the tube insertion needs to be protected to prevent necrosis (Urden et al, 2002). Once the balloons are deflated, they are usually left in place for 24 hours while the patient is monitored for rebleeding.

Portosystemic Shunt

Management of bleeding varices inevitably begins with pharmacologic agents and sclerotherapy. For patients with uncontrolled bleeding, a portosystemic shunt may be considered (Altman, 1999). The purpose of the surgery is to divert blood flow away from the liver and toward the systemic circulation. Shunts are categorized as selective, nonselective, or partial. Partial shunts allow the most effective preservation of portal blood flow. Although rebleeding is usually avoided, the long-term survival rates are not good because of the patient's compromised status before surgery (Savides & Jensen, 2000).

Transjugular Intrahepatic Portosystemic Shunt

The transjugular intrahepatic portosystemic shunt (TIPS) may be used when bleeding is not controlled by ligation or sclerotherapy (Ziegler, 2000). Catheterization of the hepatic vein is done, preferably through the right internal jugular vein. Using fluoroscopy, the clinician directs a needle into a branch of the portal vein along an intrahepatic tract and cauterization of the midhepatic vein is completed. The intrahepatic tract is dilated, and a stainless steel stent holds it open. The stent is delivered via a balloon catheter (Urden et al, 2002). The procedure allows a portosystemic shunt to be placed entirely within the liver. The risks include puncture site bleeding, hematoma formation, reactions to the contrast medium, fever, bacteremia, encephalopathy, transient renal failure, subendocardial myocardial infarction, vascular injury, bile duct trauma, and stent stenosis or thrombosis (Altman, 1999). Shunt occlusion occurs in more than 50% of patients following a year (Savides & Jensen, 2000).

7. **Discuss the rationale for Mr. Eggert's vasopressin therapy, management of side effects, and nursing concerns.**

Vasopressin is a synthetic antidiuretic hormone. It is a vasoconstrictor that lowers portal venous pressure, thereby reducing venous blood flow. The lowered portal venous pressure subsequently lowers pressure in the collateral circulation, which reduces bleeding. Side effects include coronary vasoconstriction, myocardial infarction, cardiac arrhythmias, bradycardia, elevated blood pressure, decreased cardiac output, and abdominal cramps (Altman, 1999). Nitroglycerin may be given to lessen the cardiac effects (Smolen, 2001, p. 1242). Mr. Eggert must be advised to report any changes or concerns immediately to the nurse.

Altman (1999) reported that somatostatin's more limited effects result in fewer side effects. Octreotide, an analog of somatostatin, may also be used and is believed by some to be superior to vasopressin because of the lower risk of cardiac effects (Hegab & Luketic, 2001).

Propranolol, a β-blocker, is sometimes used in the management of esophageal varices. Although support for use of propranolol is greater in reducing the initial episode of bleeding, some believe that it is still advantageous to use after one episode of bleeding (Riley & Bhatti, 2001).

8. **Identify the relevant nursing diagnoses for Mr. Eggert while he is in the ICU.**

Relevant nursing diagnoses include the following:

- Acute pain
- Chronic or situational low self-esteem
- Decreased cardiac output
- Diarrhea
- Disturbed body image

- Disturbed sleep pattern
- Disturbed thought processes
- Dysfunctional family processes
- Fear
- Fluid volume deficit
- Imbalanced nutrition: less than body requirements
- Ineffective individual coping
- Ineffective role performance
- Ineffective tissue perfusion: gastrointestinal, cerebral, cardiovascular, peripheral
- Powerlessness
- Risk for aspiration
- Risk for ineffective breathing pattern
- Risk for impaired oral mucous membranes
- Risk for infection
- Risk for injury: suffocation
- Self-care deficit

9. Discuss the patient/family teaching indicated for Mr. Eggert.

Teaching areas include those related to procedures, treatments, medications, expectations of therapies, nutrition, alcohol abuse, the ICU, and lifestyle changes.

10. What special nursing considerations are prompted by Mr. Eggert's past drinking pattern?

In regard to Mr. Eggert's history of heavy alcohol use, the nurse must discuss the amount of alcohol intake and treatment strategies for elimination of alcohol. Family considerations are of utmost importance in this area. The nurse must offer emotional and psychologic support to Mr. Eggert related to his fears of not surviving and his treatment regimen.

11. Discuss the psychosocial aspects of the care of Mr. Eggert and his family.

Mr. Eggert and his family may or may not have acknowledged that he has a drinking problem. Acknowledging the drinking problem, the problems associated with his health, and the impact of these problems on the family will affect family dynamics. Common emotions Mr. Eggert and/or his family may experience are guilt and anger. It is natural for an individual and his family to grieve the loss of health and other secondary losses. Mr. Eggert may have difficulty changing his drinking behavior if his family does not support him. Family members must be evaluated for possible codependence and appropriate referrals made. Alcoholism has an impact on the entire family, not only the spouse, so consideration of the children is important.

ESOPHAGEAL VARICES

References

Altman, M. (1999). Hepatic disorders. In L. Bucher & S. Melander (Eds.), *Critical care nursing* (pp. 745-763). Philadelphia: W. B. Saunders.

Burroughs, A. K. & Patch, D. (1999). Primary prevention of bleeding from esophageal varices. www.hepatitis-central.com/hcv/liver/prevention/varices.html

Driscoll, C. (1999). Acute gastrointestinal bleed. In In L. Bucher & S. Melander (Eds.), *Critical care nursing* (pp. 725-744). Philadelphia: W. B. Saunders.

Hegab, A. & Luketic, V. (2001). Bleeding esophageal varices. *Postgraduate Medicine, 109*(2), 75-83.

Krige, J., Bornman, P., Goldberg, P., & Terblanche, J. (2000). Variceal rebleeding and recurrence after endoscopic injection sclerotherapy: A prospective evaluation in 204 patients. *Archives of Surgery, 135,* 1315-1326.

Riley, T. & Bhatti, A. (2001). Preventive strategies in chronic liver disease: Part II. Cirrhosis. *American Family Physician, 64,* 1735-1740.

Ross, V. (2001). Assessment of nutrition and the digestive system. In J. Black, J. Hawks, & A. Keene (Eds.), *Medical-surgical nursing,* ed 6 (pp. 638-660). Philadelphia: W. B. Saunders.

Savides, T. & Jensen, D. (2000). Severe gastrointestinal hemorrhage. In W. Shoemaker, S. Ayres, A. Grenvik, & P. Holbrook (Eds.), *Textbook of critical care* (pp. 1609-1616). Philadelphia: W. B. Saunders.

Smolen, D. (2001). Management of clients with hepatic disorders. In J. Black, J. Hawks, & A. Keene (Eds.), *Medical-surgical nursing,* ed 6 (pp. 1219-1260). Philadelphia: W. B. Saunders.

Urden, L. D., Stacy, K. M., & Lough, M. E. (2002). (Eds). *Thelan's critical care nursing: Diagnosis and management* (4th ed.). St Louis: Mosby.

Zeigler, F. (2000). Managing patients with alcoholic cirrhosis. *Dimensions of critical care nursing, 19*(2), 23-30.

ENDOCRINE
ALTERATIONS

22

Adrenal Crisis

Colleen R. Walsh, RN, MSN, ONC, CS, ACNP-C

CASE PRESENTATION

Joseph Elliott, age 42 years, was admitted to the intensive care unit (ICU) following an acute exacerbation of his long-standing asthma. Mr. Elliott had been helping his neighbor install fiberglass insulation in the attic of his home when he had difficulty breathing and he did not improve with use of inhaled β_2-agonists. Several nebulized inhalation treatments in the emergency department (ED) with albuterol did not resolve his acute bronchospasms and his oxygen saturation (SaO_2) remained at 88% despite supplemental oxygen via face mask.

The arterial blood gases in the ED were:

pH	7.32
PO₂	54 mm Hg
PCO₂	57 mm Hg
HCO₃⁻	32 mmol/L

He was intubated with an 8 mm endotracheal tube in the ED and placed on a ventilator. His home medications included budesonide (Pulmicort) 800 µg two puffs bid and prednisone 2.5 mg orally every other day.

On his admission to the ICU, Mr. Elliott's skin was warm and red. He was placed on a theophylline drip at 0.55 mg/kg/hr for 12 hours then had the dose decreased to 0.39 mg/kg/hr. He was also receiving hydrocortisone 100 mg IV q8h. The ventilator settings were as follows:

Tidal Volume (V$_T$)	700 ml
FiO₂	35%
SIMV Rate	10

Physical exam revealed coarse, faintly heard rhonchi through all lung fields, and he had strong 2+ peripheral pulses.

His laboratory values and vital signs immediately after admission were as follows:

BP	126/80 mm Hg
HR	120 bpm

The editor would like to thank Anne G. Denner for her contribution to this chapter in the second edition of *Case Studies in Critical Care Nursing*.

Temperature	37° C (98° F)
Na$^+$	140 mmol/L
K$^+$	5 mmol/L
Cl$^-$	100 mmol/L
Glucose	128 mg/dl

Twenty-four hours after admission, Mr. Elliott's pulmonary status improved enough for his extubation, which he tolerated without acute decompensation. His Sao$_2$ remained greater than 92% on 1 L nasal cannula and he was transferred to the general medical unit.

The next morning, however, Mr. Elliott complained of feeling so tired and weak that he was almost unable to stand up to urinate. At 6 AM, his vital signs were as follows:

BP	90/60 mm Hg lying; 65/36 mm Hg standing
HR	120 bpm
Respirations	24 breaths/min
Temperature	38.3° C (101° F)

Blood was sent to the laboratory for electrolyte analysis, and a bolus of 200 ml of 0.5 normal saline (NS) was administered. After this bolus at 6:20 AM, his vital signs were as follows:

BP	90/60 mm Hg
HR	130 bpm
Respirations	20 breaths/min

Laboratory results included the following:

Na$^+$	136 mmol/L
K$^+$	6 mmol/L
Cl$^-$	90 mmol/L
Glucose	60 mg/dl
HCO$_3^-$	20 mmol/L

A second physical assessment of Mr. Elliott at this time revealed vague abdominal pain and nausea. His lungs were clear with only faint, scattered rhonchi. He noted that this was not the first time he had experienced these symptoms. He recalled having had these same feelings about a month ago but thought it was the flu. An immediate electrocardiogram showed sinus tachycardia and peaked T waves. At 7 AM, another set of electrolyte measurements was ordered in addition to a cortisol level. One ampule of 50% dextrose in water was given, and Mr. Elliott's IV infusions were changed to 5% dextrose in water at a rate of 200 ml/hr.

The 7 AM laboratory results included the following:

Na$^+$	132 mmol/L
K$^+$	5.8 mmol/L
Cl$^-$	88 mmol/L
Glucose	66 mg/dl
HCO$_3^-$	18 mmol/l
Cortisol	2.6 mg/dl

Mr. Elliott was given dexamethasone (Decadron) 4 mg IV as a bolus with an additional 4 mg given every 8 hours until completion of the cosyntropin (Cortrosyn) test. Laboratory data and vital signs at 3 PM were as follows:

BP	110/70 mm Hg
HR	100 bpm
Respirations	22 breaths/min
Temperature	38.3° C (101° F)
Na$^+$	135 mmol/L

K+	5.5 mmol/L
Cl-	98 mmol/L
Glucose	150 mg/dl
HCO₃-	22 mmol/L

A rapid screening test using cosyntropin was ordered. Serum cortisol levels measured at 30, 60, and 90 minutes were 2.2, 2.6, and 2 mg/dl, respectively. The serum aldosterone level at 90 minutes was 2 ng/dl, and the plasma adrenocorticotropic hormone (ACTH) level was 227 pg/ml.

Mr. Elliott's feelings of fatigue soon began to subside, intravenous medications were regulated to equivalent oral dosages, he was restarted on his budesonide inhaler within 2 days, and he was discharged. Mr. Elliott's discharge diagnoses were listed as:

1. Chronic asthma with acute exacerbation
2. Acute respiratory failure requiring mechanical ventilation
3. Adrenal crisis

ADRENAL CRISIS

QUESTIONS

1. What are the precipitating factors that have caused Mr. Elliott's short-term situation? Describe the pathophysiologic mechanisms involved in the precipitation of an adrenal crisis.

2. What are the characteristic signs and symptoms of an adrenal crisis?

3. Differentiate primary adrenal insufficiency from secondary adrenal insufficiency.

4. Describe the components of the axis involving the hypothalamus, anterior pituitary, and the adrenal cortex. What major secretions are produced by each component, and what is the secretion's effect on the other components of the axis (i.e., stimulate or inhibit)?

5. The adrenal cortex secretes both glucocorticoids and mineralocorticoids. Describe the controlling mechanism of the primary mineralocorticoid aldosterone. How did this mechanism affect Mr. Elliott's 7 AM electrolyte values?

6. Describe the physiologic functions of endogenous cortisol in the body. Which functions were not being performed as evidenced by Mr. Elliott's 6:20 AM and 7 AM laboratory results and vital signs?

7. What other hormones have been shown to interact with the renin-angiotensin-aldosterone system (RAAS) and control aldosterone levels and functions? What other hormones interact with cortisol to affect its physiologic function? What are the effects?

8. Define the stimulation test and the suppression test. Describe the mechanism used in Mr. Elliott's diagnosis. Compare the normal hormone values involved in the hypothalamic-pituitary-adrenal axis (HPA) with Mr. Elliott's values.

9. Discuss how the diagnosis of Addison's disease (primary adrenal insufficiency) is made.

10. What are the goals of treatment for adrenal crisis?

11. What are the primary nursing considerations for patients with adrenal crisis?

12. Identify potential medications for the future treatment of Mr. Elliott's potential adrenal insufficiency. What are their functions and potential adverse reactions?

13. What concepts regarding his disease should Mr. Elliott know before leaving the hospital? List the critical events that might precipitate another crisis.

ADRENAL CRISIS

QUESTIONS AND ANSWERS

1. **What are the precipitating factors that have caused Mr. Elliott's short-term situation? Describe the pathophysiologic mechanisms involved in the precipitation of an adrenal crisis.**

An adrenal crisis requires some type of trigger or stressor such as surgery, trauma, infection, or acute withdrawal of glucocorticoids (Barkley, 2001). Mr. Elliott had several factors contributing to his present situation. He had asthma that required chronic inhaled corticosteroids as well as oral prednisone. Increased levels of both glucocorticoids (primarily cortisol) and mineralocorticoids (primarily aldosterone) are needed for the body to adapt to the stress (Coursin & Wood, 2002).

Corticotropin-releasing hormone (CRH) from the hypothalamus eventually prompts release of ACTH from the anterior pituitary gland. ACTH then stimulates release and synthesis of cortisol from the adrenal cortex. Cortisol mobilizes amino acids from skeletal muscle and generally enhances the liver's capacity for gluconeogenesis as well as enhances normal immune activity and maintenance of cardiovascular integrity (Coursin & Wood, 2002). It also influences fat, carbohydrate, and protein metabolism (Preuss, 2001). The autonomic nervous system's craniosacral outflow also responds to stressors by causing release of norepinephrine and epinephrine, which stimulate hepatic glycogenolysis, lipolysis, and gluconeogenesis (Piano & Huether, 2002). These catecholamines also cause vasoconstriction, which in the kidney probably initiates release of renin, stimulating the RAAS. Antidiuretic hormone (ADH, also called *vasopressin*) is released from the hypothalamus and posterior pituitary during periods of stress. Both aldosterone and ADH attempt to conserve water and electrolytes to sustain a sufficient vascular volume (Piano & Huether, 2002).

When the adrenal glands are unable to produce sufficient quantities of the needed hormones, fluid and electrolyte imbalances, decreased plasma glucose levels, and hypotension lead to the potentially life-threatening situation of adrenal crisis (Jones & Huether, 2002). This can also occur when the negative feedback loop is suppressed due to exogenous steroid use (Jones & Huether, 2002).

2. **What are the characteristic signs and symptoms of an adrenal crisis?**

Severe hypotension and vascular collapse are the hallmarks of an adrenal crisis (Ferri, 2001). Symptoms usually present in patients with adrenal insufficiency are weakness, fatigue, and anorexia. In addition, gastrointestinal symptoms such as nausea, vomiting, abdominal pain or cramping, and diarrhea are often present (Ferri, 2001; Rivers et al, 2001).

Hypoglycemia, hyponatremia, hypovolemia, and hyperkalemia that occur in primary insufficiency contribute to the symptoms just described. Other symptoms include malaise, personality changes, arthralgias, and myalgias. With primary insufficiency, presenting symptoms might include salt craving, coagulopathies, weight loss, vitiligo, and a history of acquired immunodeficiency syndrome or recent surgery (Ferri, 2001).

In patients with chronic primary adrenal insufficiency, hyperpigmentation in the buccal mucosa, skin creases, and nonexposed skin areas may be noted. The hyperpigmentation is caused by excess plasma ACTH levels in the absence of cortisol, the endogenous negative feedback factor for the hypothalamus (Hadley, 2000; Jones & Huether, 2002).

It has been shown that a portion (the first 13 amino acids) of the ACTH molecule is identical to melanocyte-stimulating hormone (MSH). MSH normally increases skin pigmentation. Hadley (2000) also states that the heptapeptide sequence (-Met-Glu-His-Phe-Arg-Try-Gly-) is probably responsible for the melanotropic activity of ACTH.

Patients with secondary insufficiency do not necessarily have the hallmark signs of hyponatremia, hypovolemia, and hyperkalemia because the secretion of mineralocorticoid is not significantly affected. Additional symptoms often seen with secondary adrenal insufficiency include cold intolerance and hair loss as a result of hypothyroidism. Patients with secondary adrenal insufficiency will also lack the hyperpigmentation seen with the primary insufficiency. In the case of secondary insufficiencies, the entire anterior pituitary may be hypofunctioning, producing a variety of symptoms (Ferri, 2001; Preuss, 2001; Jones & Huether, 2002).

3. Differentiate primary adrenal insufficiency from secondary adrenal insufficiency.

Adrenal insufficiency may be primary or secondary. Primary insufficiency usually occurs from a progressive destruction of the adrenal gland. Primary insufficiency is uncommon but results in a deficiency of both glucocorticoids and mineralocorticoids. Clinical signs may not be evident until 90% of the gland has been destroyed (Jones & Huether, 2002). Primary insufficiency may be caused by an autoimmune or idiopathic atrophy (McConnell, 2002). Another important antibody that has been shown to correlate with primary adrenal insufficiency is the phospholipid antibody (Vlot et al, 2001). Adrenal autoantibodies appear in 50% to 70% of patients who have idiopathic atrophy (Ferri, 2001; Preuss, 2001).

Although tuberculosis is a rare cause of Addison's disease in the United States and Europe, it is still a major cause in Japan (Rubin & Farber, 1999). Other causes for primary insufficiency include leukemia, amyloidosis, histoplasmosis and sarcoidosis, hemorrhage from trauma, anticoagulation therapy and sepsis, metastasis, and a congenital absence of the ACTH response (Ferri, 2001; Jones & Huether, 2002). Drugs account for a small number of cases of adrenal crisis. Ketoconazole (Nizoral) and aminoglutethimide (Cytadren) may decrease steroid production, whereas phenytoin (Dilantin), barbiturates, and rifampin (Rifadin) cause increased steroid degradation. Each, then, may contribute to an adrenal crisis.

Adrenal hemorrhage leading to adrenal insufficiency is seen as a side effect of medical intervention. Patients receiving anticoagulant therapy (i.e., patients with acute myocardial infarction receiving anticoagulant therapy) may have concomitant adrenal hemorrhage. The incidence of adrenal hemorrhage from patients with sepsis is variable but is seen more commonly in children with severe meningococcal (Waterhouse-Friderichsen syndrome) or pneumococcal septicemia (Preuss, 2001).

Secondary adrenal insufficiency is usually associated with glucocorticoid deficiency and results from an abnormality in the hypothalamic-pituitary-adrenal axis (HPA) function (Hadley, 2000; Nelson et al, 2002). Secondary insufficiency is associated with reduced or absent ACTH secretion. A common cause of reduced or suppressed ACTH production is prolonged steroid administration for diseases of a nonendocrine origin (Nelson et al, 2002). Other causes of secondary insufficiency include pituitary tumors and infarction, hypophysectomy, irradiation of the pituitary gland, and infection.

Aldosterone deficiency is uncommon in secondary adrenal insufficiency because aldosterone's release in the body is in response to the RAAS. With normal levels of aldosterone, fluid and electrolyte imbalances are not usually seen with secondary adrenal insufficiency. Exogenous suppression of the hypothalamohypophysial-adrenal axis is generally classified as a secondary adrenal insufficiency. One source noted that 30% of patients in one ICU took steroids or had a condition requiring glucocorticoids (Rivers et al, 2001).

Two rare types of familial hypocortisolism are adrenoleukodystrophy and adrenomyeloneuropathy (Ronghe et al, 2002). These are X-linked genetic abnormalities that if undiagnosed can lead to severe neurologic disturbances (Ronghe et al, 2002).

The two types of insufficiency are differentiated using stimulation and suppression tests, which are discussed in question 8. Primary insufficiency is more serious because of the endogenous lack of a portion of the checks and balances of the negative feedback system.

4. Describe the components of the axis involving the hypothalamus, anterior pituitary, and the adrenal cortex. What major secretions are produced by each component, and what is the secretion's effect on the other components of the axis (i.e., stimulate or inhibit)?

The hypothalamus produces CRH, which stimulates release of ACTH from the anterior pituitary or adenohypophysis. ACTH is derived from a much larger molecule called *proopiomelanocortin* (POMC). Included in the fragments cleaved from POMC are ACTH, MSH, β-endorphin, and β-lipotropin (Clark, 2002; Piano & Huether, 2002). ACTH specifically stimulates the middle region of the adrenal cortex. This region is called the *zona fasciculata* and secretes mainly glucocorticoids. The inner zone, called the *zona reticularis*, is also stimulated somewhat by ACTH, but the zona reticularis secretes only the relatively weak adrenal sex steroids (Hadley, 2000).

ACTH stimulates the zona fasciculata of the adrenal cortex to secrete glucocorticoids, the primary one being cortisol or hydrocortisone. Cortisol accounts for about 95% of the glucocorticoid activity, but the other 5% is stimulated by cortisone and corticosterone. The glucocorticoids provide negative feedback to the hypothalamus and anterior pituitary to inhibit the production of CRH and ACTH, respectively (Piano & Huether, 2002). This is typical of the negative feedback pattern shown by many other hormones.

5. The adrenal cortex secretes both glucocorticoids and mineralocorticoids. Describe the controlling mechanism of the primary mineralocorticoid aldosterone. How did this mechanism affect Mr. Elliott's 7 AM electrolyte values?

Aldosterone is the primary mineralocorticoid secreted by the outer layer of the adrenal cortex, the zona glomerulosa. Although three different mineralocorticoids are secreted by the adrenal cortex, the most important one is aldosterone, which accounts for about 95% of the mineralocorticoid activity (Piano & Huether, 2002). The other major mineralocorticoid of the adrenal cortex is 11-deoxycorticosterone (Piano & Huether, 2002). Aldosterone plays an important role in the maintenance of extracellular fluid volume and electrolyte balance. It helps maintain control of blood pressure as a result of the RAAS. The RAAS is stimulated when the body perceives a decrease in normal plasma volume. This decrease in plasma volume is detected by the renal afferent arterioles, which stimulate the juxtaglomerular (JG) cells of the juxtaglomerular apparatus (JGA) in the kidney to secrete renin. The JGA consists of JG cells and special chemoreceptor cells of the distal convoluted tubule called the macula densa (Hadley, 2000; Jones & Huether, 2002). Renin converts a plasma protein called *angiotensinogen* to angiotensin I. The angiotensin I (nonactive form) is converted to angiotensin II by an angiotensin-converting enzyme found in the lungs. Angiotensin II is one of the most powerful vasoconstrictors known. Not only does angiotensin II cause vasoconstriction, it also stimulates the adrenal cortex to produce aldosterone. The aldosterone causes increased reabsorption of sodium and its accompanying expansion of the extracellular fluid compartment (Piano & Huether, 2002).

Mr. Elliott's 7 AM laboratory results were as follows:

Na^+	122 mmol/L
K^+	6.8 mmol/L
Cl^-	88 mmol/L
HCO_3^-	18 mmol/L

Two mechanisms have complicated the situation. Mr. Elliott already had borderline secondary adrenal insufficiency due to his chronic steroid use for his asthma, and he required mechanical ventilation for his acute bronchospasms. These factors increased his need for extra cortisol due to the increased physiologic stress (Rivers et al, 2001).

Because of lack of aldosterone, Mr. Elliott is hyponatremic. Aldosterone maintains sodium levels and normally does so at the expense of the intracellular cation potassium. This is why, in the absence of aldosterone, hyperkalemia results. Recall that the sodium-potassium pump is necessary for the transport of those ions. Note that the anions chloride and bicarbonate are also reduced to maintain the normal state of a neutral charge. Mr. Elliott is also experiencing an abnormal anion gap. This is calculated by subtracting total known contributing anions from cations, which, in this case, gives $122 + 6.8 - (88 + 18) = 23$. When potassium is used, any value greater than 15 is probably abnormal (Ferri, 2001).

6. Describe the physiologic functions of endogenous cortisol in the body. Which functions were not being performed as evidenced by Mr. Elliott's 6:20 AM and 7 AM laboratory results and vital signs?

In 1936, Hans Selye published his paper "A Syndrome Produced by Diverse Nocuous Agents." This syndrome was later referred to as the general adaptation syndrome (GAS). GAS is characterized by three stages: (1) an initial alarm reaction, (2) resistance, and finally, (3) exhaustion (Hadley, 2000). These actions describe the sympathoadrenal system's response to stress. Much of the response is brought about by an increase in circulating catecholamines. However, adrenal glucocorticoids are also essential for the body's response to stress (Hadley, 2000; Piano & Huether, 2002).

Glucocorticoids are produced by the zona fasciculata of the adrenal cortex under the regulation of ACTH from the anterior pituitary (Hadley, 2000; Piano & Huether, 2002). Under normal stimuli, cortisol is released in a diurnal pattern, with peaks in the morning and dips in the evening. Stress alters this secretion rhythm. Glucocorticoids affect carbohydrate, lipid, and protein metabolism. Glucocorticoids increase free fatty acids and amino acid release from tissues. Their action is antagonistic to insulin, and excessive secretion of glucocorticoids predisposes people to diabetes mellitus.

Cortisol probably suppresses the inflammatory reaction by inhibiting release of mediators of inflammation such as kinins, histamine, and prostaglandins. Cortisol also decreases proliferation of T lymphocytes and killer cell activity and decreases the production of complement. It stimulates appetite, decreases serum calcium, sensitizes the arterioles to the effects of the catecholamines, and increases the glomerular filtration rate (Piano & Huether, 2002). The effect on the arterioles helps to maintain the blood pressure.

Cortisol assists in the maintenance of normal excitability of the myocardium and central nervous system and helps maintain emotional stability and personality. Cortisol also aids in insulin production to counterbalance the glucocorticoid-induced effects of hyperglycemia (Piano & Huether, 2002).

When the body is exposed to a stressful situation, the hypothalamus senses this stress and secretes CRH. CRH promotes release from the anterior pituitary gland of ACTH, which then stimulates the release of cortisol by the adrenal cortex. Cortisol aids in the body's adaptation to stress in three ways. First, cortisol increases glycogenesis in hepatic tissue. Second, cortisol inhibits the release of kinins, which participate in the antiinflammatory response. Third, cortisol augments the release of catecholamines from the adrenal medulla and increases blood pressure (Preuss, 2001).

Mr. Elliott experienced the classic signs of acute adrenal insufficiency (crisis), which include hypotension, dehydration, weakness, and tachycardia. The cardiovascular system is affected by lack of cortisol in that it has lost its vascular tone, as evidenced by orthostatic hypotension. Mr. Elliott's blood pressure dropped to 65/36 mm Hg when he stood up. Although his urine osmolality was unavailable, he was probably dehydrated because of lack of aldosterone.

Preuss (2001) stated that because of the vagueness of the symptoms of early acute adrenal insufficiency, a high degree of suspicion would be required to make an early diagnosis. Orthostatic hypotension and tachycardia are almost always present. The hypotension is caused by the loss of responsiveness of the vascular system to the catecholamines, whereas the tachycardia is produced in response to the loss of vascular fluids and a drop in cardiac output. This loss stems from aldosterone deficiency, which leads to fluid and electrolyte loss, especially sodium.

7. What other hormones have been shown to interact with the renin-angiotensin-aldosterone system (RAAS) and control aldosterone levels and functions? What other hormones interact with cortisol to affect its physiologic function? What are the effects?

Research has confirmed that atrial natriuretic hormone (ANH) is also important in the regulation of aldosterone and sodium and water metabolism (Clark, 2002). ANH is produced by the atrial cardiocytes and is a polypeptide hormone with 28 amino acids. It produces diuresis and sodium loss (natriuresis) by inhibiting aldosterone and inhibiting release of renin and ADH from the posterior pituitary. Also, it relaxes vessels, possibly by antagonizing angiotensin II (Hadley, 2000).

Cortisol has "permissive action" with many other hormones. *Permissive action* is a term used in endocrinology to indicate that a hormone "just has to be present in the vicinity for another hormone to carry out its action." This is the role of cortisol with the catecholamines. Cortisol's absence leads to vascular collapse and death. It is essential for synthesis within the sympathetic nerve terminals and for reuptake from the cleft. Cortisol also decreases the rate of degradation by catechol-*O*-methyltransferase. In addition, cortisol's action on fat mobilization is really its effect on the ability of catecholamines to mobilize fats. Again, cortisol seems to be necessary for the activation of enzymes involved in lipid mobilization (Hadley, 2000).

There is also neural regulation and regulation by certain vitamins and antioxidants. In addition, a relatively new potential regulator has been isolated from human pheochromocytoma tumor and is called *adrenomedullin*. It is described as a hypotensive polypeptide, and it appears to play an important role in fluid and electrolyte balance and cardiorenal regulation (McCance, 2002).

8. Define the stimulation test and the suppression test. Describe the mechanism used in Mr. Elliott's diagnosis. Compare the normal hormone values involved in the hypothalamic-pituitary-adrenal axis (HPA) with Mr. Elliott's values.

Dynamic tests of endocrine function provide information beyond that obtained from measurements of single hormones or even of hormone pairs. These tests are based on either stimulation or suppression of endogenous hormone production. The ultimate functional test of endocrine function is to demonstrate a normal response in target tissues to physiologic or stressful stimuli in vivo.

Stimulation tests are used when hypofunctioning is suspected. A tropic hormone is administered to test the capacity of a target gland to increase hormone secretion. Response is measured in plasma as an increased concentration of target hormone. One example is when ACTH is given intramuscularly (IM) or intravenously (IV) when the adrenal cortex is malfunctioning (McConnell, 2002).

Suppression tests are used to assess suspected hyperfunctioning. They also determine whether the feedback mechanism is intact. A hormone or other inhibitory compound is administered, and suppression of the target substance is measured. For example, dexamethasone is used to assess hyperfunctioning of the pituitary in the secretion of ACTH (Jones & Huether, 2002).

Several problems exist with this type of testing, including the age of the person, the need for several subsequent stimulation tests to elicit a normal response, and the inherent rhythmicity of cycles. In addition, many drugs might interfere with the dynamic testing.

There are several types of stimulation tests available for use to test the hypothalamo-hypophysial-adrenal axis. These tests are the cosyntropin test and a prolonged ACTH stimulation test, which involves collection of a 24-hour urine sample (Ferri, 2001). During this test, the patient who was in a crisis situation is treated with dexamethasone, which does not interfere with the stimulation test. The single-dose metyrapone test is useful when secondary adrenal insufficiency is strongly suspected. Metyrapone is an inhibitor of the enzyme needed to convert 11-deoxycortisol to cortisol (Pagana & Pagana, 2002).

Initial diagnosis of Mr. Elliott's problem involves administration of an ACTH stimulation test or cosyntropin, which is a synthetic derivative of ACTH. It should rapidly stimulate cortisol and aldosterone production. During the procedure blood is drawn to determine a base level of cortisol (ACTH and aldosterone can also be measured). Then 0.25 mg of cosyntropin is injected IV or IM. Repeat samples of blood are drawn at 30, 60, and 90 minutes to determine the diagnosis. In this case, Mr. Elliott demonstrated a blunted or absent response, indicating adrenal suppression from exogenous administration of steroid. His long-term use of inhaled corticosteroids, plus the addition of oral prednisone, made him a likely candidate for adrenal insufficiency due to the added stressor of the acute exacerbation of his asthma. For many years it was thought that inhaled corticosteroids had little or no effect on the HPA axis, but recent studies and case presentations have demonstrated a significant effect that can lead to adrenal crisis (Caballero-Fonseca et al, 2002; Nelson et al, 2002).

A normal response to ACTH should increase plasma cortisol to at least 6 mg/dl above the baseline. The normal morning level of cortisol is 5 to 23 mg/dl or 138 to 635 nmol/L. The normal value for aldosterone is 0.015 µg/dl or 15 µg/dl. Values for ACTH range from 9 to 52 pg/ml or 2 to 11.5 pmol/L (Pagana & Pagana, 2002). Mr. Elliott's cortisol and aldosterone levels are too low, and his ACTH level is slightly elevated, indicating a diagnosis of at least acute adrenal insufficiency.

9. **Discuss how the diagnosis of Addison's disease (primary adrenal insufficiency) is made.**

Although Mr. Elliott does not have primary adrenal insufficiency, knowing how to diagnose Addison's disease is important. Many patients with Addison's disease also have some other sort of autoimmune disorder such as type 1 diabetes mellitus, rheumatoid arthritis, or inflammatory bowel disease. His response to the ACTH stimulation test was indicative of an adrenal-deficient state. The question is whether it was only temporary, truly acute, and induced by the 15 mg of prednisone per day for 3 weeks or whether the prednisone actually was masking the onset of true primary insufficiency. According to Pagana and Pagana (2002), when the ACTH level exceeds 250 pg/ml, primary adrenal insufficiency or Addison's disease is suspected. When the rapid ACTH test results are abnormal, a longer ACTH test should be performed for a conclusive diagnosis. The fact that Mr. Elliott's ACTH level did not exceed 250 pg/ml indicated that his was not primary, but rather secondary, adrenal insufficiency.

Bronze skin tones indicate primary adrenal insufficiency. This hyperpigmentation, caused by excess ACTH, accompanies primary states but does not accompany the secondary states or those induced by exogenous steroid administration (Preuss, 2001).

Generally more than 80% of the adrenal gland must be destroyed before the onset of symptoms of Addison's disease. Sometimes the hyperpigmentation appears before other symptoms appear (Preuss, 2001). The knuckles, knees, elbows, and mucous membranes are the first areas affected by the hyperpigmentation. The patient then complains of fatigue, weakness, irritability, anorexia, and depression.

10. **What are the goals of treatment for adrenal crisis?**

There are three main goals for treatment of the patient with adrenal crisis. The first goal is replacement of fluid volume and correction of electrolyte imbalances. This may require IV administration of as much as 5 L of fluid in the first 12 to 24 hours. Hyperkalemia often responds to volume expansion and glucocorticoid replacement (Preuss, 2001). Medications should be administered to reestablish high blood levels of the adrenal steroids as the second goal. Hormonal replacement may be dexamethasone (Decadron) 4 mg IV bolus, then 4 mg every 8 hours until the quick ACTH test can be completed. Another common treatment is hydrocortisone succinate (Solu-Cortef) 100 mg IV push as a bolus with a continuous infusion of hydrocortisone over the next 24 hours. In Mr. Elliott's case, fludrocortisone (Florinef) should also be given as a single daily dose of 0.05 to 0.30 mg. The third goal is identification and correction of the underlying illness that leads to increased stress. Once Mr. Elliott's acute exacerbation of asthma resolves, his need for supplemental corticosteroids will decrease.

Complications seen with glucocorticoid therapy are delayed wound healing, hyperglycemia, metabolic acidosis, and fluid retention (Preuss, 2001). The body's immune system is blunted as well, leaving the person more prone to serious systemic infections (Preuss, 2001).

11. What are the primary nursing considerations for patients with adrenal crisis?

One nursing diagnosis for the patient in adrenal crisis is fluid volume deficit and electrolyte imbalance. The patient may experience as much as 20% depletion of fluid volume during the crisis. The severity of fluid depletion makes restoration of fluid and electrolyte balance the primary goal (Ferri, 2001).

During the acute phase of the illness, the severity of symptoms associated with the illness makes emotional support and a calm attitude valuable in helping reduce stress. Once the crisis is over, knowledge deficit of the disease process and long-term care becomes a nursing diagnosis priority (Preuss, 2001). Exploring the role of stress in precipitating a crisis and identifying ways to avoid emotional and physical stress should occur. Knowledge regarding long-term corticosteroid use is also critical. Medication doses must not be missed, and during times of extreme stress, the patient should also consult the heath care provider for possible supplemental doses and should be encouraged to wear a Medic-Alert bracelet.

12. Identify potential medications for the future treatment of Mr. Elliott's potential adrenal insufficiency. What are their functions and potential adverse reactions?

Hydrocortisone is a glucocorticoid that has effects similar to cortisol. It is also antiinflammatory and immunosuppressive. At high dosages it has mineralocorticoid effects. The initial dose is 100 to 300 mg IV as a bolus, and then 100 mg every 8 hours in a continuous infusion is often prescribed. The main side effects include vertigo, headache, fluid and electrolyte disturbances, hypertension, congestive heart failure, and impaired wound healing. There may also be a tendency for a cushingoid appearance (Jones & Huether, 2002).

Cortisone acetate (Cortone) is also used in the treatment of adrenal crisis. It is given as an individualized dosage of 50 mg IV every 12 hours. Its actions are the same as those of hydrocortisone.

Dexamethasone is used during the cosyntropin test. It is given as a 4 mg IV bolus and then 4 mg IV every 8 hours until the test is complete. Its side effects are the same as those of hydrocortisone.

Fludrocortisone is used as a mineralocorticoid. It increases sodium reabsorption in renal tubules and potassium and hydrogen excretion. Its side effects include increased blood volume, edema, and hypertension. It may precipitate congestive heart failure, headaches, and weakness (Clark, 2002).

13. What concepts regarding his disease should Mr. Elliott know before leaving the hospital? List the critical events that might precipitate another crisis.

Mr. Elliott's instructions should include the signs and symptoms of insufficiency. His awareness of these facts is essential if he is to cope with his steroid-dependent chronic asthma. Patients must adjust their dosage for mild illnesses and must maintain regular contact with their physicians. Patients also must inform all of their health care professionals about their medications, including inhalers. Patients with Addison's disease should wear a Medic-Alert bracelet. Mr. Elliott should obtain and carry with him a traveling kit containing cortisone acetate, prednisone, or deoxycorticosterone acetate for self-injection.

Mr. Elliott should have a firm understanding of what type of stressors could potentially precipitate another episode of adrenal crisis. One example is a visit to a dental office. Other stressors include surgery, cold, fever, flu, or even emotional stress. Patients should consult their health care provider if any questions or concerns arise.

ADRENAL CRISIS

References

Barkley, T. W. (2001). Primary adrenocortical insufficiency (Addison's disease). In T. W. Barkley & C. M. Myers (Eds.), *Practice guidelines for acute care nurse practitioners* (pp. 470-473). Philadelphia: W. B. Saunders.

Caballero-Fonseca, F., Sanchez-Borges, M., & Todd, G. R. G. (2002). Adrenal suppression related to inhaled corticosteroids revisited. *Chest, 122*(3), 1103-1104.

Clark, J. M. (2002). Endocrine anatomy and physiology. In L. D. Urden, K. M. Stacy, & M. E. Lough (Eds.), *Thelan's critical care nursing: Diagnosis and management* (4th ed., pp. 831-839). St Louis: Mosby.

Coursin, D. B. & Wood, K. E. (2002). Corticosteroid supplementation for adrenal insufficiency. *Journal of the American Medical Association, 287*(2), 236-240.

Ferri, F. F. (2001). Endocrinology. In F. F. Ferri (Ed.), *Practical guide to the care of the medical patient* (5th ed., pp. 212-288). St Louis: Mosby.

Hadley, M. E. (2000). *Endocrinology* (4th ed.). Upper Saddle River, NJ: Prentice-Hall.

Jones, R. E. & Huether, S. E. (2002). Alterations of hormonal regulation. In K. L. McCance, & S. E. Huether (Eds.), *Pathophysiology: The biological basis for disease in adults and children* (4th ed., pp. 624-669). St Louis: Mosby.

McCance, K. L. (2002). Structure and function of the cardiovascular and lymphatic system. In K. L. McCance & S. E. Huether (Eds.), *Pathophysiology: The biological basis for disease in adults and children* (4th ed., pp. 930-979). St Louis: Mosby.

McConnell, E. A. (2002). Myths and facts about Addison's disease. *Nursing, 32*(8), 79.

Nelson, H. S., et al. (2002). A comparison of methods for assessing hypothalamic-pituitary-adrenal (HPA) activity in asthma patients treated with corticosteroids. *Journal of Clinical Pharmacology, 42*(3), 318-322.

Pagana, K. & Pagana, T. (2002). *Mosby's manual of diagnostic and laboratory tests* (2nd ed.). St Louis: Mosby.

Piano, M. R. & Huether, S. E. (2002). Mechanisms of hormonal regulation. In K. L. McCance, & S. E. Huether (Eds.), *Pathophysiology: The biological basis for disease in adults and children* (4th ed., pp. 597-623). St Louis: Mosby.

Preuss, J. M. (2001). Adrenal emergencies. *Topics in Emergency Medicine, 24*(4), 1-14.

Rivers, E. P., et al. (2001). Adrenal insufficiency in high-risk surgical ICU patients. *Chest, 119*(3), 889-897.

Ronghe, M. D., et al. (2002). The importance of testing for adrenoleucodystrophy in males with idiopathic Addison's disease. *Archives of Disease in Childhood, 86*(3), 185-189.

Rubin, E. & Farber, J. L. (1999). *Pathology* (3rd ed.). Philadelphia: Lippincott-Raven.

Vlot, A. J., van der Molen, A. J., Muis, M. J., & Fijnheer, T. (2001). Antibodies that stop the adrenals in their tracks. *The Lancet, 358*(9279), 382-383.

23

Syndrome of Inappropriate Secretion of Antidiuretic Hormone

Colleen R. Walsh, RN, MSN, ONC, CS, ACNP-C

CASE PRESENTATION

Mrs. Julie Mills, a 77-year-old white woman, was transported to the emergency department (ED) by the local emergency medical service unit after falling at home. She was alert and oriented to time, place, and person and complained of severe right hip pain. Radiographs taken in the ED revealed a comminuted right femoral neck fracture, and an orthopedic consultation was obtained. She had a history of borderline hypertension and had remained well controlled on hydrochlorothiazide 25 mg/day orally. Because of Mrs. Mills's history of chronic airflow limitation as a result of long-standing asthma, it was believed that total hip arthroplasty (THA) performed under spinal anesthesia would allow for early ambulation and lessen the chances that she would develop significant pulmonary problems after surgery. In addition, early ambulation would also protect her from developing complications of immobility such as deep vein thrombosis (DVT), pulmonary thromboembolism, and skin breakdown from prolonged bed rest. Her medical workup in the ED included a chest radiograph, electrocardiogram (ECG), complete blood count (CBC), metabolic profile (Chem 7), and pulse oximetry. The results obtained were as follows.

The chest x-ray film did not show evidence of acute pulmonary processes although the diaphragm was slightly flattened consistent with long-standing asthma.

The ECG showed normal sinus rhythm with a rate of 84 without evidence of ischemia or axis deviation.

The CBC showed the following:

WBCs	9400/mm^3
RBCs	3.9 × 10^6/mm^3
Hgb	12.1 g/dl
Hct	39%

Chem 7 results were as follows:

Glucose	92 mg/dl
BUN	18 mg/dl
Creatinine	1.1 mg/dl
Na$^+$	130 mmol/L
K$^+$	4.2 mmol/L
CO$_2$	37 mmol/L
Cl$^-$	97 mmol/L
Pulse Oximetry	94% with room air

Vital signs were as follows:

BP	154/92 mm Hg
Pulse	84 bpm
Respirations	18 breaths/min
Temperature	37° C (98.6° F)

Home medications included albuterol (metered-dose inhaler) as needed for her asthma, hydrochlorothiazide 25 mg/day orally for her borderline hypertension (HTN), ibuprofen as needed for arthritis and paroxetine (Paxil) 20 mg/day orally, which was started 10 days before admission for treatment of situational depression caused by the death of her husband 6 months previously. She denied any food or medicine allergy.

Mrs. Mills was taken from the ED to the operating room, where she underwent successful right THA. She tolerated the procedure well, and after an uneventful course in the postanesthesia care unit, she was transferred to the orthopedic unit in stable condition. Per the THA clinical pathway, Mrs. Mills had an intravenous (IV) solution of 5% dextrose in half-normal saline (D_5NS) at 100 ml/hr running into a peripheral line, a Hemovac drain to self-suction from the right hip incision, bilateral thigh-high elastic stockings with sequential compression devices, and an abduction pillow between her legs. She was also given a morphine sulfate patient-controlled analgesia (PCA) pump with a basal rate of 1 mg/hr with an as-needed dose of 1 mg every 10 minutes.

On postoperative day 1, Mrs. Mills was lethargic and confused to time and place but oriented to person, and it was believed that she was having an adverse reaction to the morphine sulfate, which was discontinued. She was slightly more alert later in the day and was able to be out of bed to the chair as per the clinical pathway. She was slightly nauseated with decreased oral intake, and her IV infusion rate was increased to 125 ml/hr. During the evening her physical assessment revealed pulmonary inspiratory and expiratory wheezes with rhonchi, and the physician was notified. Pulse oximetry revealed arterial blood oxygen saturation (SaO_2) of 89% with room air, and nebulized aerosol treatments with albuterol were ordered. These did not relieve her wheezes and her SaO_2 continued to be 88% despite the addition of 2 L of oxygen via nasal cannula. She was transferred to the intensive care unit (ICU) for monitoring of her acute exacerbation of asthma.

INTENSIVE CARE UNIT

On admission to the ICU she was given ventilatory assistance with a 40% face mask, and blood was immediately drawn for testing. The data revealed the following:

Na^+	116 mmol/L
K^+	3.5 mmol/L
Cl^-	86 mmol/L
BUN	9 mg/dl
Glucose	126 mg/dl
Creatinine	0.8 mg/dl
Hgb	9.1 g/dl
Hct	27%

Immediate serum and urine osmolality tests were ordered and revealed the following:

Serum Osmolality	243 mOsm/kg
Urine Osmolality	541 mOsm/kg (serum osmolality + 100)

A pulmonary artery (Swan-Ganz) catheter was inserted to measure fluid and cardiac status. IV fluids were changed to 3% sodium chloride at 150 ml/hr. Furosemide (Lasix) 80 mg IV push was given. Mrs. Mills then received demeclocycline (Declomycin) 250 mg four times daily. She remained confused and lethargic, but her respiratory wheezes improved after three albuterol treatments and her SaO_2 improved to 95%.

Twenty-two hours later, laboratory data were as follows:

Na$^+$	132 mmol/L
K$^+$	3.2 mmol/L
Cl$^-$	98 mmol/L
Serum Osmolality	275 mOsm/kg
Urine Osmolality	400 mOsm/kg (serum osmolality + 100)

At this time, her IV infusion was changed to 5% dextrose in normal saline at 50 ml/hr. Over the next 24 hours Mrs. Mills was weaned off the oxygen; was alert and oriented to time, place, and person; and had the following vital signs:

BP	130/78 mm Hg
Pulse	100 bpm
Respirations	20 breaths/min
Temperature	37.3° C (99.2° F)

A fluid restriction of 1200 mg/day was prescribed. The demeclocycline was continued, and furosemide 40 mg twice daily was started. After 2 days she was transferred back to the orthopedic unit, where she continued to recover from her THA, and on postoperative day 9 she was transferred to a rehabilitation center, where she remained symptom free and eventually returned home independent in all activities of daily living.

SYNDROME OF INAPPROPRIATE SECRETION OF ANTIDIURETIC HORMONE

QUESTIONS

1. Define syndrome of inappropriate secretion of antidiuretic hormone (SIADH).

2. Describe the role of antidiuretic hormone (ADH) in water regulation.

3. Explain the pathophysiology associated with SIADH.

4. Identify the common symptoms associated with SIADH.

5. Explain the effects of SIADH on the major organs.

6. Discuss laboratory studies that are pertinent in diagnosing and treating SIADH.

7. Identify the common causes of SIADH.

8. Discuss two other sodium disorders that must be differentiated from SIADH.

9. Discuss why elderly patients are more prone to developing SIADH.

10. Discuss the medical management of SIADH.

11. Discuss the pharmacologic treatment for SIADH.

12. Describe the role that hemodynamic monitoring would have in the treatment of patients with SIADH.

13. Discuss the factors that contributed to the development of SIADH in Mrs. Mills.

14. Identify pertinent nursing diagnoses for Mrs. Mills.

15. Discuss the nursing care required for Mrs. Mills.

SYNDROME OF INAPPROPRIATE SECRETION OF ANTIDIURETIC HORMONE

QUESTIONS AND ANSWERS

1. **Define syndrome of inappropriate secretion of antidiuretic hormone (SIADH).**

   SIADH is a group of symptoms that occurs when antidiuretic hormone (arginine vasopressin) is secreted in the absence of osmotic or physiologic stimuli. These stimuli include:

   > 1. Increased serum osmolality
   > 2. Decreased plasma volume
   > 3. Hypotension (Ferri, 2001)

   A decrease in plasma osmolality normally inhibits ADH production and secretion. SIADH is characterized by fluid retention, dilutional hyponatremia, hypochloremia, concentrated urine, and lack of intravascular volume depletion (Jones & Huether, 2002). SIADH is characterized by normal to increased blood volume in normoproteinemic, nonedematous, and hyponatremic patients with normal renal and endocrine function (Han & Cho, 2002; Jones & Huether, 2002).

2. **Describe the role of antiduretic hormore (ADH) in water regulation.**

   ADH regulates the body's water balance. It is synthesized in the hypothalamus and stored in the posterior pituitary gland. When released into the circulation, it acts on the kidney's distal tubules and collecting ducts, increasing their permeability to water. This decreases urine volume because more water is being reabsorbed and returned to the circulation (Piano & Huether, 2002). It also serves to produce more concentrated urine (Barkley, 2001; Piano & Huether, 2002).

   The secretion of ADH is primarily modulated by the osmoreceptors of the hypothalamus. These osmoreceptors are stimulated by increased serum osmolality (Crowley, 2001). The serum osmolality is maintained at a normal set point of 280 mOsm/kg, and when plasma osmolality increases, the rate of ADH secretion also increases (Piano & Huether, 2002).

   Another mechanism controlling the release of ADH is a change in the intravascular volume. Mechanoreceptors in the left atrium, as well as the carotid and aortic arches, are sensitive to changes in intravascular volume. When blood volume rises, pressure on the mechanoreceptors increases. This stimulus prevents ADH release, so urine output increases and blood volume returns to normal levels. Volume losses of 7% to 25% stimulate ADH release. The kidney then conserves fluid, and this increases blood volume (Piano & Huether, 2002).

   If too much ADH is released, SIADH results. If not enough ADH is released at the appropriate time, diabetes insipidus (DI) results. DI decreases water reabsorption and results in elevated serum osmolality and a low urine osmolality (Bennett, 1999; Jones & Huether, 2002).

3. **Explain the pathophysiology associated with SIADH.**

   In SIADH, ADH continues to be released in the presence of below-normal serum osmolality, when normally its secretion is inhibited. This results in a simultaneous urine osmolality that is more than that of serum. Dilutional hyponatremia occurs from an increase in tubular reabsorption of water. The retention of water leads to expanded plasma volume. This increase in extracellular fluid causes an increase in the glomerular filtration rate and increases renal excretion of sodium (Crowley, 2001; Oh, 2002; Jones & Huether, 2002). The expansion of the plasma volume also inhibits the release of renin and aldosterone (Huether, 2002a). Aldosterone is a mineralocorticoid that is released by the adrenal cortex in the presence of angiotensin II. It directly regulates sodium balance because of the sodium-water relationship. Because sodium in solution exerts osmotic pressure (water-pulling effect), water follows low sodium in physiologic proportional amounts. As a result of this sodium-water relationship, aldosterone secretion also indirectly regulates water balance. The primary target tissue for aldosterone is the renal tubular epithelium. Aldosterone secretion is stimulated by a series of events that occurs in response either to decreased sodium levels in the extracellular fluid or to an increased sodium load in the renal tubular fluid (Huether, 2002a; Saeed et al, 2002).

Renin acts enzymatically on the inactive plasma protein angiotensin I. Angiotensin I is further decreased by angiotensin-converting enzyme, which seems to be produced in the lung and secreted into the blood. The converting enzyme catalyzes the reaction in which angiotensin I is changed to angiotensin II (Huether, 2002a).

Angiotensin II causes vasoconstriction of many blood vessels and increases selective blood flow to the kidney. If serum sodium concentration is low and blood volume is above normal, the efferent arteriole is constricted. Efferent arteriolar constriction causes the effective filtration pressure in the glomerulus to be raised, which increases glomerular filtration and urinary output. If serum sodium levels are low and blood volume is normal or low, angiotensin II causes constriction of the afferent arteriole. Blood flow to the glomerulus is then diminished, and effective filtration pressure is low, which decreases glomerular filtration and urinary output. This action preserves vascular volume while restoring the sodium concentration. At the same time, angiotensin II stimulates the release of the aldosterone from the adrenal cortex (Huether, 2002a).

Aldosterone exerts its effects primarily on the distal convoluted tubules of the nephrons. The major effect is the reabsorption of filtered sodium in exchange for excretion of potassium. This effect appears to be mediated via indirect activation of the sodium-potassium pumps in the tubular epithelial membranes. Osmotic water reabsorption passively occurs at the same time in response to sodium reabsorption. This response constitutes a physiologic coping mechanism during volume depletion or sodium depletion states (Oh, 2002).

The release of aldosterone is inhibited in SIADH because of the expansion of plasma volume; therefore potassium levels may fluctuate because the secretion of potassium is influenced by aldosterone. When the kidney under the influence of aldosterone reabsorbs sodium, potassium is usually secreted. However, the aldosterone secretion and sodium reabsorption are inhibited in SIADH. Therefore potassium secretion will be diminished and potassium levels may increase, but this is rare. Hypokalemia can be seen in patients with excessive vomiting or use of diuretics and is associated with metabolic alkalosis (Milionis & Liamis, 2002). Hypochloremia is also caused by inhibition of aldosterone secretion. Aldosterone indirectly regulates chloride homeostasis through its effect on sodium. Aldosterone causes sodium to be actively reabsorbed by renal tubular epithelium, and chloride follows passively because of the electrical attraction of cations and anions. However, in SIADH, sodium is not being reabsorbed into the circulation but is being secreted into the urine. According to the sodium-chloride relationship, chloride will not be reabsorbed, which leads to hypochloremia (Huether, 2002b).

The differential diagnosis between hyponatremia caused by SIADH and a modest decrease in serum sodium is that in the latter, sodium is conserved so that the urine sodium level should be less than 10 to 15 mmol/day. In contrast, in SIADH the urine sodium level is high because of natriuresis (Milionis & Liamis, 2002).

4. Identify the common symptoms associated with SIADH.

Early symptoms of SIADH include headache, weakness, anorexia, muscle cramps, and weight gain. As the serum sodium level decreases, the patient experiences personality changes, hostility, sluggish deep tendon reflexes, nausea, vomiting, diarrhea, and oliguria. Confusion, lethargy, and Cheyne-Stokes respirations herald impending crisis. When the serum sodium level drops below 110 mmol/L, seizures, coma, and death may occur (Ferri, 2001; Saeed et al, 2002).

The severity of the symptoms is directly related to the serum sodium levels and underlying medical conditions that may have precipitated the SIADH (Ferri, 2001; Saeed et al, 2002). The rapidity in the decline of the sodium levels also influences the presentation of symptoms, with more severe, life-threatening symptoms occurring with a rapid decline in the sodium level (Han & Cho, 2002).

5. Explain the effects of SIADH on the major organs.

The central nervous, cardiac, and respiratory systems are affected by water intoxication. The primary cause of cerebral edema, the central nervous system effect, is the shift of the intracellular fluid, leading to symptoms of increased intracranial pressure. With the rapid depletion of serum sodium in hypotonic hyponatremias, brain cells exhibit compensatory changes in cell volume by exporting solutes (sodium, potassium, and organic acids) and inactivating osmoles (Han & Cho, 2002). The neurologic findings in SIADH are consistent with water intoxication or free water in the vascular system. As a result of serum dilution of sodium by the excess free water, the osmolality of the serum decreases. The brain, which has a higher osmolality, attracts and draws water from the serum into the brain cells, causing cerebral edema (Han & Cho, 2002).

A major complication of symptomatic or severe hyponatremia, which is defined as a level less than 115 mEq/L, is central pontine myeloinolysis (CPM). This is a process by which there is central nervous system demyelation, which causes permanent neurologic deficits or death (Han & Cho, 2002). The physiology of this process is not fully understood, but research has shown that it is the correction of the hyponatremia, not the hyponatremia itself, that causes these changes (Han & Cho, 2002). There are some data that suggest a certain subset of patients are more prone to developing CPM. Postoperative women who are menstruating, elderly women taking thiazide diuretics, children, psychiatric patients, and malnourished or alcoholic patients are at a higher risk of developing CPM (Han & Cho, 2002).

Alterations in cardiac output are associated with hyponatremia and increased circulating intravascular volume. The patient will experience weight gain without evidence of edema, and the patient's blood pressure and pulse may be elevated in response to the increased circulating volume (Han & Cho, 2002). Respiratory assessment findings may include crackles in the lungs as a result of fluid volume excess and central nervous system suppression of the natural respiratory drive. Hypoxemia has been associated with worse outcomes in patients with SIADH because hypoxemia is an underlying cause of SIADH in critically ill patients. Gastrointestinal tract involvement is again related to the hyponatremia and is manifested by nausea, vomiting, and diarrhea (Jones & Huether, 2002). Renal manifestations of SIADH include decreased urine output related to the effects of ADH on the kidney to conserve water (Jones & Huether, 2002).

6. Discuss laboratory studies that are pertinent in diagnosing and treating SIADH.

Many laboratory values are helpful in diagnosing SIADH. The most important concept for the practitioner to remember is that adrenal, renal, and thyroid disorders that often manifest as SIADH must be excluded (Ferri, 2001; Han & Cho, 2002; Milionis & Liamis, 2002). Thyroid function and cosyntropin stimulation tests can be used to determine whether these are the cause of the hyponatremia (Milionis & Liamis, 2002). The serum sodium level is decreased to less than 130 mEq/L, as is the serum osmolality (<280 mOsm/kg). The serum osmolality (normally 285 to 285 mOsm/kg) can be calculated using the following formula (Oh, 2002):

$$\text{Osmolality} = 2(\text{Na}^+ \text{ mmol/L}) + \text{glucose mmol/L} + \text{BUN mmol/L}$$

The urine osmolality is inappropriately elevated (>150 mOsm/kg). The blood urea nitrogen (BUN) level is usually less than 10 mg/dl with a low plasma uric acid level of less than 4 mg/dl (Milionis and Liamis, 2002; Saeed et al, 2002). This not only is dilutional in nature but also results from increased urea and uric acid clearances in response to the volume-expanded states (Saeed et al, 2002). Chloride levels are also below normal in proportion to the serum sodium. Urine-specific gravity is increased with very concentrated urine. Urine osmolality can be greater than 100% of the serum osmolality. Another diagnostic test, plasma ADH, will demonstrate elevated levels. Specific tests may be ordered to diagnose the underlying cause of SIADH.

An important concept for the practitioner to understand is that hyponatremia can be the result of the accumulation of solutes, such as glucose and mannitol that are restricted to the extracellular fluid. Increased extracellular osmolality causes a water shift from the cell in order to achieve osmotic equilibrium. Thus hyponatremia develops as a result of dilution of the extracellular sodium (Oh, 2002).

The following is the formula for correcting serum sodium values in patients with hyperglycemia (Ferri, 2001):

$$Na^+_{euglycemic} = \text{measured } Na^+ + 0.028 \text{ (glucose } -100).$$

Example:

$$Na^+ = 122 \text{ mEq/L} + 0.028(396 - 100) = 122 + 0.028(296)$$

$$= 122 + 8.288 = \text{corrected } Na^+ 130.288$$

7. Identify the common causes of SIADH.

Almost any physiologic abnormality can result in SIADH. The important goal of treatment is to correct the SIADH and then identify any underlying disease process.

Specific body system causes are as follows:

Central Nervous System

Central nervous system causes:

- Encephalitis
- Meningitis
- Acute psychosis
- Delirium tremens
- Head trauma
- Brain abscesses
- Brain tumors
- Cavernous sinus thrombosis
- Acute intermittent porphyria
- Multiple sclerosis
- Subdural or subarchnoid hemorrhage
- Hydrocephalus
- Guillain-Barré syndrome (Hyponatremia, 2003)

Cardiovascular System

- Hypotension
- Hypovolemia
- Congestive heart failure
- Decreased left atrial filling pressures

Hypotension, hypovolemia, and redistribution of plasma into the interstitial space all trigger baroreceptor-mediated release of arginine vasopressin (Huether, 2002b). Congestive heart failure can also trigger baroreceptors in the right atrium, and decreased left atrial filling pressure stimulates ADH release (Brashers, 2002).

Pulmonary System

- Pneumonia
- Lung abscesses
- Tuberculosis
- Aspergillosis
- Chronic obstructive pulmonary disease
- Bronchogenic carcinoma (Hyponatremia, 2003)

Renal/Hepatic Causes

Hypoproteinemic states such as cirrhosis and nephrosis can stimulate release of ADH, and these disorders limit the excretion of free water (Huether, 2002a). Chronic renal insufficiency and renal failure cause the glomerular filtration rate to fall, and the absolute volume of filtrate reaching the distal sites decreases (Huether, 2002a). As renal function decreases, the maximal amount of free water that can be excreted also decreases, and even minimal increases in water intake may lead to hyponatremia (Huether, 2002a). Hyponatremia without hypoosmolality can occur with elevated triglyceride levels, genitourinary irrigations, or azotemia (Huether, 2002a).

Hematologic/Oncologic Causes

- Lung cancer
- Pancreatic cancer
- Thymoma
- Lymphoma
- Mesothelioma
- Bladder cancer
- Prostate cancer
- Leukemia
- Hodgkin's disease (Hyponatremia, 2003)

Psychogenic Causes

Psychogenic polydipsia can occur in psychiatric patients who consume large volumes of water, often exceeding 10 L/day. Normal intravascular volume is maintained through the renal secretion of sodium. This is not true in SIADH and can be corrected with water restrictions, but patients will have low serum sodium levels with suppressed ADH levels (Huether, 2002b).

Pharmacologic Therapy

Many drugs have been identified as contributing directly or indirectly to the development of SIADH. These drugs can be divided into two categories: those that stimulate ADH production and those that potentiate ADH action (Okuda et al, 1999). For this discussion they will be grouped together because the end point is for the nurse to recognize that many types and classifications of drugs can cause SIADH.

- Vasopressin (ADH)
- Desmopressin
- Oxytocin
- Cyclophosphamide
- Clofibrate
- Monoamine oxidase inhibitors
- Tricyclic antidepressants
- Phenothiazines
- Carbamazepine
- Vinca alkaloids

- Chlorpropamide
- Nonsteroidal antiinflammatory drugs (NSAIDs)
- Colchicine
- Barbiturates
- Thiazide diuretics
- Haloperidol
- Bromocriptine
- General anesthesia
- Nicotine
- Narcotics, opioid derivatives
- Lorcainide (Neligan, 2002; Hyponatremia, 2003)

Surgical Procedures

Postoperative hyponatremia is caused by surgical stress, which stimulates ADH secretion in most patients. This promotes water retention for up to 5 days after surgery, leading to SIADH. Women are more often affected than men because of their smaller intravascular fluid volumes and sex-related hormonal factors (Lane & Allen, 1999). Premenopausal women can demonstrate symptoms of SIADH with serum sodium levels as high as 128 mmol/L, whereas postmenopausal woman do not usually exhibit symptoms until the serum sodium level reaches 120 mmol/L, although this varies depending on the rapidity of the change in sodium levels (Lane & Allen, 1999).

The risk of hyponatremia is especially significant in women receiving routine infusions of isotonic dextrose. After surgery, patients metabolize glucose almost immediately, so these isotonic solutions are in effect hypotonic (Lane & Allen, 1999; Oh, 2002). Volumes of isotonic solutions as low as 3 to 4 L over 2 days may cause convulsions, respiratory arrest, permanent brain damage, and death in women who were healthy before admission (Lane & Allen, 1999; Oh, 2002).

The postoperative setting is especially conducive to the development of SIADH. Pain, narcotics, hypoxemia, hypotension, and positive-pressure ventilation all increase the risk of SIADH (Neligan, 2002).

Four major clinician-mediated factors have been identified as contributing to SIADH: (1) failing to recognize those patients at high risk, (2) confusing early symptoms of hyponatremia with postoperative sequelae, (3) disregarding the dangers of routine infusions of hypotonic solutions, and (4) attributing serious neurologic symptoms of hyponatremic encephalopathy to other conditions such as stroke (Lane & Allen, 1999; Saeed et al, 2002). Patients at risk for developing SIADH should be identified before surgical procedures and appropriate monitoring instituted.

8. **Discuss two other sodium disorders that must be differentiated from SIADH.**

In many patients, especially those with traumatic brain injuries (TBIs), it is imperative that electrolyte balance be monitored closely. Diuretics used to control increased intracranial pressure can create significant fluid and electrolyte imbalances (McQuillan & Mitchell, 2002). There are two mechanisms by which this occurs. Physiologic stress activates the neurohormonal response and excess amounts of adrenocorticotropic hormone (ACTH), aldosterone, and ADH are released, with the net result being sodium and water retention. Brain injury can cause fluid and electrolyte imbalances directly by causing increased or decreased amount of ADH being released or by causing excessive sodium and water loss (McQuillan & Mitchell, 2002). The three most common pathologic sequelae of TBI are:

- Diabetes insipidus
- SIADH
- Cerebral salt wasting

Table 23-1	**Clinical Manifestations and Treatment of Neurogenic DI, Syndrome of Inappropriate ADH, and Cerebral Salt Wasting**		
Parameter	**Diabetes Insipidus**	**Syndrome of Inappropriate ADH**	**Cerebral Salt Wasting**
Urine specific gravity	Low	Elevated	Elevated
Urine osmolality	Low	Increased	Increased
Urine sodium	Low in relation to serum	Elevated	Elevated
Serum osmolality	Elevated	Decreased	Decreased
Serum sodium	Elevated	Decreased	Decreased
Clinical manifestations	Hypovolemia, dehydration Intensive thirst (if mechanism is not impaired) Large volumes of poorly concentrated urine Aqueous Pitressin administration causes urine osmolality increase of 9% or more	Euvolemic or hypervolemic Usually low urine output, low BUN Muscle cramps, weight gain without edema, lethargy, confusion, personality change, irritability, sluggish deep tendon reflexes, anorexia, nausea/ vomiting, diarrhea, abdominal cramps, fatigue, headache, restlessness Severe signs—coma, seizures, death	Hypovolemia, dehydration Increased BUN High urine output Net sodium loss

Treatment	Replete fluid volume
	• Hypotonic fluids usually indicated
	• Administer fluid to replace urine output and insensible losses
	• Administer exogenous ADH:
	  • Aqueous Pitressin— commonly used in critical phase
	  • Pitressin tannate in oil
	  • 1-Deamino, 8-D-arginine vasopressin (dDAVP, desmopressin)
	  • Nasal lysine vasopressin
		Fluid restriction
		For severe symptoms:
		  Give hypertonic saline solution
		  Diurese with furosemide (Lasix)
		  Give demeclocycline (Declomycin) to produce renal resistance to ADH
			Replete salt and fluid volume

BUN, Blood urea nitrogen.

These conditions have some similarities and the clinician needs to fully evaluate the laboratory data in order to distinguish each of these syndromes.

See Table 23-1 for the clinical manifestations and treatments for these syndromes.

9. Discuss why elderly patients are more prone to developing SIADH.

The incidence of adverse drug reactions (ADRs) increases with age. Until recently, elderly people, especially those with multiple medical problems, have been excluded from most clinical drug trials (Pollock, 1999). That has left a gap in the literature concerning the actual causes of ADRs, but several theories have been postulated: drug metabolism via the cytochrome P450 isoenzyme pathway may be slower in the elderly; the elderly person's homeostatic mechanisms may be decreased; the anticholinergic properties of many medications may lead to increased thirst with increased water intake; and catecholamine activity encourages the release of ADH (Pollock, 1999).

Another factor that possibly contributes to the development of SIADH is the polypharmacy required by elderly patients to control chronic disease (Pollock, 1999). The use of thiazide diuretics is known to increase the risk of development of SIADH (Neligan, 2002; Hyponatremia, 2003). A careful patient history and review of the medications patients take may help alert clinicians to the possibility of SIADH. Because of the prevalence of orthopedic injuries in many patients with SIADH, many resulting from hyponatremic encephalopathy, it is recommended that elderly patients with acute orthopedic injuries be screened for hyponatremia (Lane & Allen, 1999).

10. Discuss the medical management of SIADH.

The primary treatment of mild SIADH is fluid restriction to reverse hyponatremia (Ferri, 2001; McQuillan & Mitchell, 2002; Oh, 2002). The amount of fluid restriction is driven by the severity of the hyponatremia. As serum sodium levels return to normal, fluid intake may be increased to equal urine output plus insensible loss. Sodium intake should be increased by no more than 1 to 2 mmol/L/hr or 10 to 20 mmol/L/day (Barkley, 2001; Oh, 2002; Saeed et al, 2002). Too-rapid correction can lead to seizures, coma, and death (Barkley, 2001; Han & Cho, 2002).

If the SIADH is thought to be drug related, the drug responsible must be identified and stopped (Pollock, 1999). If the drug identified is an antidepressant, the drug should be stopped and the hyponatremia should be corrected. The drug may then be restarted at a lower dosage with frequent monitoring of electrolyte levels (Pollock, 1999).

Hypertonic IV fluids should be initiated if there are neurologic symptoms suggesting cerebral edema (Barkley, 2001; McQuillan & Mitchell, 2002; Saeed et al, 2002). A 3% saline solution causes water to be excreted from the cells and reduces the brain cell edema. Extreme caution is needed when using this hypertonic solution because rapid infusion can cause cerebral osmotic demyelination syndrome (Lane & Allen, 1999; Han & Cho, 2002). Serum sodium levels should be monitored at least every 2 hours (Lane & Allen, 1999). Once the sodium level returns to normal, a normal saline solution (0.9% NaCl) should be used with a potassium replacement to prevent hypokalemia. A high-sodium diet can also be ordered to increase the sodium levels. The calculations for volume and infusion rate correction are as follows (Konick-McMahon, 1999b):

Volume of 3% saline = 0.6 × weight (kg) × (desired Na – current Na)/3 mmol/L
Infusion rate = volume of 3% saline rate of correction/(desired Na – current Na)

Another equation that can be used to calculate infusion rates of hypertonic saline is 1 ml/kg/hr, and a volumetric infusion pump is used to prevent accidental overinfusion (Clark, 2002).

11. Discuss the pharmacologic treatment for SIADH.

The standard drug therapy for SIADH includes furosemide (Lasix) and demeclocycline. Lithium carbonate can also be used if ADH antagonism is needed (Barkley, 2001; Ferri, 2001). Furosemide is used to reduce the circulating intravascular volume by producing diuresis. Because large volumes of urine will be excreted, electrolytes, especially potassium, should be monitored closely (Han & Cho, 2002).

Demeclocycline also may be used. Demeclocycline is a tetracycline derivative that interferes with ADH's antidiuretic action and causes nephrogenic DI. The normal dose is 1 g given in four divided doses daily. This drug has the potential for nephrotoxic side effects; therefore it is imperative that electrolyte levels, especially BUN and creatinine, be monitored closely. Patients with cirrhosis have a higher risk of developing renal compromise if given demeclocycline (Oh, 2002).

There are several new therapies currently in clinical trials. These are vasopressin receptor antagonists, which act by antagonizing the action of both endogenous and exogenous ADH. By blocking the effects of AD, these agents can induce water diuresis in the absence of alteration in the glomerular filtration rate or solute excretion (Han & Cho, 2002). These drugs are classified as "aquaretics," but are not available at this time for general use (Han & Cho, 2002).

12. **Describe the role that hemodynamic monitoring would have in the treatment of patients with SIADH.**

An arterial line would be helpful in monitoring the patient's blood pressure on an ongoing basis to evaluate cardiac output and peripheral resistance. A pulmonary artery (Swan-Ganz) catheter could be used to evaluate the ability of the heart to handle volume changes. The right atrial pressure measures preload (pressure generated at the end of diastole), which reflects the volume delivered to the heart. Because a change in the right atrial filling pressures is one of the precipitating factors in the development of SIADH, this would be an important measurement to track. The pulmonary capillary wedge pressure measures afterload (resistance to ejection after systole), another important measure of volume status. Many of these patients already have pulmonary artery catheters in place for monitoring of the underlying disease process that stimulated the development of SIADH. In that case, monitoring the trends is an important nursing consideration.

13. **Discuss the factors that contributed to the development of SIADH in Mrs. Mills.**

Mrs. Mills had many factors that caused her to develop SIADH. The following are the major contributors:

- Mrs. Mills's age of 77
- Her preoperative sodium level of 130 mmol/L, which was not investigated or corrected before surgery
- Her history of asthma
- The hydrochlorothiazide she was taking for her baseline HTN
- The use of an isotonic/hypotonic IV solution of D_5NS over several days because of her nausea and vomiting
- The use of morphine sulfate PCA, which her postoperative confusion was attributed to but again, not fully investigated
- The recent addition of paroxetine, which can cause hyponatremia (usually within 10 days after the start of therapy), to her medication regimen (Neligan, 2002)
- Mrs. Mills's acute episode of bronchospasms secondary to her asthma, which resulted in hypoxemia

14. **Identify pertinent nursing diagnoses for Mrs. Mills.**

- Fluid volume excess related to a compromised regulatory mechanism and intravenous fluid overload
- Altered thought processes related to cerebral edema
- Alteration in nutrition: less than body requirements related to anorexia, nausea, vomiting
- High risk of injury related to confusion and postoperative THA status
- Knowledge deficit related to diagnosis and treatment
- Impaired physical mobility related to THA
- Self-care deficits: partial in bathing, dressing, and toileting related to postoperative status and confusion
- Potential for neurovascular compromise related to THA
- Impaired gas exchange related to bronchospasms secondary to asthma
- Anxiety related to hospitalization and discontinuation of antidepressant/antianxiety medication

15. Discuss the nursing care required for Mrs. Mills.

Continual assessment of Mrs. Mills's condition is imperative. Vital signs should be monitored closely, with physical assessment data correlating with the hemodynamic parameters being monitored. Neurologic assessment should be done hourly during the critical part of the disease process. Serum sodium levels should be obtained at least every 2 hours during hypertonic saline infusions (Konick-McMahon, 1999; Ferri, 2001). Seizure precautions should be instituted. Accurate hourly measurement of intake and output, including Hemovac drainage, provides valuable information on volume status. Daily weighing is important in assessing fluid status.

Because nutrition may be a problem, skin protection should be incorporated into the care plan. The elastic stockings and sequential compression devices should be removed three times daily for skin care and inspection. Good oral hygiene is important because the patient will have fluid restrictions. Preventing nausea and vomiting with use of antiemetics is helpful because electrolyte balance will be difficult to maintain.

As part of the THA critical pathway, abduction of Mrs. Mills's legs with an abduction pillow should be maintained at all times to prevent hip dislocation. She should not sit with her hips flexed greater than 60 degrees, and an elevated toilet seat should be obtained. Mrs. Mills should be turned to her affected side to prevent dislocation of her prosthesis because her body weight will act as a splint to prevent dislocation.

Prevention of DVT is a major component of the care for Mrs. Mills. The low-molecular-weight heparin should be administered as ordered, and if warfarin is used, careful monitoring of the bleeding studies is essential. Mrs. Mills should be assisted with her active and passive range-of-motion exercises, including dorsiflexion and circumduction of both her feet, and quadriceps and gluteal setting exercises. She should receive assistance to get out of bed to the chair. Physical and occupational therapy consultations should be obtained to assist with procurement of assistive devices.

Patient teaching should be an ongoing part of nursing care. The nurse should work with Mrs. Mills and her family to ensure that they understand the treatment plan, the rationale for the plan, and the expected outcomes. One of the most important aspects of Mrs. Mills's teaching is to instruct her to notify other physicians, especially dentists, that she has an artificial hip joint. Prophylactic antibiotics should be given before any dental work, including cleaning, to prevent infection of the new joint from oral bacteria.

SYNDROME OF INAPPROPRIATE SECRETION OF ANTIDIURETIC HORMONE

References

Barkley, T. W. (2001). Syndrome of inappropriate antidiuretic hormone. In T. W. Barkley & C. M. Myers (Eds.), *Practice guidelines for acute care nurse practitioners* (pp. 477-479). Philadelphia: W. B. Saunders.

Bennett, M. (1999). Fluid and electrolytes N205 nursing care of the adult I. Retrieved March 3, 2003, from www.indstate.edu/nurs/mary/fluid98/outlinee.htm.

Brashers, V. L. (2002). Alterations of cardiovascular function. In K. L. McCance & S. E. Huether (Eds.), *Pathophysiology: The biological basis for disease in adults and children* (4th ed., pp. 980-1047). Philadelphia: W. B. Saunders.

Clark, J. M. (2002). Endocrine alterations. In L. D. Urden, K. M. Stacy, & M. E. Lough (Eds.), *Thelan's critical care nursing: Diagnosis and management* (4th ed.). Philadelphia: Mosby.

Crowley, L. V. (2001). The endocrine glands. In L. V. Crowley (Ed.), *An introduction to human disease: Pathophysiology and pathophysiology correlations* (pp. 645-679). Sudbury, MA: Jones and Bartlett.

Ferri, F. F. (2001). Syndrome of inappropriate antidiuretic hormone. In F. F. Ferri (Ed.), *Practical guide to the care of the medical patient* (5th ed., pp. 244-247). St Louis: Mosby.

Han, D. E. & Cho, B. (2002). Therapeutic approach to hyponatremia. *Nephron, 92*(Suppl), S9-S12.

Huether, S. E. (2002a). Structure and function of the renal and urologic systems. In K. L. McCance & S. E. Huether (Eds.), *Pathophysiology: The biological basis for disease in adults and children* (4th ed., pp. 1170-1190). Philadelphia: W. B. Saunders.

Huether, S. E. (2002b). The cellular environment: Fluids and electrolytes, acids and bases. In K. L. McCance & S. E. Huether (Eds.). *Pathophysiology: The biological basis for disease in adults and children* (4th ed., pp. 85-114). Philadelphia: W. B. Saunders.

Hyponatremia (n.d.). Retrieved March 3, 2003, from www.homestead.com/emguidemaps/files/hyponatremia.html

Jones, R. E. & Huether, S. E. (2002). Alterations in hormone regulations. In K. L. McCance & S. E. Huether (Eds.), *Pathophysiology: The biological basis for disease in adults and children* (4th ed., pp. 624-668). Philadelphia: W. B. Saunders.

Konick-McMahon, J. (1999). Fluid, electrolyte, and acid-base abnormalities. In P. Logan (Ed.), *Principles of practice for the acute care nurse practitioner* (pp. 226-235). Stamford, CT: Appleton & Lange.

Lane, N. & Allen, K. (1999). Hyponatremia after orthopaedic surgery: Ignorance of the effects of hyponatremia is widespread and damaging. *British Medical Journal, 318*(7195), 1363-1364.

McQuillan, K. A. & Mitchell, P. H. (2002) Traumatic brain injuries. In K. A. McQuillan, et al. (Eds.), *Trauma nursing: From resuscitation through rehabilitation* (3rd ed., pp. 395-461). Philadelphia: W. B. Saunders.

Milionis, H. J. & Liamis, G. L. (2002). The hyponatremic patient: A systematic approach to laboratory diagnosis. *Journal of the Canadian Medical Association, 166*(8), 1056-1065.

Neligan, P. (2002). Syndrome of inappropriate antidiuretic hormone: Causes. Retrieved March 3, 2003, from www.ccmtutorials.com/problems/explore/name/siadh.htm.

Oh, M. S. (2002). Pathogenesis and diagnosis of hyponatremia. *Nephron, 92*, S2-S8.

Okuda, T., Kurokawa, K., & Papadakis, M. A. (1999). Fluid and electrolyte disorders. In L. M. Tierney, S. J. McPhee, & M. A. Papadakis (Eds.), *Current medical diagnosis and treatment* (38th ed., pp. 838-862). Stamford, CT: Appleton & Lange.

Piano, M. R. & Huether, S. E. (2002). Mechanisms of hormonal regulation. In K. L. McCance & S. E. Huether (Eds.), *Pathophysiology: The biological basis for disease in adults and children* (4th ed., pp. 579-623). Philadelphia: W. B. Saunders.

Pollock, B. G. (1999). Adverse reactions of antidepressants in elderly patients. *The Journal of Clinical Psychiatry, 605*, 4-7.

Saeed, B. O., Beaumont, D., Handley, G. H., & Weaver, J. U. (2002). Severe hyponatremia: Investigation and management in a district general hospital. *Journal of Clinical Pathology, 55*(12), 893-897.

24

Diabetic Ketoacidosis

Colleen R. Walsh, RN, MSN, ONC, CS, ACNP-C

CASE PRESENTATION

Dennis Bowman, a 39-year-old, 63 kg (140 lb) African American, was admitted to the hospital with diabetic ketoacidosis (DKA). After arrival at the emergency department, he had multiple episodes of vomiting. Mr. Bowman said he had been vomiting for the past 2 days and admitted to skipping several doses of insulin recently. He mentioned that he had feverish feelings at home and reported an occasional cough.

Mr. Bowman's assessment revealed pain throughout all abdominal quadrants, with "cramping" reported in all four abdominal quadrants. He was extremely lethargic and difficult to arouse at times. He complained of severe thirst. His skin was extremely dry. An electrocardiogram showed a sinus tachycardia at 120 bpm. His lungs were clear bilaterally, but respirations were deep and rapid. There was an acetone smell to Mr. Bowman's breath.

Mr. Bowman denied alcohol and illicit drug use and could recall no drug or food allergies. He did report that his father and two aunts have type 1 diabetes.

Mr. Bowman's psychosocial history revealed the following pertinent information. He works part-time as a janitor and intends to start a second job but only for 2.5 hours a week. He stated, "I'm on a fixed income, and my medicine runs out sometimes." During the past year Mr. Bowman had been admitted to the hospital with the diagnosis of DKA on March 2, June 29, and November 8. In addition, he had failed to keep his follow-up appointments on July 18 and November 23. Mr. Bowman's diagnostic data were as follows:

BP	124/80 mm Hg
HR	122 bpm
Respirations	32 breaths/min
Temperature	35.8° C (96.3° F)

Hematologic studies showed the following:

Hgb	14.6 g/dl
Hct	58%
Cl⁻	95 mmol/L
Creatinine	4.9 mg/dl
Cholesterol	338 mg/dl
BUN	52 mg/dl

The editor would like to thank Anne Denner for her contribution to this chapter in the second edition of *Case Studies in Critical Care Nursing*.

Ca^{++}	8.8 mmol/L
Glucose	560 mg/dl
Phosphorus	6.8 mg/dl
Acetone	Moderate
Na$^+$	126 mmol/L
AST (SGOT)	248 U/L
K$^+$	5.3 mmol/L
CK	34/35 IU/L
LDH	38 U/L
Alkaline Phosphatase	132 U/L

Arterial blood gas values were as follows:

pH	7.09
Pco$_2$	20 mm Hg
Po$_2$	100 mm Hg
Sao$_2$	98% (room air)
HCO$_3^-$	7.5 mmol/L

Urine tests showed the following:

Specific Gravity	1.015
Glucose	4+
Ketones	4+
Nitrates	0
Leukocytes	Few
RBCs	Many

Mr. Bowman's home medications were 16 U of 70/30 insulin in the morning and 12 U of 70/30 insulin in the evening.

DIABETIC KETOACIDOSIS

QUESTIONS

1. The hormones involved in intermediary metabolism, exclusive of insulin, that can participate in the development of diabetic ketoacidosis (DKA) are epinephrine, glucagon, cortisol, growth hormone, and thyroid hormone. Describe first the pertinent physiology of each hormone and then how each participates in the development of DKA.

2. What is insulin's function in the body? What is the most significant basic defect in the development of DKA? Describe the interplay of factors necessary for the development of DKA.

3. List the classic signs and symptoms of DKA.

4. What is an anion gap? Calculate Mr. Bowman's anion gap. Why is the anion gap important to calculate and follow in the treatment of DKA?

5. Mr. Bowman's pH of 7.09 indicates severe acidosis. Discuss Mr. Bowman's arterial blood gas values in regard to acid-base balance.

6. Discuss the possibility of an infection in Mr. Bowman's case and the effect sepsis or infection would have on a diabetic patient.

7. What are the goals of treatment for patients with DKA?

8. Identify Mr. Bowman's abnormal laboratory values and describe the treatment modalities used with a patient with DKA in regard to these values.

9. What are the major complications associated with DKA and its treatment?

10. Review Mr. Bowman's history and laboratory values to determine the complications of diabetes to which Mr. Bowman is most predisposed.

11. Mr. Bowman's current insulin regimen is 16 U of 70/30 insulin in the morning and 12 U of 70/30 insulin in the evening. Discuss Mr. Bowman's insulin coverage and its adequacy. Include the essential aspects of intensive insulin therapy.

12. What nursing considerations are important in planning Mr. Bowman's discharge?

DIABETIC KETOACIDOSIS

QUESTIONS AND ANSWERS

1. **The hormones involved in intermediary metabolism, exclusive of insulin, that can participate in the development of diabetic ketoacidosis (DKA) are epinephrine, glucagon, cortisol, growth hormone, and thyroid hormone. Describe first the pertinent physiology of each hormone and then how each participates in the development of DKA.**

   Catecholamines, cortisol, glucagon, and growth hormone (GH) are insulin counterregulatory hormones. They antagonize insulin by increasing glucose production (Piano & Huether, 2002; Clark, 2002a; Anonymous, 2000b).

   Glucagon is produced by the α-cells of the pancreas and by a number of cells that line the gastrointestinal (GI) tract (Piano & Huether, 2002). Glucagon increases blood glucose by stimulating glycogenolysis and glyconeogenesis in the liver. Glucagon is also an antagonist to insulin. A major effect of glucagon that adds to the development of DKA is the stimulation of lipolysis, which has a ketogenic effect on the metabolism of free fatty acids in the liver (Piano & Huether, 2002).

   The catecholamines (adrenaline, or epinephrine [E], and noradrenaline, or norepinephrine [NE]) are secreted by the adrenal medulla and by adrenergic nerve fibers. E and NE are important mobilizers of stored energy (Piano & Huether, 2002; Clark, 2002b). They mobilize lipid from adipose cells and glucose from extrahepatic sources. E, NE, and glucagon favor the synthesis of glucose by the liver by promoting release of fatty acids, promoting gluconeogenesis, and inhibiting β-oxidation of fatty acids (Piano & Huether, 2002). The catecholamines are known for their effects on all body systems in the so-called fight-or-flight response to physiologic stressors, and together with the nervous system, account for the physiologic changes noted during times of stress (Piano & Huether, 2002).

   In the physiologically intact animal, catecholamines inhibit insulin secretion by stimulating β-adrenergic receptors. This tends to accentuate the metabolic actions of catecholamines (Anonymous, 2000a).

   These three hormones oppose the anabolic effects of insulin and activate the enzyme systems for lipolysis and glycogenolysis (Jones & Huether, 2002). They also promote gluconeogenesis of amino acids; therefore, if there is little or no insulin, the catecholamines and glucagon effectively increase the glucose level, increased release of fatty acids, and ketogenesis (Jones & Huether, 2002).

   Glucocorticoids are produced by the adrenal cortex under the stimulation of adrenocorticotropic hormone (ACTH), which is produced by the anterior pituitary gland (adenohypophysis). The main glucocorticoid in the human is cortisol. Cortisol's action on intermediary metabolism is best understood if its action is applied in response to stressors such as starvation, disease, or other stimuli that cause significant amounts of ACTH to be secreted (Piano & Huether, 2002; Clark, 2002a). Under these circumstances, cortisol first affects the body's stores of fat. As fat becomes depleted, protein is selected as the next source of energy for the body. The action of glucocorticoids on glucose-6-phosphatase is necessary to provide needed levels of glucose for the brain (Piano & Huether, 2002).

   Cortisol protects the organism against glycogen breakdown until protein wastage is so far advanced that hypoglycemia ensues. At that time, glucagon and the catecholamines stimulate glycogenolysis to ensure sufficient glucose for the central nervous system (brain and spinal cord). The interaction of these hormones results in a hyperglycemia that is commonly called *steroid* diabetes.

   Similar mechanisms, if not countered by insulin, will increase the glucose level as seen in DKA. Consider the importance of these diabetogenic mechanisms when the patient with diabetes has an infection or inadvertently omits insulin injections.

GH, which is secreted by the anterior pituitary, has a role in intermediate metabolism because some of its actions are carried out by insulin-like growth factors. GH is diabetogenic, and its mode of action is thought to be by increasing liver glucogenolysis and increased fat mobilization (Piano & Huether, 2002). It is stimulatory to insulin secretion but has also been shown to reduce the sensitivity of insulin in the peripheral tissues (Piano & Huether, 2002).

Increased insulin secretion may be indirect and caused by the hyperglycemia resulting from reduced glucose uptake by the peripheral tissues. GH promotes growth in that it stimulates transport of amino acids into the cell, incorporation of amino acids into protein, and inhibition of gluconeogenesis (Piano & Huether, 2002).

It has been determined clinically that there is an inverse relation between insulin responsiveness and GH levels. That is, with high exogenous GH dosages or in acromegaly, one would expect to find a relative glucose intolerance and an insulin resistance.

The last hormones affecting the body's use of glucose are the thyroid hormones. The thyroid hormones (triiodothyronine [T_3] and tetraiodothyronine or thyroxine [T_4]) are produced in response to thyroid-stimulating hormone (TSH) secreted by the anterior pituitary (Gill, 2000; Piano & Huether, 2002; Clark, 2002b). The stimulus for TSH is thyrotropin-releasing hormone, which is produced by the hypothalamus. T_3 is the primary thyroid hormone involved in intermediary metabolism (Piano & Huether, 2002). Its main function is focused on respiratory oxygen consumption. At physiologic levels, T_3 is thought to regulate oxygen consumption indirectly by stimulating outward flow of sodium ions. Some dose-dependent net catabolic and anabolic effects on the organism are caused by the thyroid hormones. At lower dosages, T_3 favors anabolism and growth in general, as well as lipogenesis and protein synthesis. At higher levels, the effects are catabolic and lead to higher heat production, increased adenosine triphosphate generation, and depletion of cellular forms of energy. In patients with thyrotoxicosis, one could anticipate high levels of glucose as a result of T_3's stimulatory effect on gluconeogenesis and glycogenolysis (Jones & Huether, 2002). In addition, increased lipolysis will increase glycerol and fatty acid fragments, which can effectively raise glucose levels. All these factors, working together and in the absence of insulin, cause DKA to develop.

These same factors may result in the insulin resistance seen in patients with severe DKA. Even low-dose insulin treatment in patients with DKA results in circulating levels of insulin 4 to 15 times higher than normal. Factors contributing to insulin resistance include high levels of free fatty acids, the presence of high concentrations of counterregulatory hormones, acidosis, and even the hydrogen ion itself. It appears that acidosis interferes with insulin action not only by affecting hormone receptor action but also by inhibiting glycolysis at the 6-phosphofructokinase step (Gill, 2000).

Other endocrine conditions associated with glucose intolerance include primary hyperaldosteronism, carcinoid tumors, and prolactinomas. Central obesity is also considered to be a major cause of insulin resistance, leading to hyperglycemia.

2. **What is insulin's function in the body? What is the most significant basic defect in the development of DKA? Describe the interplay of factors necessary for the development of DKA.**

The β-cells of the pancreas synthesize insulin from the precursor, proinsulin (Piano & Huether, 2002). Insulin facilitates the rate of glucose uptake by the cells of the body, and when binding to its receptor, receptor tyrosine kinase (RTK), causes a series of reactions that result in activation of proteins, especially glucose transporter 4 (GLUT4). Translocation of GLUT4 causes a 10- to 20-fold increase in glucose uptake into the body's cells (Piano & Huether, 2002).

Insulin is an anabolic hormone that promotes the synthesis of proteins, carbohydrates, lipids, and nucleic acids (Piano & Huether, 2002). It increases amino acid uptake by muscle and synthesis of proteins from amino acids, especially in the liver. Insulin decreases protein catabolism and is called *anabolic* because it increases transfer of glucose from blood to the tissues (Piano & Huether, 2002).

In the liver, insulin increases uptake of glucose, stimulates synthesis of glycogen and fatty acids, and suppresses gluconeogenesis, glycogenolysis, and ketogenesis. The net effect of insulin in tissue is to inhibit lipolysis, protein breakdown (proteolysis) and stimulate protein synthesis, resulting in stimulation of cellular metabolism. Although insulin has multiple effects, its major function is to decrease blood glucose (Piano & Huether, 2002).

The absolute or relative lack of insulin is the most significant basic defect in the development of DKA. The person with DKA is most often a known diabetic, usually one with type 1 diabetes mellitus, who has failed to administer sufficient insulin either because of noncompliance, financial inability to buy insulin, or lack of education. Usually, the patient has omitted insulin during a mild GI upset (Ferri, 2001). Occasionally there is a relative lack of hormones because of increases in some of the counterregulatory hormones. The cause for a relative lack of insulin should be determined, even in cases of known noncompliance such as Mr. Bowman's. Common causes of relative decreases include trauma, sepsis, surgery, pancreatitis, cerebrovascular accident, alcoholism, certain drugs, and myocardial infarction (Jones & Huether, 2002; Anonymous, 2003b). Other causes might include infections of the sinuses, teeth, urinary bladder, and gallbladder and perirectal abscesses. Emotional factors and stress, especially in children, are thought to play a role as well (Jones & Huether, 2002; Anonymous, 2000b).

3. List the classic signs and symptoms of DKA.

Any person of any age who is seen with the following symptoms should be suspected of having diabetes and DKA: hyperglycemia, ketosis, altered mental status ranging from drowsiness to coma, weight loss, blurred vision, thirst, polyuria, polydipsia, enuresis, abdominal pain, nausea, or vomiting (Ferri, 2001; Anonymous, 2003b). Other symptoms include tachycardia, orthostatic hypotension, tachypnea, and Kussmaul's respirations. Included also are weakness, anorexia, poor skin turgor, and dry mucous membranes. An important clinical finding is hypothermia. Patients who have infection as a precipitating cause of DKA may be normorthermic or hypothermic due to peripheral vasodilation. Hypothermia is a poor prognostic sign (Anonymous, 2000b).

The final diagnosis of DKA can be made with the following laboratory values (Sherwin, 2000; Ferri, 2001).

Glucose	>350 mg/dl
pH	<7.30
HCO_3^-	usually <15 mEq/L
Anion Gap	High
Ketones	Positive
BUN/creatinine	Demonstrate serious dehydration
Serum Ca^{++}	Magnesium and phosphorus may be significantly depressed as well

Marked leukocytosis may be present in the absence of infection (Ferri, 2001; Clark, 2002b; Anonymous, 2000b).

Some signs of DKA result from the effect that DKA has on hemoglobin function. The molecule 2,3-diphosphoglycerate (2,3-DPG) regulates the functional activity of hemoglobin. Decreased levels of 2,3-DPG increase the affinity of hemoglobin to oxygen, and the hemoglobin is unable to supply oxygen to the cells. One factor that decreases the level of 2,3-DPG is an inadequate supply of phosphate. Therefore the combination of acidosis and dehydration results in inadequate perfusion of peripheral tissues. If the phosphate level is low, phosphate administration is required during the treatment of DKA (Barkley, 2001; Ferri, 2001; Clark, 2002b; Anonymous, 2000b). Phosphate enables 2,3-DPG levels to be restored and normalizes hemoglobin function.

4. **What is an anion gap? Calculate Mr. Bowman's anion gap. Why is the anion gap important to calculate and follow in the treatment of DKA?**

Anion gap is a test that measures the differences between the sum of the sodium (Na^+) and potassium (K^+) ion concentrations (the measured cations), and the sum of the chloride (Cl^-) and bicarbonate (HCO_3^-) concentrations (the measured anions) (Fischbach, 2000). The normal anion gap is 12 to 14 mmol/L (Fischbach, 2002). If the potassium concentration is used in the calculation, the normal anion gap is 16 ± 4 mEq/L or mmol/L (Fischbach, 2000a). This difference reflects the other concentrations of other anions that are present in the extracellular fluid but are not routinely measured and include phosphates, sulfates, ketone bodies, lactic acid, and proteins (Fischbach, 2000a). However, in the case of DKA, the main contributors to the anion gap are the ketoacids, including β-hydroxybutyric acid and acetoacetic acid.

Several estimations of the anion gap can be made. One formula for the anion gap is as follows:

$$Na^+ \cong [Cl^-] + [HCO_3^-]$$

Substituting Mr. Bowman's laboratory values reveals the following:

$$126 \cong (95 + 7.5) = 23.5$$

Note that the normal anion gap should not be greater than 12.

Mr. Bowman's anion gap is dangerously high, and it must be observed closely during treatment. The proper treatment will allow narrowing of the anion gap to within normal limits.

5. **Mr. Bowman's pH of 7.09 indicates severe acidosis. Discuss Mr. Bowman's arterial blood gas values in regard to acid-base balance.**

The P_{CO_2} is calculated as follows:

$$6\,mmol/L \times 1.5 = 9 + 8 = 17\,mm\,Hg$$

Mr. Bowman's calculated P_{CO_2} of 17 mm Hg is not equal to the last two numbers of the pH value of 7.09; therefore Mr. Bowman's disturbance is probably not a pure or simple metabolic acidosis (Fischbach, 2000b). However, if an acid-base map is used to plot Mr. Bowman's values of pH of 7.09 and actual P_{CO_2} of 14 mm Hg, these data are consistent with simple metabolic acidosis (Brashers, 2002).

It is not uncommon for people to have mixed disturbances (Anonymous, 2000). People with DKA often have a combination of two or three separate types of acid-base disorders. They may have the anion gap acidosis caused by excretion of β-hydroxybutyrate dehydrogenase and acetoacetate until there is volume depletion and there can be no more excretion. If patients are able to maintain some oral intake, they may develop a hyperchloremic nonanion gap acidosis (Anonymous, 2000). They may also have developed a lactic acidosis due to dehydration and poor perfusion.

The data given here are insufficient to determine the cause of Mr. Bowman's possible mixed acidosis. A blood lactate value (normal is about 1.8 mmol/L or 18 mg/dl) or acetoacetate value might be helpful for positive confirmation.

6. **Discuss the possibility of an infection in Mr. Bowman's case and the effect sepsis or infection would have on a diabetic patient.**

Mr. Bowman may have some type of acute inflammation in progress. He felt feverish for a few days. The fever could just be a result of the dehydration (Anonymous, 2000). If indeed Mr. Bowman did have an infection, neither the infection nor its source could be confirmed because of inadequate laboratory data (no differential available). Plausible sites that must be investigated include the teeth and sinuses. No bowel hyperactivity or other GI problems were noted. In addition, there were few white cells in the urine, which probably ruled out kidney or bladder infections. He could have had pancreatitis, but again there was no increased amylase value that could help verify that. In addition, there was no tenderness or rebound over the abdomen. However, some of his other enzyme levels (aspartate amino-transferase and alkaline phosphatase) were elevated, which could indicate generalized inflammatory responses or tissue degradation. The elevated alkaline phosphatase could, however, be indicative of obstructive liver disease. Again, no laboratory data were present to validate that. It is known that liver function results could be elevated as a result of hemo-concentration from the severe dehydration (Anonymous, 2000b).

7. **What are the goals of treatment for patients with DKA?**

The goals of managing DKA include the following (Clark, 2002b, p. 858):

1. Reverse dehydration.
2. Restore the insulin-to-glucagon ratio by promoting cellular use of glucose, reducing the counterregulatory hormone glucagon, and breaking the ketotic cycle.
3. Treat and prevent circulatory collapse.
4. Replenish electrolytes.
5. Investigate precipitating factors.

Fluid replacement should be started immediately for patients with DKA. These patients are dehydrated and hypovolemic and have fluid deficits of up to 12 L, although the usual deficit is 4 to 8 L (Barkley, 2001; Ferri, 2001; Clark, 2002a). Therefore a rapid expansion of intravascular volume is imperative. This can be accomplished by an initial infusion of 1 to 2 L of one-half normal saline or normal saline in the first 1 to 2 hours (Barkley, 2001; Ferri, 2001). For adults, the amount given is determined by the amount of dehydration. In general, this is about 1 to 2 L in the first 1 to 2 hours. The expected amount of fluid resuscitation can be up to 8 L in a 24-hour period (Barkley, 2001).

Insulin administration protocols vary from hospital to hospital. The goal of insulin therapy is to reverse the absolute or relative lack of insulin. The most widely used insulin therapy for treatment of DKA is as follows (adapted from Barkley, 2001; Ferri, 2001):

1. Patient receives loading dose IV bolus of 1.5 to 2 U/kg/hr of regular insulin in normal saline (NS). The concentration is usually mixed so as to deliver units per hour that are equal to drops per hour. This avoids serious medication errors (Ferri, 2001).
2. Monitor serum glucose every hour $\times$ 4 then every 2 to 4 hours.
3. The goal is to decrease serum glucose levels by 80 mg/dl/hr.
4. There is usually a decrease in serum glucose initially because of rehydration, but if the serum glucose level is not dropping as expected, the rate of insulin infusion is usually doubled.
5. As the serum glucose approaches 250 mg/dl, the rate of infusion is decreased to 1 to 2 units/hr and continues until electrolytes and fluid status have normalized.
6. Subcutaneous regular insulin is usually given 30 to 60 minutes prior to discontinuation of the insulin drip and glucose levels continue to need monitoring at the minimum of every 4 hours.
7. Once the patient is able to eat regular food, neutral protamine Hagedorn (NPH) insulin is administered before breakfast, and often split dosing is used, with two thirds of the maintenance dose given in the morning and the remaining daily dose given in the evening. Regular insulin is given before meals and at bedtime based on serum glucose levels using a standard sliding scale.

Once the serum glucose nears 200 mg/dl, the intravenous infusion fluid should be changed to one containing 5% dextrose. The dextrose is needed to replenish the glucose stores that have been depleted because muscle and liver gluconeogenesis has been suppressed (Barkley, 2001; Clark, 2002a). It is also important to prevent hypoglycemia from the exogenous administration of insulin, and it prevents cerebral edema (Clark, 2002a). This can occur when the acidosis is corrected and the Na^+ gains access into the cells and draws water into cell, increasing cell volume (Clark, 2002a).

The main electrolyte replacement concerns potassium. The patient often is seen, as was Mr. Bowman, with hyperkalemia. The potassium level represents extracellular potassium and only indirectly reflects intracellular potassium, which is of far greater significance. The body can lose 300 to 500 mEq of K^+ during an acute episode of DKA (Ferri, 2001). The body deficit of intravascular potassium may be much greater.

A widely accepted algorithm for potassium replacement is:

Initial Serum K^+ Level (mEq/L)	Suggested K^+ replacement (mEq/KCl/L)
	No KCl added to first liter of IV hydrating
>5.3	solution
5.0-5.3	10
4.5-5.0	20
4.0-4.5	30
3.5-4.0	40
<3.5	>40

(Data from Ferri, 2001, p. 228)

An important consideration when replacing potassium is the patient's renal status Potassium should be given cautiously to renal patients.

Another interesting phenomenon noticed in patients with DKA is electrocardiographic changes. Although total body potassium concentrations may be considerably depleted in DKA, plasma concentrations at presentation are usually normal or high. The accompanying acidosis (which causes potassium ions to leave cells), insulin deficiency, and renal impairment all contribute to hyperkalemia. Treatment with insulin and rising pH stimulates the entry of extracellular potassium, leading to a fall in extracellular concentrations (Moulik et al, 2002).

Hyperkalemia has profound effects on myocardial conduction and repolarization, thus changing the appearance of the electrocardiogram. There is peaking of the T waves and occasionally shortening of the QT interval. The ST segment may essentially disappear and becomes part of the proximal limb of the T wave. The P wave diminishes in amplitude progressively and essentially disappears when the serum K^+ level exceeds 7.5 mEq/L (Moulik et al, 2002).

Often intraventricular conduction delays occur with widening of the QRS and often resembles a right bundle branch block (RBBB). A sine wave may appear in the patient with end-stage hyperkalemia (Moulik et al, 2002).

Whether it is due to acidosis or other electrolyte abnormalities, often the electrocardiogram demonstrates ST segment elevation, thus mimicking a myocardial infarction. Clinicians should always work up a patient in DKA who has an abnormal electrocardiogram. A full cardiology exam is warranted because many patients with diabetes mellitus have "silent" myocardial infarctions and do not present in the usual fashion because of blunted pain receptors due to diabetic neuropathy. Thrombolytic therapy should not be instituted unless there is clear serum laboratory data, such as positive troponin and creatine kinase-myocardial band (CK-MB) levels (Moulik et al, 2002).

To prevent complications from treatment of DKA, weight and vital signs are obtained at admission and an indwelling catheter is used for tracking fluids. Blood glucose and potassium levels should be monitored at least hourly. Cardiac monitoring throughout the course of treatment is essential. Hemodynamic monitoring (right atrial pressure and pulmonary capillary wedge pressure) may be necessary in patients with preexisting cardiac disease to evaluate fluid resuscitation. Prevention of cerebral edema and pulmonary edema is also important (Barkley, 2001; Clark, 2002).

8. Identify Mr. Bowman's abnormal laboratory values and describe the treatment modalities used with a patient with DKA in regard to these values.

Mr. Bowman's sodium level was low at 126 mmol/L, and the potassium level was high at 5.3 mmol/L. Chloride was low at 95 mmol/L. Sodium and chloride were low because of the vomiting and polyuria. Potassium was high because potassium moves from the intracellular compartment to the extracellular compartment in an exchange for the hydrogen ions (metabolic acidosis). Potassium levels drop as a result of vomiting and polyuria. Once insulin therapy is initiated, potassium returns to the cell (Clark, 2002a).

There is often concern expressed at the low sodium levels found in patients with DKA. This hyponatremia is a result of the elevated glucose, and the clinician can calculate the corrected Na^+ by using the following formula:

$$Na^+_{euglycemic} = measured\ Na^+ + 0.028\ (patient's\ glucose - 100)\ (Ferri, 2001)$$

Therefore Mr. Bowman's actual corrected sodium level was actually 126 + 13.9 = 139.9, which is well within normal limits.

Mr. Bowman's calcium level was borderline low at 8.8 mmol/L, and his phosphorus level of 6.8 mg/dl was high. It has been shown that high phosphate levels can precipitate hypocalcemia and hypomagnesemia. Therefore close monitoring of calcium, magnesium, and phosphate is strongly recommended as the electrolyte therapy is instituted. However, it is now recommended that phosphate and magnesium levels be allowed to correct themselves, if possible. If phosphorus is required, phosphorus and potassium therapy should begin simultaneously, using potassium phosphate. Excessive phosphate repletion could lead to hypocalcemia; therefore serum phosphate and calcium levels should be observed carefully (Clark, 2002a).

If patients have severe acidosis, (pH < 7.0) or HCO_3^- should be initiated. In severe acidosis, the body uses bicarbonate to buffer the high concentration of ketoacids that results when insulin is unavailable to promote glucose entry into the cell. Bicarbonate should be administered with extreme caution because excessive bicarbonate replacement may lead to hypokalemia. If bicarbonate is administered, it should be given slowly and should not be given as a bolus (Barkley, 2001; Ferri, 2001; Latif et al, 2002).

Hypomagnesemia occurs in many people with diabetes, primarily because of unregulated excessive glucosuria. In general, an inverse relation exists between magnesium levels and glycosuria. In addition, mobilization of fats and protein catabolism are responsible for further magnesium deficits. Therefore patients with DKA often have extreme magnesium deficits (Clark, 2002b). However, the laboratory value for magnesium was unavailable for Mr. Bowman.

9.   What are the major complications associated with DKA and its treatment?

Barkley (2001) and Ferri (2001) state that the major complications associated with DKA primarily are initial hyperkalemia, late or initial hypokalemia, late hypoglycemia, cerebral and pulmonary edema, and acute renal failure. Hypokalemia is potentially lethal and must be avoided. Brain edema is rare in the adult but occurs more often in children. Neurologic signs should be assessed frequently to prevent its effects. Acute renal failure is caused by severe depletion of body fluids and/or necrosis of the renal papillae. This results in acute tubular necrosis from prerenal hypoperfusion.

Other significant complications include:

- Cardiac arrhythmias caused by electrolyte disturbances and acidosis
- Shock, caused by severe hypovolemia, infection, or cardiac dysfunction
- Hypoglycemia
- Myocardial infarction
- Acute pancreatitis (Ferri, 2001)

10.   Review Mr. Bowman's history and laboratory values to determine the complications of diabetes to which Mr. Bowman is most predisposed.

Mr. Bowman's blood urea nitrogen and creatinine levels were high, which sometimes occurs in DKA. However, the presence of blood in his urine was undoubtedly associated with the DKA. Mr. Bowman's creatinine level of 4.9 mg/dl could have been caused by dehydration, or ketoacids interfering with the measurement, but could also reflect prior damage to the kidneys. If urine output is normal, a creatinine level of 2 to 3 mg/dl should rapidly return to normal. No laboratory measure of albumin was ordered, even though this value would have been helpful. Hypertension and (micro)albuminuria have been described as the most sensitive markers of renal involvement in diabetic patients (Ferri, 2001). Mr. Bowman's blood pressure during the current DKA episode is 124/80 mm Hg, which, although not in the hypertensive range, is relatively high for a person in the dehydrated state. Current therapy for prevention of nephropathy includes administration of angiotensin-converting enzyme (ACE) inhibitors such as enalapril (Vasotec) or captopril (Capoten) (Anonymous, 2000b).

Annual screening for microalbuminuria and aggressive treatment of hypertension with ACE inhibitors are recommended by the American Diabetes Association (ADA) (Anonymous, 2000b). Other complications that, although not apparent with Mr. Bowman, may become a problem include:

- Cardiovascular diseases including hyperlipidemia and hypertriglyceridemia
- Infections
  - Skin and soft tissue
  - Nasal mucosa
  - Ears
  - Lungs
  - Gallbaldder
  - Urinary tract
  - Vagina
  - Retinopathy
  - Neuropathy
  - Peripheral neuropathy
  - Autoimmune (Ferri, 2001)

11. **Mr. Bowman's current insulin regimen is 16 U of 70/30 insulin in the morning and 12 U of 70/30 insulin in the evening. Discuss Mr. Bowman's insulin coverage and its adequacy. Include the essential aspects of intensive insulin therapy.**

Adults should receive insulin at 0.5 to 1.5 U/kg/day. Lower ranges are for adults who have hyperglycemia but no ketones, whereas higher dosages are used for patients with DKA. Intensive insulin therapy improves control of diabetes. According to the ADA, intensive insulin therapy reduces retinopathy, microalbuminuria, and clinical neuropathy and allows better glycosylated hemoglobin (hemoglobin A_{1c}) values to be achieved (Anonymous, 2000b).

Using the aforementioned ranges and calculating Mr. Bowman's probable needs for insulin reveal the following: if the lowest value is used (0.5 U/kg/day), 140 lb must be converted to kilograms by dividing by 2.2, which yields 63.6 kg × 0.5 U/kg/day = 31.8 U/day of insulin. This is the minimum dose Mr. Bowman should receive according to the intensive insulin therapy guidelines.

Mr. Bowman is receiving only 28 U, so he is not receiving sufficient insulin coverage, even if he did not have the possible acute inflammatory process and was taking his insulin. Mr. Bowman probably should be receiving at least 1 U/kg/day, approximately 64 U. According to the intensive insulin therapy regimen, insulin should initially be administered in four injections with 35% being given before breakfast, 22% before lunch, 28% before supper, and 15% before bedtime. Therefore Mr. Bowman's injections should be 22 U before breakfast, 14 U before lunch, 18 U before supper, and 10 U at bedtime. This regimen should be accompanied by blood glucose monitoring four times a day and compliance with a low-fat, low-sodium, low-protein diabetic diet. The low-fat diet is suggested because of Mr. Bowman's high cholesterol level. The low-sodium, low-protein diet is beneficial because of Mr. Bowman's predisposition to nephropathy. Mr. Bowman should also be consuming a high-fiber diet with approximately 40 g of fiber per day, which will reduce his glucose values and cholesterol and triglyceride levels (Anonymous, 2000b).

After Mr. Bowman's blood glucose level has stabilized, his insulin schedule can be altered so that he receives two thirds before breakfast and one third of his injection before supper. His 70/30 premixed insulin will continue to work well for this intensive insulin therapy.

For intensive insulin therapy, multiple injections or continuous subcutaneous pumps and multiple blood glucose monitoring (BGM) tests per day are required. Regimens suggest three to five BGM tests per day for intensive insulin therapy, whereas only three are suggested for conventional therapy (Anonymous, 2000b).

Exercise is another important aspect of intensive insulin therapy. Patients are encouraged to exercise to prevent hypoglycemia and are further advised to use injection sites most distant from the muscles that will be most active (Anonymous, 2003b).

12. What nursing considerations are important in planning Mr. Bowman's discharge?

With Mr. Bowman's cooperation, future complications from type 1 diabetes can be reduced by 50% to 70% by intensive insulin therapy (Anonymous, 2000b). The diabetes support team needs Mr. Bowman's cooperation to maintain strict control over his diabetes. The nurse must work with Mr. Bowman to develop a health contract that is realistic and geared toward his concept of health. Mr. Bowman must understand the dangers of elevated glucose levels, know the signs and symptoms of hyperglycemia and hypoglycemia, and be able to verbalize interventions for both. The nurse, dietitian, and Mr. Bowman should discuss his present eating habits and decide what changes can be made. An exercise plan should also be discussed. Finally, Mr. Bowman should be informed of local support groups who can help him maintain a regimen of care that will provide an optimum outcome.

The hypoglycemia common to intensive insulin therapy can be handled nutritionally by using the glycemic index of foods. Foods are ranked from 0 to 110 based on postprandial glucose responses (Bell & Forse, 1999). Foods with different glycemic indices (GIs) should be eaten together to avoid the pitfalls of hypoglycemia. Foods with the highest GIs (>90) include most breads, corn chips, and most potatoes. Those with intermediate GIs (70 to 90) include oatmeal, sweet potatoes, and most cookies. Most pasta, nuts, barley, and cracked wheat have lower GIs (<70) according to Bell and Forse (1999).

Other considerations to keep in mind during the discharge component are the psychosocial implications of a disease such as diabetes. These patients will have lifelong consequences caused by this illness. Patients who present with DKA are also at times thought to be "noncompliant," when in actuality they have tried to successfully deal with their illness. It must be remembered how difficult it can be for people to accept something that threatens their lives, requires extensive changes in lifestyle, and imposes a financial burden. The stresses of diabetes are significant for individuals and their families.

One factor that until recently has not been researched is the issue of monetary ability to buy the necessary medical supplies and insulin. A recent study by Booth and Hux (2003) revealed that lower-income diabetic patients had a 40% increase in hospitalization for DKA and other complications compared with patients who were able for pay for all supplies and physician office visits. Nurses caring for patients with diabetes mellitus and DKA should consult Social Services as soon as possible in order to mobilize resources to assist these patients and their families. Cost is an important factor when looking at long-term compliance.

DIABETIC KETOACIDOSIS

References

Anonymous (2000a). Hospital admission guidelines for diabetes mellitus. *Diabetes Care: American Diabetic Association: Clinical practice guidelines* (Suppl), p. S118.

Anonymous (2000b). Hyperglycemic crises in patients with diabetes mellitus. *Diabetic Care: American Diabetes Association: Clinical practice guidelines* (Suppl), pp. S1109-S117.

Barkley, T. W. (2001). Diabetic emergencies. In T. W. Barkley & C. M. Myers (Eds.), *Practice guidelines for acute care nurse practitioners* (pp. 453-459). Philadelphia: W. B. Saunders.

Bell, S. J. & Forse, A. (1999). Nutritional management of hypoglycemia. *The Diabetes Educator 25*(1), 41-47.

Booth, G. L. & Hux, J. E. (2003). Relationship between avoidable hospitalizations for diabetes mellitus and income level. *Archives of Internal Medicine, 16*(1), 101-106.

Brashers, V. L. (2002). Structure and function of the pulmonary system. In K. L. McCance & S. E. Huether (Eds.), *Pathophysiology: The biological basis for disease in adults and children* (4th ed., pp. 1082-1104). St Louis: Mosby.

Clark, J. M. (2002a). Endocrine anatomy and physiology. In L. D. Urden, K. M. Stacy, & M. E. Lough (Eds.), *Thelan's critical care nursing: Diagnosis and management* (4th ed., pp. 831-839). St Louis: Mosby.

Clark, J. M. (2002b). Endocrine disorders and therapeutic management. In L. D. Urden, K. M. Stacy, & M. E. Lough (Eds.), *Thelan's critical care nursing: Diagnosis and management* (4th ed., pp. 851-888). St Louis: Mosby.

Ferri, F. F. (2001). Endocrinology. In F. F. Ferri (Ed.), *Practical guide to the care of the medical patient* (5th ed., pp. 212-288). St Louis: Mosby.

Fischbach, F. (2000). Anion gap. In F. Fischbach (Ed.), *A manual of laboratory and diagnostic tests* (6th ed., pp. 1004-1007). Philadelphia: Lippincott.

Gill, G. N. (2000). Endocrine diseases. In L. Goldman & J. C. Bennett (Eds.), *Cecil textbook of medicine* (21st ed., pp. 1179-1189). Philadelphia: W. B. Saunders.

Jones, R. E. & Huether, S. E. (2002). Alterations of hormonal regulation. In K. L. McCance & S. E. Huether (Eds.), *Pathophysiology: The biological basis for disease in adults and children* (4th ed., pp. 624-669). St Louis: Mosby.

Latif, K. A., Friere, A. X., Kitabchi, A. E., Umpierrez, G. E., & Qureshi, N. (2002). The use of alkali in severe diabetic ketoacidosis. *Diabetes Care, 25*(11), 2113.

Moulik, P. K., Nethaji, C., & Khaleeli, A. A. (2002). Misleading electrocardiographic results in patients with hperkalemia and diabetic ketoacidosis. *British Medical Journal, 325*(7376), 1346-1347.

Piano, M. R. & Huether, S. E. (2002). Mechanisms of hormonal regulation. In K. L. McCance & S. E. Huether (Eds.), *Pathophysiology: The biological basis for disease in adults and children* (4th ed., pp. 597-623). St Louis: Mosby.

Sherwin, R. S. (2000). Diabetes mellitus. In L. Goldman & J. C. Bennett (Eds.), *Cecil textbook of medicine* (21st ed., pp. 1263-1285). Philadelphia: W. B. Saunders.

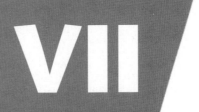
MULTISYSTEM ALTERATIONS

25

Multiple Organ Dysfunction Syndrome

Colleen R. Walsh, RN, MSN, ONC, CS, ACNP-C

CASE PRESENTATION

Mr. Walters, a 67-year-old white man, was admitted to the hospital with abdominal pain. History on admission revealed that Mr. Walters had a history of diverticulitis with intraabdominal abscess formation and underwent a partial sigmoid colectomy with delayed anastomosis 2 years ago. He denied any further problems and stated he had been having regular bowel movements until 2 days before admission. His medical history also included splenectomy after a motor vehicle accident that occurred when Mr. Walters was 47 years old. His vital signs on admission were:

BP	100/53 mm Hg
HR	105 bpm
Respirations	28 breaths/min
Temperature	36.3° C (97° F)

He appeared to be in acute distress. Breath sounds were equal and bilateral through all lung fields. Heart tones were normal. The abdomen was flat with absent bowel sounds and diffusely tender to palpation. There was no rebound tenderness. There were no palpable masses or abnormal pulsations. His Glasgow Coma Scale (GCS) score was normal (15).

Laboratory data at admission were the following:

Hgb	12.5 g/dl
Hct	38.6%
WBCs	$4.34 \times 10^3/mm^3$
Platelets	$210,000/mm^3$
Na$^+$	136 mmol/L
K$^+$	4.5 mmol/L
Cl$^-$	101 mmol/L
CO$_2$	25 mmol/L
Glucose	189 mg/dl
BUN	39 mg/dl
Creatinine	1.8 mg/dl
Bilirubin	0.4 mg/dl
Alkaline Phosphatase	56 U/L
AST (SGOT)	31 U/L

| **LDH** | 140 U/L |
| **Albumin** | 2.3 g/dl |

The patient was given intravenous fluids and pain medications after admission to the hospital. A computed tomography scan (CT) of the abdomen showed adhesions surrounding the jejunum with near total constriction of the proximal large bowel. He was immediately taken to surgery, where ischemic colon with perforation and abscess was noted. The patient underwent an emergency total colectomy, lysis of adhesions, ileostomy, and irrigation of the peritoneal cavity. A pulmonary artery catheter was inserted to monitor his hemodynamic status. He remained intubated after surgery and was taken to the intensive care unit (ICU) in serious condition. His vital signs on admission to ICU were:

BP	82/60 mm Hg (MAP 68)
HR	123 bpm
Temperature	38.8° C (101.8° F)
CVP (RAP)	8
PAP	38/18
PCWP	15
CO/CI	4.2/2.6

Ventilator settings were as follows:

Fio$_2$	50%
SIMV Rate	10
V$_T$	700 ml

Arterial blood gas (ABG) values were as follows:

pH	7.41
Pco$_2$	35 mm Hg
Po$_2$	123 mm Hg
HCO$_3^-$	23 mmol/L

On the second postoperative day the patient's respiratory status stabilized and the endotracheal tube was removed. Dopamine was continued at 5 μg/kg/min, and as Mr. Walters's blood pressure stabilized, the dopamine was titrated and then discontinued.

On the fourth postoperative day Mr. Walters's condition deteriorated, requiring reintubation and mechanical ventilation. His hemoglobin and hematocrit also dropped significantly, requiring a blood transfusion of 2 units of packed red blood cells. He did not want to be using the ventilator and continually tried to extubate himself. His GCS score decreased to 13. On postoperative day 4, diagnostic data after blood was transfused were the following:

Hgb	7.1 g/dl
Hct	21.7%
WBCs	14.4 × 10^3/mm^3
Platelets	5000/mm^3
Na$^+$	128 mmol/L
K$^+$	5.6 mmol/L
Cl$^-$	102 mmol/L
CO$_2$	32 mmol/L
Glucose	90 mg/dl
BUN	32 mg/dl
Creatinine	225 mg/dl
Bilirubin	1.1 mg/dl
Alkaline Phosphatase	69 U/L
AST (SGOT)	120 U/L
LDH	580 U/L

Albumin	1.8 g/dl

Vital signs and hemodynamic values were the following:

BP	90/64 mm Hg (MAP 70)
HR	130 bpm
Temperature	38.9° C (102° F)
CVP (RAP)	10
PAP	42/30
PCWP	15
CO/CI	3.8/2.1

Ventilator settings were as follows:

Fio_2	60%
SIMV Rate	10
V_T	700 ml
PEEP	5 cm H_2O

ABG values were as follows:

pH	7.32
Pco_2	57 mm Hg
Po_2	54 mm Hg
HCO_3^-	32 mmol/L

By postoperative day 10, Mr. Walters showed worsening signs of respiratory and liver failure. Triple antibiotic therapy continued, yet Mr. Walters's temperature continued to spike at 38.9° C (102° F) throughout his hospitalization. Multiple cultures were obtained, yet all showed no growth.

After consultation with Mr. Walters's family and in view of the patient's previous wishes regarding ventilatory support, the ventilator was removed. Mr. Walters died shortly thereafter.

MULTIPLE ORGAN DYSFUNCTION SYNDROME

QUESTIONS

1. Define the evolution of multiple organ dysfunction syndrome (MODS).

2. List etiologic factors for and discuss the incidence of MODS. What are some theories or hypotheses for the cause of MODS?

3. Describe the primary and secondary classifications of MODS. Which classification of MODS has Mr. Walters developed? Identify any predictors of mortality or significant manifestations associated with the classifications. Approximate Mr. Walters's mortality risk.

4. What pathophysiologic changes occur with MODS?

5. How is the release of oxygen-free radicals, tumor necrosis factor (TNF), and interleukin-1 (IL-1) related to the development of MODS?

6. What special considerations are there with children and elderly patients who are predisposed to MODS? What were Mr. Walters's predisposing factors?

7. Identify assessment findings and effects of MODS on individual organ systems.

8. Discuss collaborative management measures for MODS.

9. What are the nursing diagnoses for the patient with MODS?

10. What ethical considerations play a role in the diagnosis of MODS?

11. What are the future trends for the treatment of MODS?

MULTIPLE ORGAN DYSFUNCTION SYNDROME

QUESTIONS AND ANSWERS

1. Define the evolution of multiple organ dysfunction syndrome (MODS).

Multiple organ failure (MOF), the precursor to MODS, has been described since the mid-1970s and is a separate entity from single organ failure. *MOF* is the failure of two or more organ systems. MOF is a result of malignant intravascular inflammation, which is often associated with infection or sepsis (Carlson, 1999). In the late 1980s, research on MOF revealed that organ failure can also occur in the absence of infection with disorders such as shock, tissue injury, ischemic conditions with necrotic tissue, burns, acute renal failure, acute pancreatitis, severe trauma, major surgery, and acute respiratory distress syndrome (Carlson, 1999; Biffle & Moore, 2000; Parillo, 2000; Baldwin & Morris, 2002). Subsequently, MOF became a less accepted universal definition for organ failure. The 1991 consensus conference of the Society of Critical Care Medicine and the American College of Chest Physicians suggested that the term *multiple system organ failure (MOF)* be replaced with *multiple organ dysfunction syndrome (MODS)*. The reason for this suggestion was that MOF denotes actual organ failure, which is not actually the case (Baldwin & Morris, 2002). The new term is considered more appropriate because organs such as the heart, lungs, and kidneys show signs of dysfunction but do not actually fail.

MODS is the result of a systemic inflammatory response syndrome (SIRS), which results from the injury and implies an ongoing physiologic phenomenon rather than the presence or absence of organ failure (Carlson, 1999). The SIRS may directly result in MODS or may be a result of sepsis. Although no widely accepted definition of MODS exists, the definition of MODS that was developed at the 1991 consensus conference states that:

> "MODS is the presence of altered organ function in an acutely ill person such that homeostasis cannot be maintained without intervention. Primary MODS is the direct result of a well-defined insult in which organ dysfunction occurs early and can be directly attributable to the insult itself. Secondary MODS develops as consequence of a host response and is identified within the context of SIRS" (as cited in Baldwin & Morris, 2002, p. 1492).

2. List etiologic factors for and discuss the incidence of MODS. What are some theories or hypotheses for the cause of MODS?

Etiologic or Risk Factors for MODS

According to Baldwin and Morris (2002) and Urden and colleagues (2002), etiologic or predisposing factors for MODS include the following:

- Age 65 years or older
- Baseline organ dysfunction such as renal insufficiency
- Immunosuppressive therapy such as steroids
- Bowel infarction
- Coma on admission
- Inadequate, delayed resuscitation
- Malnutrition
- Multiple blood transfusions (more than 6 units per 12 hours)
- Age of packed red blood cells infused during the first 6 hours postinjury
- Persistent infectious focus
- Preexisting chronic disease, such as cancer or diabetes mellitus
- Presence of hematoma
- Significant tissue injury
- Complications of multiple trauma with prolonged highly invasive surgical procedures, perfusion deficits, and hemorrhagic shock

- Burns
- Sepsis
- Tissue hypoxemia
- Acute pancreatitis
- Ruptured aneurysm

The incidence of MODS is increasing because patients with chronic illnesses and/or severe trauma are surviving longer. Despite advances in the management of severely traumatized or ill patients, the mortality has been the same for the past 20 years and is thought to be the leading cause of ICU-related deaths (Marshall, 2001; Baldwin & Morris, 2002; Urden et al, 2002). Mortality for patients with MODS is between 45% and 55% for failure of two organ systems; greater than 80% for those when three or more organ systems fail; and almost 100% if the failure of the three organs lasts for more than 4 days (Baldwin & Morris, 2002). A study cited by Carlson (1999) described a simple scoring system, based on dysfunctional systems found on the first day of a critical care stay, that could accurately predict mortality approximately 75% of the time.

Theories or Hypotheses for the Cause of MODS

Several hypotheses have been proposed that are thought to explain the development of MODS after major trauma, surgery, and sepsis. These include unrecognized flow-dependent oxygen (O_2) consumption, ischemia, gut-barrier failure, and activation of the inflammatory cascade (Helgeby, nd).

The following are theories regarding the cause of MODS:

1. Uncontrolled infection evidenced by persistent infections, nosocomial infections, and endotoxemia
2. Systemic inflammation evidenced by activation of the inflammatory cytokines such as IL-6, IL-8, TNF, and increased capillary permeability
3. Immune paralysis evidenced by nosocomial infections, increased antiinflammatory cytokine levels (IL-10), and decreased human leukocyte antigen (HLA)-DR expression
4. Tissue hypoxia evidenced by increased lactate levels
5. Microvascular coagulopathy and endothelial activation evidenced by increased procoagulant activity, decreased anticoagulant activity, increased von Willebrand factor, soluble thrombomodulin, and increased capillary permeability
6. Dysregulated apoptosis (preprogrammed cell death) evidenced by increased epithelial and lymphoid apoptosis, and decreased neutrophil apoptosis
7. Gut-liver axis evidenced by infection with gut organisms, endotoxemia, and Kupffer cell activation (adapted from Marshall, 2001, p. S100).

3. **Describe the primary and secondary classifications of MODS. Which classification of MODS has Mr. Walters developed? Identify any predictors of mortality or significant manifestations associated with the classifications. Approximate Mr. Walters's mortality risk.**

Primary and Secondary Classifications of MODS

Primary MODS is the direct result of a well-defined organ insult in which organ dysfunction occurs early and can be related to an identifiable insult (Carlson, 1999; Baldwin & Morris, 2002). *Secondary MODS* is organ dysfunction that develops days after admission. It is the result of an excess inflammatory response in organs distant from the original injury or insult (Carlson, 1999; Baldwin & Morris, 2002). It is thought that the organ trauma is due to the host response to a second insult, and that insult can be very minor. But in the setting of an already primed inflammatory response, the effects can be disastrous (Baldwin & Morris, 2002). It appears that Mr. Walters had developed secondary MODS in response to the persistent SIRS-to-sepsis process over several days postoperatively. The clinical manifestations of SIRS-to-sepsis process associated with MODS are described in Table 25-1 (Carlson, 1999).

Table 25-1	*Clinical Manifestations of SIRS Associated with MODS*
Clinical Manifestation	**Description**
Temperature	>38° C (100.4° F) or <36° C (96.8° F)
Heart rate	>90 bpm
Respiratory rate	>20 breaths/min
Paco$_2$	<32 mm Hg (hyperventilation)
White blood cell count	>12,000/mm^3 or <4000/mm^3 or >10% immature (band) forms

Table 25-2	*Organ-Specific Descriptors Correlating with MODS Mortality*				
	Score				
System	**0**	**1**	**2**	**3**	**4**
Respiratory (Po/Fio$_2$ ratio)	>300	266-300	151-225	76-150	≤75
Renal (serum creatinine)	≤100	101-200	201-350	351-500	>500
Hepatic (serum bilirubin)	≤20	21-60	61-120	121-240	>240
Cardiovascular (PAR=HR × RAP/MAP)	≤10	10.1-15	15.1-20	20.1-30.0	>30
Hematologic (platelet count)	>120	81-120	51-80	21-50	≤20
Neurologic (Glasgow Coma Scale)	15	13-14	10-12	7-9	≤6

Reprinted with permission from Alspach, J. G. (Ed.). (1998). *American Association of Critical-Care Nurses: Core curriculum for critical care nursing* (5th ed.). Philadelphia: WB Saunders.

Predictors of Mortality or Significant Manifestations Associated with MODS

Several MODS scoring systems have been developed in order to assist clinicians with predicting outcomes in critically ill patients. Several of these scoring systems are specific to MODS in trauma patients, whereas others are more general in nature (Sommers, 1998; Vary et al, 2002). Some of these systems are dependent on physiologic parameters from other scoring systems, such as the Injury Severity Score (ISS), Acute Physiology and Chronic Health Evaluation (APACHE II and III), and acute respiratory distress syndrome (ARDS) score, and it is this variability that makes accurate prediction of mortality difficult (Baldwin & Morris, 2002).

Organ-specific descriptors correlating with mortality from MODS are described in Table 25-2 (Piper & Sibbald, 1997; Sommers, 1998). The descriptor score in relation to mortality is as follows:

- Score of 9 to 12: mortality 25%
- Score of 13 to 16: mortality 50%
- Score of 17 to 20: mortality 75%

Mr. Walters's approximate mortality score was 14 based on his data on postoperative day 4. A score of 14 places him in the 50% mortality category.

4. What pathophysiologic changes occur with MODS?

The pathophysiology of MODS must be looked at from several perspectives. The role of the SIRS cannot be overemphasized, and the role of septic shock is also complicit in the development of MODS (American College of Chest Physicians [ACCP] & Society of Critical Care Medicine [SCCM], 1992; Baldwin & Morris, 2002). Septic shock can be considered a component of the SIRS, and begins as an infection that progresses to bacteremia, then sepsis, then severe sepsis, then septic shock, and finally MODS (Baldwin & Morris, 2002; Fitch & Gossage, 2002). The development of MODS must be viewed as a progression from primary to secondary MODS.

In primary MODS the initial organ injury can be traced to a definable physiologic insult. Usually this insult is ischemia or impaired infusion from shock, trauma, tissue necrosis, or infection (Baldwin & Morris, 2002; Urden et al, 2002). This hypoperfusion is often not clinically evident, but the resultant activation of the stress response is initiated, and large amounts of stress hormones, especially catecholamine, are released (Baldwin & Morris, 2002; Fitch & Gossage, 2002). Inflammatory and stress responses are not nearly as evident in secondary MODS, but in primary MODS it is thought that the neutrophils and macrophages are "primed" by the inflammatory cytokines (Marshall, 2001; Baldwin & Morris, 2002; Fitch & Gossage, 2002). This priming leads to the exaggerated responses found in secondary MODS if further insult occurs (Baldwin & Morris, 2002).

The following is the sequence of events in **primary** MODS:

A. Initial organ insult or injury
B. Activation of resident macrophages/neutrophils
C. Local/mild systemic inflammation/stress response and "priming" of neutrophils and macrophages by cytokines

If further insult occurs, the sequence of events in **secondary** MODS is:

A. Primed macrophages release multiple mediators including:
   1. TNF and IL-1
   2. Endothelial damage throughout body from effects of TNF and IL-1
B. Activation of the plasma cascades in response to endothelial damage
   1. Complement cascade
      a. Anaphylatoxins C3a and C5a, which cause vasodilation by releasing histamine and promoting degranulation of neutrophils
      b. Important triggers in the exaggerated inflammatory response
   2. Kallikrein-kinin cascade
      a. Results in production of bradykinin, which causes vasodilation and decreased systemic vascular resistance (SVR)
   3. Coagulation cascade
      a. Results in microvascular thrombosis, which causes decreased microvascular circulation and further ischemic damage to organs
   4. Fibrinolytic cascade
      a. Unbalanced cascade that ends with net procoagulation state that can lead to disseminated intravascular coagulation (DIC) with pooling of clotting factors in the microvascular bed
C. Massive systemic inflammatory response develops as a result of the release of the cytokines and other inflammatory mediators
   1. Results in release of highly active neutrophils that undergo oxidation that releases oxygen- free radicals that are extremely toxic to vascular endothelium
      a. Oxygen-free radicals form toxic oxygen species that attack deoxyribonucleic acid (DNA) and cause cell membrane peroxidation that leads to tissue necrosis.
D. Neutrophils also cause release of:
   1. Protease, which directly damages endothelial cells and causes increased capillary permeability and organ damage
   2. Platelet activating factor (PAF), which causes further endothelial damage and increases number of active phagocytes, which continue the unrelenting SIRS
   3. Arachidonic acid metabolites: prostaglandins, especially prostaglandin (PGI_2), thromboxanes, especially thromboxane A_2 (TXA_2) and leukotrienes
      a. TXA_2 is a potent vasoconstrictor and PGI_2 is potent vasodilator, and the resultant release of excess amounts of these substances causes an unequal distribution of blood flow to organs.

E. Macrophages release more than 30 inflammatory mediators that perpetuate the unregulated inflammation in secondary MODS and affect all body systems
   1. Gastrointestinal mucosa is very sensitive to effects of inflammatory mediators, and loss of the gut protective barrier due to microcirculatory failure leads to the phenomenon of translocation of bacteria.
      a. Hypothesis is that these gut bacteria promote sepsis even in the face of failure to find an infectious focus in individuals with MODS
      b. Not proven in human clinical studies, but has been substantiated in animal studies
   2. Maldistribution of blood flow is a phenomenon in which there are differences in blood flow to various organs and large and capillary beds. This leads to impaired tissue perfusion and decreased oxygen supply to the cells. The lungs, splanchnic bed, liver, and kidneys are most severely affected.
      a. This leads to hyperdynamic circulation and increased cardiac output in response to increased venous return to the heart due to shunting in the capillary beds and decreased SVR. Despite the increased cardiac output, there is a net loss of oxygen delivery to the cells due to the shunting of blood away from the capillary beds. The end result is activation of TXA_2, which causes microemboli, as well as interstitial edema, making it more difficult for oxygen to enter cells because it has to travel farther to enter the cells.
F. Hypermetabolism
   1. Initially a compensatory mechanism that utilizes carbohydrate, protein, and fat metabolism to feed the body's increased energy needs, but eventually becomes detrimental
   2. Results from neurohormonal response to stress with increased release of catecholamines, cortisol, and TNF and IL-1 and results in catabolism of proteins. This results in loss of mean body mass, increased glucose levels due to gluconeogenesis by the liver, and decreased utilization of glucose by the cells. The net result is depletion of oxygen and fuel supplies.
G. Myocardial depression is not fully understood in MODS, but is thought to be a result of the effects of myocardial depressant factor (MDF), TNF, and IL-1 on myocardial contractility. Hypoxia in myocardial cells as well as alterations in β-adrenergic receptors in myocardium result in an imbalance in oxygen supply and demand, known as supply-dependent oxygen consumption
   1. Normally the amount of oxygen delivered to a cell is what the cell needs, and there is an oxygen reserve that is used if needed. In MODS this reserve is depleted, and hypoxia occurs.
   2. Compounding the hypoxia is a physiologic process called reperfusion injury, in which once blood flow is reestablished, the formerly hypoxic tissue, which had depleted its stores of ATP and converted the enzyme xanthine dehydrogenase to xanthine oxidase, releases oxygen-free radicals that attack already damaged cells. Although the oxygen-starved cells are reoxygenated, the effects of the oxygen-free radicals cause a net loss of oxygen, leading to cellular acidosis, impaired cellular function, and multiple organ failure (adapted from Baldwin & Morris, 2002).

5. How is the release of oxygen-free radicals, tumor necrosis factor (TNF), and interleukin-1 (IL-1) related to the development of MODS?

Baldwin and Morris (2002) state that the activation of neutrophils and macrophages are major causes of the sustained inflammatory response seen in MODS. The macrophages release TNF and IL-1, and they act synergistically, but TNF appears to be the primary factor in the perpetuation of the exaggerated inflammatory response. In addition, TNF produces potent metabolic symptoms such as fever, anorexia, hyperglycemia, hypermetabolism, and weight loss (Baldwin & Morris, 2002; Urden et al, 2002).

Oxygen-Free Radicals

Oxygen-free radicals, produced in excessive amounts, have been implicated as part of the reason for cellular destruction during multisystem organ failure. Normally antioxidant enzymes are present in sufficient numbers to prevent cellular destruction. However, during conditions such as sepsis and MOF, patients have depleted their antioxidant defense system and are especially vulnerable to these destructive effects. Oxygen metabolites cause lipid peroxidation and damage cell membranes like nervous system tissue that is high in lipid content. Oxygen-free radicals cause severe injury to the endothelial vascular tissue, which leads to tissue necrosis, and activate the coagulation cascade and cause damage to DNA (Carlson, 1999; Baldwin & Morris, 2002; Urden et al, 2002).

6. **What special considerations are there with children and elderly patients who are predisposed to MODS? What were Mr. Walters's predisposing factors?**

Special Considerations with Children

MODS in children usually develops from a primary, obvious insult as described in the classification of primary and secondary MODS. MODS can be identified in most children within 24 hours of hospital admission via diagnostic criteria. Once MODS is diagnosed, aggressive interventions and treatments must occur for positive outcomes. The most common initial insult that precipitates MODS in children is hypovolemic shock, which leads to organ hypoperfusion. This again sets off the exaggerated inflammatory response seen in adult MODS. Sepsis often follows as a result of hypoperfusion of the gastrointestinal (GI) tract. Mortality is not associated with ongoing sepsis and is less than that for adults with primary MODS. However, the progression of organ failure in children varies from that seen in adults. In children organ failure usually occurs in the pulmonary, cardiovascular, and neurologic systems, compared with the pulmonary, renal, and hepatic systems in the adult (Hazinski & Jenkins, 2002).

Special Considerations with Elderly Patients

Management of elderly patients with MODS is more difficult than that of younger adult patients. Physiologic changes occur in elderly patients that cause a decrease in functional reserve and an inability to compensate during periods of stress. To meet the challenge of caring for elderly patients, it is imperative that a complete and detailed physical and psychosocial history and comprehensive physical and laboratory assessments be obtained. Prevention of MODS is the most critical consideration in elderly patients. Aggressive interventions for organ preservation, management of all infectious processes, a balance of oxygen supply and demand, and the provision of nutritional support are essential for successful treatment of MODS. It is recognized that early enteral feedings help to preserve the gut microbial barrier, thus potentially preventing the translocation of bacteria that is thought to be a major factor in the ongoing SIRS found in MODS (Baldwin & Morris, 2002; Urden et al, 2002).

Mr. Walters's predisposing factors

Risk factors for MODS include preexisting conditions such as cancer and chronic illnesses, medications (steroids and nonsteroidal antiinflammatory drugs [NSAIDs]), immunosuppression, and age older than 65 years (Baldwin & Morris, 2002; Urden et al, 2002). Mr. Walters's predisposing factors included his age of 67 years, the prior surgical abdominal procedure, and the splenectomy that had been done 20 years before this admission. The diagnosis of MODS may be difficult in elderly patients because of the delay in appearance or even absence of symptoms of infection and inflammation. Rauen and Stamatos (1997) state that the first and possibly the only clinical symptom may be a change in mental status or generalized malaise. Elderly patients with the aforementioned predisposing factors who display these subtle symptoms should undergo thorough investigation for MODS.

7. **Identify assessment findings and effects of MODS on individual organ systems.**

Clinical presentation varies from patient to patient depending on the patient's underlying health, degree of organ dysfunction, number of organs involved, and progression of time. The onset of primary MODS is difficult to discern, but the development of secondary MODS follows a well-established pattern (Baldwin & Morris, 2002).

Usually, the individual sustains an insult or injury and the first 24 hours after injury are dedicated to resuscitation and stabilization of the patient. Approximately 24 hours after the injury, subtle symptoms such as low-grade fever, tachycardia, tachypnea, dyspnea, decreased mental status, and hemodynamic changes are noted (Baldwin & Morris, 2002). See Table 25-3 for an in-depth list of common clinical manifestations in MODS.

Table 25-3   *Effects of MODS on Individual Organ Systems*

Cardiovascular System
- Tachycardia
- Ventricular arrhythmias refractory to standard intervention
- Mean arterial pressure <70 mm Hg
- Pulmonary capillary wedge pressure <12 mm Hg
- Central venous pressure <8 mm Hg
- Cardiac output >8 L/min initially; later <4 L/min
- Cardiac index >4 L/min initially; later <2.5 L/min
- Peripheral edema with bounding or diminished pulses
- S_3 heart sound with auscultation
- Skin pale and warm initially; later pale, cool, and clammy

Pulmonary System
- Bradypnea or tachypnea
- Dyspnea with increased work of breathing and cyanosis
- Crackles or wheezes with auscultation
- ABG values: PaO_2 < 60 mm Hg, $PaCO_2$ >45 mm Hg, may have metabolic acidosis, respiratory alkalosis, or both
- Decreased pulmonary compliance and ARDS requiring mechanical ventilatory assistance
- Ventilator settings: frequent FiO_2 manipulation and 5 cm H_2O of PEEP
- Chest x-ray film with diffuse infiltrates (consistent with ARDS)

Renal System
- Oliguria or anuria
- Creatinine clearance <30 ml/min
- Serum osmolarity >295 mOsm/kg
- BUN >20 mg/dl
- Serum creatinine >2 mg/dl or double the serum creatinine level on admission
- Other serum electrolytes
  - Potassium >5 mEq/L
  - Magnesium <1.5 mEq/L
  - Sodium <130 mEq/L
  - Calcium <8.5 mg/dl
  - Phosphate >4.5 mg/dl

Hematologic System
- Bleeding tendencies with petechiae or purpura
- Susceptibility to infections
- Laboratory tests
  - WBCs >10,000 mm^3 initially; <5000 mm^3 later
  - Platelets <100,000/ml
  - Hematocrit and hemoglobin levels decreased
  - Prothrombin time >25% above normal
  - Activated partial thromboplastin time >25% above normal
  - Thrombin time prolonged
  - Fibrin split products >10 µg/ml

Table 25-3   *Effects of MODS on Individual Organ Systems—cont'd*

Central Nervous System
- Altered level of consciousness with a GCS score <6
- Headache with intracranial pressure >15 mm Hg
- Respiratory depression
- Hypothermia or hyperthermia

Gastrointestinal System
- Anorexia, nausea, vomiting
- Bleeding tendencies with stress ulcers and hematemesis
- Ileus with nasogastric output >600 ml/24 hr
- Diarrhea or constipation
- Guaiac-positive nasogastric output and stool
- Jaundice
- Laboratory tests
  - Bilirubin >2.0 mg/dl
  - Albumin <2.8 g/dl
  - Liver enzymes (lactic acid dehydrogenase, aspartate aminotransferase [serum glutamic-oxaloacetic transferase]) >50% above normal
  - Hyperglycemia initially and hypoglycemia later

8. Discuss collaborative management measures for MODS.

No definitive therapy exists for MODS. The goal of most treatments is supporting each dysfunctional organ system. However, treatment must be individualized for the whole patient because interventions for one system may cause harm to another system (Baldwin & Morris, 2002).

Baldwin and Morris (2002) and Urden and associates (2002) identify the following treatments for the medical treatment of MODS:

1. Early detection of the syndrome is essential.
2. Eliminate or control the initial source of infection.
3. Avoid a second insult if possible.
   a. Aggressively débriding necrotic tissue, draining abscesses, reducing the number of invasive procedures, and removing hematomas is of utmost importance in controlling infection.
4. Prevention and control of nosocomial infection are imperative.
5. Early reduction of long-bone fractures and surgical repair of injured tissue is important (adapted from Baldwin & Morris, 2002, p. 1498).

The goals of therapy are:

1. Control infection.
2. Provide adequate tissue oxygenation.
3. Restore intravascular volume.
4. Support function of individual organs (adapted from Baldwin & Morris, 2002, p. 1498).

Prevent and Control Infection

Prevention and control of infection must be given a high priority in the medical treatment and nursing care of patients with MODS. Prophylactic antibiotics should be considered once cultures are done on blood, sputum, urine, and invasive catheter tips. If fever continues with antibiotic therapy, antipyretics and a hypothermia blanket may be necessary. Other measures to prevent infection include maintenance of skin integrity, impeccable oral hygiene, and screening of visitors with active infections (Carlson, 1999).

Gastrointestinal tract function is essential in prevention of sepsis and MODS. As previously discussed, the gut hypothesis has not been proven in human trials to be a contributing factor in the development of MODS, but early enteral feedings can positively impact outcomes in MODS. The patient in the second stage of the stress response should receive 25 to 30 kcal/kg of nutritional support (Surline, 2001). The goal is to maintain a positive nitrogen balance without overfeeding. The use of the Harris-Benedict equation in determining basal energy expenditure (BEE) is important in determining nutritional needs of severely ill patients (Surline, 2001). The BEE can be calculated using the following formula:

Women: BEE = 655 + (9.6 × wt in kg) + (1.7 × ht in cm) − (4.7 × age in years)
Men: BEE = 66 + (13.7 × wt in kg) + (5 × ht in cm) − (6.8 × age in years)

Based on the number of physiologic stressors such as fever, fractures, burns, surgery, and so on, the kcal/kg requirements increase. Close monitoring of the patient's physiologic condition is essential to modify the nutritional plan as needed. Monitoring gastric output for color and amount as well as gastric alkalization with H_2-blockers and antacids is essential for complete GI stabilization.

Provide Adequate Oxygenation

Adequate oxygenation of tissues is another difficult task in patients with MODS. Carlson (1999) supports early aggressive ventilation, often with positive end-expiratory pressure (PEEP) that is aimed at keeping the PaO_2 greater than 80 mm Hg. Collaboration among nurses and respiratory therapists to institute aggressive pulmonary toilet for maximum air exchange is important. Close monitoring of oxygenation with ABG values, oximetry, or oximetric pulmonary artery catheters is required in patients with MODS. The use of paralytic agents such as vecuronium (Norcuron) with sedation may be necessary when an acceptable PaO_2 value cannot be reached. Propofol (Diprivan) is another agent that may be ideal for patients with MODS who are undergoing mechanical ventilation (Carlson, 1999).

In normal physiologic states, the oxygen consumption (VO_2) is fairly constant, and is independent of oxygen delivery (DO_2). This steady state is maintained unless DO_2 becomes seriously impaired, and then the relationship becomes one of supply-dependent oxygen consumption (Urden et al, 2002). In MODS/SIRS, the patient often develops supply-dependent oxygen consumption, and he or she becomes dependent on DO_2 rather than VO_2 (Urden et al, 2002, p. 959). This leads to oxygen debt, and tissue hypoxia results. Frequent measures of arterial lactic acid can assist clinicians in determining how severe this tissue hypoxia is (Urden et al, 2002, p. 959).

Many therapies have been used in attempts to improve oxygen delivery and reduce oxygen demand. Some of these therapies include:

- Maintaining supranormal DO_2 levels
- Sedation
- Mechanical ventilation
- Temperature and pain control
- Rest
- Prone positioning
- Lateral rotation positioning
- Increasing preload or decreasing afterload
- Extracorporeal membrane oxygenation (ECMO)
- Inhaled nitrous oxide via mechanical ventilation (adapted from Urden et al, 2002, p. 959)

To date there are no strong conclusive data supporting the use of recombinant human erythropoietin I in patients with MODS (Haslett, 1999). Maintaining adequate hemoglobin is important, and the use of red blood cell transfusions is the recommended method to increase hemoglobin levels. Despite adequate hemoglobin for oxygen carrying, unfortunately oxygen delivery to the tissues is impaired due to the microembolization that is the hallmark of MODS (Baldwin & Morris, 2002).

Support Appropriate Circulating Volume to Maximize Heart Pumping Effectiveness

Cardiovascular support, continuous cardiac monitoring, and antiarrhythmic therapy are other important areas of collaborative treatment of MODS. These interventions go hand in hand with hemodynamic monitoring and maintenance of fluid balance. Establishing an appropriate balance of circulating volume is challenging in patients with MODS. The use of aggressive invasive monitoring of hemodynamic values is the foundation for restoration of function and stabilization of both cardiovascular and renal systems. Using pulmonary artery monitoring to evaluate and adjust preload, afterload, inotropic agents, and blood oxygen content is vital to successfully maintaining cardiopulmonary status. Fluid resuscitation with crystalloid or colloid remains a debate; it should be administered with caution to avoid fluid overload. The use of diuretics and low-dose dopamine may be necessary to support renal function. Consideration must be given to adequately balancing fluids and supporting renal function. It may be necessary to initiate continuous renal replacement therapy (CRRT) and/or high-volume hemofiltration (HVHF) to nonselectively remove mediators of sepsis that perpetuate the SIRS (Reiter et al, 2002). If blood loss is significant, administration of blood products should be considered. The main complication from fluid resuscitation is pulmonary and peripheral edema. Edema is an expected consequence and is not necessarily considered a sign of intravascular volume overload (Carlson, 1999).

Support the Patient and Family

Support of the patient with MODS and the family dealing with MODS is a final and important medical and nursing collaborative measure. Because of the high mortality and use of costly available medical resources, the patient with MODS presents many ethical dilemmas. Patients and families need frequent and clear information related to progress and plan of care (Carlson, 1999). An aggressive versus a conservative approach to treatment has been shown to influence mortality (Fitch & Gossage, 2002). Because many of these patients are unable to articulate their wishes, the decision to discontinue treatment falls to the family. Advanced directives and living wills play an important role and can be used to convey the patient's wishes.

9. **What are the nursing diagnoses for the patient with MODS?**

Nursing diagnoses for MODS are numerous and may cover an entire list of problems with a high rate of occurrence or actual problems depending on the organ systems involved. Sommers (1998), Carlson (1999), and Urden and colleagues (2002) provided an extensive list of nursing diagnoses for the patient with MODS, which includes but may not be limited to the following:

- Alteration in tissue perfusion related to decreased cardiac output
- Alteration in cardiac output related to alterations in preload
- Alterations in cardiac output related to alterations in afterload
- Fluid volume deficit or excess related to fluid resuscitation requirements and third spacing
- Impaired gas exchange related to ventilation/perfusion mismatch and/or intrapulmonary shunting
- Ineffective airway clearance
- High risk for infection
- Alteration in nutrition: less than body requirements related to hypermetabolic state
- Alteration in skin integrity
- Impaired mobility
- Anxiety and/or fear

- Pain
- Ineffective thermoregulation
- Impaired communication
- Ineffective family coping

10. What ethical considerations play a role in the diagnosis of MODS?

Early in the course of the illness, Mr. Walters expressed a desire not to be intubated and to "let me just die." Despite Mr. Walters's wishes, he received many life support interventions. The question arises whether treatment was aggressive enough. The all-or-nothing philosophy applies to MODS. Conservative middle-of-the-road treatment of MODS increases mortality (Fitch & Gossage, 2002). The issue of advance directives, such as living wills and durable power of attorney, will continue to play an important role in today's health care environment. It is important that nurses be prepared to inform patients of the existence of advance directives and to assist them in developing their own before becoming critically ill and facing the possibility of not having their wishes carried out.

The role of the hospital's ethics committee cannot be overemphasized in caring for critically ill patients. When conflict exists within the family, the patient's expressed wishes, and medical treatments, the ethics committee can bring all concerned parties together to reach a resolution of the conflict that falls within accepted biolegal and bioethic standards. Nurses caring for patients with MODS should be aware of their institution's ethics committee and learn the process of how to access and use the committee's expertise.

Other ethical considerations for these patients are the rationing of health care dollars for expensive therapies and the futility of care (Clermont et al, 2001). Families and health care workers will face the fact that rehabilitation after recovery of the patient with MODS is costly, involving months of care before the patient achieves a functional level. Quality versus quantity of life issues may need to be addressed.

11. What are the future trends for the treatment of MODS?

There are several exciting new trends on the horizon in the treatment of MODS. The most promising is the use of continuous infusion of activated protein C (APC), also known as drotrecogin (Xigris). The basic mechanisms of action of APC are thought to result in a modulation of the inflammatory and coagulation pathways, as well as decreasing the suppression of fibrinolysis (Hinds, 2001). These hypotheses are supported by observations that:

1. Reduced levels of ACP are found in most patients with sepsis and are associated with an increased risk of death.
2. Giving APC was associated with greater decreases in the plasma D-dimer levels than in a placebo group during the first 7 days after the infusion was initiated, indicating a reduction in the generation of thrombin.
3. Treatment with APC decreased inflammation indicated by decreases in interleukin-6 levels. This finding confirms the known antiinflammatory activity of APC (Hinds, 2001).

Unfortunately, the cost of APC is prohibitive and the use of committees to determine appropriateness of patient selection is becoming more common (Clermont et al, 2001). There are also drawbacks to the use of APC in some clinical settings because it is known that excessive bleeding can occur in patients with predisposing conditions such as:

1. Gastrointestinal ulceration
2. Traumatic injury of a blood vessel
3. Highly vascular organ damage
4. Significant alteration in coagulation indicators such as prothrombin time and decreased platelet count to less than 30,000 mm^3 (Healy, 2002)

Other new therapies that are showing promise are:

1. The use of low-dose hydrocortisone over a 7-day period to suppress the immune system
2. Tissue factor pathway inhibitor (TFPI) that interrupts the clotting cascade at both the intrinsic and extrinsic pathways
3. Anti-TNF antibody to decrease the effects of the inflammatory mediators (Shulman, 2002)
4. Antithrombin III, also an important anticoagulant; levels of antithrombin III have been shown to be decreased in sepsis and MODS (Carlet, 2001)

MULTIPLE ORGAN DYSFUNCTION SYNDROME

References

American College of Chest Physicians/Society of Critical Care Medicine Consensus Conference Committee (1992). Definitions for sepsis and organ failure and guidelines for the use of innovative therapies in sepsis. *Critical Care Medicine, 20*(6), 864-870.

Baldwin, K. M. & Morris, S. E. (2002). Shock, multiple organ dysfunction syndrome, and burns in adults. In K. L. McCone & S. E. Huether (Eds.), *Pathophysiology: The biological basis for disease in adults and children* (4th ed., pp. 1483-1512). Philadelphia: W. B. Saunders.

Biffle, W. L. & Moore, E. E. (2000). Role of the gut in multiple organ failure. In W. C. Shoemaker, S. M. Ayres, A. Grenvik, & P. R. Holbrook (Eds.), *Textbook of critical care* (4th ed., pp. 1627-1635). Philadelphia: W. B. Saunders.

Carlet, J. (2001). Immunological therapy in sepsis. *Intensive Care Medicine, 27*, S93-S103.

Carlson, K. (1999). Multiple organ dysfunction syndrome. In L. Bucher & S. Melander (Eds.), *Critical care nursing* (pp. 1070-1087). Philadelphia: W. B. Saunders.

Clermont, G., et al. (2001). The effects of recombinant human activated protein C on hospital costs and resource use in severe sepsis. *American Journal of Critical Care Medicine, 163*, A802-A806.

Fitch, S. J. & Gossage, J. R. (2002). Optimal management of septic shock: Rapid recognition and institution of therapy are crucial. *Postgraduate Medicine, 111*(3), 53-57.

Haslett, C. (1999). *Davidson's principles and practice of medicine* (18th ed.). Edinburgh: Churchill Livingstone.

Hazinski, M. F. & Jenkins, M. E. (2002). Shock, multiple organ dysfunction syndrome, and burns in children. In K. L. McCance & S. E. Huether (Eds.), *Pathophysiology: The biological basis for disease in adults and children* (4th ed., pp. 1513-1539). Philadelphia: W. B. Saunders.

Healy, D. P. (2002). New and emerging therapies for sepsis. *The Annals of Pharmacotherapy, 36,* 648-654.

Helgeby, A. (nd). Multiple organ failure: Finding the issue. *Centrum for Gastroenterlogisk Forskning.* Retrieved from the world wide web on January 11, 2003. www.cgf.gu.se/fourapportaneman.html.

Hinds, C. J. (2001). Treatment of sepsis with activated protein C. *British Medical Journal, 323*, 881-882.

Marshall, S. J. (2001). Inflammation, coagulopathy, and the pathogenesis of multiple organ dysfunction. *Critical Care Medicine, 29*(7) (Suppl), S599-S106.

Parillo, J. E. (2000). Approach to the patient in shock. In L. Goldman & J. C. Bennett (Eds.), *Cecil textbook of medicine* (21st ed., pp. 495-502). Philadelphia: W. B. Saunders.

Piper, R. & Sibbald, W. (1997). Multiple organ dysfunction syndrome: The relevance of persistent infection and inflammation. In A. Fein, et al. (Eds.), *Sepsis and multiorgan failure* (pp. 189-207). Baltimore: Williams & Wilkins.

Rauen, C. & Stamatos, C. (1997). Caring for geriatric patients with MODS. *American Journal of Nursing, 97*(5), 16bb-16ii.

Reiter, K., D'Intini, V., Bordoni, V., & Baldwin, I. (2002). High-volume hemofiltration in sepsis: Theoretical basis and practical applications. *Nephron, 92*(2), 251-259.

Shulman, K. (2002). Current drug treatment of sepsis. *Hospital Pharmacist,* (9), 97-101.

Sommers, M. (1998). Multisystem. In J. Alspach (Ed.), *American association of critical-care nurses: Core curriculum for critical care nurses* (5th ed., pp. 715-798). Philadelphia: W. B. Saunders.

Surline, M. N. (2001). Nutritional considerations. In T. W. Barkley & C. Myers (Eds.), *Practice protocols for acute care nurse practitioners* (pp. 780-789). Philadelphia: W. B. Saunders.

Urden, L. D., Stacy, K. M., & Lough, M. E. (2002). Systemic inflammatory response syndrome and multiple organ dysfunction syndrome. In L. Thelan (Ed.), *Thelan's critical care nursing: Diagnosis and management* (4th ed., pp. 947-963). St Louis: Mosby.

Vary, T., McLean, B., & VonRueden, K. T. (2002). Shock and multiple organ dysfunction syndrome. In K. A. McQuillan, K. T. VonRueden, R. L. Hartsock, M. B. Flynn, & E. Whalen (Eds.), *Trauma nursing: From resuscitation through rehabilitation* (3rd ed., pp. 173-200). Philadelphia: W. B. Saunders.

26

Sepsis/Septic Shock

M. Lynn Rodgers, RNC, MSN, CCRN, CNRN, ACNP-BC

CASE PRESENTATION

Emergency Department

John Budd, a 72-year-old, arrived in the emergency department unconscious, with stab wounds to the upper-right abdomen and lower-right chest that were sustained in his home while fighting off a burglar. The paramedics secured two large-bore intravenous (IV) catheters in his right and left antecubital spaces and infused lactated Ringer's solution wide open in both sites. An endotracheal tube was inserted, and ventilation with a resuscitation bag at 100% oxygen was begun. Medical antishock trousers (MAST) were in place. Pressure dressings to both wounds were secured.

A 5-cm (2-inch) stab wound to his right lower chest and a 7.5-cm (3-inch) stab wound to his upper-right abdomen were inspected. Chest tubes were inserted into the upper-right and lower-right midaxillary regions. Immediately, 500 ml of red drainage returned via the lower chest tube. His heart rate (HR) was 125 bpm, and the monitor showed sinus tachycardia without ectopy. His blood pressure (BP) was 70/50 mm Hg. Inserting a Foley catheter resulted in drainage of 400 ml clear, dark yellow urine. After infusion of more than 2000 ml of lactated Ringer's solution, Mr. Budd was sent to surgery, still in a hypotensive state. Preoperative body weight was 74 kg (165 lb).

Surgical Intervention

During surgery, a right thoracotomy and right abdominal laparotomy were performed. The right chest wound was explored, and a lacerated intercostal artery was ligated. Exploration of his upper-right abdominal wound revealed more extensive damage. The liver and the duodenum were lacerated. Extensive hemorrhage and leaking of intestinal contents were apparent after opening the peritoneum. Mr. Budd's injuries were repaired, the peritoneal cavity was irrigated with antibiotic solution, and incisional sump drains were placed in the duodenum.

During the 4-hour surgery, Mr. Budd received 6 U of blood and an additional 3 L of lactated Ringer's solution. A pulmonary artery catheter (PAC) and right radial arterial line were inserted.

Intensive Care Unit: Immediately after Surgery

When Mr. Budd arrived in the surgical intensive care unit (ICU), he was receiving ventilatory support. Ventilator settings were as follows:

Assist	mode
Rate	12
Fio_2	60%
V_T	800 ml

Vital signs and hemodynamic parameters immediately after surgery were the following:

BP	92/52 mm Hg
HR	114 bpm
Respirations	12 breaths/min
Temperature	36.2° C (97.2° F)
PAP	20/8 mm Hg
PCWP	6 mm Hg
CVP	4 mm Hg
CO	5 L/min
CI	2.9 L/min/m^2
SVR	1040 dynes/sec/cm^{-5}

Arterial blood gas values were normal. Except for a white blood cell (WBC) count of $13.6 \times 103/mm^3$ and a hemoglobin level of 10 g/dl, Mr. Budd's other laboratory values were within normal limits.

ICU: Postoperative Day 1

Mr. Budd remained drowsy and received ventilatory support for 24 hours. His pain was controlled by IV morphine sulfate. The nasogastric tube (NGT) continued to drain large amounts of green fluid, and an incisional duodenal sump tube drained large amounts of greenish brown fluid. His chest and abdominal dressings remained dry. Breath sounds were diminished on the right side but clear on the left. His chest tubes continued to drain small amounts of bloody fluid. Urine output was 40 to 60 ml/hr. His abdomen was slightly firm and distended, and he had no bowel sounds.

ICU: Postoperative Day 2

Mr. Budd's condition remained stable until his second postoperative day. At this time he became difficult to arouse but did respond to commands. His respirations were 28 breaths/min, shallow, and labored. His urine output dropped to 20 ml/hr. His skin became warm, dry, and flushed. Other clinical data included the following:

BP	80/50 mm Hg
HR	132 bpm
Temperature	36.2° C (97.2° F)
PAP	14/7 mm Hg
PCWP	4 mm Hg
CVP	2 mm Hg
CO	8 L/min
CI	4.7 L/min/m^2
SVR	560 dynes/sec/cm^{-5}
WBCs	22,000/mm^3
Glucose	270 mg/dl

Culture and sensitivity reports from wound drainage indicated gram-negative bacilli. Appropriate IV antibiotics were administered, as well as IV hydrocortisone and naloxone (Narcan). A pharmacy consultation to formulate and calculate nutritional needs was done, and total parenteral nutrition was started. To prepare for the suspected hyperdynamic phase of septic shock, infusion of lactated Ringer's solution was increased to 150 ml/hr, and dopamine at 5 µg/kg/min was started with a concentration of 200 mg/250 ml of 5% dextrose in water (D5W).

ICU: Postoperative Day 6

By the sixth postoperative day, Mr. Budd's condition had deteriorated dramatically. His skin was cool, mottled, and moist. His sclerae were yellow tinged. He no longer responded to stimuli. A norepinephrine (Levophed) drip infused at 6 µg/min with a concentration of 4 mg/250 ml of D5W, along with a dopamine drip at 2 µg/kg/min was begun. His monitor showed sinus tachycardia with short runs of ventricular tachycardia. ST-segment elevation, T-wave inversion, and the development of Q waves over most of the anterior V leads on his electrocardiogram (ECG). A 75 mg bolus of lidocaine was given followed by a continuous infusion at 2 mg/min with a concentration of 2 g/500 ml of D5W. His breath sounds revealed crackles throughout his chest. Urinary output was only 3 to 5 ml/hr and was grossly bloody. His abdomen was enlarged and firm. His abdominal suture lines had dehisced, and the peritoneum could be seen. The duodenal sump and NGT drainage started to turn red. All arterial and venous puncture sites began oozing blood. Further clinical data included the following:

BP	70/52 mm Hg
HR	140 bpm
Respirations	14 breaths/min
Temperature	35.8° C (96.4° F)
PAP	44/26 mm Hg
PCWP	24 mm Hg
CVP	8 mm Hg
CO	2 L/min
CI	1.1 L/min/m^2
SVR	2000 dynes/sec/cm^{-5}

Other abnormal laboratory results included the following:

pH	7.14
Pco_2	49 mm Hg
Po_2	46 mm Hg
Sao_2	85%
HCO$_3^-$	12 mmol/L
Lactic Acid	3.0 mEq/L
Na$^+$	152 mmol/L
K$^+$	5.9 mmol/L
Creatinine	3.4 mg/dl
Amylase	290 U/L
Lipase	3.9 U/L
ALT (SGOT)	100 U/L
AST (SGPT)	82 U/L
FDP	39
Platelets	75,000/mm^3
PT	22 sec
PTT	98.5 sec
Fibrinogen	130 mg/dl
CK	640 U/L
Troponin I	>50

Final Developments

Despite attempts to reduce afterload with sodium nitroprusside (Nipride) and increase contractility with dobutamine (Dobutrex), Mr. Budd's hemodynamic status failed even further. When his cardiac rhythm deteriorated into ventricular fibrillation, resuscitation efforts were unsuccessful. An autopsy revealed several small abscessed areas in the lung, acute hepatic failure, multiple hemorrhagic areas, and an acute myocardial infarction (MI).

SEPSIS/SEPTIC SHOCK

QUESTIONS

1. Discuss the magnitude of bacteremia and sepsis in hospitalized patients and the relationship between these two diagnoses.

2. What are the risk factors for infection and development of septic shock? Identify those that applied to Mr. Budd.

3. Discuss the rationale for use of a PAC in monitoring septic shock.

4. What organisms most commonly cause septic shock? In which sites is infection most often seen?

5. What pathophysiologic processes occur with septic shock? What are the effects of these processes on the patient's vascular tank, volume, and pump?

6. Discuss clinical, laboratory, and therapy changes that occurred on Mr. Budd's second postoperative day.

7. What is the rationale for each of the following therapeutic modalities ordered for Mr. Budd on the second postoperative day?

> IV rate increased to 150 ml/hr
> Dopamine 5 μg/kg/min
> Steroids
> Naloxone IV infusion
> Total parenteral nutrition

8. Discuss the clinical changes that occurred during Mr. Budd's sixth postoperative day.

9. What is the rationale for each of the following therapeutic modalities ordered on the sixth postoperative day? How many milliliters per hour should be infused for each drug listed?

> Norepinephrine 6 μg/min
> Dopamine 2 μg/kg/min
> Lidocaine 2 mg/kg/min

10. What are the reasons for the changes in the following hemodynamic parameters noted on the sixth postoperative day?

> SVR
> CO/CI
> PCWP

11. Interpret Mr. Budd's blood gas levels on the sixth postoperative day.

12. Why are the renal, liver, and pancreatic laboratory values reported on the sixth postoperative day abnormal?

13. What complications do the hematologic laboratory values suggest?

14. What would account for the ECG changes described?

15. Mr. Budd's liver was lacerated during the stabbing. What effect, if any, did this have on his eventual outcome?

16. Describe the differences in the parameters below between hyperdynamic or warm septic shock and hypodynamic or cold septic shock.

	Hyperdynamic	**Hypodynamic**
LOC		
BP		
HR		
Respirations		
Pulse Pressure		
Skin		
SVR		
CO/CI		
Urine Output		

17. How do elderly patients manifest symptoms of sepsis?

18. What antimicrobial and antiendotoxin therapies should be instituted in sepsis?

19. What does the future hold for therapy in septic shock?

SEPSIS/SEPTIC SHOCK

QUESTIONS AND ANSWERS

1. **Discuss the magnitude of bacteremia and sepsis in hospitalized patients and the relationship between these two diagnoses.**

    In 1992 the American College of Chest Physicians (ACCP) and the Society of Critical Care Medicine (SCCM) developed standardized definitions for sepsis and related conditions with the continuum extending from bacteremia, sepsis, and severe sepsis to finally septic shock. These organizations defined bacteremia as the presence of live bacteria in the bloodstream. Bacteremia does not always create systemic complications or lead to sepsis. *Systemic inflammatory response syndrome (SIRS)* is a systemic reaction to infection as evidenced by two or more of the following (Parrillo, 2000; Munford, 2001):

Temperature	>38° C (100.4° F) or <36° C (96.8° F)
HR	>90 bpm
Respiratory Rate	>20/min or $Paco_2$ <32 mm Hg
WBC count	>12,000/mm^3 or <4000/mm^3 or >10% band forms

    In December 2001, the ACCP, SCCM, American Thoracic Society, and European Society of Intensive Care Medicine met and expanded this list of signs and symptoms to include chills, decreased urine output, decreased skin perfusion, poor capillary refill, skin mottling, decreased platelet count, petechiae, hypoglycemia, and unexplained change in mental status.

    When a confirmed systemic response to infection is associated with SIRS, sepsis has developed. Sepsis can be caused by pathogens other than bacteria, such as fungi, viruses, and protozoa (Munford, 2001). Mortality is highest, however, when sepsis is associated with confirmed bacteremia. Regardless of the causative organism, sepsis can result in systemic complications that occur as circulating chemical mediators released by the inflammatory response compromise the patient's cardiovascular system (Cunha, 2003). Severe sepsis occurs when hypoperfusion, hypotension, and organ dysfunction develop. If hypotension and perfusion abnormalities, lactic acidosis, oliguria, and acute onset of mental deterioration occur despite aggressive fluid resuscitation and inotropic therapy, septic shock is present (Munford, 2001).

    Septic shock is the most common cause of deaths in the ICU and the thirteenth leading cause of death in the United States (Devine & Cunnion, 2000). Each year sepsis develops in 400,000 to 800,000 patients, resulting in septic shock in 200,000 patients (Jones & Bucher, 1999; Parrillo, 2001). The economic burden of sepsis and septic shock is extensive, estimated at $16.7 billion annually in the United States (Ely et al, 2003). The incidence of death from sepsis has actually increased over the past 15 years despite the development of advanced treatments and new antibiotics (Munford, 2001). Increased virulence of organisms, mutated antibiotic-resistant organisms, weakened host resistance, and the aging of our population are all factors in the losing battle against sepsis (Chambers, 2003). Mortality from sepsis is reported to be 20% to 50%, and death from septic shock is estimated to be 40% to 70% or higher (Devine & Cunnion, 2000; Munford, 2001). Unfortunately 60% to 79% of all deaths from sepsis occur in the geriatric population (Ely et al, 2003).

2. **What are the risk factors for infection and development of septic shock? Identify those that applied to Mr. Budd.**

    Risk factors for infection and development of septic shock are patient and/or treatment related (Urden et al, 2002). Patient-related risk factors include burns, trauma, malnutrition, leukemia, age older than 70 years or newborn, debilitating diseases (especially chronic lung disease, cardiovascular disease, diabetes mellitus, or renal or liver failure), pregnancy, sleep deprivation, immunocompromised states, and response to physiologic and psychologic stressors. Most cases of sepsis originate from microbes that usually do not cause disease in hosts with normal immune defenses (Munford, 2001). Treatment-related risk factors include foreign body insertion, drugs (especially immunosuppressives, cytotoxins, and antibiotics), artificial airways, surgery, immobility, and hospital understaffing. Mr. Budd had the following risk factors: IV infusion, endotracheal tube, chest tube, Foley catheter, PAC and right radial arterial line, abdominal trauma, age older than 70 years, and leaking of gastrointestinal contents into the peritoneum.

3. **Discuss the rationale for use of a PAC in monitoring septic shock.**

A PAC is often used for monitoring patients with severe septic shock and is helpful for differentiating the type of shock. Munford (2001) suggests that invasive interventions such as a PAC may actually contribute to increased morbidity and mortality in patients with septic shock and should not be used routinely. Cardiovascular and metabolic abnormalities can be readily determined from the hemodynamic profile obtained from the PAC. Appropriate pharmacologic, medical, and nursing treatments can be determined by careful analysis of this information. Monitoring the patient's response further assists in adjusting treatment for maximal response.

Septic shock has two distinct phases: hyperdynamic and hypodynamic (Urden et al, 2002). Initially a hyperdynamic response occurs. During this phase, systemic vascular resistance (SVR) is decreased. An increase in cardiac muscle contractility also develops as a compensatory mechanism. The decrease in SVR and increase in cardiac contractility result in abnormally high cardiac output (CO) and cardiac index (CI). In addition, pulmonary artery and capillary wedge pressures (PAWP and PCWP, respectively) can be below normal because of the venous vasodilatation and decreased venous return.

During the hypodynamic phase of septic shock, compensatory mechanisms begin to fail. Fluid escapes the vascular tree into the tissues because of an increase in capillary permeability. Sympathetic nervous system stimulation causes profound vasoconstriction. The heart muscle itself is depressed, and contractility decreases. Hypotension then results from decreased intravascular volume, increased SVR, and decreased cardiac contractility. CO and CI are decreased; however, PAWP and PCWP are increased. Treatment is guided by the hemodynamic information that a PAC provides. With this information, the patient's chances of survival are increased (Urden et al, 2002).

4. **What organisms most commonly cause septic shock? In which sites is infection most often seen?**

Bacteria are the most common causes of septic shock. In the past, gram-negative bacteria were overwhelmingly the organisms most likely to cause septic shock, specifically *Escherichia coli, Klebsiella, Enterobacter, Serratia, Pseudomonas aeruginosa, Bacteroides,* and *Proteus.* Incidence of gram-negative sepsis is at 40% to 50% (Parrillo, 2000; Munford, 2001). However, the incidence of sepsis caused by gram-positive bacteria such as *Staphylococcus aureus, S. epidermidis, Streptococcus pyrogenes, Listeria,* and pneumococcal pathogens has risen to almost equal that of gram-negative bacteria and is reported at 25% to 31% (Parrillo, 2000; Munford, 2001).

In 1998, a 40-year review of the literature by Friedman, Silva, and Vincent revealed interesting historical information concerning septic shock. Before 1990, the primary source of infection in sepsis was the abdomen. From 1991 through 1997 this source had changed to the chest, with the abdomen becoming the second most common site. The urogenital system has remained the third most common site of infection in sepsis; however, in the elderly it is the most common site of sepsis (Ferri, 2001).

5. What pathophysiologic processes occur with septic shock? What are the effects of these processes on the patient's vascular tank, volume, and pump?

Once a microbial infection develops, a general but complex inflammatory response develops, resulting in increased capillary permeability and blood flow (Urden et al, 2002). These responses allow immunologic cells to migrate toward the site of infection, begin phagocytic actions, and activate the complement system. Once the complement system is activated, more WBCs come to the site of the infection and as many as 40 inflammatory mediators are released. Cytokines are one of the primary mediators that signal other cells to release additional mediators such as tumor necrosis factor-α (TNF-α) interleukin (IL)-1, IL-6, IL-8, interferon, leukotrienes, histamine, bradykinin, prostaglandins, thromboxane A_2, serotonin, nitric oxide, arachidonic acid, platelet-activating factor (PAF), oxygen-free radicals, and myocardial depressant factor (Parrillo, 2000; Munford, 2001). If the invading organism is a gram-negative bacterium, endotoxins are also released, which further stimulate the production of these inflammatory mediators (Jones & Bucher, 1999).

Sepsis also results in complex coagulopathies. Inflammatory mediators, previously described cause activation of intrinsic and extrinsic clotting pathways. Thrombosis, intravascular fibrin deposits, and bleeding develop. Inhibitory pathways of protein C and protein S are impaired or depleted, and clotting increases. Fibrinolysis is decreased due to increases in plasminogen activator inhibitor levels. Coagulation factors are depleted, and bleeding worsens. Disseminated intravascular coagulation (DIC) may result (Munford, 2001),

The three major effects of septic shock within the cardiovascular system are (1) vasodilatation, (2) maldistribution of blood volume, and (3) myocardial depression. Two interacting factors result in vasodilatation in septic shock (Carpati et al, 1999; Munford, 2001). First, a loss of vascular reaction to sympathetic nervous system stimulation occurs and, second, production of substances from the endothelial lining relaxes the vascular smooth muscle layer of the vessels (Urden et al, 2002). Profound dilation in the arterial and venous circulation results, and decreases in SVR and preload develop. Initially, compensation occurs by an increase in CO. However, tissue perfusion continues to decrease due to maldistribution of blood flow and impaired cardiac function (Parrillo, 2000).

Maldistribution of blood flow develops as a consequence of blood volume displacement from intravascular areas to extracellular spaces. Although septic shock is usually associated with vasodilatation, pulmonary, renal, hepatic, splenic, and pancreatic vasoconstriction occurs with associated organ dysfunction. Increased capillary permeability allows serum to migrate into the interstitial spaces. Parenchymal edema in the pulmonary, cardiac, and renal vascular beds results in functional failure of these organs. The interstitial fluid shift also depletes the circulating volume and increases blood viscosity. Blood flow becomes sluggish, WBCs and platelets accumulate, and microemboli develop. Vascular occlusion and inadequate tissue perfusion progress. Anaerobic metabolism with elevations in lactic acid levels leads to metabolic acidosis. Hotchkiss and colleagues (1999) postulated that cellular stress response during septic shock results in down-regulation or hibernation of the cell with a shift to fetal gene expression. Through these actions the cell reverts to a lower energy-using state and avoids death. Unfortunately only enough energy is produced to keep the individual cells alive but not enough to continue whole organ function. Multiorgan failure eventually results.

Although the exact mechanism of the septic inflammatory response is unclear, various mediators are thought to depress the function of the myocardium. Some findings suggest that microvascular and myocyte damage depresses the myocardial function and affects the responsiveness of the myofilament to calcium. Other studies found evidence that the myocardium is hyporesponsive to catecholamines because of impaired β-adrenergic receptor stimulation of cyclic adenosine monophosphate. Still other researchers found indirect evidence of specific myocardial depressant substances (Carpati et al, 1999). Regardless of the mechanism, the depressed myocardium meets no resistance in the profoundly vasodilated systemic vascular bed. Thus CO and CI initially are maintained and often are increased.

In summary, the common cardiovascular patterns demonstrated initially in septic shock consist of high CO, low SVR, decreased left ventricular ejection fraction, a dilated left ventricle, and a normal or increased stroke volume. Death is usually a result of hypotension, which results from a progressively increasing SVR, a perpetual decrease in CO, and eventual multiple organ system failure. Management of septic shock must include (1) eliminating the primary site of infection with surgical drainage or antimicrobials, (2) aggressively treating the cardiovascular, respiratory, and other organ dysfunction of failure, and (3) inhibiting septic mediators.

6. **Discuss clinical, laboratory, and therapy changes that occurred on Mr. Budd's second postoperative day.**

Difficult to Arouse

Difficult to arouse is an early cardinal sign of systemic infection and inflammatory response to circulating endotoxins. In a patient with sepsis, the level of consciousness continues to deteriorate with impending shock as a result of decreased cerebral perfusion (Parrillo, 2000). Those with prior neurologic deficits and who are elderly are more likely to experience more pronounced neurologic effects (Munford, 2001).

Respiration 28 breaths/min, shallow and labored

The lungs become a target organ as septic shock progresses. Circulating endotoxins cause deterioration of the patient's pulmonary status, as the initial pulmonary response to endotoxins creates bronchoconstriction. Pulmonary edema as a result of increased capillary permeability occurs. Tachypnea is also an early cardinal sign of systemic infection, hypoxemia, and physiologic stress (Munford, 2001).

Urine output decreased to 20 ml/hr

As renal blood flow in the patient in septic shock is reduced, urine output decreases. Antidiuretic hormone and aldosterone are released to increase intravascular water and sodium in an attempt to maintain CO and renal blood flow, often with no success. Acute tubular necrosis from capillary injury and hypotension contribute to renal failure. In addition, aminoglycoside antibiotics, frequently effective in sepsis, are nephrotoxic.

Warm, dry, flushed skin

In the early stages of septic shock, vasoactive mediators create a flushed appearance because of peripheral vasodilatation. This early stage is known as *hyperdynamic* or *warm septic* shock (Urden et al, 2002).

BP 80/50 mm Hg

Hypotension commonly is caused by the vasodilatation when cardiac compensation fails.

HR 132 bpm

Tachycardia is another early cardinal sign of a systemic infection and inflammatory response. An increase in heart rate is also a compensatory mechanism to maintain perfusion and CO (Urden et al, 2002).

Temperature (36.2°C) (97.2°F)

Fever is one of the cardinal signs of infection and inflammation. However, over one third of patients with sepsis may be normothermic or hypothermic (Munford, 2001).

CI 4.7 L/min/m^2; SVR 560 dynes/sec/cm^{-5}

The initial hyperdynamic pattern of septic shock consists of high CI as a result of low SVR. Toxic bacterial endotoxins are thought to decrease the vasomotor tone of the blood vessels by activating the release of endorphins and histamine and the complement system.

WBCs 22,000/mm³

Leukopenia is an early finding in an immunocompromised patient with sepsis. However, as sepsis progresses, the inflammatory response signals the bone marrow to accelerate leukocyte synthesis and release. Consequently, the WBC count will increase to more than 10,000/mm³. In addition abnormalities in neutrophils can develop, inducing toxic granulations, Döhle-Amato bodies, or cytoplasmic vacuoles (Munford, 2001).

Glucose level 270 mg/dl

The reaction of the adrenal cortex to shock is to release glucocorticoids. The glucocorticoids release glucagon. Glucagon stimulates the conversion of glycogen to glucose (glycolysis) and gluconeogenesis in the liver. Therefore, the serum glucose level may be elevated. Regulating glucose levels with insulin infusion can reduce morbidity and mortality (Ely et al, 2003).

Culture and sensitivity reports indicate gram-negative bacilli

Gram-negative bacteria are the organisms that account for 60% of sepsis in adults. Gram-positive bacteria are the causative organisms 35% of the time, with fungi and other organisms at 5% (Chambers, 2003). Three blood cultures from different sites should be obtained before starting antimicrobials. Up to 20% to 40% of blood cultures for sepsis from a single site will be negative. Three different samples increase the chance of finding organisms by 95% (Chambers, 2003).

7. **What is the rationale for each of the following therapeutic modalities ordered for Mr. Budd on the second postoperative day?**

IV Rate Increased to 150 ml/hr

Restoration of adequate intravascular volume is an important aspect of patient care during episodes of hypotension. Vasodilatation during sepsis dramatically decreases preload and afterload. The vascular tree is too large for the circulating volume. The circulating volume is also further decreased because increased capillary permeability allows fluid to escape into interstitial spaces (Munford, 2001).

Dopamine 5 µg/kg/min

The severe vasodilatation developing during the hyperdynamic phase of septic shock must be addressed. Low-dose dopamine increases cardiac output and renal blood flow, creates a moderate pressor effect, and improves cardiac performance (Ferri, 2001).

Steroids

Use of corticosteroids is controversial and should be reserved for patients in septic shock who have a suspected or documented adrenal insufficiency. These patients more likely have refractory hypotension (Munford, 2001). According to Briegel and associates (1999) infusion of steroids reduced the length of vasopressor therapy and resulted in earlier resolution of organ dysfunction related to sepsis. Mortality of patients with sepsis or septic shock who receive corticosteroids may not be significantly reduced and in some cases may be higher owing to development of secondary infections.

Naloxone (Narcan) IV infusion

Naloxone is a narcotic antagonist generally used to reverse the respiratory depression caused by narcotics. As described by Jones and Bucher (1999), naloxone is now given to patients with severe septic shock before compensatory mechanisms cease. Its primary action is to block opioid receptors and other receptors that mediate vasodilatation. Levels of endogenous endorphins and myocardial depressant factor are reduced, thereby combating vasodilatation and decreased contractility.

Total parenteral nutrition

Because of the disruption of Mr. Budd's gastrointestinal system, tube feedings were not feasible. Nutrition via parenteral means was required. Uehara and colleagues (1999) studied resting energy expenditure during the first week after onset of severe sepsis and found it drastically increased to 40% greater than normal. Further findings indicated that activity energy expenditure increased by three to four times normal requirements. Finally, overall total energy expenditure can increase to 50 to 60 kcal/kg/day with severe sepsis.

8. **Discuss the clinical changes that occurred during Mr. Budd's sixth postoperative day.**

As described by Parrillo (2000), the following clinical changes occur as septic shock progresses.

Cool, Mottled, Moist Skin

The skin indicates the change from hyperdynamic (warm) to hypodynamic (cold) septic shock. This is a poor prognostic sign for the patient because it indicates failure of the compensatory mechanisms.

Yellow Sclerae

As chemical mediators continue to shunt blood to various organs, the patient's liver and kidneys become hypoperfused. Hyperbilirubinemia and jaundice are common clinical indicators that the liver is adversely affected. In addition, Mr. Budd's liver was lacerated during his injury.

ECG Changes—Sinus Tachycardia with Short Runs of Ventricular Tachycardia

Sinus and ventricular tachycardia indicate further myocardial damage from the circulating endotoxins and the decreased CO. Because the kidneys are hypoperfused, the patient may be experiencing acute renal failure. The K^+ level of 5.9 mmol/L could suggest acute renal failure or adrenal insufficiency and is probably responsible for the ventricular tachycardia (Ferri, 2001). The 12-lead ECG indicated a massive anterior wall MI.

BP 70/52 mm Hg, CO 2 L/min, CI 1.1 L/min/m², PAP 44/26 mm Hg, PCWP 24 mm Hg, SVR 2000 dynes/sec/cm⁻⁵, CVP 8 mm Hg

Mr. Budd's hemodynamic changes are classic indications of the hypodynamic phase of septic shock. Afterload is drastically increased, and contractility is decreased. Multisystem failure is imminent (Ely et al, 2003).

Respirations 14/min, Congested Breath Sounds

Mr. Budd's respiratory assessment indicates further deterioration of respiratory status caused by circulating endotoxins, pulmonary edema, and left ventricular failure (Urden et al, 2002).

Temperature 35.8° C (96.4° F)

The low temperature is another indication that septic shock has progressed from hyperdynamic to hypodynamic (Devine & Cunnion, 2000).

Abdomen Large and Firm, Wound Dehiscence

Because of increased capillary permeability, accumulation of inflammatory fluids, and cardiac failure, ascites is present. The increased intraabdominal pressure and poor healing produced wound dehiscence.

9. **What is the rationale for each of the following therapeutic modalities ordered on the sixth postoperative day? How many milliliters per hour should be infused for each drug listed?**

   Norepinephrine 6 µg/min = 22.5 ml/hr

   Norepinephrine is indicated for hemodynamically significant hypotension unresponsive to other vasopressors.

   Dopamine 2 µg/kg/min = 11.25 ml/hr

   Dopamine at 1 to 3 mg/kg/min dilates the renal and mesenteric vessels. Norepinephrine constricts the renal and mesenteric vessels, and adding low dosages of dopamine counteracts some of this effect.

   Lidocaine 2 mg/kg/min = 30 ml/hr

   Lidocaine was started to decrease the ventricular irritability, which is evidenced by the ventricular tachycardia and most likely is caused in part by the K^+ level of 5.9 mmol/L.

10. **What are the reasons for the changes in the following hemodynamic parameters noted on the sixth postoperative day?**

    SVR

    The SVR increased from 560 to 2000 dynes/sec/cm^{-5}. Clinically the SVR represents the resistance against which the left ventricle must pump to eject its volume. This elevation indicates a change from hyperdynamic to hypodynamic septic shock (Urden et al, 2002).

    CO and CI

    The CO decreased from 8 to 2 L/min, and the CI decreased from 2 to 1.1 L/min/m^2 on the sixth postoperative day. Because CO represents the amount of blood pumped by the ventricle in 1 minute, it can be concluded that an increase in SVR will decrease the CO and CI. A drop in CO and CI indicates that hypodynamic septic shock has developed (Munford, 2001).

    PCWP

    The PCWP increased from 4 to 24 mm Hg, indicating an increase in the pressure in the left side of the heart. This could be from the ventricular dilation and decreased ejection fraction that occur in late septic shock and from the release of various chemical and hormonal mediators that depress myocardial function.

11. **Interpret Mr. Budd's blood gas levels on the sixth postoperative day.**

    Mr. Budd's blood gas levels indicate metabolic and respiratory acidosis. Lactic acidosis caused by increased oxygen debt from abnormal cellular metabolism is a common finding in patients with septic shock. During the progression of septic shock, a ventilation-perfusion mismatch also develops as chemical mediators create pulmonary interstitial edema and a maldistribution in pulmonic blood flow. In addition, localization of activated neutrophils in the microvasculature of the pulmonary system is thought to contribute to the sepsis-induced pathologic lung damage (Munford, 2001).

12. **Why are the renal, liver, and pancreatic laboratory values reported on the sixth postoperative day abnormal?**

    As described by Urden and colleagues (2002), the kidneys, liver, brain, and lungs are the organs most frequently affected by septic shock. As renal blood flow is reduced, urine output decreases, and the body is unable to eliminate waste products. Acute renal failure ensues. As chemical mediators continue to shunt blood to various organs, the liver and pancreas become hypoperfused. Shock liver and acute cholestatic jaundice are common. DIC is an ominous complication that occurs most often in sepsis caused by gram-negative organisms.

Sepsis increases procoagulant effects, early fibrinolysis, and plasminogen activator inhibitor 1 protein and decreases antithrombin III anticoagulation activity (Jones & Bucher, 1999). Laboratory results of liver function and clotting factors reflect development of DIC. The increased lactic acid level is also significant because this indicates the severity of perfusion failure and oxygen debt and is associated with impending death.

13. What complications do the hematologic laboratory values suggest?

Possible complications based on the hematologic laboratory values include acute renal and hepatic failure, DIC, adult respiratory distress syndrome, and acute MI (Gawlinski et al, 1999).

14. What would account for the ECG changes described?

Mr. Budd's ECG changes could indicate an acute anterior wall MI. This diagnosis can be made by the ST-segment elevation, T-wave inversion, and diagnostic Q waves evident in the V anterior chest leads. His elevated creatinine kinase, troponin I, and aspartate amino-transferase levels verified the diagnosis (Urden et al, 2002).

15. Mr. Budd's liver was lacerated during the stabbing. What effect, if any, did this have on his eventual outcome?

Patients at greatest risk for development of septic shock are those who have sustained open wounds, open fractures, massive tissue injury, or significant head injury. The lacerated liver was directly related to the acute hepatic failure noted on the autopsy.

16. Describe the differences in the parameters below between hyperdynamic or warm septic shock and hypodynamic or cold septic shock.

Jones and Bucher (1999) and Urden and associates (2002) summarized the differences in the hyperdynamic and hypodynamic stages of septic shock as follows:

	Hyperdynamic	Hypodynamic
LOC	Mental cloudiness	Continued deterioration
BP	Normal to just below baseline	Profound hypotension
HR	Bounding pulses, tachycardia	Thready pulse, tachycardia
Respirations	Decreased rate or mild respiratory distress	Decreased rate with severe respiratory complications
Pulse Pressure	Normal to wide	Narrow
Skin	Warm, dry	Cool, moist, mottled
SVR	Decreased	Increased
CO/CI	Increased	Decreased
Urine Output	Normal	Decreased

17. How do elderly patients manifest symptoms of sepsis?

Many elderly patients demonstrate blunted responses to sepsis. Temperature elevations may only be primary to secondary, or hypothermia may develop. Elevations in WBC counts may not occur; however, a shift to the left may be seen, indicating an increase in the number of immature cells. Cell-mediated immunity is also decreased as evidenced by a decrease in T-cell production. Elderly patients also demonstrate a decrease in physiologic reserve. Cardiovascular compensatory mechanisms are decreased because the usual response to catecholamine release with tachycardia and vasoconstriction does not readily occur in elderly patients. Colonization of the lungs with infective organisms with resulting pneumonia is more common and occurs more quickly in elderly patients with sepsis. Nonspecific signs and symptoms such as delirium, decreased functional status, anorexia, vomiting, incontinence, urinary frequency or oliguria, or hypotension may be present. The most common presenting symptom of sepsis in elderly patients, although nonspecific and elusive, is a sudden mental status change. This vague picture of sepsis in elderly patients accounts for delayed treatment, increased severity of sepsis, and resulting high mortality (Munford, 2001).

18. What antimicrobial and antiendotoxin therapies should be instituted in sepsis?

Selection of antimicrobials should be based on site of infection and causative organism. Antimicrobials such as imipenem (Primaxin), polymycin B, and meropenem. Other effective antiendotoxin therapies have recently been developed. Drotrecogin (Xigris) is an activated protein C drug that interferes with microvascular coagulation. Interference with clotting in the coagulation cascade is thought to decrease the multiorgan damage that results in death. It also has antiinflammatory and profibrinolytic properties (Ely et al, 2003). It is costly ($8600 for 4 days of treatment) and is reserved for the most severe cases of sepsis. Cost effectiveness is less when long-term life expectancy is poor. The recent Recombinant Human Activated Protein C Worldwide Evaluation in Severe Sepsis Study (PROWESS) demonstrated, however, that signs and symptoms of SIRS decrease and morbidity and mortality from multiorgan dysfunction syndrome is decreased with use of drotrecogin (Ely et al, 2003).

19. What does the future hold for therapy in septic shock?

Research on septic shock therapy is targeted at neutralizing or preventing damage from the many inflammatory mediators. Development and testing of several endotoxin antibodies such as IL-1 receptor agonists, anti-TNF antibodies or binders, and PAF receptor antagonists are in progress. Drugs to alter host response to endotoxins, to bind endotoxins, and control inflammatory mediators are under investigation (Munford, 2001). Medications that decrease stimulation of the complement pathway such as C1 esterase inhibitor and heparin are being used. Coagulation control using such substances as heparin, antithrombin III, heroin, protein C, or thrombomodulin demonstrates some effectiveness against DIC, which is a prevalent complication of severe septic shock. The use of pentoxifylline and monoclonal antibodies to decrease leukocyte adherence has produced mixed clinical outcome results. Defense boosting with antiproteases, antioxidants, growth hormone, and vaccines is being explored (Urden et al, 2002).

      Because of the complex nature of the body's inflammatory response, the ability of researchers to influence the course of sepsis and septic shock remains disappointing. The dose and timing of various interventions may be crucial. Many researchers too narrowly focus their approach on only single-agent therapies when multiple agents may need to be considered for an optimal outcome. In addition, much has been written on the medical-ethical consequences of the specific therapies for sepsis (Morris, 2003). Several of the potential treatments are extremely costly, and insurance plans may refuse payment. At what price do we treat the patient with sepsis? How can we as a society get the best value for our health care dollars?

      Withholding proven medical treatment on the basis of financial reimbursement presents several ethical issues (Cunha, 2003). Some interventions may actually increase morbidity and mortality in some patients. Much is yet to be learned about the treatment of this devastating disease process. Truly, treatment of sepsis and septic shock will remain a medical research priority and an ethical dilemma in the 21st century.

SEPSIS/SEPTIC SHOCK

References

Briegel, J., Forst, H., Haller, M., Schelling, G., Killer, E., et al. (1999). Stress doses of hydrocortisone reverse hyperdynamic septic shock: A prospective, randomized, double-blind, single-center study. *Critical Care Medicine, 27*(4), 723-732.

Carpati, C. M., Astiz, M. E., & Rackow, E. C. (1999). Mechanisms and management of myocardial dysfunction in septic shock. *Critical Care Medicine, 27*(2), 231-232.

Chambers, H. F. (2003). Infectious diseases: Bacterial and chlamydial. In L. M. Tierney, S. J. McPhee & M. A. Papadakis (Eds.), *2003 Current medical diagnosis and treatment.* New York: Lange Medical Books/McGraw-Hill.

Cunha, B. A. (2003). Bacteremia and sepsis. In R. E. Rakel & E. T. Bope (Eds.), *Conn's current therapy 2003.* Philadelphia: W. B. Saunders.

Devine, M. A. & Cunnion, R. E. (2000). Sepsis syndrome. In R. M. Wachter, L. Goldman, & H. Hollander (Eds.), *Hospital medicine.* Philadelphia: Lippincott Williams & Wilkins.

Ely, E. W., Kleinpell, R. M., & Goyette, R. E. (2003). Advances in the understanding of clinical manifestations and therapy of severe sepsis: An update for critical care nurses. *American Journal of Critical Care, 12*(2), 120-133.

Ferri, F. F. (2001). *Practical guide to the care of the medical patient.* St Louis: Mosby.

Friedman, G., Silva, E., & Vincent, J. (1998). Has the mortality of septic shock changed with time? *Critical Care Medicine, 26*(12), 2078-2086.

Gawlinski, A., McCloy, K., Caswell, D., & Quinones-Baldrich, W. J. (1999). Cardiovascular disorders. In A. Gawlinski & D. Hamwi (Eds.), *Acute care nurse practitioner clinical curriculum and certification review.* Philadelphia: W. B. Saunders.

Hotchkiss, R. S., Swanson, P. E., Freeman, B. D., Tinsley, K. W., Cobb, J. P., et al. (1999). Apoptotic cell death in patients, with sepsis, shock, and multiple organ dysfunction. *Critical Care Medicine, 27*(7), 1230-1251.

Jones, K. M. & Bucher, L. (1999). Shock. In L. Bucher & S. Melander (Eds.), *Critical care nursing.* Philadelphia: W. B. Saunders.

Morris, P. E. (2003). Meeting unmet needs in patients with sepsis: the role of drotrecogin alfa (activated). *American Journal of Critical Care, 12*(2), 94-97.

Munford, R. S. (2001). Sepsis and septic shock. In Braunwald, E. (Ed.), *Harrison's principles of internal medicine.* New York: McGraw-Hill.

Parrillo, J. E. (2001). Shock syndromes related to sepsis. In E. Goldman, L. Bennett, & J. Claude (Eds.), *Textbook of internal medicine* (21st ed.). Philadelphia: W. B. Saunders.

Uehara, M., Plank, L. D., & Hill, G. L. (1999). Components of energy expenditure in patients with severe sepsis and major trauma: A basis for clinical care. *Critical Care Medicine, 27*(7), 1295-1302.

Urden, L. D., Stacy, K. M., & Lough, M. E. (Eds.) (2002). *Thelan's critical care nursing: Diagnosis and management* (4th ed.). St Louis: Mosby.

27

Burns

Ann H. White, RN, PhD, MBA, CNA

Kevin Lewis, 21 years old, was involved in an industrial fire. Mr. Lewis was welding a steel structure when a spark from his torch ignited a barrel of flammable material that was inadvertently placed in his work area. Mr. Lewis sustained full-thickness burns over the upper half of his chest and circumferential burns to both arms. He also sustained superficial partial-thickness burns to his face, neck, and both hands. His entire abdomen, upper half of his back, and front of his upper legs sustained deep partial-thickness burns.

He was transported to a small community hospital where two intravenous (IV) lines were started, a Foley catheter and nasogastric tube were inserted, and humidified oxygen at 3 L/min was started through a nasal cannula. He was given mannitol 12.5 g IV before being transported to a major burn center. Vital signs immediately before transport were as follows:

BP	136/84 mm Hg
HR	96 bpm
Respirations	24 breaths/min
Temperature	37.2° C (99° F) (oral)

Mr. Lewis's preburn weight was 72 kg (160 lb). He was received in the burn unit 4 hours after sustaining the burn injury. At admission to the burn unit, Mr. Lewis was alert and oriented, and his vital signs were as follows:

BP	140/90 mm Hg
HR	110 bpm
Respirations	24 breaths/min
Temperature	36.1° C (97° F) (oral)

Mr. Lewis's lungs were clear in all fields on auscultation, and he had an occasional productive cough of a small amount of carbon-tinged sputum. His voice was becoming hoarse. No bowel sounds were heard, and the nasogastric tube was draining dark yellow-green liquid. Peripheral pulses were obtained with a Doppler stethoscope because they could not be palpated manually. The Foley catheter was draining burgundy-colored urine. Urine output totaled 280 ml since the insertion of the Foley catheter 4 hours before. Fluid resuscitation efforts since the burn injury included 4 L of lactated Ringer's solution through the

IV lines. The following laboratory results were determined after Mr. Lewis's arrival in the burn unit:

Complete blood count

WBCs	$12 \times 10^3/mm^3$
RBCs	$34.8 \times 10^6/mm^3$
Hgb	12.8 g/dl
Hct	52%

Arterial blood gases (on 3 L of oxygen)

pH	7.37
Pco_2	35 mm Hg
Po_2	105 mm Hg
HCO_3^-	18 mmol/L
Sao_2	99%

SMAC 20

Na^+	151 mmol/L
K^+	5.2 mmol/L
Cl^-	112 mmol/L
BUN	22 mg/dl
Creatinine	1.6 mg/dl

Additional bloodwork

Myoglobin (RIA)	90 ng/ml
Carboxyhemoglobin	6%

Urinalysis revealed the following:

Specific Gravity	1.040
Glucose	+1
Ketones	Trace
Blood	Trace
Protein	Trace

The burn unit physician performed a fiberoptic bronchoscopy, which showed minimal redness of the glottis and no edema. Escharotomies were performed on both arms immediately after admission to the burn unit. Mr. Lewis was bathed, his scalp was shaved, and his burns were dressed in occlusive silver sulfadiazine (Silvadene) dressings. His burns were then dressed twice a day with silver sulfadiazine. The following regimen was prescribed: ranitidine (Zantac) 150 mg IV push every 12 hours; antacid 30 ml every hour instilled through a nasogastric tube and clamped for 15 minutes for the first 48 hours after the burn; and morphine sulfate 3 mg IV push every hour as needed for pain.

Bowel sounds returned on day 3, the nasogastric tube was removed, and a high-calorie, high-protein diet was begun. On day 5 of the hospital stay, Mr. Lewis was taken to surgery for the first of a series of surgical procedures to excise and graft the areas of full-thickness injury with split-thickness autografts. The donor sites included his buttocks and the backs of his legs. Mr. Lewis was discharged from the hospital after a 65-day hospital stay with follow-up and rehabilitation scheduled.

BURNS

QUESTIONS

1. Discuss the pathophysiology of burns, including the classification of burn depth and severity of burn injury.

2. Using the rule of nines and the Lund and Browder chart, calculate the percentage of total body surface area (TBSA) burned. Based on the TBSA percentage and depth of burn, how would you classify Mr. Lewis's burn?

3. Describe the initial assessment and stabilization of a burn victim at the scene of the injury and in the emergency department.

4. Describe the three phases of burn physiology, including a discussion of the effects on the following systems during the emergent and acute phases: cardiovascular, respiratory, immune system, gastrohepatic, genitourinary, and neurologic.

5. Based on Mr. Lewis's preburn weight, use the Parkland formula to calculate the fluid requirement for adequate resuscitation.

6. What significance, if any, would the administration of mannitol have on fluid resuscitation?

7. What assessment findings would indicate myoglobinuria? Describe the treatment protocol for myoglobinuria.

8. What assessment findings are critical to establishing the presence of an inhalation injury? Which of Mr. Lewis's assessment findings warrant concern?

9. Describe the treatment protocol of a burn patient with an inhalation injury or a suspected inhalation injury.

10. What is the purpose of escharotomies?

11. Discuss pain management in the treatment protocol for the patient with a burn injury.

12. Using the Curreri formula for nutrition, calculate Mr. Lewis's nutritional needs. Discuss the need for a high-calorie, high-protein diet.

13. Discuss burn wound care and dressing techniques. Include the types of topical antimicrobial agents commonly used in wound care, listing advantages and disadvantages of each.

14. Describe the types of biologic and synthetic dressings used in wound care.

15. Discuss the use of autografts and the nursing care required.

16. Describe the appropriate care for donor sites.

17. Discuss the splinting/positioning required for Mr. Lewis to maintain use of his extremities and upper body.

18. List the nursing diagnoses, outcomes, and interventions appropriate for the care of the patient with a burn injury during the emergent and acute phases of burn physiology.

19. Discuss the psychosocial aspects of caring for the patient with a burn injury and the impact on the patient's support system.

BURNS

QUESTIONS AND ANSWERS

The skin is the largest organ of the human body and consists of two layers: the epidermis and dermis (Huether, 2002). The epidermis is composed of avascular cells that act to protect the body from the environment. The dermis contains the structures of the skin, including blood vessels, glands, hair follicles, nerves, and capillaries that bring nourishment to the epidermis and sensory fibers. The skin serves to maintain body temperature, control evaporation and fluid loss, produce vitamin D, and protect the body against the environment (Huether, 2002). A burn injury results in the loss of all or portions of the epidermis and dermis and the associated functions.

Experts estimate that 1.25 million people in the United States sustain a burn injury each year with approximately 50,000 to 70,000 people hospitalized for a burn injury annually (Kagan, 2000; Cohen & Moelleken, 2003). A burn injury, although directly affecting the skin, also has dramatic effects on every system in the body.

1. Discuss the pathophysiology of burns, including the classification of burn depth and severity of burn injury.

A burn injury results in the coagulation of cellular proteins in the cells of the skin. The denaturation of protein is produced by the heat or actual contact from a thermal, chemical, electrical, or radiation exposure (Greenfield, 1999). The coagulation of the cellular proteins leads to irreversible cell injury with local as well as systemic inflammatory responses. At the local level, the cells are devitalized, resulting in loss of the sodium-potassium pump and release of free radicals, and the protein is destroyed (Cornwell, 2001). Systemic response to a burn injury results in the release of cell and inflammatory mediators including bradykinin, histamine, prostaglandins, tumor necrosis factor, interferon, and interleukins (Cohen & Moelleken, 2003). The release of these substances leads to increased capillary permeability and alteration of the cell membrane resulting in cell death.

Types of Burns

Thermal burn

A thermal burn is a heat-related injury produced through exposure to hot liquids, steam, flames from a fire, or direct contact with some heat source. This exposure disrupts the function of the skin and its appendages. The extent or severity of this disruption depends on the length of contact time with the heat source, extent of tissue exposed to the heat source, and ability of the heat source and tissue to dissipate the heat (Greenfield, 1999).

Chemical burn

A chemical burn causes denaturation of the protein through actual contact of the chemical with the skin. The extent of the damage depends on the chemical, the chemical's action, the concentration of the chemical, and the length of contact of the chemical with the skin (Baldwin & Morris, 2002). The chemical will continue to burn the skin until totally removed from the body.

Electrical burn

Although electrical burns account for only about 5% of all of the burns sustained, these burns have a much higher mortality rate than the other types of burns because of the severity of the tissue damage (Greenfield, 1999). Electrical injuries may result from exposure to high-voltage power lines or faulty electrical wiring. Lightning is also a form of an electrical burn (Cornwell, 2001). There may be minimal damage to the skin, but the structures under the skin, including muscles, nerves, blood vessels, and bones, may sustain extensive damage because of the amount of heat produced as the electrical current passes through the body.

Table 27-1	*Classification of Burn Depth*			
		Partial Thickness		
	Superficial	**Superficial**	**Deep**	**Full Thickness**
Morphology	Destruction of epidermis (no other layers involved)	Destruction of epidermis and minimal dermis	Destruction of epidermis and dermis; skin appendages (e.g., hair follicles) intact	Destruction of epidermis and dermis; loss of skin appendages and possible loss of subcutaneous tissue
Skin function	Intact	Absent	Absent	Absent
Tactile and pain sensors	Intact	Intact	Diminished	Absent
Blisters	May be present after 24 hr	Fluid-filled blisters appear immediately after injury	Usually not present, eschar formation	Not present, eschar formation
Appearance of wound	Redness of area with local edema	Moist, pink, or mottled red	Mottled with areas of waxy white, dry surface; absence of blanching	Thick, leathery eschar; white, cherry red, or brown-black; blood vessels may be thrombosed
Healing time	3-5 days	21-28 days	30+ days	Will not heal
Scarring	None	Low incidence; may be influenced by genetic predisposition	High incidence due to slow healing; may be influenced by genetic predisposition	High incidence; depends on time of grafting and surgical techniques used

Modified from McCance, K. & Huether, S. (2002). *Pathophysiology: The biologic basis for disease in adults and children* (4th ed., p. 1500), St Louis: Mosby.

Radiation burn

Radiation burns may result from exposure to radiation therapy as a treatment modality for certain types of cancer or industrial exposure to certain types of equipment (Cornwell, 2001). These burns are typically localized, and damage depends on the amount of radiation exposure. Sunburn, due to prolonged exposure to ultraviolet rays, can also be identified as a form of radiation burn (Cornwell, 2001).

Classification of Burn Depth

Traditionally burns have been classified as first, second, and third degree. Today, burns are described as superficial, partial thickness, and full thickness. Table 27-1 describes each type of burn and the common characteristics of each.

Severity of Burn Injury

The American Burn Association (ABA) established guidelines to determine the severity of the burn injury. These guidelines rate a burn as minor, moderate, or major, depending on the person's age, areas of the body involved in the burn injury, and the TBSA burned (Cornwell, 2001). A minor burn for adults usually has a small surface area (less than 10% to 15% of the TBSA), with no involvement of the face, hands, feet, or perineum, and can

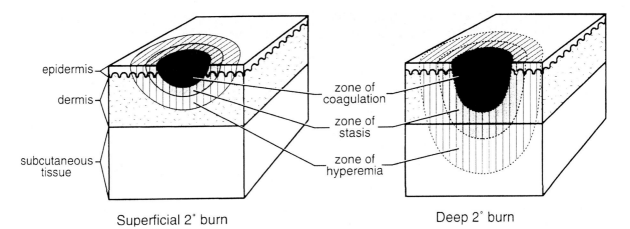

Figure **27-1**   A diagrammatic rendition of Jackson's three zones of burn injury. If the zone of stasis progresses to necrosis, the potential for conversion of partial-thickness injury to full-thickness injury exists. *(From Williams, G. [2002]. Pathophysiology of the burn wound. In D. N. Herndon [Ed.], Total burn care [2nd ed.]. London: W. B. Saunders.)*

be treated in the home environment. A moderate burn injury has a larger surface area (usually 15% to 25% of the TBSA), including partial- and full-thickness burns. A major burn has a TBSA of more than 25% of the TBSA, including partial- and full-thickness burns. Any burns involving parts of the face, hands, feet, or perineum are included in this category. Electrical burns and inhalation injuries regardless of TBSA percent are also considered major burns. Moderate and major burn injuries should be treated in a burn center or a critical care area with expertise in the care of patients with burns.

Three concentric zones of injury and their impact on the severity of the burn injury have also been described (Greenfield, 1999). The *zone of hyperemia* is the least damaged area and typically heals in 3 to 5 days. The *zone of stasis* is the area in which tissue perfusion is compromised. If resuscitative methods are effective in returning tissue perfusion, the tissue may survive. The *zone of coagulation* is the area of permanent burn injury that is characterized by cellular death. Figure 27-1 depicts the three concentric zones of a burn injury.

2. **Using the rule of nines and the Lund and Browder chart, calculate the percentage of total body surface area (TBSA) burned. Based on the TBSA percentage and depth of burn, how would you classify Mr. Lewis's burn?**

The two methods most commonly used to determine the TBSA of the burn injury are the rule of nines and the Lund and Browder chart (Cornwell, 2001). To ensure adequate fluid resuscitation, an accurate estimate of the TBSA must be obtained. Only partial- and full-thickness burns are calculated as part of the burn injury.

The rule of nines is most commonly used at the site of the burn injury by emergency medical technicians or paramedics and in the emergency department. This method quickly provides an estimate of the TBSA so that fluid resuscitative efforts can begin. It should be noted here that because of differences in proportion of body surface areas, two forms of the rule of nines are available. One form should be used for adults and a second form for children. The form used in this case presentation is for adults only.

The Lund and Browder method is a more accurate estimate of the burn injury, but it takes longer to complete. This method is used in most burn centers because a more accurate determination of the burn injury is needed. Many times the burn percentage or depth of burn will need to be changed 24 to 48 hours after the burn injury due to eschar removal and resolution of the huge fluid shifts initially seen in the first 24 hours of the burn injury. The Lund and Browder method provides a means to revise the chart as necessary to accurately reflect the burned percentage.

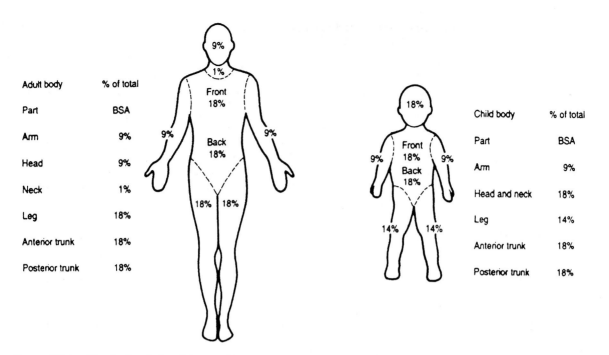

Adult body	% of total
Part	BSA
Arm	9%
Head	9%
Neck	1%
Leg	18%
Anterior trunk	18%
Posterior trunk	18%

Child body	% of total
Part	BSA
Arm	9%
Head and neck	18%
Leg	14%
Anterior trunk	18%
Posterior trunk	18%

Figure **27-2**   The "rule of nines" is useful in estimating the extent of burn injury. Note the differences between adults and children. BSA, Body surface area. *(From Micak, R.P. & Buffalo, M.C. [2002]. Pre-hospital management, transportation, and emergency care. In D. N. Herndon [Ed.],* Total burn care *[2nd ed.]. London: W. B. Saunders.)*

Figures 27-2 and 27-3 depict the rule of nines and the Lund and Browder charts. Based on the information provided in the case presentation, Mr. Lewis sustained a 65% TBSA burn. According to the ABA classification of burn injuries, Mr. Lewis sustained a major burn injury because of the amount of TBSA involved in the burn and the location of the burns around the neck and face.

3. Describe the initial assessment and stabilization of a burn victim at the scene of the injury and in the emergency department.

The care received at the site of the burn injury is critical. The basic concern at the scene of a burn injury is to stop the burning process. With a thermal burn, the flames must be extinguished and the clothing and jewelry removed. Articles of clothing should be removed if there is concern that the clothing may be smoldering and continuing to burn the injured person. If the clothing is embedded in the burn, trying to remove the clothing may not be warranted (Wiebelhaus & Hansen, 2001). With a chemical burn, the victim must be removed from the source of the chemical agent. Any clothing that came in contact with the chemical agent should be removed immediately. If safe, any dry chemical may be brushed off prior to irrigation. Once that is accomplished, copious amounts of water should be used to flush the chemical from the skin. In most cases, trying to find an antidote for the chemical is not advised (Greenfield, 1999). While the antidote is being sought, the chemical continues to burn the skin and valuable time is lost. The victim of an electrical injury should be removed from the source of the electricity as soon as possible. A major concern during this effort is to keep the rescuer from becoming a part of the circuit and sustaining an electrical injury as well.

Wiebelhaus and Hansen (2001) developed a protocol for the immediate management of burns that includes removing the person from the fire; tending to the trauma maintaining airway, breathing, and circulation (ABCs) and observing for life-threatening injuries; address airway and breathing needs first followed by maintaining circulatory status. A quick assessment of level of consciousness using an AVPU mnemonic was suggested and includes

BURN ESTIMATE AND DIAGRAM
AGE vs AREA

Area	Birth 1 yr.	1-4 yr.	5-9 yr.	10-14 yr.	15 yr.	Adult	2°	3°	Total	Donor Areas
Head	19	17	13	11	9	7				
Neck	2	2	2	2	2	2				
Ant. Trunk	13	13	13	13	13	13				
Post. Trunk	13	13	13	13	13	13				
R. Buttock	2¹/₂	2¹/₂	2¹/₂	2¹/₂	2¹/₂	2¹/₂				
L. Buttock	2¹/₂	2¹/₂	2¹/₂	2¹/₂	2¹/₂	2¹/₂				
Genitalia	1	1	1	1	1	1				
R. U. Arm	4	4	4	4	4	4				
L. U. Arm	4	4	4	4	4	4				
R. L. Arm	3	3	3	3	3	3				
L. L. Arm	3	3	3	3	3	3				
R. Hand	2¹/₂	2¹/₂	2¹/₂	2¹/₂	2¹/₂	2¹/₂				
L. Hand	2¹/₂	2¹/₂	2¹/₂	2¹/₂	2¹/₂	2¹/₂				
R. Thigh	5¹/₂	6¹/₂	8	8¹/₂	9	9¹/₂				
L. Thigh	5¹/₂	6¹/₂	8	8¹/₂	9	9¹/₂				
R. Leg	5	5	5¹/₂	6	6¹/₂	7				
L. Leg	5	5	5¹/₂	6	6¹/₂	7				
R. Foot	3¹/₂	3¹/₂	3¹/₂	3¹/₂	3¹/₂	3¹/₂				
L. Foot	3¹/₂	3¹/₂	3¹/₂	3¹/₂	3¹/₂	3¹/₂				
						TOTAL				

Cause of Burn _____

Date of Burn _____

Time of Burn _____

Age _____

Sex _____

Weight _____

BURN DIAGRAM

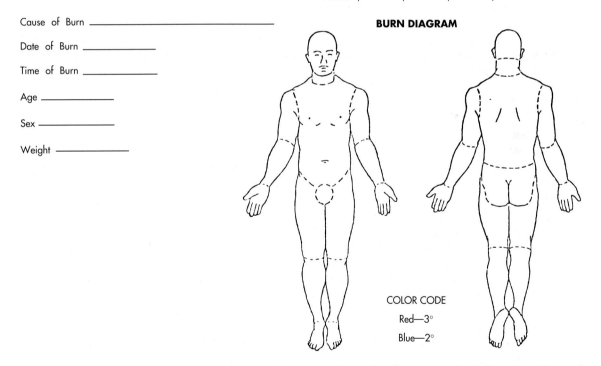

COLOR CODE

Red—3°

Blue—2°

Figure **27-3**   This is the burn diagram based on the Lund and Browder chart using the Berkow formula to take into account the anatomic and age differences in body size. Regional differences in body surface are calculated based on age. This diagram is also used to map the patient's extent of injury and color code depth of injury for partial-thickness and full-thickness burns. *(Courtesy Intermountain Burn Center, University of Utah.)*

A (Alert and orients), V (responds to Verbal stimuli), P (responds to painful stimuli only), and U (Unresponsive) (Wiebelhaus & Hansen, 2001, p. 3). Once critical life-threatening issues are managed, further information can be obtained using the AMPLE history approach. AMPLE asks questions about Allergies, all types of Medications, Past medical history, Last meal, and Event about the injury (Wiebelhaus & Hansen, 2001, p. 3).

A burn victim should receive the same management as any other trauma victim. Maintaining the ABCs is paramount, followed by an assessment of any other types of injury. Evaluation of circulatory status includes checking the peripheral pulses to ensure adequate perfusion to all the extremities. A burn victim is usually alert and oriented. If there is a change in the person's mental status or if the person is disoriented or confused, other types of injury must be investigated.

Once the burn victim's condition is stabilized, he or she should be transported to the closest facility. If the burn injury is moderate or major, the preference is to transport the person to a burn center. When the burn victim reaches the emergency department or burn center, a thorough head-to-toe assessment should be conducted (Cornwell, 2001). A complete history, including allergies, current medications, immunizations (current tetanus), and drug and tobacco use, should be completed. Baseline laboratory data should also be collected. The initial results may be normal but it is necessary to compare subsequent lab results as the patient progresses through the phases of the burn injury. The emergency department of a hospital without a burn center should be in immediate contact with a burn center to coordinate transporting the burn victim to the center and to provide effective treatment of the burn injury.

4. **Describe the three phases of burn physiology, including a discussion of the effects on the following systems during the emergent and acute phases: cardiovascular, respiratory, immune system, gastrohepatic, genitourinary, and neurologic.**

The first phase of burn physiology is the emergent, or shock phase. This phase typically lasts 24 to 48 hours and is a crucial period for the patient. The second phase begins when diuresis is noted and lasts until wound closure. This phase is referred to as the acute, or fluid resuscitation phase. The third and last phase is the rehabilitation phase. This phase should begin immediately after the burn injury to help maintain or restore function and cosmetic appearance so the patient can function in society (Cornwell, 2001).

Emergent, or Shock Phase

During the emergent phase the patient experiences a type of hypovolemic shock. This shock is the result of increased capillary permeability, which permits the shift of fluid from the plasma to the interstitial spaces. Direct cell damage increases capillary permeability, permitting the escape of large amounts of fluid, electrolytes, protein, and debris. Changes in capillary permeability begin within 30 minutes of the thermal injury, and fluid and electrolyte losses peak within 6 to 8 hours of the burn injury and usually persist for up to 24 hours after the injury (Greenfield, 1999). In addition, the fluid regulators, including the osmotic and hydrostatic pressures and the sodium pump, are lost. The cumulative effect of the loss of these regulatory mechanisms is hypovolemic shock, also referred to as *burn shock*. These rapid fluid shifts affect every system in the body.

Cardiovascular System

The cardiovascular system responds to the hypovolemic shock by attempting to compensate for the massive loss of fluid. Catecholamines are released, decreasing cardiac output and increasing peripheral resistance in an attempt to increase the fluid volume in the vascular system. Ultimately, if fluid resuscitation efforts are not initiated, cardiac output is further decreased and there is hemoconcentration of blood cells with diminished perfusion to major organs (Greenfield, 1999).

Respiratory System

The respiratory system may sustain an inhalation injury (see questions 8 and 9). Even if an inhalation injury is not sustained, lung compliance may decrease as a result of the extensive injury, and pulmonary care similar to that required for an inhalation injury may be necessary (Cornwell, 2001).

Immune System

In the immunologic system, the mechanical barrier response and the cellular immune response are lost. Loss of the mechanical barrier means a loss of the body's ability to protect itself from invading organisms. Immediately after the injury, the arachidonic acid cascade and the inflammatory cytokine cascade are activated (Greenfield, 1999). Changes in the leukocytes, neutrophils, and macrophages are also noted (Baldwin & Morris, 2002). The final result is that the body loses powerful mechanisms to protect itself from invading organisms. Infection is one of the greatest concerns in a patient with a burn injury. Because of colonization of bacteria on the burn wound itself and loss of the defense mechanisms to fight against this colonization, a massive infection can develop in a patient with a burn injury.

Gastrohepatic System

The gastrohepatic system responds to a burn injury by shutting down, which results in the development of a paralytic ileus. This response probably is a result of the decrease in perfusion of this system and the endocrine response to the trauma (Greenfield, 1999). Another concern is the development of stress ulcers. With the neurologic and endocrine responses to injury (release of catecholamines, etc.), burn patients are at high risk for the erosion of the gastric and intestinal lining.

Genitourinary System

The genitourinary system responds by decreasing kidney function through secretion of antidiuretic hormone and renal vasoconstriction. The body attempts to use compensatory mechanisms to offset the hypovolemia. In this case, the kidneys may be compromised because of the extensive loss of fluid volume in the vascular system. Adequate fluid resuscitation to maintain effective kidney function is vital.

Neurologic System

Burn patients should typically be alert and oriented. If the burn victim is confused or disoriented, identifying the cause of this decrease in level of consciousness is imperative. Assessment findings should include ruling out other injuries including a possible head injury, hypovolemia, and the potential for inhalation of drugs or noxious gases/substances that may have altered the person's response (Hilton, 2001).

Acute, or Fluid Resuscitation Phase

The second phase of burn physiology is the acute, or fluid resuscitation phase. This phase begins when the return of fluid control effects diuresis. The eschar begins to separate, and the focus of care turns to the preparation of the wound for healing or grafting. The cardiovascular system begins to stabilize because capillary permeability decreases, and fluid shifts are less severe. Cardiac output and lymphatic system functions return to normal. The respiratory system may be prone to development of pulmonary edema or pneumonia because of the massive fluid shifts and hospitalization. Patients with previous cardiovascular or pulmonary disease are more likely to develop respiratory problems. The patient remains immunosuppressed, and all efforts to prevent any type of infection should continue.

The gastrohepatic system begins to function, which leads to the concern for adequate nutritional intake. An additional concern is the development of stress ulcers. Careful monitoring of the gastric contents, stool, and any emesis for blood is imperative. The use of antacids and histamine-receptor antagonists to prevent the occurrence of stress ulcers is critical. Renal function should return. However, careful monitoring of kidney function is imperative as the body attempts to excrete waste products and debris from the burn injury. Renal failure is a possibility at this stage as well.

Rehabilitation Phase

The rehabilitation phase focuses on the return of the patient to his or her previous roles and responsibilities in society. With adequate fluid resuscitation efforts and care in the first two stages, the systems will have stabilized by the time the patient enters the third phase.

5. **Based on Mr. Lewis's preburn weight, use the Parkland formula to calculate the fluid requirement for adequate resuscitation.**

The Parkland formula permits the calculation of fluid needs for the first 24 hours immediately after the burn injury (Hilton, 2001). However, this formula calculates the fluid need of crystalloids only:

> 4 ml of isotonic volume replacement × kg of body weight × % TBSA burned
> (exclude superficial burns)

Mr. Lewis's fluid need based on 65% TBSA burned is 4 ml × 72 kg × 65% TBSA = 18,720 ml of fluid in the first 24 hours. Half the fluid (9360 ml) should be infused during the first 8 hours after the burn. This time is calculated from the *time of the actual burn injury,* not from the time the patient is first seen by medical personnel (Hilton, 2001). Therefore it is essential that the critical care nurse know the actual time of the injury and the amount of fluid that has been infused before the patient arrives in the unit. (Note: For this case, 4 L had been infused thus far, and a total of 9.36 L must be infused. The nurse has 4 hours to infuse the remaining 5.36 L.) The remaining half of the fluid requirement is then infused over the next 16 hours.

Lactated Ringer's solution without dextrose is the crystalloid solution most often used to provide a balanced salt solution. Because a burn injury affects the fluid and electrolyte balance of the body, the amount and type of IV fluid is important. In the first 24 hours after a burn injury, the capillary permeability is increased and the selectivity is decreased (Cornwell, 2001). Because of these physiologic changes in the capillary seal, large amounts of fluid shift from the intravascular space, leading to the loss of osmotic pressure and with it the body's ability to pull fluid back into the intravascular space. These changes lead to hypovolemic shock and massive edema. Additional fluid is lost through the burn injury itself in the form of wound drainage and evaporation.

The destruction of the cells in a burn injury also leads to a loss of electrolytes during the first 24 hours. The loss of sodium and potassium is of greatest concern. The sodium loss is the result of the fluid shifts and the cellular destruction. Potassium is lost into the extracellular fluid because of the cellular destruction.

Replacement therapy focuses on maintenance of the patient's condition until the capillary permeability and selectivity are restored. As stated earlier, lactated Ringer's solution is the IV solution of choice because the composition of this solution closely resembles the composition of the fluid being lost. Table 27-2 compares the composition of lactated Ringer's solution and the extracellular fluid.

The use of colloids (albumin or fresh frozen plasma) during the first 24 hours continues to be controversial. As capillary integrity is restored, colloids may be infused to aid in the reestablishment of the fluid regulators, including osmotic and hydrostatic pressures. However, colloids are not usually infused until after the first 24 hours or the patient is considered "capillary sealed" (capillary integrity has been restored) (Baldwin & Morris, 2003). Each burn unit will have an accepted fluid resuscitation protocol to maintain the cardiovascular status.

Table 27-2	*Comparison of Ringer's Lactated Solution and Extracellular Fluid*	
Electrolyte	**Lactated Ringer's Solution (mmol/L)***	**Extracellular Fluid (mmol/L)†**
Na^+ (mmol/L)	130	135-145
K^+ (mmol/L)	4	3.5-5.5
Cl^- (mmol/L)	109	96-106
HCO_3^- (mmol/L)	28	20-30

Modified from Lewis, S., Heitkemper, M., & Dirksen, S. (Eds.). (2000). *Medical-surgical nursing*, St Louis: Mosby.
*Normal value ranges may differ slightly between clinical laboratories.
†Plus 80 to 100 ml of free water per liter.

An important consideration when calculating fluid requirements for the patient with a burn injury is to understand that these formulas are guidelines. The patient's urine output and vital signs must be monitored carefully with the age and response of the patient taken into consideration. The rate of fluid administration must be adjusted according to the patient's needs.

Hourly urine output is the most valuable parameter to assess the adequacy of fluid resuscitation and renal perfusion. Hourly outputs should range from 0.5 to 1 ml/kg of body weight for adults (Hilton, 2001). Typically this results in an hourly output of 30 to 50 ml of urine. If no prior renal disorder is present, hourly outputs less than 0.5 ml/kg may indicate hypovolemia.

6. **What significance, if any, would the administration of mannitol have on fluid resuscitation?**

Mannitol functions as an osmotic diuretic to increase water excretion by osmotic action (Horne & Bond, 2000). Mannitol is administered to maintain urinary output adequate to prevent acute renal failure during trauma such as a burn injury. Also, osmotic diuretics are sometimes recommended when there is evidence of myoglobinuria, which necessitates the flushing of the kidneys to prevent sludging and possible acute tubular necrosis (Greenfield, 1999). The major problem with this treatment approach is the absolute need for accurate measurement of hourly urine output. As presented in question 5, careful monitoring of the patient with a burn injury is required to ascertain fluid resuscitation needs. Hourly urine outputs are the major parameter in this monitoring. If an osmotic diuretic is administered, the burn unit staff treating the patient has no way of knowing if the urine output is a result of adequate fluid resuscitation or infusion of the osmotic diuretic.

Typically osmotic diuretics should be used only as a last resort in an attempt to protect the kidneys. Adequate fluid resuscitation should maintain kidney functioning. If assessment findings support the presence of myoglobinuria, the amount of IV fluids administered should be increased first to flush out the kidneys and prevent sludging of the myoglobin. If forced diuresis is attempted, the patient must be monitored carefully for fluid overload, especially elderly patients and those with previous cardiac or renal diseases.

7. **What assessment findings would indicate myoglobinuria? Describe the treatment protocol for myoglobinuria.**

Myoglobin is a pigment released when muscle tissue is damaged and may be evident with large thermal or electrical burn injuries. Myoglobin is a fairly large molecule that the body attempts to excrete through the kidneys. However, myoglobin has a tendency to sludge in the kidneys. If inadequate amounts of urine are produced, sludging may occur. Acute tubular necrosis may result from the kidneys' inability to remove the myoglobin.

Assessment findings that would indicate the presence of myoglobin in the urine include the TBSA of the burn, the type of burn injury, and the color of the urine produced. Urine that contains myoglobin is usually a burgundy to rust color. Mr. Lewis sustained a large (65%) TBSA thermal burn. Also when Mr. Lewis arrived at the burn unit, the color of his urine was burgundy. Both assessment findings indicate a high possibility for the presence of myoglobin in the urine.

Two treatment protocols are available to ensure adequate urine output to flush the myoglobin from the kidneys. The first option is adequate fluid resuscitation. With a possibility of myoglobin in the urine, the hourly output should be greater than 30 ml to ensure the flushing of the kidneys. The urine output may need to be increased to 100 ml/hour to protect the kidneys (Laskowski-Jones, 1999). Patient response to the fluid resuscitation must also be monitored. The patient's cardiovascular, respiratory, and renal systems must be able to withstand the amount of fluids required to sustain the target hourly urine output.

A second option is the use of osmotic diuretics. Mannitol, administered intravenously with the dosage based on body weight, is usually the drug of choice. The decision to administer an osmotic diuretic must be made cautiously because it destroys the validity of the hourly urine output measurement.

8. **What assessment findings are critical to establishing the presence of an inhalation injury? Which of Mr. Lewis's assessment findings warrant concern?**

The extent of pulmonary injury depends on the heat of the inhaled gases, the agent inhaled such as steam or smoke, the concentration of toxic substances in the agent inhaled, and the length of exposure to the agent (Schiller, 2000). Inhalation injuries are typically observed within the first 12 to 24 hours after the burn injury (Morgan et al, 2000). Respiratory insufficiency may develop 48 to 72 hours after burn injury (Schiller, 2000).

Inhalation injuries can be classified according to the location of the injury relative to the glottis (Greenfield, 1999). Upper airway inhalation injuries (above the glottis) should be suspected if there are obvious burns to the face, neck, or upper chest. The potential for an inhalation injury is increased if the burn injury is sustained in an enclosed space. A lower airway inhalation injury is a direct burn below the glottis and usually results from inhaling heated air or steam. An inhalation injury below the glottis is rare because of the ability of the trachea to dissipate heat and the reflex action of the vocal cords to close off the lower airway when they are exposed to toxic air. Smoke inhalation, which is often the cause of death in burn-related injuries, typically results in carbon monoxide or cyanide toxicity. The fire also consumes the oxygen, and hypoxia may occur if the burn victim is in an enclosed space and/or trapped.

Edema formation may also lead to airway obstruction and respiratory distress. The edema may be the result of an actual burn to the tissues in the airway or may result from fluid resuscitation efforts, especially if the face, neck, and chest are involved in the burn.

The following clinical indicators increase the risk of a possible inhalation injury (Greenfield, 1999):

- A burn injury sustained in an enclosed space
- Burns to the face, neck, and chest*
- Singed nasal hair or eyebrows
- Carboniferous material in mouth
- Carboniferous sputum*
- Carboxyhemoglobin level more than 10%
- Wheezing
- Hoarseness*
- Deep, labored respirations
- Altered level of consciousness

*These indicators were observed with Mr. Lewis.

- Cough
- Tachypnea

9. Describe the treatment protocol of a burn patient with an inhalation injury or a suspected inhalation injury.

Monitoring of the respiratory status of a patient with a burn injury is critical and should take priority over all other concerns. The basic ABCs of survival must be met first, as with any trauma patient. Monitoring of the respiratory system and the treatment protocols include the following:

- Assess the respiratory rate, rhythm, and quality frequently.
- Monitor arterial blood gas (ABG) and carboxyhemoglobin values periodically.
- Deliver humidified oxygen. The type of delivery system used depends on the extent of the inhalation injury. It can vary from a nasal cannula to intubation and ventilator support if the inhalation injury is severe. Delivery of 100% humidified oxygen through a non-rebreather mask or ventilator promotes oxygenation and excretion of carbon monoxide (Wiebelhaus & Hansen, 2001).
- Perform pulmonary hygiene efforts including positioning, coughing and deep breathing, incentive spirometry, or ultrasound nebulizers.
- Elevate the head of the bed at least 30 to 40 degrees unless contraindicated by another condition.
- Obtain chest x-ray films.
- Use fiberoptic bronchoscopy to directly visualize the airway.
- Obtain a xenon-133 ventilation-perfusion lung scan: xenon-133 is injected intravenously with serial scans done to monitor the clearance of the xenon by the lungs. Xenon is usually washed out of the alveoli within 90 seconds. Care should be taken with these results. Previous history of chronic obstructive pulmonary disease (COPD) or infection may cause a false positive (Greenfield, 1999).
- Perform escharotomies if chest expansion is compromised. Escharotomies may be necessary if there is extensive burn injury to the anterior or posterior trunk. If eschar is present, the respiratory effort and therefore ventilation may be compromised. Escharotomies on both sides of the chest through the midaxillary line may aid in decreasing the respiratory effort.

Initially, the chest x-ray film, ABG values, and carboxyhemoglobin findings may appear normal. The initial results become baseline data for comparison with subsequent laboratory results. Serial studies can identify deterioration of the pulmonary function. Fiberoptic bronchoscopy can accurately diagnose 100% of inhalation injuries (Greenfield, 1999).

10. What is the purpose of escharotomies?

Escharotomies are incisions made through the eschar to allow for swelling without compromising tissue perfusion. An eschar is typically thick and leathery, allowing little expansion if there is swelling under it. If the burn is circumferential and eschar is present, the swelling from the burn injury itself and the swelling associated with fluid resuscitation can compromise the arterial blood flow to the area.

The incisions should extend through the eschar down to the subcutaneous fat to allow adequate separation of the edges of the incision and to relieve the pressure from the swelling. Incisions are made in the midlateral or midmedial line, moving from the proximal to the distal end of the involved extremities. The locations of the incisions are critical to prevent causing trauma to nerves, tendons, joints, and the vascular structure. The incisions may be performed at the bedside because there is no pain sensation in these types of burn injuries. Antimicrobial agents should be applied after the incisions are made to delay colonization of bacteria (Cornwell, 2001).

With or without escharotomies, peripheral blood flow should be assessed based upon unit protocol. Peripheral pulses in all involved extremities should be assessed by manual palpation or with the use of a Doppler stethoscope. Manual palpation may be difficult due to swelling in the extremity, which then will require the use of an ultrasound system to hear the pulsations. Changes in assessment findings should be reported immediately.

11. Discuss pain management in the treatment protocol for the patient with a burn injury.

Pain management is a major concern in the care of the patient with a burn injury. Continual monitoring of both the physical and emotional pain experienced by these patients during all phases of the burn injury is important. Many believe that anyone experiencing a full-thickness burn does not have pain because of the loss of pain sensors in the burned tissue. However, total full-thickness burns are rare. There is usually a mixture of partial- and full-thickness burns. Because the pain sensors are intact with partial-thickness burns, the patient may experience severe pain. Initially because of the massive edema resulting from the burn and fluid resuscitation efforts, only IV pain medication such as morphine should be administered. Massive edema compromises the absorption of the pain medication if it is given intramuscularly or subcutaneously. Once the patient enters the acute and rehabilitation phases, other routes of administration of pain medication can be considered. Alternative methods of pain management should also be considered. For example, guided imagery has been used very successfully for some patients with burn injuries.

Initial interventions for pain should include small doses of IV narcotic medications such as morphine by IV push or patient-controlled anesthesia pump. After the first 24 to 48 hours, other forms of pain medication may be used, including oral doses of morphine or meperidine and transcutaneous doses of fentanyl (Greenfield, 1999). Medication other than narcotics may aid in pain control after the initial 48 hours. Anxiolytics such as diazepam (Valium) and lorazepam (Librium) may decrease the anxiety associated with the anticipation of painful dressing changes. Diphenhydramine (Benadryl) and hydroxyzine (Atarax) may also be used to decrease the itching associated with wound healing (Greenfield, 1999). Careful assessment of the patient must be made so that adequate management if pain and anxiety is accomplished without altering sensorium.

12. Using the Curreri formula for nutrition, calculate Mr. Lewis's nutritional needs. Discuss the need for a high-calorie, high-protein diet.

Many formulas have been developed to calculate caloric requirements. The Curreri formula is used to establish the number of calories required by the patient with a burn injury (Cornwell, 2001). The formula estimates only the number of calories and does not address the percentage of proteins, fats, and carbohydrates the patient requires.

$$(25 \text{ kcal} \times \text{weight [kg]}) + (40 \times \text{TBSA}) = \text{total calories}$$

Mr. Lewis's caloric need per day would be calculated as follows:

$$(25 \text{ kcal} \times 72 \text{ kg}) + (40 \times 65\%) = 4400 \text{ kcal}$$

Nutritional support becomes paramount once the condition of the patient with a burn injury has stabilized. Hypermetabolism that is directly proportional to the extent of the burn injury results. The basal metabolic rate may double or triple in a patient with a 40% or greater TBSA burn injury (Ramzy et al, 1999).

Because of the high metabolic rate and the need for a positive nitrogen balance to promote healing, a diet high in calories and protein is essential. Once the patient's condition is stabilized, nutritional intake must begin. If the patient cannot consume enough calories orally, enteral feedings may be required to meet the extensive nutritional needs. These include oral supplements or continuous feedings through a nasoenteric (intestinal) tube. Specific types of feedings and tubes used for enteral therapy depend on the condition of the patient, the anticipated time of nutritional support required to meet the metabolic needs, and the risk of aspiration. The protein intake per day for the patient with a burn injury can range from 1.6 to 3.2 g/kg of body weight. For Mr. Lewis, this would result in an intake of 115 to 230 g of protein per day.

Some of the latest research is being conducted on decreasing the metabolic rate after a burn injury through the use of anabolic hormone therapy (Ramzy et al, 1999). By decreasing the hypermetabolism, adequate nutrient for healing will be available, and there is a decrease in the amount of lean protein mass lost because the burn victim cannot keep up with the metabolic needs. Further research is necessary in this area.

13. Discuss burn wound care and dressing techniques. Include the types of topical antimicrobial agents commonly used in wound care, listing advantages and disadvantages of each.

With the loss of integrity of the skin and the colonization of bacteria in the burn wound and under eschar, management of the burn wound becomes imperative (Cornwell, 2001). If a wound becomes infected, consequences such as conversion of a partial-thickness to full-thickness wound may occur, healing may be delayed, and the wound infection can lead to septic shock and death.

Five goals of burn wound care include closing the wound as soon as possible, supporting the development of granulation tissue, cleaning the wound for grafting, reducing scar formation and contractures, and providing patient comfort (Greenfield, 1999). The first step in the process of burn wound care is wound cleansing. Hydrotherapy is begun as soon as possible to promote meticulous cleansing and wound débridement. The type of hydrotherapy depends on the infection control policies of the unit and the condition of the patient. Some patients are placed in a Hubbard tank or are given a shower. Typically hydrotherapy is completed at least daily but may be performed more often if ordered by the burn unit team. The goal is to wash all areas carefully, being sure to thoroughly remove all antimicrobial agents previously placed on the burn wound. Also, any eschar that is beginning to separate may be removed with forceps and scissors. All hair should be shaved around the burn wound to decrease the chance of infection (Kagan, 2000).

Hydrotherapy can be a painful ordeal for the patient. Adequate premedication is required. The actual time of the hydrotherapy (usually 30 minutes or less) should be monitored carefully to prevent hypothermia. Heat lamps may be used to decrease the amount of heat lost by the patient. During hydrotherapy, the wound must be assessed continually for color and appearance: the presence of eschar and healing as seen by budding of the skin; presence of drainage, including odor, color, and amount; and any exposed deep tissue such as tendons and bone (Greenfield, 1999).

Once the wound is cleansed, an antimicrobial agent is applied. These agents are the best method to control burn wound sepsis and to reduce the number of bacteria colonizing in the wound. The agents ideally will also restrain colonization of bacteria to a level that the body can control through its internal defense mechanisms. The three most commonly used antimicrobial agents are listed in Table 27-3. Selection of an antimicrobial agent depends on the wound depth, location, condition, and specific organism isolated, which are established by wound culture (Cornwell, 2001).

There are two methods of dressing a burn wound. The first method is the open method. An antimicrobial cream is applied with a sterile glove with no dressing applied. This approach allows direct visualization of the wound, less discomfort for the patient during wound care, and simplicity in wound care. However, the patient may experience hypothermia, may further traumatize the wound, or may have psychologic difficulty looking at the wound.

A second method is the closed method, in which dressings are applied to the wound. Antimicrobial cream is applied to the wound using a sterile glove or is coated on a gauze pad and laid on the wound, which is then covered with an additional dressing. If a solution is used, the dressing is saturated and placed on the wound and covered with additional

Table 27-3	*Characteristics of Topical Antimicrobial Agents*		
Agent	**Activity**	**Advantages**	**Disadvantages**
Mafenide acetate cream 11.2% (Sulfamylon)	Broad-spectrum activity against gram-positive and gram-negative organisms Persistent activity against *Pseudomonas*	Good eschar penetration because of high solubility	Pain for 20-30 min after application Possible metabolic acidosis from hyperventilation Occasional hypersensitivity
Silver sulfadiazine cream 1% (Silvadene)	Activity against gram-negative and gram-positive organisms	Painless application Effectiveness against yeasts	Rare hypersensitivity Poor eschar penetration Transient leukopenia (rare)
Silver nitrate 0.5% soaks	Effectiveness against a wide spectrum of pathogens, including fungal infections	No contribution to ongoing allergic reactions in toxic epidermal necrolysis Decreased evaporative heat loss from dressings	Limited joint motion Equipment and environment staining Poor eschar penetration

From Bucher, L., and Melander, S. (1999). *Critical care nursing*, p. 1059. Philadelphia: W. B. Saunders.

dressings. These dressings should be wrapped distal to proximal with no two burn surfaces touching each other. The advantages of this type of dressing are limitation of fluid loss through evaporation, débridement of the wound when the dressings are removed, absorption of the exudate from the wound, and patient comfort. Disadvantages of this type of dressing are the discomfort experienced by the patient during dressing changes and the warm, moist environment created under the dressings.

14. Describe the types of biologic and synthetic dressings used in wound care.

Biologic dressings are used as temporary wound coverings until autografts are available. Reasons that biologic dressings aid in the management of burn wounds include the following:

- Decreasing bacterial proliferation on the wound
- Preventing necrosis of viable elements in the dermis
- Preventing wound desiccation
- Assisting in control of evaporation of fluid and heat loss through the open wound
- Decreasing protein loss in fluid exudate
- Decreasing patient's pain
- Protecting exposed structures such as blood vessels, tendons, and nerves
- Stimulating healing and preparing the wound bed for autograft skin
- Facilitating joint motion (Winfrey et al, 1999)

The most commonly used biologic and synthetic dressings are described in Table 27-4. New forms of dressings and débridement material are on the market. Each of these new products has properties that aid in the débridement and healing of burn injuries. Burn centers will continue to investigate and develop wound management care that will promote healing, decrease scarring, and decrease the threat of infection.

Table 27-4	*Common Biologic and Synthetic Dressings*
Type of Dressing	**Definition**
Biologic dressing	Temporary wound cover of human or animal species tissue
Allograft (homograft)	Temporary wound cover composed of a graft of skin transplanted from another human, living or dead
Xenograft (heterograft) skin	Used as a temporary wound cover to promote healing; a graft of skin, usually pigskin, transplanted between animals of different species
Biosynthetic dressing	A wound covering composed of both biologic and synthetic materials
Temporary skin substitute (Biobrane)	A bilaminar wound dressing composed of nylon mesh enclosed in a collagen derivative with a silicone rubber outer membrane; permeable to some antibiotic ointments
"Artificial skin" (Integra)	A wound dressing composed of two layers: (1) a "dermal" layer made of animal collagen that interfaces with an open wound surface; (2) an "epidermal" layer made of polymeric silicone (Silastic) that controls water loss from the dermis and acts as a bacterial barrier; the dermal layer biodegrades within several months and is reabsorbed; the epidermal layer may be removed and replaced with autograft skin when appropriate

15. Discuss the use of autografts and the nursing care required.

With a full-thickness burn, healing and reepithelialization are not possible. As a result, an autograft using viable skin from the patient is the only option for covering the wound. For the autograft to "take," the wound itself must be pink, firm, and free of exudate or eschar, which is accomplished through wound cleansing and débridement. Once the wound is ready for the graft, the patient is taken to surgery, where the autograft is obtained. Autografts may be split thickness, full thickness, pedicle flaps, or free flaps, depending on the area of the body requiring the autograft (Kagan, 2000). Most autografts are split-thickness grafts to cover the wound early. Sheet grafts are used over the face and if the burn area is small. If the area requiring coverage is large, the autograft is meshed so that it can cover a larger surface area. The autograft can be meshed by a ratio of 1:1.5 to 1:4. This means that the autograft can cover 1.5 to 4 times its own surface area. Meshed grafts have a tendency to adhere better to the wound and allow exudate and debris to ooze through the open meshed areas. A ratio of 1 : 4 is typically the largest ratio used to prevent longer healing time and scarring. The graft is laid on the wound and stapled or sutured in place. Some burn units use fibrin glue to hold the autograft in place. Further investigation of this approach is needed. Once the autograph is secured to the wound, a dressing is applied and the patient is returned to the burn unit.

Another option is to develop a cultured epithelial autograft (CEA). Punch grafts of skin not involved in the burn are taken from the patient and placed in a cultured medium for up to 30 days. Once the cells reproduce, the graft is then placed on a clean area. The challenge with this approach is the amount of time required to grow sufficient cells for grafting. The CEAs have also been found to be more fragile and in some cases less likely to adhere to the wound bed (Winfrey et al, 1999).

The nurse must take special care not to disrupt the autograft. The patient may be confined to bed rest or the extremity may be immobilized with splints to promote proper positioning and to prevent disruption of the graft. The nurse must ensure proper positioning while being fully aware of the potential for other complications, such as respiratory infection and skin breakdown as a result of the immobility. An autograft "takes" when it becomes a permanent part of the wound. Blood flow through capillaries growing into the autograft is established by the third to fifth day after the graft. Wound closure is anticipated within 7 to 10 days after graft placement.

16. Describe the appropriate care for donor sites.

Selection of autograft skin donor sites is based on the location and the extent of the burn. Any site on the body, including the scalp, can potentially be used as a donor site. Once the autograft skin is obtained, the donor site must be monitored because of the creation of a partial-thickness injury. In surgery, fine-mesh gauze (either dry or impregnated with a substance such as scarlet red or a synthetic material) is placed over the donor site to promote healing and prevent further injury. On the patient's return to the burn unit, the donor site should be exposed to air. Some burn units apply a radiant heat source to the area to increase drying. Once the donor site begins to heal, usually 7 to 14 days after the graft is obtained, the gauze or synthetic material will begin to separate from the wound (Solotkin & Knipe, 2000). As this separation occurs, the material can be trimmed from the wound with scissors. The nurse must be careful to keep the donor site clean, dry, and trimmed. A donor site can be used more than once if there are no complications such as an infection. If the donor site becomes infected, it should be treated as the burn wound.

17. Discuss the splinting/positioning required for Mr. Lewis to maintain use of his extremities and upper body.

Most burn units have physical therapists and occupational therapists available to assist patients with burn injuries. In collaboration with the nursing staff, their goal is to maintain as much function as possible so that the patient can return to society. All joints should be placed in a neutral position if possible. Splints must be applied correctly. If necessary, the therapist should apply the splints or provide in-service training for nurses on the application of splints (Cornwell, 2001). Footboards or shoes are used to prevent footdrop. Early ambulation requires coordination of the nursing staff and physical therapist to provide the optimal environment for the patient to accomplish this goal. Pain management that allows the patient to ambulate and participate in exercises becomes an important issue.

18. List the nursing diagnoses, outcomes, and interventions appropriate for the care of the patient with a burn injury during the emergent and acute phases of burn physiology.

Solotkin and Knipe (2000) created a nursing care plan identifying the most common nursing diagnoses for a patient with a burn injury. Although many nursing diagnoses may be important for this type of patient, this care plan presents the most common interventions (Table 27-5).

19. Discuss the psychosocial aspects of caring for the patient with a burn injury and the impact on the patient's support system.

Burn injuries are some of the most devastating injuries to sustain. An individual's identity and self-image are directly related to his or her appearance. Disfigurement from burns to the face can be especially difficult for the patient. The nurse must constantly assess the patient and the support system available through family or friends. This assessment includes identifying feelings of guilt, abandonment, pain, loss, and fear. In addition, the patient may experience anxiety, sleep deprivation, and disorientation (Badger, 2001). The nurse can encourage the patient, family, and friends to verbalize their concerns and provide them with appropriate information. Also, a referral to a social worker, psychologist, or chaplain may be necessary to provide additional psychosocial or spiritual support.

Table 27-5	*Nursing Care Plan for Resuscitative and Acute Care Phase of the Patient with a Major Burn Injury*	

Nursing Diagnosis	Outcome	Interventions
Ineffective airway clearance or impaired gas exchange related to tracheal edema or interstitial edema secondary to inhalation injury and manifested by hypoxemia and hypercapnia	Po_2 >90 mm Hg, Pco_2 <40 mm Hg, O_2 saturation >95% Respirations 16-20 min Clear mentations Ability to mobilize secretions Clear to white secretions Absence of dyspnea and increased work of breathing with appropriate positioning	Assess respiratory rate and character qh, breath sounds q4h, and level of consciousness qh. Evaluate need for chest escharotomy during fluid resuscitation. If patient is not intubated, assess for stridor, hoarseness qh. Monitor oxygen saturation qh; obtain and evaluate ABC values prn. Administer humidified oxygen as ordered. Cough and deep breathe qh while awake. Suction q1-2h or prn; monitor sputum characteristics and amount. Schedule activities to avoid fatigue and dyspnea. Turn q2h to mobilize secretions. Assist with obtaining chest x-ray film as ordered.
Fluid volume deficit secondary to fluid shifts and evaporate loss of fluids from the injured skin	Hourly urine output: 30-50 ml; 1 ml/kg—children <30 kg body weight; 75-100 ml—electrical injury Stable vital signs Clear sensorium	Titrate calculated fluid requirements in first 48 hr to maintain acceptable urinary output. Obtain and evaluate urine specific gravity and sugar and acetone q2h. Monitor vital signs qh until hemodynamically stable. Monitor mental status qh for at least 48 hr. Obtain and record daily weights. Record hourly intake and output measurements and evaluate trends. Monitor laboratory values for first 48 hr and then as required by patient status.
High risk for impaired vascular perfusion in extremities with circumferential burns manifested by decreased or absent peripheral pulses	Absence of tissue injury in extremities secondary to inadequate perfusion related to vascular compression from edema	Check peripheral pulses qh for 72 hr by palpation or ultrasonic flowmeter; evaluate sensation of pain and capillary refill in extremities.

Continued

Table 27-5	**Nursing Care Plan for Resuscitative and Acute Care Phase of the Patient with a Major Burn Injury—cont'd**

Nursing Diagnosis	Outcome	Interventions
		Notify physician of changes in pulses, capillary refill, or pain sensation; be prepared to assist with escharotomy or fasciotomy.
Alteration in comfort: acute pain related to burn trauma	Able to identify factors that contribute to pain Verbalizes improved comfort level Physiologic parameters return to normal Adequate respirations and hemodynamic stability after administration of narcotic analgesia	Evaluate upper extremities. Medicate before bathing, dressing changes, major procedures, prn. Reduce anxiety; explain all activities before initiating them; talk to patient while performing activities; assess need for analgesic or anxiolytic medication; use nonpharmacologic pain-reducing methods as appropriate. Monitor and document response to analgesics or other interventions.
High risk for infection related to loss of skin, impaired immune response, invasive therapies	Absence of infected burn wounds Vital signs stable Laboratory values within normal limits Negative results from sputum, blood, and urine cultures	Assess burn wound and invasive catheter sites. Assess and document characteristics of urine and sputum q8h. Obtain wound, sputum, urine, and blood cultures as ordered. Assess and record temperature and vital signs q1-4h as appropriate. Provide protective isolation appropriate to method of wound care. Provide wound care with antimicrobial topical agents as ordered.
Impaired skin integrity related to burn wound, or consequences of immobility	No evidence of progressive burn wound or donor site injury Burn wound or donor site healing and skin graft adherence within appropriate time frames	Assess and document: skin over pressure areas, burn wounds, donor sites, pressure points under splints, dependent area of unburned skin. Pad pressure areas: heels, elbows, sacrum, scapulas, and burned ears. Check circulation distally and digits in splinted extremities. Promote drying of donor sites as appropriate; keep heat lamps at a safe distance to prevent injury.

Table 27-5	*Nursing Care Plan for Resuscitative and Acute and Phase of the Patient with a Major Burn Injury—cont'd*	
Nursing Diagnosis	**Outcome**	**Interventions**
		Immobilize skin graft sites for 5-7 days after grafting to promote graft adherence.
High risk for aspiration *R/T; hypoactivity of gastrointestinal tract	No aspiration of gastric contents No respiratory complications from aspirations	Insert and maintain nasogastric tube to low suction until bowel sounds return. Auscultate for bowel sounds q4h. Test stools and gastric contents for pressure of blood. Administer histamine blockers and antacids as ordered.
High risk for nutritional deficit related to increased metabolic demands due to wound healing	Consumption of daily requirement of nutrients, based on formulas for appropriate calorie calculation Positive nitrogen balance Progressive wound healing	Monitor weights every day or biweekly. Assess abdomen, bowel sounds q8h. Record all oral intake. Activate enteral, parenteral feeding protocol as appropriate prn. Provide adaptive devices to facilitate self-feeding.
High risk for hemorrhage related to presence of a stress ulcer	No occurrence of stress ulcer while in hospital	Assess all stools, emesis, and residual of the tube feedings for blood. Monitor hemoglobin and hematocrit levels. Administer histamine blockers and antacids as ordered. Auscultate abdomen and monitor for bowel sounds and pain. Encourage oral diet as soon as possible.
High risk for hypothermia related to loss of skin or external cooling	Rectal and core temperature is 37.2° to 37.8° C (99°-100° F)	Monitor and document rectal and core temperature q1-2h.
High risk for ineffective patient and family coping related to acute stress of critical injury and potential life-threatening crisis; alteration in family processes related to critical injury	Patient or family verbalize goals of treatment regimen Patient or family demonstrate knowledge of support systems that are available Patient or family able to express concerns and fears Patient or family coping functional and realistic for phase of hospitalization, family processes at precrisis level	Support adaptive and functional coping mechanisms. Use interventions to reduce patient fatigue and pain. Promote use of group support session for patients and families. Orient patient and family to unit and support services and reinforce information frequently. Involve patient and family in treatment goals and plan of care.

BURNS

References

Badger, J. (2001). Burns: The psychological aspect. *American Journal of Nursing, 101*(11), 38-41.

Baldwin, K. & Morris, S. (2002). Shock, multiple organ dysfunction syndrome, and burns in adults. In K. McCance & S. Huether (Eds.), *Pathophysiology: The biological basis for disease in adults and children* (4th ed., pp. 1499-1508). St Louis: Mosby.

Cohen, R. & Moelleken, B. (2003). Disorder due to physical agents. In L. Tierney, S. McPhee, & M. Papadakis (Eds.), *Current medical diagnosis and treatment* (42nd ed., pp. 1543-1547). New York: Lange Medical Books.

Cornwell, P. (2001). Management of clients with burn injury. In J. Black, J. Hawks, & A Keene (Eds.), *Medical surgical nursing* (6th ed., pp. 1331-1359). Philadelphia: W. B. Saunders.

Greenfield, E. (1999) Burns. In L. Bucher & S. Melander (Eds.), *Critical care nursing* (pp. 1036-1069). Philadelphia: W. B. Saunders.

Hilton, G. (2001). Thermal burns. *American Journal of Nursing, 101*(11), 32-34.

Horne, M. & Bond, E. (2000). Fluid, electrolyte, and acid-base imbalances. In S. Lewis, M. Heitkemper, & S. Dirksen (Eds.), *Medical-surgical nursing* (5th ed., pp. 323-351). St Louis: Mosby.

Huether, S. (2002). Structure, function, and disorders of the integument. In K. McCance & S. Huether (Eds.), Pathophysiology: the biological basis for disease in adults and children (4th ed., pp. 1434-1437). St Louis: Mosby.

Kagan, R. (2000). Evaluation and treatment of thermal burns. [Electronic version]. *Dermatology Nursing 12*(5), 334-350, 338-44, 347-50.

Laskowski-Jones, K. (1999). Burns. In L. Bucher & S. Melander (Eds.). *Critical care nursing* (pp. 1036-1069). Philadelphia: Saunders.

Morgan, E., Bledsoe, S., & Barker, J. (2000). Ambulatory management of burns. [Electronic version]. *American Family Physician, 62*(9), 2015-2026.

Ramzy, P., Wolf, S., & Herndon, D. (1999). Current status of anabolic hormone administration in human burn injury. [Electronic version]. *Journal of Parenteral and Enteral Nutrition 23*(6), S190-S194.

Schiller, W. (2000). Burn care and inhalation injury. In A. Grenvik (Ed.), *Textbook of critical care* (4th ed., pp. 365-374). Philadelphia: W. B. Saunders.

Solotkin, K. & Knipe, C. (2000). Patients with burns. In S. Lewis, M. Heitkemper, & S. Dirksen (Eds.), *Medical-surgical nursing* (5th ed., pp. 523-550). St Louis: Mosby.

Wiebelhaus, P. & Hansen, S. (2001). Managing burn emergencies. [Electronic version]. *Dimensions of Critical Care Nursing 20*(4), 2-8.

Winfrey, M., Cochran, M., & Hegarty, M. (1999). A new technology: INTEGRA artificial skin. [Electronic version]. *Dimensions of Critical Care Nursing 19*(1), 14-20.

28

Acquired Immunodeficiency Syndrome

Connie Cooper, RN, BSN, MSN

CASE PRESENTATION

Ben Majors, a 35-year-old white man, came to the local mental health hospital complaining of impaired concentration, withdrawal from family and friends, mood swings, difficulty with his memory, fatigue, and suicidal ideation. Two months before coming to the hospital, he had moved to the area from San Francisco to be with his family.

On admission, Mr. Majors's assessment revealed he had lost 4.5 to 7 kg (10 to 15 lb) since coming to his parents' home. He has not been able to read or concentrate. His suicidal ideas involve harming himself but no specific plan. Mr. Majors's psychosocial history revealed that he was homosexual and in the mid-1980s had visited several bathhouses in San Francisco before settling down with his one close friend. Mr. Majors stated he had returned home to tell his family that his test for human immunodeficiency virus (HIV) was positive. His family told him they would stand by him. He denied the use of intravenous (IV) drugs but has used marijuana on occasion. His medical history included having had diarrhea for the past 3 weeks, night sweats, and enlarged glands in his neck and under his arms. Two of his friends recently had been told that they were HIV positive, and two other friends died from acquired immunodeficiency syndrome (AIDS). He fears he has become depressed, believes he is losing his mind, and is becoming more confused. He told the nurse he was having difficulty with tremors in his legs, which occasionally have given him problems with walking.

His admitting diagnosis was major depression—single episode; rule out AIDS dementia complex (ADC).

After Mr. Majors's psychiatrist was informed of his history, medication orders were given for fluoxetine (Prozac) and nortriptyline (Pamelor).

Current vital signs and laboratory results are as follows:

BP	134/88 mm Hg
HR	90 bpm
Respirations	20 breaths/min
Temperature	37.2° C (98.9° F) (oral)
ELISA	Positive for HIV antigens (confirmed by Western blot test)
Chest x-Ray Film	Within normal limits
RBCs	$3.5 \times 10^6/mm^3$
WBCs	$6.6 \times 10^3/mm^3$

Hgb	12.9 g/dl
Hct	36.8%
Lymphocytes	13%

After 1 week of psychotherapy and medication therapy, Mr. Majors did not show any improvement in mood, affect, or neurologic deficits. He began falling when attempting to walk, had difficulty with the Mini-Mental State Examination, and became more confused. The psychiatrist made a medical referral. Two physicians refused to accept the referral. Finally an oncologist accepted Mr. Majors's case. Two days later Mr. Majors was transferred to the oncology unit. More tests were ordered.

Results for a complete blood count with differential were the following:

RBCs	$5.5 \times 10^6/\text{mm}^3$
WBCs	$4.4 \times 10^3/\text{mm}^3$
Hgb	12.7 g/dl
Hct	38.9%
Lymphocytes	11%
Monocytes	3%

The lymphocyte subset results were the following:

Total Lymphocyte Count	$411/\text{mm}^3$
Absolute B-cell Count	$99/\text{mm}^3$
Absolute T-cell Count	$206/\text{mm}^3$
Helper:Suppressor Ratio ($CD4^+$:$CD8^+$)	0.07

Routine chemistry results were the following:

Na^+	137 mmol/L
Glucose	120 mg/dl
Creatinine	0.8 mg/dl
Albumin	2.6 g/dl
BUN	9 mg/dl
Total protein	6.3 g/dl
K^+	3.7mmol/L
Cl^-	100 mmol/L
CO_2	26 mmol/L

Results of other tests were the following:

VDRL	Negative
Hepatitis B serology	Negative
Viral Load	230,000 copies/ml
Stool Culture	*Salmonella*
CT Scan	Mild brain atrophy and white matter changes

Once Mr. Majors was transferred to a medical floor, treatment with abacavir/zidovudine/lamivudine (Trizivir) and ampicillin (Ampicin) for *Salmonella* infection was begun. During Mr. Majors's hospitalization, his assessment revealed no previous opportunistic diseases. He reported that his first symptoms were night sweats, diarrhea, and difficulty with his memory. Difficulty walking began shortly thereafter. His respiratory status began to change. On day 9, he developed a nonproductive cough, dyspnea, chills, and a few crackles in the base of his lungs. The physician was informed of changes, and orders included oxygen via mask at 40%, a chest x-ray film, and a second CD4+ count. The chest x-ray examination revealed bilateral infiltrates. A flexible fiberoptic bronchoscopy revealed *Pneumocystis carinii* pneumonia (PCP). Mr. Majors was treated with IV pentamidine. On day 13, his respiratory status worsened. There were indications of respiratory failure, and a decision had to be made about intubation and mechanical ventilation. Mr. Majors had difficulty with

Table 28-1   *Vital Signs*

	Day					
	4	**7**	**9**	**13**	**14**	**15**
BP (mm Hg)	112/72	154/82	132/84	132/62	112/72	130/84
HR (bpm)	112	112	112	120	112	90
Respirations (breaths/min)	20	22	26	36	40	35
Temperature						
° C	36.7-37.2	36.7-37.2	37.2-37.8	37.8-38.9	38.9-39.4	36.7-37.2
° F	98-99	98-99	99-100	100-102	102-103	98-99

BP, Blood pressure; *HR,* heart rate.

Table 28-2   *Laboratory Results*

	Day				
	7 (room air)	**9 (40% O$_2$)**	**13 (100% O$_2$)**	**14 (40% O$_2$)**	**15 (room air)**
pH	7.48	7.49	7.45	7.48	7.46
Pco$_2$ (mm Hg)	36	32	35	28	32
Pao$_2$ (mm Hg)	49	44	104	93	85
Sao$_2$ (%)	89	83	97	97	96
HCO$_3^-$ (mm Hg)	27	25	24	20	23
Mode			A/C	A/C	
Ventilation rate			17	17	
Vr			900	900	
PEEP (cm H$_2$O)			14	12	

PEEP, Positive end-expiratory pressure.

decision making and exhibited some psychomotor slowing. His family was kept informed of his physical condition. Mr. Majors wanted his family to help him make this difficult decision. Considering the quick onset of his symptoms and change in condition, the family chose admission to the intensive care unit (ICU) and mechanical ventilation. He was admitted to the ICU. Treatment with IV ampicillin and IV hydrocortisone was initiated.

Within 2 days, Mr. Majors was afebrile and was weaned from the ventilator. His respiratory rate had fallen from 40 to 25 breaths/min, and his respiratory distress had lessened. Mr. Majors was then transferred back to the medical unit, receiving oxygen via nasal cannula. A third CD4$^+$ cell count was 190/mm^3. Tables 28-1 and 28-2 show diagnostic data at Mr. Majors's return to the medical unit.

After his return to the medical unit, Mr. Majors was treated for oral candidiasis with nystatin (Nyaderm) and ketoconazole (Nizoral). His skin tests indicated complete failure of delayed hypersensitivity reactions, and AIDS was diagnosed. After 1.5 weeks of IV trimethoprim-sulfamethoxazole (TMP-SMZ; Bactrim), Mr. Majors was weaned from oxygen and discharged.

After discharge from the hospital, Mr. Majors was treated with Retrovir (zidovudine), 300 mg; abacavir, 300 mg; lamivudine, 150 mg; and oral TMP-SMZ.

ACQUIRED IMMUNODEFICIENCY SYNDROME

QUESTIONS

1. What factors put Mr. Majors at risk for HIV infection/AIDS?

2. What tests are used to screen for HIV infection?

3. What laboratory tests are done to help determine treatment for HIV infection/AIDS?

4. What clinical indicators would be used to determine whether Mr. Majors has major depression or ADC?

5. What is the difference between HIV infection and AIDS?

6. When is it appropriate to offer antiretroviral therapy to an HIV-positive patient?

7. What clinical indicators confirmed that Mr. Majors's HIV infection had progressed to AIDS?

8. Describe the symptoms of PCP.

9. What symptoms and pulmonary diagnostic findings in Mr. Majors's case indicated the need for transfer to the ICU?

10. Mechanical ventilation and ICU admission for a person with AIDS is controversial. Why was Mr. Majors admitted to the ICU?

11. What treatments did Mr. Majors receive in the ICU to ensure a successful outcome? Include medications for HIV infection such as highly active antiretroviral therapy (HAART) and PCP prophylaxis.

12. What are some of the nursing interventions that will help Mr. Majors with his psychosocial and physiologic needs?

13. When assigned to a patient with HIV infection, what personal feelings or concerns should be acknowledged?

14. Are the ICU nurses at an increased risk of acquiring AIDS from patients who receive mechanical ventilation?

15. What is the recommended protocol for occupational exposure to HIV?

ACQUIRED IMMUNODEFICIENCY SYNDROME

QUESTIONS AND ANSWERS

1. **What factors put Mr. Majors at risk for HIV infection/AIDS?**

    Mr. Majors's history revealed that he was homosexual and had had many sexual partners. Researchers have agreed that the greatest risk of exposure to HIV in a homosexual man comes from anal sexual intercourse and sexual practices with multiple sexual partners (Ungvarski & Flaskerud, 1999). Such sexual practices cause trauma to the rectal mucosa, which increases the chances of transmission of the HIV virus and other sexually transmitted diseases.

2. **What tests are used to screen for HIV infection?**

    It is important to do a health history and physical assessment along with gathering diagnostic data (Douglas, 1999). Two tests are used to screen for HIV infection: enzyme-linked immunosorbent assay (ELISA) and Western blot. Exposure to HIV elicits an antigen-antibody reaction and creates antibodies. These antibodies are then detected by the screening tests. The Western blot is a confirmatory test after a positive ELISA (Ungvarski & Flaskerud, 1999). The presence of the antibody indicates that the person is infected and is infectious. The incubation period for AIDS is wide.

    The ELISA was first developed to screen the blood supply before transfusion. The Western blot is more specific than the ELISA. It confirms that the antibody in question is specifically reactive with HIV by detecting antibody reactivity to individual components of the virus (Ungvarski & Flaskerud, 1999).

    Other tests available to detect HIV infection include abnormal helper to suppressor ratio (less than 1.0), and white blood cell count with differential looking for leukopenia and thrombocytopenia (Sole et al, 2001). The HIV rapid tests are also available and are licensed by the U.S. Food and Drug Administration (FDA). The rapid test can provide results in 30 minutes. This test is important in the situation of occupational exposure when immediate treatment decisions need to be made (Ungvarski & Flaskerud, 1999).

3. **What laboratory tests are done to help determine treatment for HIV infection/AIDS?**

    Lymphocytes are mononuclear white blood cells (WBCs) that are critical in immune defense. Two major classes of lymphocytes are B cells and T cells. Humoral immunity is the B-cell response to harmful antigens. Humoral immunity protects the body by circulating antibodies that are produced by the B cells. The creation of antibodies helps a person's system fight infections. When the B cells are activated, they release large amounts of immunoglobulins (antibodies). Cellular immunity is immune protection resulting from the direct action of cells of the immune system (Stine, 2003). Key cell types are phagocytes and lymphocytes.

    CD4$^+$ T-lymphocyte counts are used to stage the client's immune system in response to infection and provide an indication for antiretroviral therapy and prophylaxis (Douglas, 1999). Data indicate a strong relationship between plasma HIV ribonucleic acid (RNA) levels and CD4$^+$ T-cell counts in terms of risk of progression to AIDS in patients (Department of Health and Human Services [DHHS], 2002).

    Viral load or viral burden is a more direct method of measuring HIV activity. Viral load or HIV RNA in plasma will allow the clinician to more accurately assess the amount of HIV activity that is taking place in the body. Viral load tests help the clinician determine prognosis, the need for antiretroviral treatment, and the patient's response to antiretroviral treatment (Ungvarski & Flaskerud, 1999; DHHS, 2002). The DHHS (2002) recommends that CD4$^+$ lymphocyte count and plasma HIV RNA be performed on two occasions to ensure accuracy.

4. What clinical indicators would be used to determine whether Mr. Majors has major depression or ADC?

A patient with major depression usually complains of depressed mood, diminished interest or pleasure in activities, appetite changes with weight changes (up or down), insomnia or hypersomnia, fatigue or loss of energy, inability to concentrate, feelings of worthlessness or guilt, psychomotor agitation or retardation, and thoughts of death or suicide. The presence of any five of these symptoms, lasting for at least 2 weeks, is a clinical indication of a major affective disorder that requires intervention. According to Ciesla and Roberts (2001) patients who are HIV positive are twice as likely to suffer from major depressive disorders than patients who are HIV negative. It is important to take a careful history to determine symptoms and situational crises that could precipitate the symptoms. Assessment of suicidal ideation is important at the time of the initial interview. Any precipitating factors such as bereavement, reactions to medication, or thyroid problems should be ruled out. Nurses in acute care or mental health settings must be aware of the psychosocial and neuropsychiatric aspects of HIV disease. It may be necessary to manage the case of a patient who has anxiety or depression associated with a new diagnosis of HIV infection or AIDS or a patient who may be manifesting dementia associated with AIDS (Flaskerud & Ungvarski, 1999).

HIV is capable of invading brain tissue. Neurologic symptoms have been reported in approximately 40% to 70% of all patients with AIDS, with 10% having manifestations of neurologic involvement at the time of diagnosis (Flaskerud & Ungvarski, 1999). According to Douglas (1999) and Stine (2003), the early manifestations of ADC are decreased memory, forgetfulness, inability to concentrate, apathy, slowness in thinking, depressed mood, agitation, unsteady gait, tremor, clumsiness, motor weakness, and psychotic features. HIV-positive patients are often aware of the changes in their neurologic well-being, which may lead to an adjustment disorder with fear, anxiety, or depression. Late symptoms may include loss of speech, great fatigue, muscle weakness, bladder and bowel incontinence, headache, seizures, and finally death (Stine, 2003). "Approximately 95% of patients with ADC have HIV antibodies in their cerebral spinal fluid" (Stine, 2003, p. 194).

Mr. Majors had symptoms that fit both categories. The most significant symptom that precipitated the transfer to a medical unit was the change in his ambulation status. It is important to avoid medications that have anticholinergic side effects because these can cause delirium, including hallucinations, confusion, and sometimes agitation. The medications of choice include zidovudine, lamivudine, psychostimulants, and antidepressants (Douglas, 1999).

5. What is the difference between HIV infection and AIDS?

The terms *HIV infection* and *AIDS* are not synonymous. AIDS is used to indicate only the most severe diseases or clinical conditions observed in the continuum of illness related to infection with the retrovirus HIV type 1 (HIV-1) (Flaskerud & Ungvarski, 1999).

The definition and classification system for HIV infection was revised and published in December 18, 1992, by the Centers for Disease Control and Prevention (CDC). The CDC classifies HIV infection according to CD4$^+$ T-lymphocyte counts and clinical conditions associated with HIV infection (CDC, 1992). The HIV virus affects the CD4$^+$ T-lymphocyte cell. "Plasma HIV RNA level was predictive of an increased risk of opportunistic infections [OI] independent of T$_4$ cell count, which also is predictive of OI risk. This information confirms that maintaining control of viral replication may be a critical component of preventing OIs in HIV-infected persons" (Stine, 2003). The compromised immune system allows opportunistic organisms to invade the body, which normally would be able to defend it from these invaders.

The HIV/AIDS classification system emphasizes the clinical importance of the CD4$^+$ lymphocyte count in the categorization of HIV-related clinical conditions (CDC, 1992). The definition includes all infected people with CD4$^+$ counts of less than 200/mm^3 and patients with three additional opportunistic infections: pulmonary tuberculosis, invasive cervical cancer, and recurrent bacterial pneumonia (Douglas, 1999).

According to the CDC (1992) revised classification system, counts of CD4$^+$ T lymphocytes are placed in the following three categories:

1. Category 1: ≥500/µl
2. Category 2: 200-499/µl
3. Category 3: ≤200/µl

These categories guide clinical and therapeutic management of adolescents and adults with HIV infections. The CD4$^+$ T-cell count classification presents a continuum for HIV disease. The continuum ranges from an asymptomatic stage to advanced HIV disease.

The asymptomatic stage is manifested by an acute primary HIV infection, an asymptomatic condition, or persistent generalized lymphadenopathy (CDC, 1992). As many as 90% of patients with HIV infections have severe flulike symptoms 1 to 3 weeks after infection. These symptoms may last for 1 to 2 weeks. During this time their HIV antibody test results are usually negative, although they do have a steady decline in their CD4$^+$ T-lymphocyte count and an increase in viral RNA (Flaskerud & Ungvarski, 1999). The HIV antibody test results usually become positive 2 to 18 weeks after infection.

The early symptomatic stage develops when CD4$^+$ T-cell counts drop to around 500/µl (Ungvarski & Flaskerud, 1999). Clinical conditions that could occur at this stage include candidiasis, herpes zoster, pelvic inflammatory disease, and peripheral neuropathy (CDC, 1992).

The late symptomatic stage begins when a patient's CD4$^+$ T-lymphocyte cell count drops below 200/µl (Flaskerud & Ungvarski, 1999). A patient may develop life-threatening infections and cancers. The infections usually are treatable. At this point the stage of infection reflects the CDC criteria for AIDS. The last stage of HIV infection is the advanced HIV disease stage. The patient's CD4$^+$ T-cell count has dropped to less than 50/µl (Ungvarski & Flaskerud, 1999). Once this level has been reached, death is likely within 1 year.

6. When is it appropriate to offer antiretroviral therapy to an HIV-positive patient?

After reviewing the stages of HIV/AIDS, a question to be answered is when is the right time to offer antiretroviral therapy to patients with established HIV infection? The Department of Health and Human Services places HIV-positive patients in two categories: asymptomatic infection and symptomatic disease (wasting, thrush, or unexplained fever for more than 2 weeks) including the AIDS definition of 1992 (DHHS, 2002). For people in the second category, such as Mr. Majors, it is felt that they should be offered antiretroviral therapy. A complete medical workup should be done for patients including CD4$^+$ count and HIV RNA. There is evidence that starting treatment for asymptomatic patients with CD4$^+$ cell counts <200 cells/mm^3 reduces their chances of progressing to AIDS. For patients with CD4$^+$ counts >200 cells/mm^3, recommendations are done according to individual patient's circumstances. In the "MultiCenter AIDS Cohort Study (MACS) it was demonstrated that the 3-year risk of progressing to AIDS was 38.5% among patients with 201-350 CD4$^+$ cell count compared to 14.3% for patients with CD4 counts >350" (DHHS, 2002, p. 7).

7. What clinical indicators confirmed that Mr. Majors's HIV infection had progressed to AIDS?

Laboratory findings in the diagnosis of AIDS include a positive HIV antibody test, decreased WBC and lymphocyte counts, depressed CD4$^+$ T-cell count, an abnormal CD4$^+$:CD8 ratio, and an RNA viral load (Douglas, 1999; Ungvarski & Flaskerud, 1999; DHHS, 2002). According to the CDC's definition and classification of the disease, Mr. Majors's disease progressed from HIV infection to AIDS when his CD4$^+$ count dropped below 200/µl. Mr. Majors also had three opportunistic diseases: PCP, *Candida* infection of the oral mucosa, and *Salmonella* infection of the gastrointestinal tract.

8. Describe the symptoms of PCP.

People infected with HIV eventually have at least one episode of PCP when the CD4$^+$ cells fall below 200/µl (Valenti, 2002). Statistics indicate that as many as 75% to 80% of patients with AIDS will have PCP. *Pneumocystis carinii* was originally classified as a protozoan, but today new data suggest that *P. carinii* is more closely related to fungi. *P. carinii* is a simple fungus that is found in the lungs of humans, rats, cats, dogs, and several other animals. Most children develop antibodies to *P. carinii* at an early age. *P. carinii* is not considered a serious pathogenic organism unless a person is severely immunocompromised. In PCP, the alveoli fill with proteinaceous material that contains cysts and trophozoites. Air distribution into alveoli filled with *P. carinii* is impaired (Ungvarski & Flaskerud, 1999). Stringer and associates (2002) suggest that the organism that causes *P. carinii* pneumonia be renamed *Pneumocystis jiroveci* because of DNA findings. The initials PCP will remain the acronym.

Symptoms associated with PCP include fever; high respiratory rate (>30 breaths/min); dyspnea on exertion then at rest; normal or abnormal chest examination results; normal breath sounds or minimal rales; cyanosis around the mouth, nailbeds, and mucous membranes; dry, nonproductive cough (unless the patient is a smoker); and thrush, which indicates immunosuppression (Ungvarski & Flaskerud, 1999; Stine, 2003).

9. What symptoms and pulmonary diagnostic findings in Mr. Majors's case indicated the need for transfer to the ICU?

Mr. Majors's symptoms after his transfer to the medical unit included dyspnea, fever, and nonproductive cough. His chest x-ray examination showed minimal infiltrates in both lobes. Oxygen was necessary for his hypoxia. His vital signs were within normal limits except for his temperature. Mr. Majors required admission to the ICU when his worsening respiratory status became life threatening. Because of his diminished respiratory function, he required intubation and mechanical ventilation.

10. Mechanical ventilation and ICU admission for a person with AIDS is controversial. Why was Mr. Majors admitted to the ICU?

The primary reason for patients with PCP to be admitted to the ICU is for mechanical ventilation related to respiratory failure. Infection with *P. carinii* destroys lung tissue, and repeated infections decrease functioning lung surface area and cause mechanical problems in mobilizing secretions (Ungvarski & Flaskerud, 1999). Endotracheal tube placement allows for better oral hygiene and positive pressure ventilation forced through the endotracheal tube (Urden et al, 2002). Studies indicate that survival rate is higher for patients with a first episode of PCP than for those with subsequent episodes. PCP is being diagnosed sooner and is being treated more effectively (Flaskerud & Ungvarski, 1999). With early treatment most patients with AIDS survive their first bout with PCP.

This was Mr. Majors's first episode of PCP. His CD4$^+$ count was below 200/µl but not significantly. There is a wide range of indications for critical care for patients with HIV infections. Patients who receive prophylaxis treatment for PCP present about 14.5% of the time with PCP as the primary OI infection, compared with 46% of patients without prophylaxis who present with PCP as their primary OI. In a retrospective study by Gill and colleagues (1999), it was found that 36% of HIV-positive patients admitted to the ICU had PCP. In another study by Bedos and associates (1999), among the 34 patients admitted to the ICU for PCP who required mechanical ventilation, 76% died. It was also found in the Bedos study that approximately 100% of those who delayed mechanical ventilation for more than 3 days died within a 3 month period.

11. What treatments did Mr. Majors receive in the ICU to ensure a successful outcome? Include medications for HIV infection such as highly active antiretroviral therapy (HAART) and PCP prophylaxis.

The results from the flexible fiberoptic bronchoscopic examination indicated PCP. This in turn alerted the physician to begin IV pentamidine. Pentamidine was chosen because Mr. Majors was receiving Trizivir and high-dose IV TMP-SMZ, which could potentially cause bone marrow depression (DHHS, 2002). Bone marrow depression is also a side effect of AZT. When Mr. Majors's status did not improve, ampicillin and hydrocortisone were added. His oral candidiasis was treated with ketoconazole.

For his HIV status Mr. Majors is being treated with AZT, 3TC, and indinavir. When nucleoside analog reverse transcriptase inhibitors (NRTIs) are incorporated into the DNA of HIV during its replication phase, the NRTI terminates the replication (Ungvarski & Flaskerud, 1999). Triple NRTI regimen was chosen because it is easier to use and adhere to. It is also sparing of protease inhibitors (PI) and non-nucleoside reverse transcriptase inhibitors (NNRTI) for future use if drug resistance occurs (DHHS, 2002). The terminology used to describe combination therapy today is HAART. Monotherapy is no longer recommended. HAART has been considered a great breakthrough for treatment of HIV infection. For some patients the therapy has failed. With successful use of HAART, discontinuation of PCP prophylaxis (primary and secondary) has been possible. The criterion that must be met before the prophylaxis can be discontinued is a CD4$^+$ cell count greater than 200 cells/µl documented twice in a 1-month interval. The study by Schneider and coworkers (1999) found that patients whose CD4$^+$ cell count was greater than 200/µl could discontinue their PCP prophylaxis. (See Table 28-3 for approved medications for HIV infection and Table 28-4 for treatment and prevention of opportunistic infections.)

12. What are some of the nursing interventions that will help Mr. Majors with his psychosocial and physiologic needs?

Mr. Majors's initial admission assessment demonstrated several psychosocial needs. It is important to assess his safety both through necessary suicidal precautions and assistance with ambulation. Mr. Majors's safety should be a priority. It is also important to maintain the patient's support systems.

Potential nursing diagnoses for ADC include the following:

- Anxiety related to unknown progression of HIV/AIDS
- Ineffective coping related to depression and AIDS dementia
- ADC related to unknown progression of HIV/AIDS
- Fear related to the unknown progression of HIV/AIDS

It is necessary to design a plan of care according to assessment data and expected outcomes. For example, because Mr. Majors will have perceptual alterations, including diminishing memory, it is important to have him keep a calendar to help him follow treatment regimens. Instructions should be simple and concise.

During the time that Mr. Majors has PCP, it is important to follow care according to developed nursing diagnoses and expected outcomes.

The nursing care of a patient with ADC and PCP in the ICU depends not only on the nurses' knowledge of the physiology of the disease process but also on the psychosocial needs of the critically ill patient. The stressors that a patient faces when in the ICU include but are not limited to fear of death, threat of survival, loss of control, inability to communicate needs, and loss of dignity (Urden et al, 2002). Compliance with medication regimens is very important to stress to a patient with HIV/AIDS. Noncompliance with HIV medication can cause viral mutation and drug resistance.

Text continued on p. 428

Table 28-3   *Antiretroviral Drugs Overview**

Generic (Trade)	Adverse Events	Comments	FDA Approval Date/Manufacturer‡
Nucleoside Reverse Transcriptase Inhibitors (NRTIs)†			
zidovudine/AZT/ZDV (Retrovir)	Bone marrow suppression, anemia and/or neutropenia, gastrointestinal intolerance, headache, insomnia, asthenia	May be given with or without food. Routine dose modification is not required when coadministering fluconazole, methadone, rifampin, and valproic acid.	March 19, 1987/Glaxo SmithKline
didanosine/ddI (Videx)	Pancreatitis, peripheral neuropathy, nausea, diarrhea	Tablets are flavored and can be chewed or dissolved in water. Avoid alcohol because it could increase chances of pancreatitis.	October 9, 1991/Bristol-Myers Squibb
zalcitabine/ddc (Hivid)	Peripheral neuropathy, stomatitis	Due to the need to dose frequently this drug is seldom prescribed.	June 19, 1992/Hoffmann-La Roche
tenofovir disoproxil fumarate (Viread)	Asthenia, headache, diarrhea, nausea, vomiting, flatulence	The likelihood of drug interactions is small.	October 26, 2001/Gilead Sciences Inc.
stavudine/d4T (Zerit)	Pancreatitis, peripheral neuropathy	May be taken with or without food.	June 24, 1994/Bristol-Myers Squibb
lamivudine/3TC (Epivir)	Minimal toxicity; cough, dizziness, fatigue, stomach discomfort, headache, and trouble sleeping. Epivir has also been known to cause anemia (decreased red blood cell function), hair loss, rash, and neutropenia (decreased neutrophils, a type of white blood cell)	TMP-SMZ has shown to increase lamivudine levels.	November 17, 1995/Glaxo SmithKline
abacavir/ABC (Ziagen)	Hypersensitivity reaction, fever, rash, nausea, vomiting, malaise or fatigue, loss of appetite, sore throat, cough, shortness of breath	Patients should receive medication guide and warning card at time of prescription. May be taken with or without food.	September 17, 1998/Bristol Myers-Squibb
Non-Nucleoside Reverse Transcriptase Inhibitors (NNRTIs)			
nevirapine (Viramune)	Rash, in a small number the rash has been severe. Rare hepatitis/liver problems	May lower plasma levels of other concomitant medications.	June 21, 1996/Boehringer Ingelheim Pharmaceuticals, Inc
delavirdine (Rescriptor)	Rash, increased transaminase levels, headache	These drugs should not be taken with delavirdine: terfenadine (Seldane), astemizole (Hismanal), alprazolam, midazolam, triazolam, cisapride (Propulsid), rifabutin (Mycobutin), rifampin, phenytoin, phenobarbital, carbamazepine. Antacids and didanosine (Videx) should be taken at least an hour apart from delavirdine. The class of H₂ inhibitor medications is not recommended. May be taken with or without food.	April 4, 1997/Pfizer

Table 28-3 *Antiretroviral Drugs Overview*—cont'd

Generic (Trade)	Adverse Events	Comments	FDA Approval Date/Manufacturer†
efavirenz (Sustiva)	Rash, central nervous system symptoms, increased transaminase levels, false-positive cannabinoid test	Should be taken on an empty stomach preferably at bedtime. Avoid the following drugs: astemizole, cisapride, midazolam, triazolam, or ergot derivatives and St. John's wort.	September 17, 1998/Bristol Myers-Squibb
Protease Inhibitors (PIs)			
indinavir (Crixivan)	Nephrolithiasis, GI intolerance, nausea, increased indirect bilirubin, headache, asthenia, blurred vision, dizziness, rash, metallic taste, thrombocytopenia, alopecia, hyperglycemia, fat redistribution, lipid abnormalities	Avoid the following drugs: cisapride, ergotamine or dihydroergotamine, astemizole or terfenadine, and midazolam or triazolam.	March 13, 1996/Merck & Co., Inc.
ritonavir (Norvir)	GI intolerance, nausea, vomiting, diarrhea, paresthesia, hepatitis, pancreatitis, asthenia, taste perversion, abnormal liver enzymes and cholesterol, creatine phosphokinase (CPK) and uric acid elevations, hyperglycemia	Avoid cisapride, astemizole or terfenadine, rifabutin; herbal or natural products containing St. John's wort, pimozide, ergotamine or dihydroergotamine; amiodarone, bepridil, flecainide, propafenone, or quinidine (Quinidex, others); diazepam, clorazepate, estazolam, flurazepam, midazolam, triazolam, or zolpidem. Take with food. Ritonavir may reduce the effectiveness of birth control pills.	March 1, 1996/Abbott Laboratories
nelfinavir (Viracept)	Diarrhea, hyperglycemia, abnormal liver enzymes	Avoid terfenadine, astemizole, cisapride, triazolam, midazolam, amiodarone, quinidine, and drugs known as ergot derivatives. The interactions could be life-threatening. Rifampin reduces levels of nelfinavir. Rifabutin should not be taken with nelfinavir. Ketoconazole increases the effect of nelfinavir. Take with food approximately 12 hours apart.	March 14, 1997/Pfizer
fosamprenavir calcium (Lexiva)	Diarrhea, nausea, vomiting, headache, and rash were generally mild to moderate in severity	To be used as in combination with other antiretroviral agents. May be taken with or without food.	October 20, 2003/GlaxoSmithKline

Drug	Adverse Effects	Comments	Approval Date/Manufacturer
saquinavir (Invirase; Fortovase)	GI intolerance, nausea, diarrhea, headache, elevated transaminase levels, hyperglycemia, lipid abnormalities	Avoid astemizole, terfenadine, ergotamine, cisapride, midazolam, triazolam. Take with food, full meal.	November 7, 1997/Hoffmann-La Roche
amprenavir (Agenerase)	GI intolerance, nausea, diarrhea, headache, elevated transaminase levels, hyperglycemia, lipid abnormalities	The pharmacokinetic parameters can be altered when combined with several drugs that are typically coadministered. May be given with or without food.	April 15, 1999/Glaxo SmithKline

Fusion Inhibitors (New Classification)

Drug	Adverse Effects	Comments	Approval Date/Manufacturer
enfuvirtide (Fuzeon)	Injection site reaction (98%), Pneumonia, hypersensitivity reactions, less frequent adverse events: glomerulonephritis, thrombocytopenia, neutropenia, fever, hyperglycemia, sixth nerve palsy.	Patient education important in order to have a good understanding of the Fuzeon injection instructions. Monitor for cellulitis at injection site. Fuzeon is not a cure for HIV-1 infections. Must be taken as part of a combination antiretroviral regimen.	March 13, 2003 Roche

Combination Drugs

Drug	Adverse Effects	Comments	Approval Date/Manufacturer
lamivudine & zidovudine (Combivir)	Headache, malaise, fatigue, nausea, diarrhea, anorexia, neuropathy, insomnia, nasal signs and symptoms, musculoskeletal pain	Educate individuals who are taking this medicine that they should not drink alcoholic beverages. Patients should inform their physicians if they have blood disease, kidney or liver disease, or an inflamed pancreas before starting Combivir.	September 7, 1997/Glaxo SmithKline
abacavir, zidovudine, and lamivudine (Trizivir)	Similar to individual drugs; hypersensitivity issue with abacavir	Drugs that may alter Trizivir blood concentrations: TMP-SMZ, fluconazole, ethanol, and valproic acid. Medication guide and warning card should be given to the patient describing the hypersensitivity issue.	November 14, 2000/Glaxo Wellcome
lopinavir + ritonavir (Kaletra)	GI intolerance, nausea, diarrhea, asthenia, elevated transaminase levels, hyperglycemia, lipid abnormalities	Avoid cisapride, pimozide, flecainide, propafenone, astemizole, terfenadine, dihydroergotamine, ergonovise, ergotamine, methylergonovine, midazolam, and triazolam. Take with food.	September 15, 2000/Abbott Laboratories
tenofovir disoproxil fumarate (Viread)	Headache, pain, diarrhea, depression, and rash	Take with food, preferably a full meal that contains some fat. Possibly effective against hepatitis B virus (HBV).	October 26, 2001/Gilead Sciences, Inc.

*This is a summary of the adverse events and comments and should be used for informational purposes only. Package insert information should be referred to.

†Manufacturer provided because some companies offer compassionate care programs to help defer the cost of drug.

‡The NRTIs have a toxic effect on the liver, potentially causing lactic acidosis with hepatic steatosis.

Flaskerud, J. H., & Ungvarski, P. J. (1999). *HIV/AIDS: A guide to primary care management* (4th ed.). Philadelphia: Saunders http://www.fda.gov/oashi/aids/virals.html 12/19/2002. FDA AIDS HIV Antiviral Drugs (Nov 7, 2001). US Food and Drug Association. http://www.fda.gov/oashi/aids/stat_app.html 12/19/2002. Approved Drugs for HIV/AIDS and AIDS-related Conditions (Feb 19, 2002).

Package inserts from Pharmaceutical companies http://www.aidsmeds.com/List.htm 11/6/2003 AIDS Meds.com (Apr 23, 2003). Additional References from Package Inserts for Anti-Virals include Abbott Laboratories, Boehringer Ingelheim Pharmaceuticals, Inc., Bristol Myers-Squibb, Gilead Sciences, Glaxo

Table 28-4	HIV-Related Illnesses—Opportunistic Infections			
Disease	**Organism**	**Symptoms/Diseases**	**Treatment**	**Prevention**
		Protozoans		
Cryptosporidiosis	*Cryptosporidium*	Profuse watery diarrhea that can result in weight loss, electrolyte imbalance, and dehydration	No drug has been identified as effective on cryptosporidium. Treat symptoms and HAART.	Avoidance of ingestion of spores. Spores are found in human and animal feces and contaminated water.
Isosporiasis	*Isospora belli*	Gastroenteritis, profuse watery diarrhea, headache, malaise, fever, abdominal pain, vomiting, dehydration, and weight loss	Trimethoprim-sulfamethoxazole (TMP-SMZ)	Avoidance of infective feces and good handwashing.
Toxoplasmosis	*Toxoplasma gondii*	Alteration in mental status, seizures, motor weakness, cranial nerve disturbances, sensory abnormalities, movement disorders, encephalitis, retinitis, and disseminated intravascular coagulopathies	TMP-SMZ, dapsone, pyrimethamine, and sulfadiazine. Also treatment of symptoms such as with phenytoin for seizures.	Proper handwashing, food safety, and pet care
		Fungi		
Candidiasis	*Candida* spp.	Stomatitis/white plaques or lesions (thrush), proctitis, vaginitis, and esophagitis	Clotrimazole troches, nystatin suspension, nystatin pastilles, ketoconazole, fluconazole, miconazole, and sometimes itraconazole or amphotericin B	Preventive prophylaxis is not needed because oral *Candida* responds well to treatment. Weekly fluconazole is recommended for the prevention of vaginal candidiasis.

Coccidioidomycosis	*Coccidioides immitis*	Respiratory symptoms, along with fever, chills, weight loss, fatigue, meningitis, and dessemination	Amphotericin B and then continual treatment with oral fluconazole	Preventive prophylaxis is not recommended. People in areas that are endemic of *Coccidioides* should avoid exposure. After first exposure lifelong suppressive therapy is needed to prevent relapse.
Cryptococcosis	*Cryptococcus neoformans*	Headache, fever, lethargy, confusion, meningitis, (inflammation of spinal cord and brain), pneumonia, encephalitis, and dissemination	Itraconanzole, fluconazole, amphotericin B, in rare occasions	Prevention is avoidance of pigeon feces because the spores enter the lungs. Acquired through the respiratory tract.
Histoplasmosis	*Histoplasma capsulatum*	Pneumonia, dissemination, fever, weight loss, hepatosplenomegaly, mouth ulcers. Other symptoms will depend on organ involvement.	Fluconazole and itraconanzole show a better response than amphotericin B or ketoconazole.	Areas endemic are the middle, central and southern United States. Avoid chicken coops, disturbing soil near bird roosting areas, and cave exploration.
Pneumocystis carinii	*Pneumocystis carinii* pneumonia (PCP)	Develops over a 2- to 3-week period. Shortness of breath, fever, and a nonproductive cough	TMP-SMZ or pentamidine are the main drugs of choice. Dapsone-trimethoprim, clindamycin-preaquine and atovaquone have been studied as possible treatments.	Prevention of PCP is primary prophylaxis.

Table 28-4 HIV-Related Illnesses—Opportunistic Infections—cont'd

Disease	Organism	Symptoms/Diseases	Treatment	Prevention
Bacteria				
Mycobacterium avium-intracellulare (MAC) disease	*Mycobacterium avium-intracellulare* disease (MAC)	Dissemination, pneumonia, diarrhea, weight loss, high fever, lymphadenopathy, severe gastrointestinal disease	Clarithromycin or azithromycin plus ethambutol, rifabutin, ciprofloxacin, clofazimine, or amikacin are recommendations by the CDC.	MAC is found in the environment and difficult to prevent.
Mycobacterium Tuberculosis	*Mycobacterium tuberculosis*	Fever, weight loss, night sweats, fatigue, dyspnea, chills, hemoptysis, chest pain, meningitis, and dissemination	A four-drug regimen is recommended by CDC: isoniazid, rifampin, pyrazinamide, and either streptomycin or ethambutol.	Preventive chemotherapy
Cytomegalovirus (CMV)	Cytomegalovirus	Fever, hepatitis, encephalitis, visual loss, visual field alteration, floaters, retinitis, pneumonia, colitis, esophagitis	High-dose ganciclovir or foscarnet IV and maintenance oral ganciclovir	HIV-positive people should be evaluated for prior exposure to CMV. If seropositive for CMV, they should receive prophylaxis against the disease.
HIV encephalopathy, AIDS-dementia complex (ADC)	HIV-1	Mild neurocognitive disorder, forgetfulness	Zidovudine (AZT)	Preventive treatment is not available at this time.
Epstein-Barr virus	Oral hairy leukoplakia, B cell lymphoma, mononucleosis	Fever, malaise, pharyngeal pain, pharyngitis, adenopathy, headaches, sore throat, nausea, vomiting and splenomegaly	Bedrest, medications for fever, brief corticosteroid therapy, acyclovir may have some benefit.	Education on transmission through saliva.
Herpes simplex	Herpes simplex I and II	Mucocutaneous (mouth, genital, rectal) blisters and/or ulcers, pneumonia, esophagitis, and encephalitis	Acyclovir; IV, oral and topical, famciclovir	Education on transmission, encouragement to use latex condoms and protection during oral sex

Human papovavirus (JC virus JCV)	Progressive multifocal leukoencephalopathy	Mental deficits, visual difficulties, motor weakness, lack of coordination, speech difficulties, headaches, vertigo, and seizures	At this time no forms of therapy have been effective.	At this time there are no recommended preventive measures.
Shingles, chickenpox	Varicella-zoster	Dermatomal vesicular skin lesions (shingles) and encephalitis	Famciclovir, acyclovir, foscarnet, and analgesic for symptom (pain) relief	Avoid exposure to chickenpox. Virus is harbored in body.
Cancers				
Kaposi's sarcoma	Kaposi's sarcoma (KS)	Disseminated mucocutaneous (pink, red) papule or nodular lesions involving skin, lymph nodes, and visceral organs (lungs and gastrointestinal)	Localized radiation, cryotherapy, laser therapy, and intralesional therapy for small lesions. For progressive disease antineoplastic agent can be used.	There is a theory that KS could be associated with oncogenic virus that could be sexually transmitted. Prevention is safe sex.
Non-Hodgkin's lymphoma	Non-Hodgkin's lymphoma	Fever, night sweats, weight loss, enlarged lymph nodes. Depending on location of tumor, localized symptoms	Radiation and studies are being done on the use of radiation and systemic chemotherapy.	No current recommendations
Cervical cancer	Cervical intraepithelial neoplasia	Asymptomatic in early stages, vaginal bleeding, malodorous blood-tinged vaginal discharge; with disease progression could be abdominal, pelvic, and back pain and cervical dysplasia	Carbon dioxide laser therapy, conization, cryosurgery, cautery, and simple hysterectomy	Early treatment of cervical dysplasia; timely Pap smears for early diagnosis

US Food and Drug Administration (Feb 19, 2002). Approved drugs for HIV/AIDS and AIDS-related conditions. References: USPHS/IDSA. (2001, Nov 28) Guidelines for the prevention of opportunistic infections in person infected with human immunodeficiency virus.
US Food and Drug Administration (2002, Feb 19). Approved drugs for HIV/AIDS and AIDS-related conditions.
Ungvarski, P. J. and Flaskerud, J. H. (1999). HIV/AIDS: A guide to primary care management. 4th ed. Saunders. Philadelphia, PA.
Kirton, C. (Ed.). (2003). ANAC's *Core Curriculum for HIV/AIDS Nursing.* Thousand Oaks: Sage Publications.

13. When assigned to a patient with HIV infection, what personal feelings or concerns should be acknowledged?

These fears are going to be very individualized. It is important that the nurse addresses his or her fears related to disease transmission, homophobia, and other feelings that arise when caring for patients with HIV infection. Unfortunately it is still common in hospitals and in community settings to encounter nurses who are "afraid" to care for these patients. Individual needs should be recognized and educational programs that correct misinformation related to this disease should be developed and implemented. The latest revision of the American Nurses Association's Nurses Code is a guide for carrying out nursing responsibilities in a manner consistent with quality in nursing care and the ethical obligations of the profession. Sole and associates (2001) suggest that nurses who care for HIV-positive patients receive assistance to meet their own physical and emotional needs and to do continuing education for the nurses that may help to address their fears.

14. Are the ICU nurses at an increased risk of acquiring AIDS from patients who receive mechanical ventilation?

The incidence of medical personnel contracting AIDS from patients is quite low. The use of universal precautions by all medical personnel lessens the risk of infection. It is important to handle blood and body fluids properly. It is important to follow the CDC recommendations for prevention of HIV transmission in health care settings and to follow the Occupational Safety and Health Administration's blood and body fluid precautions.

The risk of acquiring HIV infection from needlesticks or cuts exposed to HIV-infected blood is 0.3% (1 in 300). The risk of exposure of the eyes, nose, or mouth (mucous membranes) to HIV-infected blood is 0.09% (CDC, 2001). Exposure of skin to a small amount of blood has practically no risk. It is important that ICU staff take precautions to avoid contact with blood and body fluids from all patients. As of June 2000, the CDC has received 56 documented cases and 138 possible cases of occupationally acquired HIV infection among health care workers (CDC, 2001). The United States has laws and regulations to protect the health care worker. These laws are about the implementation of needle-safe devices to reduce needlestick injuries (West, 2002). Health care workers also need to protect themselves from hepatitis C transmission.

15. What is the recommended protocol for occupational exposure to HIV?

The CDC has very specific guidelines for the follow-up of potential occupational exposure. These protocols can be found on their website at www.cdc.gov/ncidod/hip/faq.htm and include the following (CDC, 2001):

1. If the source client is seronegative for HIV and has no clinical evidence or risk for HIV infection or AIDS, no further follow-up is indicated. No postexposure prophylaxis (PEP) recommended.

2. If the source patient has AIDS, is seropositive for HIV, or refuses to be tested and has HIV risk factors, as soon as possible after the exposure, the health care worker (HCW) will be referred for baseline serologic testing for evidence of HIV. The HCW may go to the employee health or emergency room health care provider/facility of choice or may be referred to a designated laboratory/agency. This will depend on the employer's infection control policy. The HCW should be referred for postexposure counseling about the risk of infection, prevention of transmission of HIV during the follow-up period, and the need for appropriate follow-up medical care. Generally PEP recommendations are done according to the status of the patient. If the patient is asymptomatic HIV+ or has a known low viral load, the recommended PEP is the 2-drug regimen. If the patient is symptomatic HIV+ PEP should not be delayed and a 3-drug regimen is recommended.

3. Those exposed will have follow-up HIV testing at 6 weeks, 3 months, 6 months, and 12 months postexposure at a health care provider/facility of choice.

ACQUIRED IMMUNODEFICIENCY SYNDROME

References

Approved drugs for HIV/AIDS and AIDS- related conditions. (2002, Feb 19). Retrieved December 19, 2002. www.fda.gov/oashi/aids/stat_app.html.

Bedos, J. P., et al. (June, 1999). *Pneumocystis carinii* pneumonia requiring intensive care management; survival and prognostic study in 110 patients with human immunodeficiency virus. *Critical Care Medicine, 27*(6), 1109-1115.

Centers for Disease Control and Prevention. (1992). 1993 revised classification system for HIV infection and expanded surveillance case definition for AIDS among adolescents and adults. *MMWR Morbidity and Mortality Weekly Report, 41*(RR-17), 1-19.

Centers for Disease Control and Prevention. (2001). Updated U.S. public health service guidelines for the management of occupational exposure to HBV, HCV, and HIV and recommendations for postexposure prophylaxis. *MMWR Morbidity and Mortality Weekly Report, 41*(RR-11), 1-52.

Cielsa, J. & Roberts, J. (2001) Being HIV-positive could increase risk of depression. *American Journal of Psychiatry, 158*, 725-730.

Department of Health and Human Services (DHHS) and the Henry J. Kaiser Family Foundation. (Feb 4, 2002). *Guidelines for the use of antiretroviral agents in HIV-infected adults and adolescents.* Also can be found at www.hivatis.org.

Department of Health and Human Services (DHHS) and the Henry J. Kaiser Family Foundation. (July 14, 2003) *Guidelines for the use of antiretroviral agents in HIV-1 infected adults and adolescents.* Also can be found at http://aidsinfo.nih.gov/guidelines/adult/AA_071403.pdf.

Douglas, S. (1999). Human immunodeficiency virus disease. In L. Bucher & S. Melander (Eds.), *Critical care nursing.* Philadelphia: W. B. Saunders.

Gill, J. K., Greene, L., Miller, R., Pozniak, A., Cartledge, J., et al. (1999). ICU admission in patients infected with the human immunodeficiency virus—A multicentre survey. *Anaesthesia, 54*(8), 727-732.

Package inserts for antiretroviral drugs: zidovudine (AZT/ZDV/Retrovir), didanosine (ddI/Videx), zalcitabine (ddC/Hivid), tenofovir disoproxil fumarate (Viread), Stavudine (d4T/Zerit), abacavir (ABC/Ziagen), lamivudine (3TC/Epivir), nevirapine (Viramune), delavirdine (Rescriptor), efavirenz (Sustiva), indinavir (Crixivan), ritonavir (Norvir), nelfinavir (Viracept), saquinavir (Invirase/Fortovase), amprenavir (Agenerase), abacavir, zidovudine, and lamivudine (Trizivir), lamivudine and zidovudine (Combivir), lopinavir and ritonavir (Kaletra), tenofovir disoproxil fumarate (Viread).

Schneider, M. M., Borleffs, J. C., Stolk, R. P., Jaspers, C. A., & Hoepelman (1999). Discontinuation of prophylaxis for *Pneumocystis carinii* pneumonia in HIV-1–infected patients treated with highly active antiretroviral therapy. *The Lancet, 353*(9148), 201-203.

Stine, G. J. (2003). *AIDS update 2003.* Upper Saddle River, NJ: Prentice-Hall.

Stringer, J. R., Beard, C. B., Miller, R., & Wakefield, A. E. (2002). A new name *(Pneumocystis jiroveci)* for pneumocystis from humans. [Electronic version]. *Emergency Infectious Diseases 8*(9).

Sole, M. L., Lamborn, M. L., & Hartshorn, J. C. (2001). *Introduction to critical nursing* (3rd ed.). Philadelphia: W. B. Saunders.

US Food and Drug Administration. (2001, Nov 7). FDA AIDS/HIV antiviral drugs. Retrieved December 19, 2002. www.fda.gov/oashi/aids/virals.html.

Ungvarski, P. J., & Flaskerud, J. H. (1999). *HIV/AIDS: A guide to primary care management* (4th ed.). Philadelphia: W. B. Saunders.

Urden, L. D., Stacy, K. M., & Lough, M. E. (2002). *Thelan's critical care nursing diagnosis and management* (4th ed.). St Louis: Mosby.

Valenti, W. (2002). HIV Disease Management: New technologies improve outcomes and contain costs, *The AIDS Reader, 12*(2):64-66.

West, K. (2002). AIDS update: Occupational exposure and post-exposure treatment of HIV/AIDS. *Journal of Emergency Medical Service, 27*(12), 48-60.

29

Blunt Abdominal Trauma

Joan E. King, RN, PhD, ACNP, ANP

CASE PRESENTATION

Mr. Lancaster is a 35-year-old patient who was involved in a motor vehicle accident. Mr. Lancaster was wearing a seat belt and driving at a high rate of speed when he lost control of the car and hit an abutment. He was initially awake at the scene, but his level of consciousness declined while in transport to the hospital. Upon arrival, he was already intubated and he had received 2 L of normal saline.

Mr. Lancaster's medical history was noncontributory. His family history was negative for heart disease, diabetes, or cancer. Mr. Lancaster has a 15-pack-year history of smoking, and he drinks socially.

Upon arrival at the hospital, Mr. Lancaster was on a backboard with a cervical collar. His vital signs were the following:

BP	110/80 mm Hg
HR	113 bpm
Sao$_2$	95% (with 100% oxygen)

His pupils were 3 cm and equal and reacted briskly to light. Mr. Lancaster did not have Battle's sign or raccoon eyes, and no abnormalities ("step-offs") were noted over his skull or down his spine. The tympanic membranes were clear, and the trachea was midline. Examination of the chest revealed no flailing and no subcutaneous emphysema. Breath sounds were diminished in the lower lobes bilaterally. The patient was tachycardic with normal S_1 and S_2 and no murmurs, rubs, or gallops. Peripheral pulses were 2+ bilaterally. His abdomen was soft and moderately distended with hypoactive bowel sounds. There were no palpable masses and no hepatosplenomegaly. The pelvis was stable. Genitourinary examination revealed no gross hematuria. Rectal tone was normal, and stool was guaiac negative. The patient was able to move all four extremities spontaneously, but orientation to time, person, and place was difficult to assess because he had been sedated.

Initially Mr. Lancaster was taken for a computed tomographic (CT) scan, which revealed a grade III liver laceration. No splenic or renal injuries were noted. A CT scan of the head revealed no hematoma. Because of the patient's unstable condition, his spine could not be fully evaluated. Chest x-ray examination revealed bilateral pulmonary contusion with bilateral rib fractures.

His initial laboratory values after fluid resuscitation were the following:

WBCs	21.7×10^3 mm^3
PCVs	34
Platelets	217,000/mm^3

PT	21.0 sec
INR	1.7
PTT	41.9 sec
Na$^+$	135 mmol/L
K$^+$	4.2 mmol/L
CO$_2$	22 mmol/L
Cl$^-$	119 mmol/L
BUN	9 mg/dl
Creatinine	1.0 mg/dl
Glucose	170 mg/dl
AST (SGOT)	635 U/L
Bilirubin	0.9 mg/dl
Albumin	1.8 g/dl

Arterial blood gas (ABG) values were as follows:

pH	7.1
Pa$_{CO_2}$	51 mm Hg
Pa$_{O_2}$	82 mm Hg (with 100% oxygen)
Base deficit	14.4

A toxicology screen was negative for drugs, but Mr. Lancaster's blood alcohol level was 171 g/dl.

Mr. Lancaster's problem list upon admission to the trauma center was the following:

1. Blunt abdominal trauma
2. No closed head injury (CHI) as revealed by CT scan
3. Bilateral pulmonary contusions with bilateral rib fractures
4. Relative hypoxia with a Pa$_{O_2}$ value of 80 with inhalation of 100% oxygen
5. Metabolic acidosis
6. Hypovolemic shock

Mr. Lancaster was taken directly to the trauma intensive care unit, where he was given synchronized intermittent mechanical ventilation (SIMV) with positive end-expiratory pressure (PEEP) and pressure support (PS). A pulmonary artery (PA) catheter, nasogastric tube (NGT), and Foley catheter were inserted. Because of his hyperchloremia, his fluid infusions were changed from normal saline to lactated Ringer's solution. His acidosis was treated with three runs of sodium bicarbonate. Over the next 12 hours Mr. Lancaster's abdomen became very firm and distended, with less than 300 ml of drainage from the NGT. In addition, his peak inspiratory pressure (PIP) rose from 35 to 60 mm Hg, and his bladder pressure rose to 35 mm Hg.

At this time, his vital signs were as follows:

BP	100/80 mm Hg
HR	130 bpm
Respirations	14 breaths/min

The diagnosis of abdominal compartment syndrome (ACS) was made. Mr. Lancaster was immediately taken to the operating room, and a decompression celiotomy was performed. At that time, the laceration on the right dome of the liver was assessed and packed. No other injuries were noted, but the small bowel was edematous and distended. Because of the edema, the abdomen could not be closed, and the intestines were covered with a sterile towel and a large sterile transparent dressing was placed over the wound.

When Mr. Lancaster was returned to the trauma unit, vital signs were the following:

PIP	35 mm Hg
BP	120/64 mm Hg
HR	112 bpm
PAP	50/27
CI	5.5 L/min/m^2
EF	40%
EDVI	98 ml/m^2

His ventilator settings were the following:

SIMV rate	14
Respirations	14 breaths/min
V$_T$	750 ml
Fio$_2$	40%
PEEP	10 cm H$_2$O
PS	5
Sao$_2$	97%
Svo$_2$	83%

Antibiotics (gentamicin and trovafloxacin/alatrofloxacin [Trovan]) were started with fentanyl (Sublimaze) for pain control. Peptic ulcer prophylaxis with famotidine (Pepcid) was begun. Because of his pulmonary contusions and the need to control his respiratory status, Mr. Lancaster was given conscious sedation using lorazepam (Ativan).

Two days after his initial surgery, Mr. Lancaster returned to the operating room for reexploration of his abdomen, and an assessment of his liver laceration. When the packing was removed, hemostasis had been maintained and there was no necrosis of the liver or any signs of active bleeding. On day 6 he was returned to the operating room, and his abdominal fascia was closed using stay sutures. The skin was not closed because the wound had been open for 6 days, and instead the wound was packed with sterile wet to dry dressings. Other significant events that occurred included the start of enteral feedings on day 3 with progression to 90 ml of Perative every hour by day 5. On day 6 Mr. Lancaster underwent a tracheotomy, and weaning from the ventilator began on day 8. Nineteen days after Mr. Lancaster was in the accident, he was transferred to a rehabilitation facility, where he required only supplementary oxygen through a tracheotomy collar with minimal suction every 2 hours.

BLUNT ABDOMINAL TRAUMA

QUESTIONS

1. What are the initial assessment priorities for a patient with blunt abdominal trauma?

2. What is meant by a secondary survey?

3. What is meant by a tertiary survey?

4. What diagnostic tests are done to evaluate and treat patients who have sustained a blunt abdominal trauma?

5. What are the management guidelines for a patient with blunt abdominal trauma?

6. What is meant by ACS?

7. What is a pulmonary contusion?

8. What other factors may be contributing to Mr. Lancaster's poor oxygenation status?

9. Why was conscious sedation used with Mr. Lancaster and does it differ from pharmacologically paralyzing a patient?

10. What other complications is Mr. Lancaster at risk for, and how should they be monitored?

11. What are the nutritional needs of a patient with a blunt abdominal trauma?

BLUNT ABDOMINAL TRAUMA

QUESTIONS AND ANSWERS

1. ### What are the initial assessment priorities for a patient with blunt abdominal trauma?

Trauma is the fourth leading cause of death in the United States (Laskowski-Jones, 1999), with the mortality rate for major liver injuries (grade IV/V) ranging between 50% and 80% (Yang et al, 2002). Blunt abdominal trauma is particularly challenging because assessment of the injuries is often difficult and injuries can be missed (Melanson & Heller, 1998). Assessment of the patient with blunt abdominal trauma can be divided into primary survey, secondary survey, and tertiary survey.

The primary survey focuses on an initial assessment of airway, breathing, and circulation and a rapid neurologic assessment to identify spinal injuries or a CHI. Airway management and oxygenation are of prime importance. This includes assessing for a patent airway, life-threatening facial injuries, the patient's ability to breathe spontaneously, and the presence and quality of breath sounds. Absent or diminished breath sounds may indicate a hemothorax or pneumothorax. Absent breath sounds with a deviated trachea are signs of a tension pneumothorax, which requires immediate management with the insertion of a chest tube or decompression with a 14- to 16-gauge needle. Further assessment of the chest for rib fractures; flail chest; sucking, open wounds; or subcutaneous emphysema should be rapidly performed. If the patient is responsive to pain, palpation of the chest anteriorly and laterally may help identify possible rib fractures (Prentice & Ahrens, 1994; Urden et al, 2002). A flail chest can be assessed by noting the paradoxic movement of the chest wall caused by multiple rib fractures in two or more places. Portable chest x-ray units provide added data about rib fractures and document the presence of a hemothorax or pneumothorax. Many patients with a pneumothorax or a flail chest may require intubation to provide ventilatory support and improve oxygenation.

Although ABG values give the most definitive assessment of the patient's respiratory status, pulse oximetry can provide a quick assessment of the patient's oxygen saturations. It should be noted that if the patient has a low hemoglobin (Hgb) level, the oxygen saturations may still be in the acceptable range (Brooks-Brunn, 1999). However, important information can still be obtained with pulse oximetry, including oxygen saturation trends and critically low saturations below 90%.

While a rapid assessment of the respiratory system is performed, the circulatory status is also assessed, including heart rate, rhythm, and blood pressure (BP). In the prehospital field, if a BP reading cannot be obtained, the following guidelines are used: (1) if a radial pulse is palpable the BP is estimated to be 80 mm Hg systolic; (2) if the radial pulse is not palpable but the femoral artery is, the BP is estimated to be 70 mm Hg systolic; and (3) if only the carotid pulse is palpable, the BP is estimated to be 60 mm Hg systolic (Laskowski-Jones, 1999). During the primary survey any overt signs of bleeding are assessed and controlled, if possible, with direct pressure.

Interventions to achieve stabilization of the circulatory system will include the administration of fluids, either normal saline or lactated Ringer's, and blood products. There is a great deal of controversy concerning the use of colloids during initial stabilization. It is important to realize that capillaries of patients in shock begin to leak fluid into the interstitial spaces as a result of increased capillary permeability. This implies that regardless of the type of fluid administered, a certain proportion will leave the circulatory system and enter the interstitial spaces. This phenomenon is called *third spacing,* and it contributes to the edema that trauma patients experience in the postresuscitation phase. Because it is believed that colloids may enhance the third spacing as a result of an increase in colloidal osmotic pressure in the interstitial spaces, crystalloids are preferred (Melio, 1998). Further controversy exists as to how much fluid should be given. Previously it was thought that because of the generalized increase in capillary permeability, during the initial resuscitation phase, patients would require 3 L of fluids to be administered for every 1 L of estimated blood loss (Jacobs, 1994). However, more current research indicates that massive fluid resuscitation may not be desirable and that it is more prudent to titrate fluid administration according to the patient's blood pressure (Armstrong, 2002; Dutton et al, 2002). Thus monitoring the BP serves as the key assessment parameter in determining the amount of fluid required.

Another factor that needs to be evaluated when determining fluid resuscitation is whether the bleeding is considered to be controlled or uncontrolled. *Controlled bleeding* refers to the ability to identify and stop the source of bleeding. *Uncontrolled bleeding* or *hemorrhage* refers to the inability to either identify or stop the source of the bleeding. According to Melio (1998), if the bleeding can be controlled, maximal fluid resuscitation is appropriate. However, if the bleeding is uncontrolled, rapid fluid resuscitation may promote additional bleeding and increase mortality. In patients with uncontrolled bleeding or hemorrhage, sufficient amounts of fluid should be administered to treat the shock, but not enough to restore full cardiovascular status and hence promote additional bleeding (Melio, 1998). Armstrong (2002) advocates for "permissive hypotension," in which the fluid resuscitation is titrated toward a lower than normal systolic blood pressure (Dutton et al, 2002).

Patients with blunt trauma must also be assessed for cardiac tamponade, especially those involved in a motor vehicle accident. Because of the frequent presence of hypotension or hemorrhagic shock, the classic Beck's triad (elevated central venous pressure [CVP], pulsus paradoxus, and decreased heart sounds) may not be evident. Melio (1998) recommends ultrasonography or echocardiography if the patient's condition is stable, and a pericardiocentesis if the patient's condition is unstable and a cardiac tamponade is suspected.

Although many trauma patients will enter the emergency department already intubated and sedated and with the cervical spine immobilized, it is important to perform a primary neurologic survey. The patient's level of responsiveness to verbal and painful stimuli should be assessed as well as the pupillary response to light and pupil size. In addition, the patient's ability to move all four extremities should be assessed quickly. At all times until the patient can have appropriate radiologic studies done to assess the cervical spine, trauma patients must be considered to have a cervical spine injury, and a cervical collar should be applied. Flexion and extension of the neck must be avoided even during intubation.

2. What is meant by a secondary survey?

As the primary survey is completed and life-threatening diagnoses are managed, the secondary survey begins. The secondary survey is a more complete and focused head-to-toe assessment of the patient. For patients with blunt abdominal trauma, the purpose of the secondary survey is to identify the extent of internal injuries. Obtaining information about the mechanism of injury is often helpful in guiding clinicians with their assessment. For patients who were involved in a motor vehicle collision, such as Mr. Lancaster, it is important to determine whether the patient was wearing a seat belt, if an air bag was activated, or if the patient was thrown from the vehicle. People who had been wearing a seat belt are often protected from CHIs but, depending on whether the patient was a passenger or the driver, will influence whether one anticipates liver or splenic injuries. A more thorough examination of the patient's abdomen, pelvis, and extremities is important during the secondary survey. Assessment of the abdomen should include auscultating for bowel sounds, percussion, and palpation. Abdominal tenderness is often difficult to assess in patients with blunt trauma, particularly if there is a CHI or if alcohol was involved. Both of these conditions diminish or alter the patient's response to pain and hence may provide misleading information about the absence of any abdominal trauma. Tests that may be performed to confirm or deny the presence of any abdominal injuries include a diagnostic peritoneal lavage (DPL), bedside ultrasonography, and an abdominal CT scan (Melanson & Heller,

1998; Urden et al, 2002). Although DPL can help detect abdominal injuries, it places the patient at risk for further injury to the iliac or mesenteric vessels and possible perforation of the intestines and bladder (Melanson & Heller, 1998). Institutional variation may exist in terms of whether ultrasonography or a CT scan is used, based on the resources available and how accessible the CT scanner is. Level I trauma centers frequently have the ability to quickly perform "traumagrams," which includes a CT scan of the head, neck, thoracic cavity, and abdomen.

Kidney and bladder injuries are also assessed during the secondary survey. Blood at the meatus and/or hematuria are indicators for additional tests to be performed to determine the extent of the injury and the definitive treatment. Hematuria is considered the hallmark of genitourinary injury. If urine tests show either microscopic or gross hematuria, subsequent diagnostic tests including a CT scan, an intravenous pyelogram, or a cystogram may be required (Ahn et al, 1998).

Additional assessments that will be made during the secondary survey include a continual assessment of cardiovascular and pulmonary function via vital signs and cardiac rhythm, and possibly echocardiography and CT scan of the thorax to assess for valvular problems, missed pneumothoraces, or missed injuries to the aorta or peripheral vasculature.

A more in-depth neurologic examination is also performed during the secondary survey, with attention being given to any skull or spinal abnormalities, usually referred to as *step-offs*. In addition, assessment of rectal tone can provide information about the integrity of the spinal nerves. Assessment for raccoon eyes (periorbital ecchymosis), Battle's sign (mastoid ecchymosis), or rhinorrhea should also be performed. The presence of any of these conditions may indicate a basilar skull fracture.

3. What is meant by a tertiary survey?

Tertiary survey refers to an additional comprehensive assessment that is done either after the patient can talk, when the patient is about to ambulate, or in some institutions within 24 hours of admission (Janjua et al, 1998). The focus of the tertiary survey is to identify previously missed injuries and to prevent possible complications caused by missed injuries. Studies have indicated great variability in the frequency of missed injuries for trauma patients, ranging from 2% to 50% (Sommers, 1995). However, patients with blunt abdominal trauma are at a higher risk for missed injuries than patients with penetrating trauma (Janjua et al, 1998). For all trauma patients, the most frequently missed injuries are musculoskeletal, with the most critically missed injury being a cervical spine injury. Although alterations in level of consciousness caused by either head injuries or drug or alcohol intake contribute to injuries being missed, hemodynamic instability and radiologic and technical errors also add to the problem. The guideline for assessing trauma patients is always to have a high degree of suspicion for missed injuries and to do frequent reassessments, looking for musculoskeletal injuries, additional pulmonary injuries (including rib fractures, cardiac and spinal injuries), and hidden abdominal injuries (Sommers, 1995; Ferrera et al, 1998). When a tertiary survey is being performed, external signs of injury should be noted, including any indication of soft tissue injury that may accompany skeletal, muscular, or nerve injury.

4. What diagnostic tests are done to evaluate and treat patients who have sustained a blunt abdominal trauma?

Routine laboratory tests performed for trauma patients include serial hematocrit measurements to assess the degree of bleeding; chemistry profiles to determine any imbalances particularly with sodium, chloride, and potassium as the result of fluid resuscitation; and serum glucose to assess for the degree of hyperglycemia that is often the result of insulin resistance caused by the trauma. The blood urea nitrogen (BUN) and creatinine levels should also be monitored to evaluate kidney function both at the time of admission and throughout the patient's hospitalization. ABG values also need to be monitored closely.

Mr. Lancaster had developed hyperchloremia caused by his metabolic acidosis and the administration of normal saline during his prehospital resuscitation. Correction of both metabolic acidosis and hyperchloremia involved administration of sodium bicarbonate and changing Mr. Lancaster's fluid infusions from normal saline, which has 154 mEq/L of both sodium and chloride, to lactated Ringer's solution, which has 130 mEq/L sodium and 107 mEq/L chloride. In addition, lactated Ringer's includes 4 mEq/L potassium, 2.7 mEq/L calcium, and 27 mEq/L lactate. Changing Mr. Lancaster's fluid infusions was beneficial in a number of ways. First, the lactate in lactated Ringer's solution is converted to bicarbonate in the absence of liver failure, and hence helps buffer the acidosis. Second, as the bicarbonate levels increase, the kidneys are able to exchange chloride ions for bicarbonate ions. Third, the lactated Ringer's solution contains less chloride. Thus the change not only addressed his hyperchloremia, but also his metabolic acidosis.

Additional tests that may be ordered are serial cardiac enzyme measurements if chest trauma is suspected. Also 12-lead electrocardiograms will help document any patterns of ischemia or injury. Toxicologic analysis of blood and blood alcohol levels are important to determine whether altered mental status is related to a CHI or to drug or alcohol use. Mr. Lancaster had a blood alcohol level of 171 g/dl. Any value greater than 100 is considered intoxication.

As previously stated, for assessment of blunt abdominal trauma, either bedside ultrasonography or an abdominal CT scan may be ordered. With the advent of new capabilities for CT scanning, abdominal CT scans have become more widely used. Numerous studies have been done that indicate the reliability of using CT scans to determine not only the area of the bleeding, but also the degree of involvement. CT scans are particularly useful in assessing solid organ damage such as liver lacerations, splenic involvement, and kidney injuries in addition to assessing injury to bone structures and the presence of either a hemoperitoneum or retroperitoneum (Melanson & Heller, 1998). CT scans are less reliable in assessing hollow organ damage such as damage to the bladder or intestines, and CT scans cannot detect whether bleeding has stopped (Melanson & Heller, 1998; Melio, 1998).

5. What are the management guidelines for a patient with blunt abdominal trauma?

The liver and spleen are the most commonly injured organs in blunt abdominal trauma. However, because of refinements in CT scanning, all patients with abdominal traumas are no longer automatically taken to the operating room for surgical treatment. Between 80% and 90% of all patients with blunt abdominal traumas are managed nonoperatively (Richardson et al, 2000). Liver injuries are graded I through VI, with grade I representing a hematoma involving less than 10% of the surface area or a laceration less than 1 cm in depth, and grade VI representing total avulsion (Box 29-1). The current trend is nonoperative management for patients who have sustained a blunt trauma to the abdomen, whose conditions are hemodynamically stable, and who have less than 500 ml of blood in the peritoneum as evidenced by CT scan. Patients managed nonoperatively necessitate frequent abdominal assessments, including noting any increase in abdominal girth and tension and the presence or absence of bowel sounds. These patients are also closely assessed for a decrease in hematocrit, hemodynamic instability, and any increase in abdominal pain (Zacharias et al, 1999). A change in any of these parameters would indicate a reevaluation of the patient and possible surgery. For patients whose conditions become hemodynamically unstable, an emergency celiotomy is performed, which is frequently referred as "damage control surgery." Damage control surgery implies a limited laparotomy focusing on the most immediate problem, rather than full corrective surgery.

Mr. Lancaster's case illustrates the newest trend in managing abdominal blunt traumas. He had sustained a grade III liver laceration. After initial fluid resuscitation, Mr. Lancaster's condition was hemodynamically stable, thus making him a candidate for nonoperative management. However, over the course of 12 hours, Mr. Lancaster's abdomen became more distended and firm, and his ventilation became increasingly difficult with peak inspiratory pressures as high as 60 mm Hg. ACS was diagnosed, and subsequently he was taken to the operating room for a decompression celiotomy.

Box 29-1   **Blunt Abdominal Trauma: Liver Injury Scale**

GRADE I
Subcapsular hematoma <10% of surface area, or
Laceration <1 cm deep

GRADE II
Subcapsular hematoma between 10% and 50% surface area, or
Intraparenchymal hematoma <10 cm wide
Laceration between 1-3 cm deep or <10 cm long

GRADE III
Subcapsular hematoma >50% or expanding, or
Ruptured Subcapsular or parenchymal hematoma
Intraparenchymal hematoma >10 cm or expanding or
Laceration >3 cm in parenchymal depth

GRADE IV
Laceration or parenchymal disruption involving 25%-75% of hepatic lobe, or
Between 1 and 33 Couinaud segments within a single lobe

GRADE V
Laceration or parenchymal disruption involving >75% of a hepatic lobe, or
>3 Couinaud segments within a single lobe, or
Juxtahepatic venous injury

GRADE VI
Hepatic avulsion

From Pachter, H. L. & Feliciano, D. V. (1996). Complex hepatic injuries. *Surgical Clinics of North America, 76*(4), 763-783.

In the past, patients who sustained abdominal injuries underwent total corrective surgery for any abdominal injuries at the time of the initial procedure. However, total corrective surgery usually involved extended operating time, which could lead to problems related to hypothermia, coagulopathies, and acidosis. As previously stated the current trend is to do only a staged laparotomy, during which the major sources of bleeding are identified and are either ligated or packed, any bowel leakage is controlled, and the patient is returned to the intensive care unit for stabilization (Zacharias et al, 1999). Often, because of the edema from the trauma itself and the fluid resuscitation, the abdomen cannot be closed and either towel clips or occlusive dressings are used to protect the abdomen. Although this places the patient at risk for infection, the risk is offset by the positive effects of preserving vascular integrity and function of the abdomen. Usually 12 to 48 hours after the initial celiotomy, the patient is returned to the operating room for surgical reexploration. There, the liver, spleen, and other organs can be assessed, and the viability of the intestines can be determined. If the edema has subsided, the abdomen may be closed at that time, or additional procedures may be required depending upon the patient's status.

6. What is meant by ACS?

ACS refers to an increase in intraabdominal pressures greater than 25 mm Hg as the result of expanding abdominal contents (Ivatury et al, 1998; Lozen, 1999; Zacharias et al, 1999). The increase in abdominal contents can be the result of bleeding within the abdominal cavity or bowel edema caused by the injury itself or fluid resuscitation (Zacharias et al, 1999). Patients who have also had an emergency celiotomy or laparotomy are also at risk for developing ACS. Although additional bleeding and edema may contribute to the development of ACS in these patients, abdominal surgical packs, used to control bleeding, also place these patients at risk for developing ACS. Regardless of the cause of ACS, the increase in abdominal pressure can produce cardiovascular instability as a result of a decrease in preload from compression of the inferior vena cava and decrease the cardiac output (CO), resulting in hypotension. The increase in intraabdominal pressures can also transmit high pressure to the ventricles, which further reduces stroke volume and subsequent CO. Rising intraabdominal pressures also transmit the pressure to the pulmonary system and restrict alveolar ventilation and can dramatically increase peak inspiratory pressures. Renal function is also compromised as a result of the reduced CO and direct compression on the kidneys. The rise in abdominal pressures also reduces urinary flow and blood flow to the intestines and abdominal organs themselves and places them at risk for ischemia. Clinical signs and symptoms of ACS include a sudden rise in peak inspiratory pressure, elevated pulmonary artery pressure, and pulmonary capillary wedge pressure (PCWP), a drop in arterial blood oxygen saturation (SaO_2), a falsely high CVP, a decrease in CO, an increase in systemic vascular resistance (SVR), and either oliguria or anuria. If a sudden rise in peak inspiratory pressures and hemodynamic instability occurs in a patient such as Mr. Lancaster, decompression of the abdomen may be done as an emergency procedure either at the bedside or in the operating room (Eddy et al, 1997). For patients in whom development of ACS is suspected but whose conditions are not profoundly hemodynamically unstable, bladder pressures may be measured to document rising intraabdominal pressures. Bladder pressures may be obtained by instilling 50 ml of sterile fluid into the bladder via a Foley catheter and then measuring the bladder pressures with a manometer. Bladder pressures of 25 mm Hg or greater usually require an emergency celiotomy (Zacharias et al, 1999).

Although relief of ACS is critical, a sudden release of abdominal pressures also poses problems. Research has indicated that as the intraabdominal pressure is released, there is a sudden drop in BP and a sudden release of toxic anaerobic by-products into the systemic circulation. This predisposes the patient to cardiovascular complications including asystole. Eddy and colleagues (1997) recommend infusing 2 L of saline mixed with mannitol and bicarbonate in order to reduce the incidence of what they define as "reperfusion syndrome" (p. 809).

7. What is a pulmonary contusion?

Although Mr. Lancaster did not sustain any trauma to his heart muscle or his aorta, he did sustain rib fractures and bilateral pulmonary contusions. *Pulmonary contusion* is a hemorrhage into the alveolar and interstitial spaces, resulting in reduced alveolar ventilation and subsequent hypoxemia. Of patients who sustain blunt trauma to the chest, 75% will have pulmonary contusions, with a 40% mortality (Prentice & Ahrens, 1994). Chest injuries that accompany pulmonary contusion are rib fractures, flail chest, hemothorax, pneumothorax, and scapula fractures, all of which place the patient at risk for bruised or injured lung parenchyma. Depending on the extent of the contusion, the patient will not only develop hypoxemia from loss of ventilated alveoli but also experience reduced pulmonary compliance and an increase in pulmonary vascular resistance. Assessment parameters include both monitoring ABGs and monitoring SaO_2. In addition, derived oxygen variables can help to determine the degree of alveolar capillary shunting. Normally, less than 5% of the total pulmonary blood flow is not oxygenated (Prentice & Ahrens, 1994). However, with pulmonary injury, the alveoli cannot be ventilated, and hence the blood flowing past those alveoli is not oxygenated. One formula that can be used to calculate the degree of alveolar-capillary shunting is to divide the arterial oxygen pressure (PaO_2) by the fraction of inspired oxygen (FiO_2): PaO_2/FiO_2. The normal value is 286 or greater. Mr. Lancaster's PaO_2 was 82 and his FiO_2 was 1. This indicates an alveolar capillary shunt of 82, which represents an extremely large shunt. Thus although Mr. Lancaster appears to have a normal PaO_2 value, it is important for clinicians to interpret the ABG values in reference to the amount of supplementary oxygen the patient is receiving. For a patient with an FiO_2 of 1 not to have an alveolar capillary shunt, the PaO_2 should be 286 or higher. Thus by correlating Mr. Lancaster's chest x-ray films, which revealed bilateral pulmonary contusions, with his ABG values and his alveolar capillary shunting, the clinician is able to assess the degree of damage to Mr. Lancaster's lungs, and the need for continual mechanical ventilation. Patients with greater than 28% pulmonary contusions require mechanical ventilation (Prentice & Ahrens, 1994). Nursing considerations for these patients include suctioning and positioning the patient to allow the good lung to receive maximum gas exchange. In some cases, this may require a semi-Fowler's position or reverse Trendelenburg or even prone position. Daily assessment of chest x-ray films and the characteristics of secretions is also important because 50% of patients who have pulmonary contusions may develop pneumonia (Prentice & Ahrens, 1994).

8. **What other factors may be contributing to Mr. Lancaster's poor oxygenation status?**

Although Mr. Lancaster's pulmonary contusion is contributing to his poor oxygenation status and his need for mechanical ventilation, trauma patients are also at risk for developing acute respiratory distress syndrome (ARDS). *ARDS* can be defined as noncardiogenic pulmonary edema. It is the accumulation of fluid in the interstitial spaces in the lungs from noncardiac causes. Often trauma is accompanied by overactivation of the systemic inflammatory immune system. This overactivation results in neutrophils and macrophages migrating to the lungs. Although neutrophils and macrophages are part of the normal inflammatory response, when they are overactivated, these cells become very destructive. Much of the destruction that accompanies the neutrophils and macrophages is from chemicals that they release and also from a cascade effect as the chemicals from the neutrophils and macrophages cause other chemicals to be released. The chemicals, or chemical mediators as they are called, include oxygen radicals, interleukin-1, tissue necrosis factor, proteases, platelet-activating factor, thromboxane, leukotrienes, and prostaglandins. These chemical mediators produce vasodilation and increase capillary permeability. The increase in capillary permeability in turn allows fluid from the vascular bed to leak into the interstitial spaces. When this process occurs in the lungs, it is called *ARDS* (discussed fully in Chapter 12). ARDS is characterized by the lungs becoming wet and boggy, and oxygen exchange is dramatically reduced. Clinically the patient's oxygen therapy is no longer effective, and a very high FiO_2 is required to maintain a PaO_2 within normal range. Because the lungs have an excess amount of fluid in the interstitial spaces, the lungs become very difficult to ventilate and high pressures develop. To help facilitate ventilation, PEEP and PS are commonly used. In addition current research also supports the use of low tidal volumes (5-6 ml/kg) in order to prevent volume trauma to the lungs (Brower, 2002). Also although Mr. Lancaster was maintained on SIMV, other modes of ventilation may be used such as inverse inspiratory/expiratory ratio, jet ventilation, and pressure-regulated, volume-controlled ventilation.

9. **Why was conscious sedation used with Mr. Lancaster and does it differ from pharmacologically paralyzing a patient?**

Because ventilation is difficult in patients who have ARDS, they often require high levels of PEEP and PS as well as a high FiO_2. High levels of both PEEP and PS are uncomfortable for the patient and may make the patient feel dyspneic. To facilitate ventilation and reduce their metabolic needs, patients may either receive conscious sedation or be pharmacologically paralyzed. For conscious sedation lorazepam (Ativan) or midazolam hydrochloride (Versed) may be used. The goal for conscious sedation is to sedate the patient sufficiently that he or she does not "fight" the ventilator. If pharmacologically paralyzing the patient is the goal cisatracurium (Nimbex) may be used. Cisatracurium is a neuromuscular blocker that produces skeletal muscle relaxation. It has a minimal effect on the cardiovascular system and no analgesic effect. The cisatracurium dose for paralysis with mechanical ventilation is 9 mg/kg/min as a continuous infusion (Wilson et al, 1998).

It is important to remember that cisatracurium does *not* alter consciousness or cerebration. Hence it is important to provide adequate pain relief and sedation because these patients are actually "awake" but paralyzed and are still aware of pain. When caring for patients who are pharmacologically paralyzed, the nurse must continually monitor their SaO_2 values and set the respiratory rate on the ventilator high enough to provide adequate minute ventilation. Failure to set the respiratory rate at the proper setting can be devastating to patients because they no longer have a respiratory drive. For Mr. Lancaster, lorazepam (Ativan) was used to produce conscious sedation and fentanyl (Sublimaze) was given for pain management. The decision was made not to chemically paralyze Mr. Lancaster, because adequate ventilation could be obtained by inducing conscious sedation.

10. What other complications is Mr. Lancaster at risk for, and how should they be monitored?

After stabilization, Mr. Lancaster was at risk for hemorrhage or rebleeding from his liver injury. Continual cardiac hemodynamic monitoring is vital. Changes in his CO, his pulmonary wedge pressures, BP, and SVR all provide data concerning his hemodynamic stability. Also because of the potential of needing high levels of PEEP to ventilate Mr. Lancaster, a pulmonary catheter was used that measured right ventricular volumes and cardiac output. This form of pulmonary catheter measures the patient's ejection fraction and cardiac output within the right ventricle and is able to provide a calculated preload measurement called the end diastolic volume index (EDVI). Research studies indicate that the EDVI correlates with the more traditional pulmonary artery occlusive pressure (POAP), but it is not subjected to the pulmonary pressure changes that accompany high levels of PEEP (Safcsak & Nelson, 1999). Hemorrhage would be manifested as a drop in CO with a drop in BP. As the body attempts to compensate and epinephrine is released, there is an accompanying increase in SVR. The SVR can be calculated from the following formula:

$$([MAP - CVP]/CO) \times 80$$

The normal SVR is between 800 and 1200 dynes/cm^{-5}.

Rebleeding or continual bleeding from internal injuries is monitored most effectively by serial hematocrit measurements. However, as previously discussed, Mr. Lancaster's grade III liver laceration continued to bleed and he developed ACS. His ACS was assessed by his sudden increase in peak inspiratory pressures and increase in bladder pressures greater than 35 cm H_2O. He was then taken to the operating room for an emergency celiotomy to relieve the pressure and control the bleeding. Because of the extent of his intestinal edema, Mr. Lancaster's abdomen was left open until the edema resolved.

Because Mr. Lancaster's abdomen was not surgically closed at the time of his first operation, he was at risk for developing an infection. White blood cell (WBC) count and temperature are important parameters to monitor to determine whether an infection has developed. Daily chest x-ray films are also important to assess whether the patient has developed pneumonia in addition to ARDS. Once a patient's temperature begins to increase, blood, urine, and sputum cultures need to be obtained to determine the origin of the infection and the type of antibiotic therapy needed.

Often patients with blunt abdominal trauma are at risk for developing sepsis. Sources of the sepsis include invasive monitoring lines, Foley catheter, pulmonary infections, and abdominal abscesses. An additional problem, called *translocation of bacteria,* may also cause sepsis (Faries et al, 1998). Bacterial translocation occurs when the villi in the intestinal wall become ischemic as a result of hypoperfusion. The ischemic villi allow bacteria from the gut to travel across the membrane into either the blood or the lymph system and seed these systems with their own native gastrointestinal (GI) flora. Steps to prevent translocation of bacteria include restoring perfusion as quickly as possible and use of the GI tract as soon as possible. Although initial tube feedings for patients with abdominal trauma will not support their nutritional needs, research has shown that 15 to 25 ml of tube feeding per hour is sufficient to keep the GI tract functional and reduce the chance of translocation of bacteria (Wachtel, 1994).

However, despite all efforts to prevent a systemic infection, many trauma patients develop septic shock. Septic shock can be differentiated clinically from hemorrhagic or hypovolemic shock by monitoring the SVR in addition to monitoring the BP, heart rate, CO, and PCWP. With septic shock, the SVR will drop. The drop in SVR is attributed to the vasodilation that accompanies the release of the bacterial toxins, especially endotoxins. Management of septic shock includes treatment of the infection as well as vasopressor therapy to maintain the BP and restore the SVR.

Early in the resuscitative phase, all trauma patients are at risk for "the trauma triad of death" (Zacharias et al, 1999). The trauma triad is hypothermia, coagulopathy, and acidosis. Because of the events surrounding the trauma and vasoconstriction caused by shock, patients often are hypothermic on arrival in the emergency department. Removal of clothing and the administration of large amounts of intravenous fluids can contribute to their hypothermia. In addition, if patients are taken to the operating room and their intestines are exposed to room air, they can lose as much as 4.6° C/hr (Zacharias et al, 1999). Administration of cool blood can also contribute to their hypothermia. Hypothermia can produce a number of negative sequelae: reduced platelet activity that can lead to the development of coagulopathies; altered respiratory status, making patients unable to compensate for rising levels of arterial carbon dioxide pressure ($PaCO_2$); and effects on the cardiovascular system that predispose patients to develop arrhythmias that are refractory to drugs such as lidocaine and procainamide (Fritsch, 1995). Coagulopathy and acidosis are additional problems that can develop as the result of the ensuing shock after the trauma. Coagulopathy can also occur as the result of massive blood transfusions.

Prevention of hypothermia and early detection of bleeding problems and acidosis are key elements in reducing the mortality associated with these conditions. Specific nursing interventions that can be used to treat these problems are first to remove all wet clothing upon admission to the hospital and keep the patient as covered and protected as possible even during primary and secondary surveys. Second, IV fluids should be warmed before administration. If large amounts of fluid and blood are needed, a rapid infuser may be used that will not only allow for the administration of fluid at a rate of 1.5 L/min, but also warm the fluids and blood. Third, warming units, head wraps, or heat shields should be used to warm the patient. To assess for any coagulopathies, the nurse should closely monitor the patient's clotting studies, including prothrombin time (PT) and partial thromboplastin time (PTT), and platelet levels. If large amounts of blood are needed, it is important to be prepared to also administer fresh frozen plasma (FFP) and platelets. Although guidelines may vary from institution to institution, one protocol recommends 2 U of FFP be administered for the first 10 U of packed red blood cells (PRBCs), and 1 U of FFP for each subsequent 5 U of RBCs (Robb, 1999). To correct the metabolic acidosis, administration of sodium bicarbonate may be required as well as reestablishment of respiratory function.

Once the patient has survived the initial resuscitative phase, bleeding problems can still occur. As previously stated, trauma patients often have overactive inflammatory immune systems, and they can develop systemic inflammatory immune response syndrome (SIRS). *SIRS* is overactivation of the inflammatory-immune system as manifested by tachycardia greater than 90, $PaCO_2$ less than 32 mm Hg, temperature either above 38° C (100.4° F) less than 36° C, and a WBC count either greater than 12,000 or less than 4000. When these signs and symptoms cannot be attributable to any other cause, the patient has developed SIRS. One of the outcomes of SIRS is the development of disseminated intravascular coagulation (DIC). DIC results in clotting in the patient's microvascular circulation and consumption of clotting factors, including platelets. The result is organ failure secondary to the microvascular clotting and bleeding secondary to the consumption of clotting factors. In addition, because of the extensive clotting, patients also have increased fibrinolytic activity and hence fibrin split product levels are elevated. DIC is a coagulopathy that is manifested by prolonged PTs and PTTs, a drop in the platelet count, and an increase in fibrin split product levels. To assess whether a patient has developed a coagulopathy either from hypothermia, massive blood transfusions, or DIC, PT and PTT and platelet levels should be measured. If DIC is suspected, fibrin split product and D-dimer levels should also be monitored (Tabatabai, 2001).

Because patients with multiple trauma, including abdominal traumas, are often immobile for an extended period, they are at risk for the development of deep vein thrombosis (DVT) and subsequent pulmonary embolus. To prevent the development of DVT, sequential compression stockings or similar devices should be used as soon as possible. These devices help maintain normal venous return and prevent venous statis. Heparin therapy should also be started. For DVT prophylaxis, Mr. Lancaster was given enoxaparin (Lovenox) on day 7. Because the calf or thigh is often the site of a DVT, nursing assessment should include monitoring for an increase in calf or thigh size and the presence of a warm, tender area. Although the absence of a positive Homans' sign does not rule out the presence of a DVT, the presence of a positive Homans' sign is considered clinically significant. Because a DVT may develop into an embolus, signs and symptoms of a pulmonary embolus should also be monitored. These signs and symptoms include dyspnea, pleuritic chest pain, a decrease in SaO_2, hypoxia, tachycardia, arrhythmias, and hypotension.

11. What are the nutritional needs of a patient with a blunt abdominal trauma?

Supporting the nutritional needs of every trauma patient is very important. As the result of the trauma, these patients are hypermetabolic and hyperglycemic and in a catabolic state. Failure to support the nutritional needs of these patients can predispose them to poor wound healing, sepsis, respiratory failure, an increased incidence of translocation of bacteria, and multisystem organ failure (Stamatos & Reed, 1994; Romito, 1995). Factors that need to be kept in mind are that the gut is the largest immune organ in the body, and failure to use the gut even on a short-term basis will result in atrophy of the intestinal villi. As previously stated, even small amounts of intestinal feeding have been shown to maintain gut integrity (Romito, 1995). Other factors that are important to consider when the body is in a catabolic state is that the body uses all muscle mass, including the diaphragm, as an energy source. Hence, while the patient is in a catabolic state, he or she has an additional risk of respiratory failure caused by a decrease in the strength of the diaphragm. Also if the patient is febrile, energy requirements increase by 7% for every 1° F increase in temperature (Stamatos & Reed, 1994).

With a stressful event, the metabolic demands of the body can be divided into two phases: the ebb phase and the flow phase. The *ebb phase* is the first 24 to 48 hours after an injury and is characterized by shunting of blood to the heart, lungs, and brain in an effort to maintain perfusion. During the ebb phase, the body's metabolism is reduced. After stabilization, the body's metabolic rate begins to climb. This is called the *flow phase* and is characterized by an increase in CO, oxygen consumption, body temperature, and catabolic activity (Stamatos & Reed, 1994).

Ideally nutritional support should be started within 24 to 72 hours of admission or at the resolution of the ebb phase (Stamatos & Reed, 1994; Romito, 1995). For the patient with abdominal trauma, it is important to assess bowel and renal function to determine whether any pancreatic injury is present. However, even if bowel function is hypoactive, small amounts of enteral feedings are recommended to preserve bowel function.

Nutritional support may include both total parenteral nutrition and enteral feedings, but enteral feedings are preferred in an effort to maintain the function of the bowel and to prevent translocation of bacteria. A number of products for enteral feeding are on the market. Mr. Lancaster was given Perative on day 3. Perative contains 1.3 kcal/ml, and it has 66.6 g of protein per liter, plus supplemental arginine, medium chain triglycerides, and omega-fatty acids. Although there are a number of ways to institute enteral feedings, one approach is to begin with 25 to 30 ml/hr and increase the amount every 6 hours until the goal is reached. Mr. Lancaster's enteral feedings were gradually increased over a 48-hour period, until finally on day 5 he was receiving 90 ml of Perative per hour.

Once enteral feedings are started it is important to monitor electrolyte, glucose, BUN, and creatinine levels as well as daily weights. Weekly laboratory studies should include a liver function panel and triglyceride levels. For long-term management, anthropometric studies, including thigh and midarm circumferences, can help monitor the patient's progress, prealbumin levels, and weight.

BLUNT ABDOMINAL TRAUMA

References

Ahn, J., Morey, A., & McAninch, J. (1998). Workup and management of traumatic hematuria. *Emergency Medicine Clinics of North America, 16*(1), 145-165.

Armstrong, B. (2002). Permissive hypotension. www.trauma.org. Compiled by Jon Hoerner. Trauma.org (7:10), October 2002.

Brooks-Brunn, J. (1999). Respiratory laboratory and diagnostic tests. In L. Bucher & S. Melander (Eds.), *Critical care nursing*. Philadelphia: W. B. Saunders.

Brower, R. (2002). Mechanical ventilation in acute lung injury and ARDS. *Critical Care Clinics, 18*(1), 1-13.

Dutton, R., MacKenzie, D., & Scalea, T. (2002). Hypotensive resuscitation during active hemorrhage: Impact on in-hospital mortality. *Journal of Trauma, 52*(6), 1141-1146.

Eddy, V., Nunn, C., & Morris, J. (1997). Abdominal compartment syndrome. *Surgical Clinics of North America, 77*(4), 801-813.

Faries, P., Simon, R., Martella, A., Lee, M., & Machiedo, G. (1998). Intestinal permeability correlates with severity of injury. *The Journal of Trauma Injury Infection and Critical Care, 44*(6), 1031-1035.

Ferrera, P., Verdile, V., Bartfield, J., Snyder, H., & Salluzzo, R. (1998). Injuries distracting from intraabdominal injuries after blunt trauma. *American Journal of Emergency Medicine, 16*(2), 145-149.

Fritsch, D. (1995). Hypothermia in the trauma patient. *AACN Clinical Issues, 6*(2), 196-211.

Ivatury, R., et al. (1998). Intraabdominal hypertension after life-threatening penetrating abdominal trauma; pro-phylaxis, incidence, and clinical relevance to gastric mucosal pH and abdominal compartment syndrome. *The Journal of Trauma Injury Infection and Critical Care, 44*(6), 1016-1023.

Jacobs, L. (1994). Timing of fluid resuscitation in trauma. *The New England Journal of Medicine, 331*(17), 1153-1154.

Janjua, K., Sugrue, M., & Deane, S. (1998). Prospective evaluation of early missed injuries and the role of tertiary trauma survey. *The Journal of Trauma, Injury, Infection and Critical Care, 44*(6), 1000-1007.

Laskowski-Jones, L. (1999). Trauma. In L. Bucher & S. Melander (Eds.), *Critical care nursing*. Philadelphia: W. B. Saunders.

Lozen, Y. (1999). Intraabdominal hypertension and abdominal compartment syndrome in trauma: Pathophysiology and intervention. *AACN Clinical Issues, 10*(1), 104-112.

Melanson, S. & Heller, M. (1998). The emerging role of bedside ultrasonography in trauma care. *Contemporary Issues in Trauma, 16*(1), 165-183.

Melio, F. (1998). Priorities in the multiple trauma patient. *Emergency Medicine Clinics of North America, 16*(1), 29-43.

Prentice, D. & Ahrens, T. (1994). Pulmonary complications of trauma. *Critical Care Nursing Quarterly, 17*(2), 24-33.

Richardson, D., Franklin, G., Lukan, J., Carrillo, E., Spain, D., et al. (2000). Evolution in the management of hepatic trauma: A 25 year perspective. *Annals of Surgery, 232*(3), 324-330.

Robb, W. (1999). Massive transfusion in trauma. *AACN Clinical Issues, 10*(1), 69-84.

Romito, R. (1995). Early administration of enteral nutrients in critically ill patients. *AACN Clinical Issues, 6*(2), 242-257.

Safcsak, K. & Nelson, L. (1999). Right heart volumetric monitoring: Measuring preload in the critically injured patient. *AACN Clinical Issues, 10*(1), 22-31.

Sommers, M. (1995). Missed injuries: A case study of trauma hide and seek. *AACN Clinical Issues, 6*(2), 187-195.

Stamatos, C. & Reed, E. (1994). Nutritional needs of the trauma patient. *Critical Care Nursing Clinics of North America, 6*(3), 501-514.

Tabatabai, A. (2001). Disorders of hemostatis. In S. Ahya, K. Flood, & S. Paranjothi (Eds.), *Washington manual*. Philadelphia: Lippincott Williams & Wilkins.

Urden, L. D., Stacy, K. M., & Lough, M. E. (Eds.) (2002). *Thelan's critical care nursing: Diagnosis and management* (4th ed.). St Louis: Mosby.

Wachtel, T. (1994). Critical care concepts in the management of abdominal trauma. *Critical Care Nursing Quarterly, 17*(2), 34-49.

Wilson, B., Shannon, M., & Stang, C. (1998). *Nurses drug guide*. Stamford, CT: Appleton & Lange.

Yang, E., Marder, S., Hasting, G., & Knudson, M. (2002). The abdominal compartment syndrome complicating nonoperative management of major blunt liver injuries: Recognition and treatment using multimodality therapy. *The Journal of Trauma, Injury, Infection and Critical Care, 52*, 982-986.

Zacharias, S., Offner, P., Moore, E., & Burch, J. (1999). Damage control surgery. *AACN Clinical Issues, 10*(1), 95-103.

30

Hypertensive Crisis/Emergency

Mary Jane Swartz, RN, MSN, APRN, BC

CASE PRESENTATION

Mildred James, a 63-year-old, came to the emergency department, at 2100 hours complaining of a severe headache. She complained of visual problems and rated her pain as a 5 (on a scale of 1 to 5). Her husband states she awoke at 0200, complaining of a severe right-sided headache. Despite taking acetaminophen (Lortab), she continued to have symptoms all day. Upon her arrival you notice some difficulty with speech. Her initial vital signs were as follows:

BP	227/130 mm Hg
Temperature	37.2° C (99° F) orally
HR	72 bpm
Respirations	24 breaths/min
Sao$_2$	98% with room air

She has a previous history of myocardial infarction, coronary artery bypass surgery several years ago, depression treated with electroconvulsive therapy, and deep vein thrombophlebitis, which required insertion of a Greenfield filter. Home medications include aspirin, niacin, metoprolol (Toprol-XL), and lorazepam (Ativan). The following are results obtained from diagnostic testing:

Glucose	151 mg/dl
BUN	20 mg/dl
Creatinine	0.8 mg/dl
Na$^+$	139 mmol/L
K$^+$	3.8 mmol/L
Cl$^-$	104 mmol/L
Ca^{++}	8.9 mmol/L
Total Protein	7.5 g/d
Albumin	4.0 g/dl
Bilirubin	0.5 mg/dl
AST	30 μ/L
ALKP	80 μ/L
CO$_2$	24 mmol/L

Electrocardiogram showed some nonspecific ST-segment changes. A computed tomography (CT) scan of the head was ordered with negative findings.

Emergency Department Treatment Record

2200	BP 248/100 right arm mm Hg
2217	enalapril (Vasotec) 1.25 mg given intravenously
2218	BP 238/100 right arm
2230	nalbuphine (Nubain) 10 mg with promethazine (Phenergan) 12.5 mg given intravenously for complaints of nausea and continued headache
2245	BP 238/100 mm Hg enalapril (Vasotec) 4 mg given intravenously
2253	BP 213/64 mm Hg left arm, morphine sulfate 1 mg given intravenously
0010	BP 216/66 mm Hg clonidine (Catapres) 0.2 mg given orally
0100	Mrs. James became unresponsive and had tonic-clonic seizure activity.
0110	lorazepam (Ativan) 10 mg intravenously
0230	BP 117/67 mm Hg
	HR 96 bpm

After Mrs. James awakened, she was transferred to the intensive care unit (ICU).

Her admitting diagnosis was hypertensive urgency, cephalgia, and new-onset seizure.

ICU Admission

After admission to the ICU, Mrs. James remained alert and oriented. She rated her headache as 1 on a scale of 1 to 10.   Her vital signs were as follows:

BP	167/68 mm Hg
Temperature	38.3° C (101° F) orally
HR	76 bpm
Respirations	24 breaths/min

At 0800 Mrs. James's blood pressure (BP) was charted as 190/70 mm Hg. At 0835 Mrs. James had a grand mal seizure, which led to respiratory arrest and a brief period of asystole. She was placed on mechanical ventilation after two attempts at intubation. Due to poor venous access, a central line was placed and an arterial line was placed in her right radial artery. She received lorazepam 2 mg intravenously. She was started on fosphenytoin (Cerebyx) 15 mg/kg loading dose, then 100 mg every 8 hours. Code team members voiced concern regarding the possibility that she may have aspirated gastric contents. Tracheal aspirate and urine for culture/sensitivity along with blood cultures were collected. She had suffered a prior episode of *Pseudomonas* pneumonia; therefore she was started on vancomycin.

Day 2

She was weaned from mechanical ventilation. Magnetic resonance imaging (MRI) of the head revealed no acute hemorrhage but more likely represented an ischemic event. Electroencephalograph (EEG) and spinal tap were normal. Echocardiogram revealed 50% left ventricular ejection fraction. She was speaking coherently and following all commands.

Day 3

Mrs. James's BP was 170/60 mm Hg. Blood sugars ranged from 101 to 129 dl. Nasogastric feedings were discontinued and she was started on clear liquids. She was placed on phenytoin (Dilantin) 200 mg twice daily. At this time the patient was transferred to the step-down unit, where her stay was uneventful.

Day 8

Mrs. James was transferred to a rehabilitation unit. Discharge medications at the time of transfer included aspirin, niacin, lorazepam, amlodipine (Norvasc), enalapril, metoprolol, phenytoin, thiamin, famotidine (Pepcid), simvastatin (Zocor), (levofloxacin (Levaquin), and vancomycin.

HYPERTENSIVE CRISIS/EMERGENCY

QUESTIONS

1. Based on her presenting symptoms and admission assessment, what other possible conditions could be contributing to her headache?

2. Which of her lab values and diagnostic tests were significant?

3. When obtaining a blood pressure reading, what factors and conditions can hinder correct assessment?

4. What clinical guidelines are established for the prevention and treatment of hypertension?

5. What is the classification system for blood pressure in adults?

6. Differentiate hypertensive emergency and hypertensive urgency.

7. What clinical manifestations may be seen in hypertensive crisis?

8. Outline the goal for treating hypertensive crisis.

9. Discuss the importance of risk factor reduction for patients diagnosed with hypertension.

10. What pharmacologic agents are recommended for the treatment of hypertensive crisis?

11. Why is the sublingual administration of nifedipine not recommended in hypertensive crisis?

12. Explain the relationship between Mrs. James's hypertensive urgency and her new onset of seizure activity.

13. What are the possible complications that can occur when a patient requires direct arterial blood pressure monitoring via arterial line?

14. List the nursing diagnoses and interventions appropriate for the care of a patient in hypertensive crisis.

HYPERTENSIVE CRISIS/EMERGENCY

QUESTIONS AND ANSWERS

1. Based on her presenting symptoms and admission assessment, what other possible conditions could be contributing to her headache?

Many conditions can mimic hypertensive crisis including encephalitis, acute anxiety with panic attacks, uremia, subarachnoid hemorrhage, head injury, brain tumor, and postictal epilepsy (Braunwald et al, 2001). Patients should be assessed for the use of monoamine oxidase inhibitors and recreational drugs such as cocaine, amphetamines, and phencyclidine (Varnon & Marik, 2001).

2. Which of her lab values and diagnostic tests were significant?

All of her lab values were normal, except her blood sugar, which was slightly elevated. The CT scan was necessary to rule out any neurologic cause such as ischemia, hemorrhage, tumor, cyst, and edema. Her electrocardiogram (ECG) showed only nonspecific ST-segment changes. The ECG should be compared with a previous tracing.

3. When obtaining a blood pressure reading, what factors and conditions can hinder correct assessment?

Several factors can interfere with correct blood pressure measurement:

- Patients should be seated or lying down with their arms bared and supported at heart level for at least 5 minutes prior to obtaining the blood pressure reading.
- Measurements of blood pressure should occur in both arms. If there is an abnormal discrepancy between readings, the physician should be notified to determine which reading to use for basis of medication as needed.
- Patients should refrain from smoking or ingesting caffeine 30 minutes prior to taking blood pressure.
- The appropriate cuff size should be utilized for the patient's arm.
- Both systolic blood pressure (SBP) and diastolic blood pressure (DSP) should be recorded. Measuring blood pressure in the supine and standing positions is desirable at times. Two or more readings separated by 2 minutes should be averaged.
- Operator error

4. What clinical guidelines are established for the prevention and treatment of hypertension?

The Seventh Report of the Joint National Committee on Prevention, Detection, Evaluation, and the Treatment of High Blood Pressure (JNC-7) is a document with guidelines that were developed using evidence-based medicine with agreement by clinicians. The report contains discussion of new pharmacologic therapies, role of managed care in the treatment of hypertension, and information from recent randomized controlled trials. The report includes a guide to help clinicians individualize treatment and strategies for special patient populations. The utilization of this document with consideration of patient comorbidities and special needs can be used to formulate a plan of care for the patient with hypertension (National High Blood Pressure Education Program, 2003).

5. What is the classification system for blood pressure in adults?

Hypertension stage 1 is defined as SBP of 140 mm Hg or greater, DBP of 90 mm Hg or greater, or taking medication to control hypertension. There is a relationship between SBP and DBP with subsequent effects upon cardiovascular health. The new JNC-7 guidelines identify normal systolic and diastolic values and include a new category titled Prehypertension (Table 30-1).

	Category	SBP mm Hg	DBP mm Hg
Normal	<120	and	<80
Prehypertension	120-139	or	80-89
Hypertension, Stage 1	140-159	or	90-99
Hypertension, Stage 2	≥160	or	≥100

Table **30-1**   *Classification of Blood Pressure (BP)*

SBP, Systolic blood pressure; *DBP*, diastolic blood pressure. From *The Seventh Report of the Joint National Committee on Prevention, Detection, Evaluation, and Treatment of High Blood Pressure* (JNC-7) (2003). Washington, DC: National Heart, Lung, and Blood Institute: www.nhlbi.nihgov.

6. **Differentiate between hypertensive emergency and hypertensive urgency.**

Hypertension crisis can be divided into two categories: emergency and urgency. Hypertension emergencies are those that require immediate blood pressure reduction. Conditions associated with hypertensive emergencies are hypertensive encephalopathy, intracranial hemorrhage, unstable angina pectoris, acute myocardial infarction, acute left ventricular failure with pulmonary edema, dissecting aortic aneurysm, or eclampsia. Hypertensive urgencies are those in which the goal is to reduce the blood pressure within a few hours. Conditions associated with hypertensive urgencies are stage 2 hypertension, which is defined as an SBP greater than or equal to 160 mm Hg or a DBP greater than or equal to 100 mm Hg, hypertension with optic disk edema, progressive target organ complications, and severe perioperative hypertension (Urden et al, 2002; National High Blood Pressure Education Program, 2003). In the clinical situation in which the patient maybe experiencing a cerebrovascular accident (ischemic stroke), the clinician should use caution in reducing the blood pressure too quickly. A sudden drop in mean arterial pressure could severely reduce cerebral perfusion pressure.

7. **What clinical manifestations may be seen in hypertensive crisis?**

Undetected hypertension is called the silent killer due to the asymptomatic presentation. Patients with hypertension are at risk for developing cerebrovascular, peripheral vascular, and renal vascular complications. In hypertensive crisis the clinician may see the following signs and symptoms:

- DBP >140 mm Hg
- Funduscopic: papilledema, hemorrhage
- Neurologic: headache, confusion, seizures, coma, visual loss
- Cardiac: cardiac enlargement, congestive failure
- Renal: oliguria, azotemia
- Gastrointestinal: nausea, vomiting (Urden et al, 2002)

8. **Outline the goal for treating hypertensive crisis.**

The initial goal in hypertensive emergencies is to reduce the arterial blood pressure by no more than 20% to 25% (within 2 minutes to 2 hours), then toward 160/100 mm Hg within 2 to 6 hours, avoiding excessive falls in pressure that may precipitate renal, cardiac, or coronary ischemia. See JNC-7 hypertension treatment algorithm (Fig. 30-1) (Urden et al, 2002; National High Blood Pressure Education Program, 2003).

9. **Discuss the importance of risk factor reduction for patients diagnosed with hypertension.**

It is necessary to use nonpharmacologic as well as pharmacologic methods for reduction of blood pressure. Overall recommendations suggest the reduction of as many risk factors as possible. Some cardiovascular risk factors can be modified by lifestyle changes, whereas

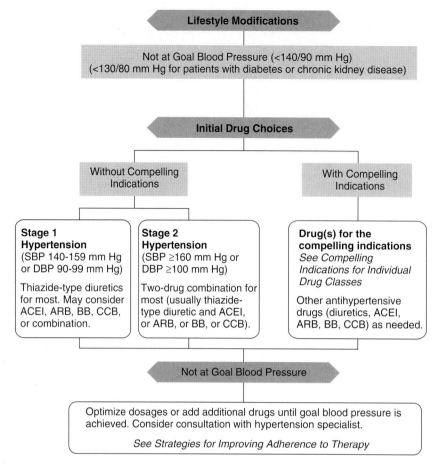

Figure **30-1** Algorithm for treatment of hypertension. (From *The Seventh Report of the Joint National Committee on Prevention, Detection, Evaluation, and Treatment of High Blood Pressure* (JNC-7) (2003). Washington, DC: National Heart, Lung, and Blood Institute: www.nhlbi.nihgov.

others cannot. You may see these identified as modifiable and nonmodifiable risk factors. With constant cardiovascular risk factor management it is possible to reduce medications that may have been necessary initially in the control of hypertension.

Major cardiovascular risk factors are:

- Smoking
- Dyslipidemia
- Diabetes mellitus
- Age older than 60
- Obesity
- Sex (men or postmenopausal women)
- Family history of heart disease: women younger than 65 or men younger than 55 years
- Target organ damage/clinical cardiovascular disease
- Heart disease
  - Left ventricular hypertrophy
  - Angina/prior myocardial infarction (MI)
  - Prior coronary revascularization
  - Heart failure

- Stroke or transient ischemic attack
- Nephropathy
- Peripheral arterial disease
- Retinopathy
- Physical inactivity
- Microalbuminuria

Identifiable causes of hypertension are:

- Sleep apnea
- Drug induced
- Chronic kidney disease
- Primary aldosteronism
- Renovascular disease
- Cushing's syndrome
- Pheochromocytoma
- Coarctation of the aorta
- Thyroid/parathyroid disease (JNC-7, 2003)

10. What pharmacologic agents are recommended for the treatment of hypertensive crisis?

Most hypertensive emergencies are treated with parenteral medication administration.

Hypertensive urgencies can be managed with the use of oral agents with rapid onset. The classification of drugs used in the management of hypertensive crisis include loop diuretics, β-blockers, angiotensin-converting enzyme (ACE) inhibitors, α$_2$-agonists, and calcium antagonists.

11. Why is the sublingual administration of nifedipine not recommended in hypertensive crisis?

The administration of nifedipine has been used as a fast-acting agent in hypertensive crisis. Nifedipine use can have serious adverse effects due to the unpredictable ability to control the rate or degree of drop in blood pressure. Excessive falls in blood pressure can lead to renal, cerebral, or coronary ischemia, which could then lead to syncope and/or seizures.

12. Explain the relationship between Mrs. James's hypertensive urgency and her new onset of seizure activity.

When DBP is greater than 140 mm Hg, there is rapidly progressive damage to the arterial vasculature and hyperperfusion to the brain under high pressure. The symptoms of hypertensive encephalopathy are probably related to cerebral edema and spasms of the cerebral blood vessels (Braunwald et al, 2001).

13. What are the possible complications that can occur when a patient requires direct arterial blood pressure monitoring via arterial line?

The arterial line is most commonly placed in the radial artery. Prior to placing an arterial line, the extremity can be assessed for circulatory adequacy using the Allen's test. The nurse should assess the arterial line frequently for the following: hemorrhage, emboli (air, clots, fibrin), vascular spasm, and infection. The nurse should assess the distal pulse, hand temperature and color, oozing around the catheter, redness, and drainage. The accuracy of the waveform reading should be correlated with a peripheral blood pressure routinely to ensure accuracy. A difference of 5 mm Hg or more between invasive and noninvasive blood pressure is common, with the direct blood pressure generally higher than the noninvasive reading. Treatment should be decided on a trend rather than a single measurement. (See Fig. 30-2 for an illustration of normal arterial waveform. See Fig. 30-3 for an illustration of a damped waveform.)

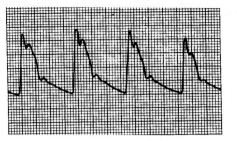

Figure **30-2**   Normal arterial waveform. Characteristics include sharp upstroke and clear dicrotic (closure of aortic valve) notch.

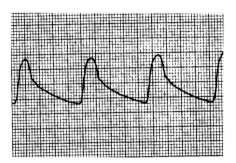

Figure **30-3**   Damped waveform caused by catheter obstruction. May be corrected if repositioned away from the arterial wall or aspiration of any visible clots.

14. List the nursing diagnoses and interventions appropriate for the care of a patient in hypertensive crisis.

Nursing diagnosis and interventions for the patient with hypertensive crisis would include the following:

Diagnoses

- Altered tissue perfusion related to elevated blood pressure
- Ineffective cerebral tissue perfusion related to vasospasm or hemorrhage
- Ineffective cerebral tissue perfusion related to acute myocardial ischemia
- Anxiety related to threat to biologic, psychologic, and/or social integrity
- Risk for fluid volume deficit and hypotension related to diuretic and antihypertensive medication

Interventions

- Continuous assessment of patient's response to treatment with frequent blood pressure readings and hemodynamic readings. Initial readings should be every 15 minutes.
- Administer antihypertensive drugs.
- Monitor ECG for arrhythmias.
- Assess for signs of increased intracranial pressure (headache, nausea, lethargy, confusion, vomiting).
- Maintain intravascular access.
- Accurate intake and output and daily weights.
- Monitor for abnormalities in laboratory values, particularly electrolytes.
- Educate patient concerning all diagnostic tests, and procedures.

HYPERTENSIVE CRISIS/EMERGENCY

References

Braunwald, E., Zipes, D., & Libby, D. (2001). *Heart disease* (6th ed.). Philadelphia: W.B. Saunders.

Chase, S. (2000). Hypertensive crisis. *RN*, 62-28.

Lewis, S., Heitkemper, M., & Dirksen, S. (2000). *Medical-surgical nursing: Assessment and management of clinical problems* (5th ed.). St Louis: Mosby. National High Blood Pressure Education Program, US Department of Health and Human Services, Public Health Service. (2003). *The Seventh Report of the Joint National Committee on Prevention, Detection, Evaluation, and Treatment of High Blood Pressure* (JNC-7). Washington, DC: National Heart, Lung and Blood Institute. www.nhlbi.nih.gov.

Urden, L., Stacy, K., & Lough, M. (Eds.) (2002). *Thelan's critical care nursing: Diagnosis and management* (4th ed.). St Louis: Mosby.

Varnon, J. & Marik, P. (2001). The diagnosis and management of hypertensive crisis. *Chest,* January 119(1):316.

Vaughan, C. & Delanty, N. (2000). Hypertensive emergencies. *The Lancet, 356*(9239), 1442-1443.

31

Drug Overdose

Linda K. Evinger, RN, MSN, C-OGNP
Katherine B. Riedford, RN, BSN, MSN, DNS

CASE PRESENTATION

Sean Christian, age 19, was brought to the emergency department (ED) by a friend. Mr. Christian was nonresponsive upon arrival. His friend stated that he discovered Mr. Christian lying on the sofa of his home and could not get a response from him. He found Mr. Christian approximately 30 minutes ago and immediately brought him to the ED. The friend related that Mr. Christian stated yesterday that the world would be better off without him. Initial assessment revealed dry, warm skin; pupils equal and constricted; patient nonresponsive to sound and touch.

Current vital signs and laboratory results are as follows:

BP	86/50 mm Hg
HR	52 bpm
Respirations	8 breaths/min
Temperature	36.9° C (98.3° F) (oral)

Toxicology Screen Results

Amphetamines—negative
Alcohol—negative
Barbiturates—negative
Benzodiazepines—negative
Cocaine—negative
Cyanide—negative
Opiates—positive
THC—negative
Phencyclidine—negative
LSD—negative
Analgesics—negative
Sedatives—negative
Major tranquilizers—negative
Stimulants—negative
Sympathomimetics—negative

Lab Results

Glucose	85 mg/dl
CBC	Within normal limits
Metabolic panel	Within normal limits
Urinalysis	Within normal limits
BUN	17 mg/dl
Creatinine	1.0 mg/dl
LDH	135 U/L
AST (SGOT)	11 U/L
ALT (SGPT)	13 U/L
Alkaline phosphatase	43 U/L
Total bilirubin	0.6 mg/dl
Albumin	4.0 g/dl

ABG abnormalities

$Paco_2$	Elevated
So_2	Decreased
Sao_2	Decreased
pH	Elevated

An intravenous drip (IV) was initiated with normal saline. Mr. Christian was intubated. A 12-lead electrocardiogram (ECG) was obtained and cardiac monitoring was continued. Drug screen results were obtained. A nagogastric tube was passed and gastric lavage was completed with activated charcoal. An initial dose of naloxone (Narcan) 2 mg was given IV. Two hours after arriving in the ED, Mr. Christian was tranferred to the intensive care unit (ICU) with an intravenous infusion of normal saline. A complete neurologic assessment was completed and a second dose of naloxone 2 mg was given IV.

DRUG OVERDOSE

QUESTIONS

1. Identify the signs and symptoms of opiate use, overdose, and withdrawal.

2. What do Mr. Christian's laboratory tests indicate about his current health status?

3. What other classifications of drugs would produce similar signs and symptoms of overdose and withdrawal?

4. What are the most common types of drug overdose seen?

5. What signs and symptoms would be found in each of the drug classifications listed in question 4?

6. What drug and its use or overdose signs and symptoms mimic other medical situations?

7. What is the rationale for using activated charcoal and naloxone (Narcan)?

8. Identify nursing diagnoses appropriate for this type of client in the ICU.

9. Discuss the short- and long-term patient/family teaching indicated for Mr. Christian.

10. What special nursing considerations are prompted by Mr. Christian's attempted suicide?

DRUG OVERDOSE

QUESTIONS AND ANSWERS

1. Identify the signs and symptoms of opiate use, overdose, and withdrawal.

Physical signs and symptoms of the use of opiates include impaired physical performance, slurred speech, constricted pupils, lethargy, mental clouding, decreased blood pressure, and decreased respiration. Psychologic symptoms include euphoria followed by anxiety, dysphoria, fear, mood changes, and impaired judgment (Black et al, 2001).

Signs of overdose may include cold and clammy skin, respiratory depression, Cheyne-Stokes respirations, dilated pupils due to anoxia, flaccid skeletal muscles, bradycardia, hypotension, extreme somnolence leading to coma, and death (Fitzgerald et al, 2000; Stuart & Laraia, 2001).

Signs and symptoms of withdrawal might include restlessness, irritability, anxiety, craving, abdominal cramping, nausea and vomiting, sweating, fever, chills, increased blood pressure, increased pulse, increased respirations, dilated pupils, tremors, muscle aches, and muscle spasms (Stuart & Laraia, 2001).

2. What do Mr. Christian's laboratory tests indicate about his current health status?

Many lab values remain within normal limits due to the limited amount of time that has passed since the opioid was ingested. The toxicology report listing only opiates as positive indication that Mr. Christian is probably not a user of drugs and that he did not take more than one drug in his suicide attempt. A blood opioid concentration is not necessary because it doesn't guide treatment decisions. The arterial blood gases (ABGs) are affected by the central nervous system (CNS) depression, resulting in a decrease in oxygen and a rise in carbon dioxide (Rakel & Bope, 2003).

One important consideration for overdose of hydrocodone is that depending on the dose, the person may suffer from fatal hepatic necrosis due to acetaminophen overdose. Acetaminophen, 500 mg, is included in each 2.5 mg, 5 mg, 7.5 mg, and 10 mg tablet of acetaminophen (Lortab). A massive overdose of acetaminophen may lead to hepatic toxicity. Consider toxicity if the ingested dose is greater than 10 g over a period of less than 8 hours. Fatalities have rarely been reported unless an overdose is more than 15 g. If overdose is suspected, treatment with N-acetylcysteine is indicated as soon as possible (Schmidt et al, 2002).

Despite the fact that acetaminophen is used safely as an analgesic on a worldwide basis, it continues to be the drug used most frequently in suicide attempts in the United States. The cost of these toxic drug ingestions is outstanding in both human suffering and costs (Gunnell et al, 2000).

3. What other classifications of drugs would produce similar signs and symptoms of overdose and withdrawal?

Other drug classifications that would produce similar signs and symptoms include the following:

Sedative hypnotics—Overdose of these drugs produces symptoms similar to those of opiates. These include confusion, somnolence, diminished reflexes, and impaired coordination. There is potential respiratory depression, shock, coma, seizures, and death. Symptoms of withdrawal from drugs in this classification include insomnia, dysphoria, abdominal and muscle cramps, nausea and vomiting, anxiety, sweating, possible convulsions, and hallucinations. Blood pressure tends to increase as with opioid withdrawal (Stuart & Laraia, 2001).

Alcohol—Overdose of alcohol also produces symptoms similar to those of opioids. These symptoms include respiratory depression, stupor, possible seizures, coma, and death. Some of the major withdrawal symptoms from alcohol include anxiety, sweating, tremors, and weakness. Patients often display agitated behaviors, nausea and vomiting, and may have hallucinations. Other symptoms include anorexia, insomnia, and vivid nightmares. With alcohol withdrawal, vital signs tend to mimic opioid withdrawal, with the patient exhibiting increased blood pressure and pulse (Stuart & Laraia, 2001).

4. What are the most common types of drug overdose seen?

The most common types of drug overdoses that are intentional include ethyl alcohol, acetaminophen, aspirin, antidepressants, stimulants, and sedative hypnotics. Suicidal poisonings make up 10% to 15% of exposure to poisons and constitute 60% to 90% of fatalities from ingestion of substances (Rakel & Bope, 2003). Generally, overdoses include multiple substances instead of only one drug.

5. What signs and symptoms would be found in each of the drug classifications listed in question 4?

According to the *Physician's Desk Reference* (2003), signs and symptoms of overdose of drugs in the aforementioned question include the following:

Alcohol—These symptoms include respiratory depression, stupor, possible seizures, coma, and death.

Acetaminophen—Symptoms to be alert for after a potential overdose include sweating, nausea and vomiting, and general malaise. Actual laboratory and clinical evidence of toxicity may not appear for 48 to 72 hours after ingestion.

Aspirin—Early signs of overdose include tinnitus, increased temperature, and hyperventilation. Severe acid-base disturbances and electrolyte imbalances may occur.

Antidepressants—Overdose produces seizures and hypotension, along with cardiac arrhythmias and central nervous system depression. The QRS is increased (Heard et al, 1999).

Stimulants—Symptoms include restlessness, confusion, hyperreflexia, tremor, rapid respiratory rate, hyperpyrexia, assaultiveness, and hallucinations. Other symptoms include headache, nausea, vomiting, diarrhea, and arrhythmias (Stuart & Laraia, 2001).

Sedative hypnotics—The symptoms include confusion, somnolence, diminished reflexes, and impaired coordination. There is potential respiratory depression, shock, coma, seizures, and death.

6. What drug and its use or overdose signs and symptoms mimic other medical situations?

Cocaine is a stimulant that causes a short period of euphoria that is the result of the blockage of the reuptake of norepinephrine and dopamine. A toxic psychosis is possible that produces symptoms of paranoia, delusions, hallucinations, possible aggression, and an extremely labile mood (Stuart & Laraia, 2001). Individuals with these symptoms may be incorrectly diagnosed as psychotic from a thought disorder or suspected of being under the influence of a drug like phencyclidine (PCP). Overdose signs and symptoms of cocaine include seizures and multiple cardiac effects. Arrhythmias, spasms of the coronary arteries, myocardial infarctions, along with extreme increases in blood pressure and temperature are possible. These may lead to cardiovascular shock and death (Stuart & Laraia, 2001). These signs and symptoms can lead to diagnoses of the cardiac problems without consideration of the use of cocaine.

7. What is the rationale for using activated charcoal and naloxone (Narcan)?

Activated charcoal is known for its adsorptive qualities. It can decrease serum drug levels in some cases particularly if given within 60 minutes of the drug's ingestion (Mokhlesi et al, 2003). Charcoal is administered after the stomach is emptied by vomiting or gastric lavage. In nonresponsive patients, protection of the airway is imperative. Aspiration of charcoal can lead to pneumonia, adult respiratory distress syndrome (ARDS), bronchiolitis obliterans, and death (Mokhlesi et al, 2003).

Naloxone (Narcan) is an opioid antagonist that quickly reverses the opioid effects of coma, hypotension, and respiratory depression. It is given IV in an initial dose of 0.2 to 2 mg, and subsequent doses may be given after 2 to 3 minutes until 10 mg total has been given (Mokhlesi et al, 2003). Because this drug is an opioid antagonist, withdrawal symptoms may occur in the long-term user.

8. Identify nursing diagnoses appropriate for this type of client in the ICU.

Relevant nursing diagnoses include the following:

- Altered family processes
- Chronic or situational low self-esteem
- Decreased cardiac output
- Disturbed body image
- Dysfunctional family processes
- Fatigue
- Fear
- Grieving
- Hopelessness
- Impaired verbal communication
- Ineffective individual coping
- Ineffective role performance
- Powerlessness
- Risk for aspiration
- Risk for ineffective breathing pattern
- Risk for injury: suffocation
- Risk for suicide
- Sleep pattern disturbance

9. Discuss the short- and long-term patient/family teaching indicated for Mr. Christian.

Short-term teaching areas include those related to procedures, treatments, medications, expectations of therapies, and the ICU. Long-term teaching areas include the identification of the areas in Mr. Christian's life that led to the suicide attempt. Other teaching areas will need to address the referral for mental health care and mental health care providers.

10. What special nursing considerations are prompted by Mr. Christian's attempted suicide?

In regard to Mr. Christian's suicide attempt, the nurse must discuss the reasons for the suicide. If Mr. Christian does not already have a mental health care provider, he will need a referral. Willingness to listen to Mr. Christian and a nonjudgmental attitude are imperative. Mr. Christian may be disappointed, upset, and angry that his attempt to kill himself was unsuccessful. Family considerations are of utmost importance in this area. The nurse must offer emotional and psychologic support to Mr. Christian's family to help them understand why he attempted suicide (if known) and what supportive measures they can provide along with community resources (Neale, 2000).

DRUG OVERDOSE

References

Black, J. M., Hawks, J. H., & Keene, A. M. (2001). *Medical-surgical nursing: Clinical management for positive outcomes.* Philadelphia: Saunders.

Fitzgerald, J., Hamilton, M., & Dietze, P. (2000). Walking overdoses: A re-appraisal of non-fatal illicit drug overdose. *Addiction Research, 8,* 327-355.

Gunnell, D., Murray, V., & Hawton, K. (2000). Use of paracetamol for suicide and nonfatal poisoning: Worldwide patterns of use and misuse. *Suicide and Life-Threatening Behavior, 30,* 313-326.

Heard, K., O'Malley, G. F., & Dart, R. C. (1999). Treatment of amitriptyline poisoning with ovine antibody to tricyclic antidepressants. *The Lancet, 354,* 1614-1615.

Mokhlesi, B., Leiken, J. B., Murray, P., & Corbridge, T. C. (2003). Adult toxicology in critical care: Part I: General approach to the intoxicated patient. *Chest, 123,* 577-592.

Neale, J. (2000). Suicidal intent in non-fatal illicit drug overdose. *Addiction, 95*(1), 85-93.

Rakel, R. E. & Bope, E. T. (2003). *Conn's current therapy 2003* (55th ed.). Philadelphia: W. B. Saunders.

Schmidt, L. E., Knudsen, T. T., Dalhoff, K., & Bendsten, F. (2002). Effect of acetylcysteine on prothrombin index in paracetamol poisoning without hepatocellular injury. *The Lancet, 360,* 1151-1152.

Sifton, D. W. (Ed.). (2003). *Physicians' desk reference.* Montvale, NJ: Thomson PDR.

Stuart, G. W. & Laraia, M. T. (2001). *Principles and practice of psychiatric nursing* (7th ed.). St Louis: Mosby.

32

Disseminated Intravascular Coagulation

Lynn Smith Schnautz, RN, MSN, CCRN, CCNS

CASE PRESENTATION

Mary Beavers, a 36-year-old white woman, is admitted to the emergency department complaining of diffuse abdominal pain rated as a 5 on a scale of 1 to 5. Mary is 1 week post cesarean section. She states that she is constipated and has had only one small bowel movement since discharge. She denies fever, chills, vomiting, urinary frequency or dysuria, and states vaginal discharge is normal.

Vital signs on admission are:

HR	114 bpm
BP	110/70 mmHg
Respirations	28 breaths/min
Temperature	(98.7° F) (37° C) orally

Mary is alert and oriented to person, place, and time. She denies headache, neck pain, neck stiffness, and/or double vision. Abdominal bowel sounds are absent. A firm distended abdomen is noted with rebound tenderness. A midline lower abdominal incision is slightly reddened and tender to touch.

Lab	Values
WBC	24,000 with 88% segs
Hgb	13.5 g/dl
Amylase	75 U/L
Lipase	302 U/L
K⁺	3.5 mmol/L

Blood cultures are obtained. Computed tomography (CT) of the abdomen reveals the following: no evidence of obstruction or perforation, dermoid cyst in the right ovary with tooth embedded in area, and a markedly enlarged uterus with large amounts of fluid in the cul-de-sac.

Past medical history includes gravida 4, para 4, three dilation and curettages (D&Cs), right knee ligament repair, and tonsillectomy.

In the emergency department (ED) she received D_5NS with 20 mEq of potassium chloride (KCl) at 250 cc/hr times 1 L, meperidine (Demerol) 100 mg IV and ampicillin sodium (Unasyn) 3 g/100 cc normal saline (NS). She is admitted to the medical/surgical floor with a diagnosis of endometritis for possible D&C.

Admission orders include the following: D$_5$NS at 125 cc/hr, patient-controlled anesthesia (PCA) morphine, and Unasyn 1.5 g IV every 6 hours.

Day 4 postadmission: White blood cells (WBCs) are 20,000 and the patient has a temperature of 102° F. Mary is taken for an exploratory laparotomy that reveals diffuse peritonitis, lysed adhesions, and débrided fibrinous areas. An appendectomy is performed with placement of a Jackson-Pratt (JP) drain, nasogastric tube, and right subclavian triple-lumen catheter. Mary complains of severe continuous postoperative pain, level 5 on scale of 1 to 5 despite multiple doses of morphine sulfate (MS). Mary is transferred to the intensive care unit (ICU).

Vital signs on admission are:

HR	114-145 bpm
BP	80-110/35-70 mmHg
Respirations	26-50 breaths/min
SaO$_2$	94%-96%
Temperature	95.7°-96.7° F (35.3° C-35.9° C)

Mary continues to complain of severe abdominal and back pain. The ICU nurse titrates MS as ordered. The nurse also notes that Mary's right hand is very cool to the touch.

Four hours after admission to the ICU Mary becomes unresponsive with no respirations, and a code blue is called for respiratory arrest. Mary is intubated and placed on a mechanical ventilator; she is hypotensive with systolic blood pressure (SBP) 50 mm Hg per Doppler. The midline anterior abdominal wall dressing is dry and intact. The JP drain contains 100 cc of dark red blood, and the right arm remains extremely cool to the touch with a palpable pulse. A fluid bolus of 500 cc NS is administered. She receives 0.5 mg of epinephrine, and dopamine is started to maintain SBP >90 mm Hg. Arterial blood gases (ABGs), a comprehensive metabolic profile, complete blood count (CBC), and D-dimer were ordered. Mary was severely acidotic and given 4 ampules of sodium bicarbonate. Lab work at this time included:

WBC	27.5 mm^3
PT	35.5
INR	7
Hgb	6.8 g/dl

The patient's husband remained present during the code blue event. The post-code diagnosis included possible pulmonary embolism (PE) and disseminated intravascular coagulation (DIC). Mary was treated with multiple infusions of packed red blood cells (PRBCs), fresh frozen plasma (FFP), and cryoprecipitate. Once stable Mary was taken for a CT scan that revealed a pleural effusion in the right lung. She was then transferred to the operating room for a right thoracoscopy with chest tube insertion, fiberoptic bronchoscopy, and right femoral arterial line placement.

During the next 3 days Mary received a total of 20 U of cryoprecipitate, 9 U of FFP, and 16 U of PRBCs, imipenem-cilastatin (Primaxin), and metronidazole (Flagyl). She showed significant improvement, and was extubated. Mary was discharged 22 days after admission.

DISSEMINATED INTRAVASCULAR COAGULATION

QUESTIONS

1. Define disseminated intravascular coagulation (diffuse intravascular coagulation, or DIC).

2. Identify the causes of DIC.

3. Explain the pathophysiology of DIC.

4. What clinical presentation will the patient with a diagnosis of DIC display?

5. Identify the key laboratory findings in the patient with a diagnosis of DIC.

6. Identify appropriate nursing diagnoses for the patient with DIC.

7. Outline the collaborative plan of care for the patient with DIC.

DISSEMINATED INTRAVASCULAR COAGULATION

QUESTIONS AND ANSWERS

1. Define disseminated intravascular coagulation (diffuse intravascular coagulation, or DIC).

DIC is defined as a catastrophic bleeding disorder characterized by thrombus formation and hemorrhage secondary to overstimulation of the normal coagulation process, resulting in a decrease in clotting factors and platelets. The syndrome may be acute or chronic (Dennison, 2000).

2. Identify the causes of DIC.

DIC has numerous causes (Table 32-1), but all are related to vascular damage with activation of plasma coagulation factors that leads to thrombin generation by the intrinsic coagulation pathway or entry of tissue thromboplastic material into the blood and generation of thrombin by the extrinsic coagulation pathway (Stein, 1998).

3. Explain the pathophysiology of DIC.

See Figure 32-1 and Table 32-2.

Table 32-1 *Causes of DIC*	
Vascular Disorders	**Neoplastic Disorders-cont'd**
Shock	Leukemia
Vasculitis	Pheochromocytoma
Giant hemangioma	
Dissecting aneurysm	**Infections**
Malignant hypertension	Bacterial
Cardiopulmonary bypass pump	Gram positive (*Staphylococcus* and *Streptococcus*)
Thoracic surgery	Gram negative (*Escherichia coli*)
Fat embolism	Viral (influenza, herpes)
	Rickettsial (Rocky Mountain spotted fever)
Hematologic/Immunologic	Protozoal (malaria)
Hemolytic blood transfusion reaction	Fungal (aspergillosis)
Massive blood transfusion	Granulomatous (tuberculosis)
Sickle cell crisis	
Thalassemia major	**Trauma**
Polycythemia vera	Multiple trauma
Anaphylaxis	Burns
Systemic lupus erythematosus	Acute anoxia
Transplant rejection	Heatstroke
Acute leukemia	Crush injury
Promyelocytic leukemia	Head injury
	Surgery
Neoplastic Disorders	**Obstetric Complications**
Pancreatic cancer	Amniotic fluid embolism
Breast cancer	Abruptio placentae
Prostate cancer	Retained dead fetus
Ovarian cancer	Eclampsia
Lung cancer	Septic abortion
Colon cancer	Induced abortion
Stomach cancer	Hydatidiform mole
Sarcoma	Acute fatty liver of pregnancy
Cancer of the urinary tract	Toxemia

Continued

Table 32-1 *Causes of DIC—cont'd*

Pulmonary
Pulmonary embolism
Adult respiratory distress syndrome (ARDS)
Fat embolism
Amniotic fluid embolism

Toxins
Snake bites
Aspirin poisoning
Allergic IV drug reactions

Miscellaneous
Decompression sickness
Amyloidosis
Heatstroke

Gastrointestinal/Accessory Organs
Necrotizing enterocolitis
Pancreatitis
Obstructive jaundice
Hepatitis
Cirrhosis
Acute hepatic failure

Prosthetic Devices
LeVeen or Denver shunt
Intraaortic balloon pump

Data from Stein, J. H. (Ed.). (1998). *Internal medicine* (5th ed.). St Louis: Mosby.

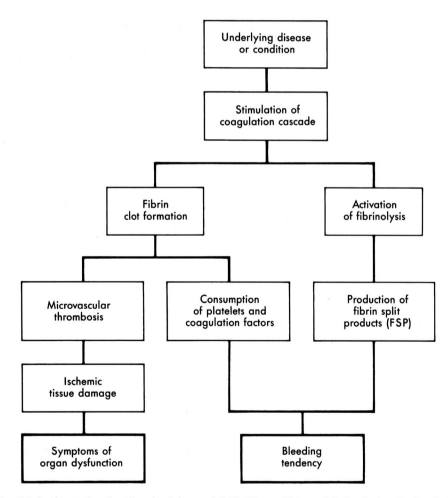

Figure **32-1** Brief schematic of pathophysiology of DIC. (From Kinney, M. R., Paska, D. R., & Dunbar, S. B. [1998]. *AACN clinical reference for critical care nursing* [4th ed.]. St Louis: Mosby.)

Table 32-2 *Pathophysiology of DIC*	
Stimulus	**Intrinsic coagulation system activation/cell or platelet damage**
	Extrinsic coagulation system activation: release of tissue thromboplastin
Clotting causes ischemia and tissue and organ necrosis	Tissue damage releases thromboplastin into circulation
	Thromboplastin converts prothrombin into thrombin
	Abundant intravascular thrombin is produced that converts fibrinogen to a fibrin clot and enhances platelet aggregation
	Excessive blood coagulation creates microvascular thrombi in the microcirculation, causing ischemia
Bleeding causes loss of hemoglobin and oxygen-carrying capacity, leading to hypoxia and ischemia	Excessive aggregation of platelets causes thrombocytopenia, and excessive blood coagulation causes depletion of clotting factors (aka consumptive coagulopathy)
	A stable clot cannot be formed at injury sites, predisposing patient to hemorrhage
Fibrinolysis causes the destruction of once-stable clots and more bleeding	Activation of plasminogen to plasmin causes lysis of preexisting clots and surface bleeding
	Naturally occurring antithrombins, which inhibit thrombin, are inactivated by plasmin
	Fibrinolysis causes production of fibrin split products (FSPs), aka fibrin degradation products (FDPs)
	Fibrin split products are normally cleared by reticuloendothelial system but overproduction overwhelms the system
	Fibrin split products act as an anticoagulant perpetuating bleeding
	• FSPs coat the platelets and interfere with platelet function
	• FSPs interfere with thrombin and disrupt coagulation
	• FSPs attach to fibrinogen, which interferes with the polymerization process necessary to form a stable clot

Data from Dennison, R. D. (2000). *Pass CCRN!* (2nd ed., p. 564). St Louis: Mosby.

4. What clinical presentation will the patient with a diagnosis of DIC display?

The patient must have a history of predisposing factors. In Mary's case, she was 1 week post-cesarean section with a diagnosis of endometritis on admission, then possible pulmonary emboli with sepsis post code. The patient will display symptoms of ischemia such as chest pain, dyspnea, and abdominal pain. Objective symptoms may include indications of decreased perfusion related to specific body systems (brain: change in level of consciousness, seizures, focal neurologic signs; cardiovascular: chest pain, ST-segment elevation or depression, hypoperfusion; pulmonary: dyspnea, chest pain, hypoxemia; genitourinary: decreased urine output, proteinuria, electrolyte imbalance; gastrointestinal: pain, diarrhea; and skin: cyanosis of toes, fingers, lips, nose, and ears; coldness; and necrosis (Hawkins, 1999; Levi, de Jonge, & van der Poll, 2001).

On admission Mary complained of abdominal pain that became progressively worse. Just before coding, Mary's right arm was noted to be extremely cool especially when compared with the left arm. Mary subsequently became lethargic and unresponsive, which later developed into a code blue event (Table 32-3) (Alspach, 1998; Levi & ten Cate, 1999).

Table 32-3	*Clinical Presentation of DIC*
Subjective	History of predisposing factors
	Symptoms related to ischemia
	Chest pain
	Dyspnea
	Abdominal pain
Objective	Indications of decreased perfusion
	Neurologic
	Change in LOC
	Focal neurologic signs
	Seizures
	Cardiovascular
	ST segment elevation or depression
	Hypoperfusion
	Pulmonary
	Dyspnea
	Hypoxemia
	Genitourinary
	Decreased urine output
	Proteinuria
	Electrolyte imbalance
	GI tract
	Abdominal pain
	Diarrhea
	Skin
	Acral cyanosis of toes, fingers, lips, nose, ears
	Mottling
	Coldness
	Necrosis
Indications of platelet dysfunction	Petechiae
	Ecchymosis
	Purpura
Indications of hemorrhage	Tachycardia
	Hypotension
	Tachypnea
	Overt bleeding
	Mucosal surface:
	Gingival bleeding
	Epistaxis
	Genitourinary
	Hematuria
	Gastrointestinal
	Hematemesis
	Hematochezia
	Melena
	Guaiac-positive stool
	Pulmonary
	Hemoptysis
	Gynecologic
	Vaginal bleeding
	Skin
	Prolonged oozing from puncture sites, IV sites, and wounds
	Bruising
	Occult bleeding
	Bleeding into joints
	Swollen joints
	Intraperitoneal bleeding
	Abdominal distention
	Rebound tenderness

Table 32-3 *Clinical Presentation of DIC—cont'd*	
Indications of hemorrhage—cont'd	Occult bleeding—cont'd
	Retroperitoneal bleeding
	Back pain
	Leg numbness
	Hypotension
	Intracranial hemorrhage
	Headache
	Change in level of consciousness
	Pupillary changes
	Retinal hemorrhage
	Visual changes
	Blurred vision
	Loss of visual fields
	Hemodynamics
	Decreased
	Right atrial pressure
	Pulmonary artery occlusive pressure
	Cardiac output
	Cardiac index

Data from Dennison, R. D. (2000). *Pass CCRN!* (2nd ed., p. 566). St Louis, Mosby. and Stein, J.H. (Ed.). (1998). *Internal medicine* (5th ed.). St. Louis: Mosby.

5. **Identify the key laboratory findings in the patient with a diagnosis of DIC.**

The key laboratory findings in a patient with DIC include thrombocytopenia of varying degrees, elevated prothrombin and partial thromboplastin times, fibrinogen degradation product levels, D-dimer, and fibrin monomer level. The patient's fibrinogen level is usually decreased (Kruse et al, 2003).

     Additional lab abnormalities may include respiratory acidosis progressing to metabolic acidosis due to lactic acidosis. Urine, stool, and sputum may all be positive for blood (Levi, de Jonge, van der Poll, & ten Cate, 2000).

6. **Identify appropriate nursing diagnoses for the patient with DIC.**

There are a multitude of nursing diagnoses for the patient with DIC. A few of the possibilities are as follows:

- Altered peripheral, cardiopulmonary, cerebral, renal tissue perfusion related to microclots and/or hemorrhage
- Risk for fluid volume deficit related to hemorrhage
- Decreased cardiac output related to alteration in preload
- Decreased cardiac output related to alteration in afterload
- Decreased cardiac output related to alteration in contractility
- Impaired gas exchange related to microclots in pulmonary circulation
- Impaired gas exchange related to ventilation/perfusion mismatching or intrapulmonary shunting
- Risk of injury related to altered clotting, prescribed therapies
- Ineffective renal tissue perfusion related to decreased renal blood flow
- Risk for infection
- Acute confusion related to sensory overload, sensory deprivation, and sleep pattern disturbances
- Pain related to ischemia, necrosis
- Anxiety related to acute change in health status
- Ineffective individual coping related to situational crisis, powerlessness, change in role
- Ineffective family coping related to critically ill family member (Dennison, 2000; Urden et al, 2002)

7. Outline the collaborative plan of care for the patient with DIC.

The collaborative plan of care is outlined in Table 32-4 (Dennison, 2000; Levi, de Jorge, van der Poll, & ten Cate, 2000; Stein, 1998).

Table 32-4 *Collaborative Plan of Care*	

1. Detect DIC early and control causative factors	A. Identify high-risk groups for clinical indications of DIC
	  1. Monitor for thrombosis or bleeding
	    a. Note petechiae, ecchymosis, acrocyanosis
	    b. Test NG aspirate or vomitus, stool, and urine for blood
	    c. Monitor oral/pulmonary secretions and gums for bleeding
	    d. Monitor peripheral pulses, capillary refill
	  2. Monitor laboratory studies for indications of DIC
	  3. Assess for clinical indications of hypoperfusion or intracranial hemorrhage
	  4. Monitor hemodynamic parameters as indicated
	  5. Insert indwelling urinary catheter to monitor hourly urine output
	B. Control underlying causative factor
	  1. Surgery
	    a. Surgical debridement
	    b. Abscess drainage
	    c. Evacuation of the uterus
	    d. Removal of tumor
	  2. Antimicrobials for infection
	  3. Antineoplastics for malignancy

2. Maintain airway, ventilation, and oxygenation	A. Administer oxygen to maintain PaO_2 of 80 mm Hg and SpO_2 of 95% unless contraindicated B. Assist with intubation and mechanical ventilation as necessary C. Suction only as necessary and with low suction to avoid trauma to the tracheobronchial mucosa
3. Correct hypovolemia, hypotension, hypoxia, and acidosis	A. Insert or ensure patency of peripheral intravenous catheter B. Administer normal saline to replace volume until type and crossmatch completed and blood available C. Administer volume replacement, inotropes, and/or vasopressors as prescribed to maintain MAP > than 60 mm Hg
4. Stop microclotting to maintain perfusion and protect vital organ function	A. Administer intravenous heparin (usually 15 U/kg/hr) as prescribed; aPTT will not be utilized to adjust dose because it is affected by DIC. Heparin prevents further thrombosis in microvasculature and prevents platelet aggregation. Dalteparin sodium (Fragmin) and

Table 32-4	***Collaborative Plan of Care—cont'd***

	enoxaparin (Lovenox) utilized for chronic DIC not acute
	B. Administer antithrombin III as prescribed; antithrombin III inhibits the action of thrombin
	C. Administer aminocaproic acid (Amicar) as prescribed; blocks fibrinolytic system so that stable clots are not degraded
	D. Administer drotrecogin alfa (Xigris) (activated protein C) as prescribed
	E. Assist with plasmapheresis
5. Stop the bleeding by supporting coagulation	A. Administer blood products as prescribed 1. FFP (contains clotting factors); used for bleeding patients with elevated PT and aPTT 2. Cryoprecipitate (contains factors VIII, XIII, and fibrinogen); used to maintain fibrinogen levels > 100 mg/dl 3. Platelets; used to maintain platelet count >50,000/mm^3 4. PRBCs; used if blood loss is significant
	B. Administer hemostatic cofactors as prescribed 1. Vitamin K; needed for liver production of several clotting factors 2. Folic acid; folic acid deficiency may cause thrombocytopenia
	C. Administer aminocaproic acid as prescribed for primary fibrinolysis
	D. Apply thrombin-soaked gauze, pressure dressings, and/or ice packs to control bleeding sites
6. Treat ischemic pain	A. Administer analgesics as prescribed
	B. Apply cold compresses for pain caused by bleeding in joints and tissues
7. Maintain skin integrity and minimize tissue trauma	A. Provide meticulous skin care 1. Turn q2h 2. Keep skin moist with lubricating lotions 3. Utilize specialized beds as needed
	B. Provide mouth care utilizing alcohol-free mouthwash and swabs
	C. Provide careful perianal care; avoid rectal temperatures and suppositories
	D. Alternate activity with rest
	E. Use an electric razor instead of straight-edge
	F. Avoid tape if possible; utilize adhesive remover to remove tape
	G. Apply local pressure to any break in skin integrity 1. Avoid intramuscular and subcutaneous injections 2. Use arterial line or saline lock for sampling

Continued

Table 32-4	*Collaborative Plan of Care—cont'd*

	a. If venous puncture is necessary; apply pressure for 3-5 minutes after procedure
	b. If arterial puncture is necessary; apply pressure for 10-15 minutes after procedure
	H. Reduce frequency of cuff BPs; an arterial line is ideal for pressure monitoring and obtaining blood specimens
	I. DO NOT give ASA or NSAIDs due to their effect on platelet aggregation
	J. Teach patient to avoid Valsalva maneuver
	K. DO NOT disturb any clot
8. Provide psychologic support and reassurance	A. Reassure patient that treatment is being provided to stop the bleeding
	B. Inquire with family regarding spiritual support
9. Monitor for complications	A. Intracerebral hemorrhage
	B. Hemorrhagic shock
	C. ARDS
	D. GI dysfunction
	E. Renal failure
	F. Infection

DISSEMINATED INTRAVASCULAR COAGULATION

References

Dennison, R. D. (2000). *Pass CCRN!* St Louis: Mosby.

Grif Alspach, J. (1998). *American Association of Critical Care Nurses: Core curriculum of critical care nursing* (5th ed.). Philadelphia: W. B. Saunders Company.

Hawkins, R. (1999). Clinical focus: Disseminated intravascular coagulation. *Clinical Journal of Oncology Nursing, 3*(3), 127-131.

Levi, M., de Jonge, E., & van der Poll, T. (2001). Rationale for restoration of physiological anticoagulant pathways in patients with sepsis and disseminated intravascular coagulation. *Critical Care Medicine, 29*(7 Suppl), S90-S94.

Levi, M., de Jonge, E., van der Poll, T., & ten Cate, H. (2000). Novel approaches to the management of disseminated intravascular coagulation. *Critical Care Medicine, 28*(9 Suppl), S20-S24.

Levi. M. & ten Cate, H. (1999). Disseminated intravascular coagulation. *The New England Journal of Medicine, 341*(8):586-592.

Kruse, J. A., Fink, M. P., & Carlson, R. W. (2003). *Saunders manual of critical care.* Philadelphia: W. B. Saunders.

Stein, J. H. (Ed.). (1998). *Internal medicine* (5th ed.). St Louis: Mosby. www.sepsis.com.

Urden, L. D., Stacy, K. M., & Lough, M. E. (Eds). (2002). *Thelan's critical care nursing: Diagnosis and management* (4th ed.). St Louis: Mosby.

33

End of Life Issues

W. Gale Hoehn, RN, MSN

CASE PRESENTATION

Emmet Steel, 64 years old, has a long history of chronic obstructive pulmonary disease (COPD), alcoholism, and osteoarthritis. He was diagnosed with inoperable non–small-cell lung cancer 3 months ago and has had two cycles of chemotherapy. Mr. Steel was admitted to the hospital 16 days ago with difficulty breathing, chronic cough, and severe shortness of breath with any exertion. He continues to require hospitalization for fever and pancytopenia. Admission chest x-ray revealed bilateral pleural effusions with greater involvement on the right, and an empyema located in the right middle lobe.

PAST MEDICAL HISTORY

Left upper extremity deep vein thrombosis (DVT) 2 years ago, right lower DVT approximately 8 months ago; gastrointestinal (GI) bleed (last episode 1 year ago); COPD (stopped smoking 2.5 years ago after 55 pack-years); occasional beer or two after work—quit at one time then drinking increased after divorce 6 years ago; hypothyroidism, gout, and allergic rhinitis. Childhood illnesses were usual and included a fracture in the right upper extremity and left elbow on different occasions.

Social History

Mr. Steel has been retired for 2 years from warehouse work as a dock loader and forklift driver. He has Medicare without supplemental insurance coverage. Mr. Steel's ex-wife and two married children are estranged; his sister is the primary caregiver but is a single parent working two jobs and raising five children under the age of 14.

Medications on admission to the hospital were:

allopurinol (Aloprim) 300 mg po qd
furosemide (Lasix) 40 mg po qd
potassium chloride (K-Dur) 10 mg po bid
levothyroxine (Levoxyl) 0.88 mg po qd
fluticasone (Flovent) 110 μg two puffs bid
ipratropium bromide/albuterol (Combivent) two puffs qid
zolpidem (Ambien) 10 mg $\frac{1}{2}$ qhs prn
oxycodone/acetaminophen (Percocet) 7.5 mg q3h prn
acetaminophen (Tylenol) 500 mg two tablets q 4-6 hr prn (temp/pain)
propoxyphene/acetaminophen (Darvocet N 100) 1 or 2 tablets q4h prn (pain)
sodium chloride (Ocean Mist nasal spray) qd prn (mucosal membrane dryness and irritation)

Medications added upon admission:

> clindamycin hydrochloride (Cleocin) 600 mg IV q8h
> vancomycin hydrochloride (Vancocin) 750 mg IV q12h
> cefepime (Maxipime) 2 g IV q8h
> oxycodone/acetaminophen (Percocet) 7.5 mg 1 tablet q3h prn (severe pain)
> promethazine (Phenergan) 12.5 mg IV q6h prn (nausea)
> diphenoxylate/atropine (Lomotil) 2.5-5 mg po q6h prn (diarrhea)
> nystatin (Mycostatin) 5 cc po qid (mucositis)
> insulin (Novolin R) (per sliding scale)

Day 10

Mr. Steel's admission was uneventful until day 10. At this time one of the two chest tubes began to be tender to touch and looked as though the tube had sclerosed. This chest tube was removed. The second chest tube continued to drain thick, gray-tinged fluid. Mr. Steel reported left arm pain with increased swelling and redness. Sonograph evaluation revealed brachial and axillary veins with thrombus noted in the left subclavian and left jugular veins. Enoxaparin (Lovenox) 1 mg/kg SQ bid and warfarin (Coumadin) 5 mg qd were added to the medication regimen.

Mr. Steel has had no visitors other than his sister, who is only able to visit for 10 to 15 minutes as her children wait downstairs. He has refused daily hygiene care for 3 days and has refused to get out of bed this morning for linen change. He remains in protective isolation and keeps the room dark. He does not watch TV and has refused visits from the hospital chaplain. Physical therapy and occupational therapy have documented that Mr. Steel is refusing assistance or treatment. Staff personnel report that Mr. Steel's behavior has not changed much from the first week of admission. His sister states he does not communicate easily and has been a "mean, sour" person all his life. Mr. Steel's pain level has progressed from 1 to 4 on scale of 0 to 5, with 5 being the worst pain he's ever had in his lower back and spine. He has refused offers from his physician for increased pain medication but nursing notes indicate he has been calling out for the last three nights asking for pain medication. The physician does not feel there is a need for antidepressants at this time and has documented that he has discussed with Mr. Steel the prognosis of his disease. He has stated in the progress notes that he has informed the patient that the disease is progressing despite aggressive treatment, but he feels he must continue treatment if Mr. Steel plans to ever leave the hospital.

Mr. Steel remains a full code and continues to deny any conversation with his physician about disease progression. The hospital's admission form states Mr. Steel does not have advance directives, power of attorney, or a health care representative. Efforts by nursing personnel to discuss these issues have been met with silence and an unspoken unwillingness to discuss advance directives.

Day 16

Today, when speaking to her brother's nurse, she conveys that she is very upset because the physician returned a call regarding her brother's prognosis and stated he was going to start total parenteral nutrition (TPN) before the start of the third cycle of chemotherapy. The sister wants the nurse to change Mr. Steel's code status to No code. The sister feels there is no need to continue with the chemotherapy. She is also very concerned about the increasing pain and confusion when she talks to her brother. She says she thinks her brother has given up and she too is just tired of the whole thing because her brother has been unable or unwilling to care for himself for the past 3 months.

END OF LIFE ISSUES

QUESTIONS

1. What are advance directives and what are the implications for nursing care?

2. Given the stage IV disease and likelihood of metastasis, what is your role as a nurse in the decision making regarding end of life issues with the patient and his sister?

3. What do you consider a priority for the optimal care and decision making for this patient?

4. What are the considerations that must be discussed before responding to the sister's request for change of code status?

5. Discuss the pros and cons of continued therapy and what role nursing can play in helping the patient in a futile situation.

6. Under what circumstances can treatment be stopped or feedings withdrawn?

7. What can be done from the nursing perspective to assist the family?

END OF LIFE ISSUES

QUESTIONS AND ANSWERS

1. What are advance directives and what are the implications for nursing care?

Nurses have a unique opportunity to implement into practice the Patient Self-Determination Act (PSDA). This can be accomplished by using the nursing process and therapeutic communications with the patient and family. Advance directives are legal documents that describe the type of care a patient may desire in the event that he or she is incapacitated and unable to make medical decisions (Urden et al, 2002). A living will is a type of advanced directive that allows the patient to document wishes concerning medical treatments at the end of life. A durable power of attorney or health care proxy is another type of advance directive that permits the patient to appoint or name a trusted person to make decisions in his or her behalf. The PSDA, implemented in 1991, mandates that the providers of health care services under Medicare and Medicaid comply with requirements for accessibility to advance directive documents. These documents are written instructions declaring the patients' wishes patients become incapacitated. Providers may not be reimbursed for services and care rendered unless mandates of the law are met (Urden et al, 2002). Responsibility for providing information to patients should be delegated to members of the health care team who have received appropriate training.

2. Given the stage IV disease and likelihood of metastasis, what is your role as a nurse in the decision making regarding end of life issues with the patient and his sister?

Stage IV disease implies that Mr. Steel's disease is terminal. Biopsy specimens are classified in terms of the cancer growth and extent of disease by the pathologist in accordance with the TNM classification system. *T* defines the evaluation of the characteristics of the primary tumor; *N* signifies the involvement of the lymph nodes; and *M* demonstrates the evidence of metastasis. These diagnostic factors are based on the knowledge and characteristics of the natural history of the disease. Utilizing the TNM classification, cancers may be categorized into stages 1 through 4, with four indicating the cancer cells are poorly differentiated and have evolved to the worst prognosis (Black et al, 2001).

In addressing end of life issues, it is essential that nurses develop an honest, trusting relationship with the patient, family members, and/or caregivers. The nursing staff must explore Mr. Steel's reluctance to discuss issues that deal with the severity of this illness and his wishes for advance directives. Kirmse (1998) supports the belief that advanced practice as well as critical care nurses must play a key role in educating patients and their families about advance directives and end of life decisions. The American Nurses Association position statement on nursing care and do-not-resuscitate decisions recommends that "the choices and values of the competent patient should always be given highest priority, even when these wishes conflict with those of health care providers and families" (American Nurses Association [ANA], 1992). This position statement clarifies the nurse's duty to educate patients and their loved ones about the various forms of advance care directives and patients' rights.

It is imperative that nurses be aware of and take an active role in developing such policies in their work setting if they do not exist. In the discussion for commonly used life support measures, advance care planning, and/or advance care directives, one will need to ask the following questions: What does Mr. Steel know about his disease and usual disease process? What does Mr. Steel expect to benefit from the chemotherapy and other aggressive treatments? What quality of life does Mr. Steel want and/or expect?

Each institution should have process mechanisms outlined in policies and protocols for resolution on end of life conflicts. Preferably, acute health care facilities should utilize the interdisciplinary ethics committee with nurse membership for recommendations in disputes or in absence of health care directives in patients who are unable to speak for themselves and may be without family or health care representation.

3. **What do you consider a priority for the optimal care and decision making for this patient?**

Communication and pain relief are key issues in this case scenario. Mr. Steel's isolation has been complicated by his immunosuppressed state as well as by his personal separation issues with his ex-wife, children, and sister. Mr. Steel does not have friends that visit or assist with his care. He has a history that implies he may have some difficulty with communication. The nurse providing his care has a duty to encourage open communication with the physician and perhaps seek the assistance of a social worker or one who is trained to assist with dysfunctional communication. Once trust has been established and the client believes that the health care team will effectively manage his pain and other symptoms, he may begin to open up and discuss his thoughts and concerns regarding illness and death. Although the goal at the onset of treatment may have been for prolongation of life, palliation with relief of pain and suffering may be the more realistic goal at this point.

Patient assessment for end of life care should focus on the relief of suffering and pain. Suffering is a physical or psychologic experience that the patient dislikes or experiences when feeling threatened. Suffering may also be termed an evaluation of the significance and meaning of pain. McCaffery and Pasero (1999) define pain for the clinical setting: "Pain is whatever the experiencing person says it is, existing whenever he says it does."

The nurse continues to be an advocate for the patient and remains available for listening in a nonjudgmental relationship. Ideally the shift of focus in care is gradual and in compliance with the patient's wishes. We do not know Mr. Steel's goals for the medical or nursing treatment of his lung cancer. The lack of this information has become an obstacle for Mr. Steel and his caregivers.

Direct communication between the patient, physician, and sister involved with the nursing staff personnel in Mr. Steel's care must be paramount to the decision making for advance care planning. In the coordination of care, the nurse can arrange an interdisciplinary care conference meeting including the physician, patient, sister, hospital chaplain, social worker, and a member of the nursing staff. The interdisciplinary team may be beneficial and effective for the exploration of Mr. Steel's values, beliefs, and wishes for a peaceful death. Decisions about life-sustaining treatment are agonizing for family and many staff members when the patient's wishes have not been documented or discussed with the physician prior to a crisis in the illness or disease (McFarland et al, 2003).

4. **What are the considerations that must be discussed before responding to the sister's request for change of code status?**

The sister is obviously overwhelmed with her own personal situations as well as trying to cope with the grief that her brother is dying. The families of terminally ill patients, when highly involved in providing care without respite, may be emotionally as well as physically exhausted. The sister could benefit from continued support from all members of the interdisciplinary health care team. The nurse will want to gently remind the sister that her brother has the right to determine his own code status. The concept of autonomy is well established in the medical and nursing literature and arises from the Greek philosophy: "In health care, autonomy can be viewed as the freedom to make decision about one's own body without the coercion or interference of others. Autonomy is a freedom of choice or a self-determination that is a basic human right" (Urden et al, 2002, pp. 19-20).

Questions as to why she feels that her brother is confused are important. The nurse realizes that a change in mental status may be an indicator of the disease sequelae. Options for the sister may include spiritual or pastoral consultation. Many hospitals have volunteer organizations that could be called upon to assist with the children so that the sister may get some counseling. It is very important for the nursing staff to be present and supportive for the sister as well as Mr. Steel. There may be opportunities within the hospital facility for the children to view a movie or be entertained while the sister and brother have some uninterrupted time together to discuss these very important issues.

5. Discuss the pros and cons of continued therapy and what role nursing can play in helping the patient in a futile situation.

Mr. Steel's cancer is not responding to the chemotherapy drugs and his immune system has been severely impaired and damaged by the disease as well as the therapeutic interventions. With the known course of this disease, aggressive treatment for Mr. Steel's case could be considered "futile." Futility in the medical sense generally refers to therapeutic interventions that are unlikely to initiate any significant benefit for the patient. Making a case for futility depends on data or the evidence documented to support the proposed outcome of the intervention. Yet from a nursing point of view, it may be morally justified to continue support through the chemotherapy treatments with all supportive measures including the TPN. It may well depend on the data and evidence of disease that determine the course of treatment and bring meaning to the word *futility*. Daniel Callahan in a Hasting report in 1991 stated that "a standard of futility compatible with the goal of avoiding an unnecessarily painful or extended death would be most valuable" (p. 6). Our health care community has yet to determine standards for futility.

The American Association of Critical Care Nurses' (AACN) position statement on withholding and withdrawing life-sustaining treatment recognizes that nurses have a crucial role in supporting a patient's choices and beliefs regarding end of life care. The statement declares that critical care nurses are to collaborate with the patient, family, physician, and other health care providers. AACN affirms that this collaboration and communication should occur in an atmosphere that supports logical discussions and concentrates on the needs and wishes of the patient (AACN, 1990).

Treatment decisions must be individualized for the patient and family members. An interdisciplinary team of health care providers can be of great value when presenting the information and usual course of the disease in such a way that Mr. Steel and his sister have all the facts, evidence, and adequate time to arrive at a decision. This patient may need assistance in determining the quality of life that he wishes as his progressive illness continues to be symptomatic and interferes with his usual activities of daily living.

6. Under what circumstances can treatment be stopped or feedings withdrawn?

Once a rigorous treatment is initiated, it is more difficult to stop as it may be in the case of Mr. Steele. Usually a written or a verbal consent is obtained and agreed upon by the physician and the patient before a chemotherapy regimen is initiated. The practice of informed consent and authorization of treatment and the patient's right to accept or refuse treatment began in the 18th century, stemming from the common law "right not to be touched without giving consent" (Urden et al, 2002, p. 38). In the case of *Scholendorff v. Society of New York Hospital*, the court determined that every adult individual with sound mind had a right to determine what should be done with their own body (Urden et al, 2002). Since then, most states have adopted informed consent statutes. In congruence with those statutes, physicians have a legal and moral duty to disclose information to facilitate decisions by the patient to accept or refuse medical treatment.

The physician usually conducts discussions of treatment preferences, but other members of the health care team participate and support the implementation of treatment decisions (Emanuel et al, 1999). In many instances it is the nurse who interprets the information or translates for the patient and family. This discussion with the nurse may occur after the initial discussion with the physician when the patient has had some time to assimilate the information and formulate questions and/or concerns.

It is essential when discussing end of life or changing treatment plans that may lead to end of life issues that the patient and family understand the language associated with life-sustaining treatments. There is a wide range of treatment/interventions that may be considered as life sustaining. These may include cardiopulmonary resuscitation (CPR), mechanical ventilation with elective intubation, dialysis, blood transfusions or blood products, artificial nutrition, hydration, antibiotics, surgery, and other invasive procedures (Emanuel et al, 1999). When goals of care have been determined by the patient and/or family, the health care team has the responsibility of implementing those goals. Discuss treatment plans with other health care team members as often and appropriate as necessary to clarify. Patients also have the right to modify their goals at any time throughout the continuum of care.

7. What can be done from the nursing perspective to assist the family?

Nurses as members of the health care team spend large amounts of time with patients and their families. The power of presence as a supportive measure of care for the patient and family is an art long recognized by the nursing profession. Many patients with cancer are aware of the caring presence of a nurse. The significance of this presence increases with the realities of dying as patients may seek the meaning of their life experiences (Stanley, 2002). It is vital that patients and their families understand that end of life care or terminal care does not mean that they will not receive adequate health care; rather, it is the focus of care that changes. Achieving quality of life at the end of life means addressing multiple dimensions that influence a patient's understanding of the disease process and subsequently the dying process. The most common fear for patients and their families may be the fear of abandonment if life-sustaining treatment is withdrawn. Anticipating the patient's needs and offering supportive care may avoid this apprehension in patients as well as their families. Attention to realistic goals for end of life care is essential in making the end of life as peaceful and dignified as possible.

END OF LIFE ISSUES

References

American Association of Critical Care Nurses, www.AACN.org. American Nurses Association, Task Force on the Nurse's Role in End of Life Decisions. (1992). *Position statements: Nursing care and do-not-resuscitate decisions.* Retrieved March 16, 2003, from http://nursingworld.org/readroom/position/ethics/etdnr.htm.

Black, J. M., Hawks, J. H., & Keene, A. M. (Eds.). (2001). *Medical-surgical nursing: Clinical management for positive outcomes* (6th ed., vol. 1). Philadelphia: W. B. Saunders.

Callahan, D. Medical futility, medical necessity. *Hastings Center Report.* (July-August 1991.)

Emanuel, L. L., von Gunten, C. F., & Ferris, F. D. (1999). *The education for physicians on end-of-life care (epec) curriculum.* Washington, DC: Author.

Kirmse, J. M. (1998). Aggressive implementation of advance directives. *Critical Care Nursing Quarterly, 21*(1), 83-89.

McFaffery, M. & Pasero, C. (1999). *Pain: Clinical manual* (2nd ed.). St Louis: Mosby, Inc.

McFarland, E., Likourezos, A., Chichin, E., Castor T., & Paris, B. (2003). Stability of preferences regarding life-sustaining treatment: A two-year prospective study of nursing home residents. *The Mount Sinai Journal of Medicine, 70*(2), 85-92.

Stanley, K. J. (2002). The healing power of presence: Respite from the fear of abandonment. *Oncology Nursing Forum, 29*(6), 935-940.

Urden, L. D., Stacy, K. M., & Lough, M. E. (Eds.) (2002). *Thelan's critical care nursing: Diagnosis and management* (4th ed.). St. Louis: Mosby.

ABBREVIATIONS

AAA Abdominal aortic aneurysm
ABG Arterial blood gas
ACE Angiotensin-converting enzyme
ACS Abdominal compartment syndrome
ACTH Adrenocorticotropic hormone
ADH Antidiuretic hormone
ADP Adenosine diphosphate
ADR Adverse drug reaction
AHA American Heart Association
ALT Alanine aminotransferase
AMI Acute myocardial infarction
ANH Atrial natriuretic hormone
aPTT Activated partial thromboplastin time
ARDS Acute respiratory distress syndrome; adult respiratory distress syndrome
ARF Acute renal failure
AST Aspartate aminotransferase
ATN Acute tubular necrosis
ATP Adenosine triphosphate
AV Atrioventricular; arteriovenous
AZT Azidothymidine
BGM Blood glucose monitoring
BP Blood pressure
bpm Beats per minute
BUN Blood urea nitrogen
CABG Coronary artery bypass graft
CAP Community-acquired pneumonia
CAPD Continuous ambulatory peritoneal dialysis
CAVHD Continuous arteriovenous hemofiltration dialysis
CBC Complete blood count
CCS Corticosteroid
CCU Cardiac care unit
CHF Congestive heart failure
CI Cardiac index
CICU Cardiac intensive care unit
CK Creatine kinase
CK-MB Creatine kinase–myocardial band
CO Cardiac output
COPD Chronic obstructive pulmonary disease
CPP Cerebral perfusion pressure
CRF Chronic renal failure
CRH Corticotropin-releasing hormone
CRRT Continuous renal replacement therapy
C&S Culture and sensitivity
CSF Cerebrospinal fluid
CT Computed tomography
CVA Cerebrovascular accident
CVC Central venous catheter

CVP Central venous pressure
CVVHD Continuous venovenous hemodialysis
D5LR 5% dextrose in lactated Ringer's solution
D5W 5% dextrose in water
DAI Diffuse axonal injury
DI Diabetes insipidus
DIC Disseminated intravascular coagulation
DKA Diabetic ketoacidosis
dl Deciliter
DVT Deep venous thrombosis; deep vein thrombosis
E Epinephrine
ECG Electrocardiogram
ED Emergency department
EDH Epidural hematoma
EF Ejection fraction
EGD Esophagogastroduodenoscopy
ELISA Enzyme-linked immunosorbent assay
EPO Erythropoietin
ES Elastic stockings
ESRD End-stage renal disease
FEV Forced expiratory volume
ft Feet
g Gram
GCS Glasgow Coma Scale
GFR Glomerular filtration rate
GH Growth hormone
GI Gastrointestinal
GIs Glycemic indices
GP Glycoprotein
HAART Highly active antiretroviral therapy
HAP Hospital-acquired pneumonia
HAV Hepatitis A virus
HBV Hepatitis B virus
HCG Human chorionic gonadotropin
Hct Hematocrit
HCV Hepatitis C virus
HCW Health care worker
Hgb Hemoglobin
HPV Human papillomavirus
HR Heart rate
HRP Hormone replacement therapy
HSV Herpes simplex virus
IABP Intraaortic balloon pump
ICP Intracranial pressure
ICU Intensive care unit
IL Interleukin
IM Intramuscular
IMV Intermittent mandatory ventilation
in Inch
INR International Normalized Ratio
IPC Intermittent pneumatic compression
IV Intravenous
IVC Inferior vena cava
IVP Intravenous push

JG Juxtaglomerular
JGA Juxtaglomerular apparatus
KS Kaposi's sarcoma
KUB Kidney, ureter, and bladder (x-ray)
LAP Left atrial pressure
LBBB Left bundle-branch block
LDH Lactate dehydrogenase
LDUH Low-dose unfractionated heparin
LMWH Low-molecular-weight heparin
LOC Level of consciousness
LR Lactated Ringer's solution
LVF Left ventricular failure
μl Microliter
MAP Mean arterial pressure
MAST Medical antishock trousers
MI Myocardial infarction
MIDCABG Minimally invasive direct coronary artery bypass graft
mm Hg Millimeters of mercury
MODS Multiple organ dysfunction syndrome
MOF Multiple organ failure
MRI Magnetic resonance imaging
MSH Melanocyte-stimulating hormone
NE Norepinephrine
NPO Nothing by mouth
NRTI Nucleoside analog reverse transcriptase inhibitor
NS Normal saline
NSAIDs Nonsteroidal antiinflammatory drugs
NSR Normal sinus rhythm
NSS Normal saline solution
NTG Nasogastric tube
PAC Pulmonary artery catheter
PADP Pulmonary artery diastolic (pressure)
PAF Platelet-activating factor
PAOP Pulmonary artery occlusive pressure
PAP Pulmonary artery pressure
PAS Pulmonary artery systolic (pressure)
PAWP Pulmonary artery wedge pressure
PCA Patient-controlled analgesia
PCV Packed cell volume
PCWP Pulmonary capillary wedge pressure
PEEP Positive end-expiratory pressure
PI Pulmonary infarction
PIP Peak inspiratory pressure
PMI Point of maximum impulse; point of maximum impulse of intensity
po Orally
POMC Pro-opiomelanocortin
PRBCs Packed red blood cells
PS Pressure support
PT Prothrombin time
PTCA Percutaneous transluminal coronary angioplasty
PTT Partial thromboplastin time
PVC Premature ventricular contraction
PVR Peripheral vascular resistance
qd Every day

RAAS Renin-angiotensin-aldosterone system
RAP Right atrial pressure
RAS Renin-angiotensin system
RBCs Red blood cells
RN Registered nurse
RVF Right ventricular failure
SDH Subdural hematoma
SIADH Syndrome of inappropriate secretion of antidiuretic hormone
SICU Surgical intensive care unit
SIMV Synchronized intermittent mandatory ventilation
SIRS Systemic inflammatory response system
SNS Sympathetic nervous system
SOB Shortness of breath
SV Stroke volume
SVR Systemic vascular resistance
T_4 Tetraiodothyronine, thyroxine
T_3 Triiodothyronine
TEE Transesophageal echocardiography
THA Total hip arthroplasty
THK Total knee replacement
THR Total hip replacement
TIA Transient ischemic attack
TLC Total lung capacity
TMP-SMZ Trimethoprim-sulfamethoxazole
TNF Tumor necrosis factor
tPA Tissue plasminogen activation
TPN Total parenteral nutrition
TSH Thyroid-stimulating hormone
VAD Ventricular assist device
VTE Venous thromboembolism
V_T Tidal volume
WBCs White blood cells
WHO World Health Organization

Page numbers followed by f indicate figures; t indicates tables; b indicates boxes.

thrombus formation and extension of existing thrombi. Heparin must be titrated for effect using activated partial thromboplastin times (aPTT). Heparin and aspirin are used together to prevent the formation of thrombus (Gurfinkel et al, 1998; Goldman & Bennett, 2000). "It is recommended that all patients who have received tPA or reteplase should receive heparin" (Cairns et al, 1998).

Enoxaparin is a new low-molecular-weight heparin (LMWH). The pharmacologic properties of LMWHs include a binding affinity for antithrombin III, antifactor IIa activity, excellent bioavailability, minimal protein binding, predictable anticoagulant response, and clinical tolerance by patients. Enoxaparin is given subcutaneously, usually at 1 mg/kg every 12 hours. The emerging role of LMWHs is to offer efficacy plus safety for the treatment of acute coronary problems and in treatment for patients who received coronary stents. This new pharmacologic antithrombic approach offers a significant reduction in rehospitalization rate, interventions, and medical costs (Gurfinkel et al, 1998; Zidar, 1998; Goldman & Bennett, 2000). Enoxaparin has the benefit of being therapeutic at the onset of administration, whereas heparin must be titrated to the aPTT for a therapeutic effect. It may take several hours to get the aPTT to the desired level.

13. Discuss the pharmacologic effects of morphine.

Catecholamines are released in response to the pain and anxiety associated with an MI. This causes an increase in heart rate and blood pressure and vasoconstriction. All of these increase the workload on the heart. Morphine can relieve anxiety, thereby reducing the catecholamine release and easing the workload on the heart. Morphine also exerts mild hemodynamic effects by increasing the venous capacitance and by reducing systemic vascular resistance. The result of both effects is a reduction in myocardial oxygen demand (Urden et al, 2002).

14. Describe what a β-blocker is and the rationale for Mr. Johnson receiving this medication.

A β-blocker acts by blocking the β-adrenergic responses to catecholamine stimulation. It can decrease heart rate, blood pressure, contractility, and myocardial oxygen demand. This sudden decrease in workload will increase the cardiac output and lessen the severity of the MI. β-blockers can interrupt evolving infarcts, limit infarct size, and decrease the incidence of ventricular arrhythmias by decreasing oxygen demand. They increase diastolic filling time and increase exercise tolerance. β-blockers are contraindicated in patients with heart failure, hypotension, bradycardia, heart block, and bronchial asthma (Alexander et al, 1998; Lessig & Lessig, 1998; Goldman & Bennett, 2000; Green 2003). For AMI, metoprolol titrate (Lopressor) 5 mg is given intravenously every 2 to 5 minutes for three doses (total 15 mg). After each bolus, vital signs must be assessed for 2 to 5 minutes. The boluses are stopped if the heart rate decreases to less than 60 bpm or systolic blood pressure drops to less than 100 mm Hg (Green, 2003).

15. Why was Mr. Johnson given lidocaine?

One of the adverse effects of a decrease in myocardial blood flow is arrhythmias. Arrhythmias can be life threatening. Tachycardias increase the oxygen demand and decrease coronary perfusion. Bradycardias can result in CHF. Heart blocks decrease coronary and systemic perfusion and can contribute to cardiogenic shock. When myocardial blood supply or oxygen decreases, myocardial tissue becomes irritable and can trigger VT. Reperfusion arrhythmias (especially PVCs) can result when the blood supply is restored after tPA or PTCA. They are so common that they are considered signs of successful reperfusion.

Previously lidocaine was used as a preventive treatment in all MI patients. It is no longer recommended as prophylactic treatment for AMIs. However, in Mr. Johnson's case, he began having VT after the PTCA restored blood supply to the myocardium (reperfusion arrhythmia). A reperfusion arrhythmia is considered a good sign, but the arrhythmias still need to be treated, especially VT. Therefore he was given a 100-mg bolus of lidocaine and a drip at 2 mg/min. Toxic effects of lidocaine include drowsiness, slurred speech, hallucinations, and seizures. These effects are potentiated in elderly patients and those with renal failure (Bucher & Melander, 1999; Goldman & Bennett, 2000).

16. tPA is a thrombolytic agent. Discuss the effects of a thrombolytic agent and why it was used for Mr. Johnson initially rather than angioplasty.

Not only are the coronary arteries closed by plaque, but the plaque also causes turbulence in them and slows the blood flow. This can cause a clot to form at that site, completely closing the artery. tPA is a human protein manufactured by genetic engineering. "Tissue plasminogen activator is one of several drugs now approved for use in certain patients having a heart attack. These drugs have the ability to dissolve the blood clots that are responsible for causing the majority of all heart attacks. Studies have shown that tPA and other thrombolytic agents can reduce the amount of damage to the heart muscle as well as the number of heart attack deaths if administered soon [within a few hours] after symptoms begin" (American Heart Association, 1999; Goldman & Bennett, 2000). The desired effect of tPA is to break up the clots that have formed in the coronary arteries. "It is strongly recommended that all patients with AMI be considered for anticoagulant therapy" (Cairns et al, 1998; Popma et al, 2002). tPA is given as a 15-mg bolus, then 0.75 mg/kg (maximum of 50 mg) over 30 minutes, followed by 0.5 mg/kg (maximum of 35 mg) over 60 minutes for a total of 100 mg over 90 minutes (Lessig & Lessig, 1998; Popma et al, 2002). Signs of reperfusion include pain relief, reperfusion arrhythmias (accelerated idioventricular rhythm, ventricular ectopy, and bradycardia), and ST-segment resolution. The side effects of tPA are related to its systemic action that breaks up any clots in the body. This is why there is a long list of contraindications for tPA.

There has been controversy about whether direct angioplasty is better than therapy with tPA. Direct angioplasty became an attractive alternative in 1993 when three small randomized trials concluded that the technique saved an estimated 40 lives per 1000 patients treated, a huge clinical advantage. However, these trials were performed at "selected hospitals with a lot of experience, involved few patients, and except in one case, used thrombolytic regimens that are suboptimal by today's standards" (GUSTO IIb, 1997). Initially, the Duke study was designed to include as many patients as possible for a lengthier period. It looked at the outcomes of 1138 patients who were given either the clot-busting drug tPA or direct angioplasty in 57 hospitals in 9 countries as part of a substudy of the GUSTO IIb clinical trial. It concluded that direct angioplasty had a "small to moderate" clinical advantage over thrombolytic drug therapy 1 month after treatment. Those same patients have now been followed for 6 months, and researchers have found that the advantage has diminished. The rate of death or second heart attack was not statistically different between the two therapies (Aversano, 1998). The Myocardial Infarction Triage and Intervention (MITI) Project Registry is the largest study published to date comparing primary angioplasty with thrombolytic therapy in AMI patients. There was no difference between in-hospital or 3-year mortality rates for patients treated with primary angioplasty and those treated with thrombolytic therapy, even after controlling for differences in baseline characteristics known to affect mortality (Aversano, 1998; Goldman & Bennett, 2000).

At present, physicians deciding which therapy to offer a patient who is eligible for either treatment should return to fundamentals established in multiple large studies. The rapid restoration of brisk antegrade coronary flow is critical in reducing mortality. If a skilled cardiologist is readily available and the patient can be treated rapidly, angioplasty may be preferable. In most situations, however, thrombolytic therapy should still be regarded as an excellent strategy of reperfusion. The important point is not to delay restoration of myocardial reperfusion in suitable candidates with either of the two attractive alternatives (GUSTO IIb, 1997; Goldman & Bennett, 2000).

Mr. Johnson was admitted late in the evening (8 PM) with severe chest pain and was already showing signs of cardiogenic shock. Therefore because the catheterization laboratory was closed for the evening, it was better time management to treat Mr. Johnson with tPA. Unfortunately tPA was not completely successful in restoring the blood supply to the myocardium, and he needed angioplasty later that evening.

17. What are the contraindications for tPA?

Contraindications for tPA include the following (Bucher & Melander, 1999; Goldman & Bennett, 2000):

- Active internal bleeding
- Intracranial neoplasm or recent head injury
- Prolonged, traumatic cardiopulmonary resuscitation
- Suspicion of aortic dissection
- Pregnancy
- History of hemorrhagic, cerebrovascular accident, or recent nonhemorrhagic cerebrovascular accident
- Recorded blood pressure greater than 200/120 mm Hg
- Trauma or surgery, that is, a potential bleeding source, within the previous 2 weeks
- Allergy to streptokinase or anisoylated plasminogen streptokinase activator complex if being considered

18. What is a PTCA?

A PTCA is an effective revascularization procedure used to increase the diameter of coronary arteries that have been stenosed by CAD and therefore to increase coronary blood flow (Lessig & Lessig, 1998). The PTCA is performed in the catheterization laboratory. Using fluoroscopy, the cardiologist inserts a catheter through the femoral or radial artery and guides it through the ascending aorta and into the ostium of the right or left coronary artery. A balloon-tipped catheter is passed into the area of blockage and the balloon is inflated for 30 to 129 seconds. This occludes the blood flow to the area of the heart supplied by this artery, and the patient may experience chest pain for the few seconds after the balloon is inflated. The balloon compresses the plaque against the artery lumina and also stretches the lumina of the artery to allow improved blood flow. The balloon may need to be deflated and reinflated several times to decrease the obstruction and open the clogged blood vessel (Lessig & Lessig, 1998; Becker, 1999; Goldman & Bennett, 2000). Progression of coronary atherosclerosis remains a significant problem after PTCA, requiring patients to make ongoing modifications in their risk factors for coronary disease and lifestyle. Research has supported the reduction in risks for CAD by positive lifestyle modifications and by drug interventions (e.g., lipid- and blood pressure–lowering therapy and aspirin therapy). Most patients need comprehensive risk factor modification plans. When patients are educated regarding lifestyle changes, achieving balance seems to be the most realistic, attainable, and satisfying approach to use (Gulanick et al, 1998).

19. What made Mr. Johnson a candidate for PTCA? What are the potential complications for a patient undergoing PTCA?

The indications for PTCA are as follows:

- Unstable or chronic angina
- AMI and post-AMI
- Postoperative angina after coronary artery bypass grafting

The ideal patient has single- or double-vessel disease with at least 50% stenosis; a lesion that is discrete; preferably proximal, noncalcific, concentric blockage located away from bifurcations; and the potential to survive emergency surgery if the procedure is complicated or fails. PTCA is contraindicated in patients with left main CAD, especially if the patient is not considered a good surgical risk, in patients with variant angina, in patients with vessels stenosed at the orifice by the aortic wall, and in patients with critical valvular disease (Lessig & Lessig, 1998; Goldman & Bennett, 2000).

Complications of PTCA include the following:

- Acute coronary occlusion, necessitating emergency surgery
- Dissection of the artery
- Reaction to contrast medium
- Bleeding or hematoma at the insertion site; retroperitoneal bleeding
- Decrease in peripheral pulses distal to the insertion site
- Vasovagal reaction at time of sheath removal
- Pseudoaneurysm of artery
- Restenosis of artery within 6 months (30% to 40%)
- A clot breaking loose and migrating to other areas causing a stroke or MI

Mr. Johnson was a candidate for a PTCA because he continued to experience pain after the thrombolytic therapy. Because of his continued pain, we can assume the atherosclerotic changes had caused blockage of a coronary artery. tPA is a "clot buster" and can be very successful in restoring adequate blood supply to the heart; however, sometimes it is not enough, and the patient continues to experience chest pain as the artery remains occluded. PTCA allows the cardiologist to compress the plaque so that blood flow resumes. Shavelle and colleagues (1999) conducted a study to see if early intervention in patients with ST-segment depression and MI, provided a benefit. The data were inconclusive that intervention within a 6- to 12-hour period had any different long-term outcomes. This study had many baseline variables with the patients. The patients tended to be male, young, smokers, and less of a cardiac history. If the mix of patients were to be different in a replicated study, so might be the morbidity and mortality outcomes.

Lundergan and associates (2002) performed a study that looked at time delay with the use of thrombolytics, and how long of a delay is too long to be beneficial. This study found that delay in time to reperfusion, measured in minutes, resulted in significant loss of ventricular function after myocardial infarction.

Holubkov and coworkers (2002) conducted a study that looked at patients 1 year after their PTCA. They found that approximately three quarters of the group receiving percutaneous coronary intervention were angina free at 1 year. Females had more symptoms than males as did subgroups that had a history of previous interventions or previous MIs.

20. What is a stent and why was it used on Mr. Johnson?

A stent is a small, circular stainless steel tube that fits on the end of the balloon-tipped catheter and is inserted into a coronary artery just after PTCA to prevent reocclusion or to help repair a dissection. Stents are also used after restenosis in patients who had undergone previous angioplasties. Evidence has shown that there is a benefit of stenting in patients in whom there was renarrowing of a coronary vessel after balloon angioplasty (Erbel et al, 1998; Topol, 1998). Holmes (1999) states, "Coronary stenting has revolutionized the practice of interventional cardiology and has arguably been as large an incremental step as the initial introduction of percutaneous transluminal coronary angioplasty." To place a stent, the guidewire with the balloon is withdrawn, and another guidewire with the stent and balloon is placed at the occlusion. Inflating the balloon causes the stent to expand and embeds it into the lumen of the artery. After the balloon is deflated and removed, the stent remains in place, keeping the artery open. Placing a stent requires that the patient had been receiving anticoagulant therapy for 6 to 8 weeks. Zidar (1998) states, "This trial (ENTICES) has demonstrated that the combination of enoxaparin (Lovenox), ticlopidine (Ticlid), and aspirin after elective stenting is a well-tolerated and effective treatment strategy to decrease ischemic complications and hemorrhagic vascular complications."

21. What do the readings from the pulmonary artery catheter tell the nurse about Mr. Johnson?

Heart function is optimal when there is a balance between myocardial oxygen demand and myocardial oxygen supply. "Cardiac output is a function of heart rate and stoke volume.